Treating Child and Adolescent Depression

Treating Child and Adolescent Depression

Editors

Joseph M. Rey, MB, BS, Ph.D., FRANZCP

Honorary Professor
Psychological Medicine
University of Sydney
Sydney, Australia

Boris Birmaher, M.D.

Professor of Psychiatry
Endowed Chair in Early Onset Bipolar Disease
University of Pittsburgh School of Medicine
Co-Director
Child and Adolescent Bipolar Services
Western Psychiatric Institute and Clinic
Pittsburgh, Pennsylvania

Wolters Kluwer | Lippincott Williams & Wilkins
Health

Philadelphia • Baltimore • New York • London
Buenos Aires • Hong Kong • Sydney • Tokyo

Acquisitions Editor: Charles W. Mitchell
Managing Editor: Sirkka E. Howes
Marketing Manager: Kimberly Schonberger
Associate Production Manager: Kevin P. Johnson
Designer: Stephen Druding
Compositor: International Typesetting and Composition

351 West Camden Street   530 Walnut Street
Baltimore, MD 21201   Philadelphia, PA 19106

Printed in the People's Republic of China

9 8 7 6 5 4 3 2 1

Library of Congress Cataloging-in-Publication Data

Treating child and adolescent depression / editors, Joseph M. Rey, Boris Birmaher.
   p. ; cm.
  Includes bibliographical references and index.
  ISBN-13: 978-0-7817-9569-2
  ISBN-10: 0-7817-9569-9
 1. Depression in children—Treatment.   2. Depression in
adolescence—Treatment.   I. Rey, Joseph.   II. Birmaher, Boris.
  [DNLM: 1. Depressive Disorder—therapy.   2. Adolescent.   3. Child.
4. Depressive Disorder—psychology.   WM 171 T7825 2009]
  RJ506.D4T76 2009
  618.92'8527—dc22

                                                                2008031235

To purchase additional copies of this book, call our customer service department at **(800) 638-3030** or fax orders to **(301) 223-2320**. International customers should call **(301) 223-2300**.

Visit Lippincott Williams & Wilkins on the Internet: http://www.lww.com. Lippincott Williams & Wilkins customer service representatives are available from 8:30 am to 6:00 pm, EST.

Sadly, unhappy children are not a new phenomenon. However, conceptualizing some of them as having a serious disorder, a major depressive disorder, in fact, is a phenomenon of the past 40 to 50 years. The interest in its existence as something related to clinical depression in adults had theoretical underpinnings. But its acceptance was born out of the hope that it was a treatable condition as its adult counterpart appeared to be.

Between 1957 and 1978, about 10,000 papers were published on the drug imipramine, mostly as an antidepressant for adult depression. The conclusion was that this drug and other tricyclic antidepressants (TCAs) were generally superior to placebo. A number of early, and now long-forgotten, child psychiatrists jumped into the fray and published case reports and open studies on antidepressants in unhappy children, often with encouraging results. I don't think it is a distortion of history to claim that by the time child psychiatrists had developed the systematic assessments needed to ascertain the presence of clinical depression reliably in children in the 1970s, there was a great deal of hope that the condition as diagnosed would be readily treated and a whole generation of youth would be spared the long-term consequences of a debilitating disorder.

Alas, we were in for a rude awakening. Instead of the hoped-for triumph, the more advanced methodology of systematic assessment and placebo-controlled trials revealed that whatever "childhood depression" was, it wasn't going to lend itself to an easy solution, at least pharmacologically. The psychological treatment of childhood depression was not quite so depressing but for a different reason. Not only were there fewer expectations for it, but also there are—even now—few manualized treatments that lend themselves for use with children (versus adolescents). Thus the differences between child and adult psychotherapy responses were less glaring. Clearly, however, another treatment approach did not appear to be the metaphorical cavalry rushing in to pick up the therapeutic pieces of the failed TCA treatment.

A number of theories were generated to explain why the TCAs appeared to be such a disappointment in children. (They are slightly less disappointing in adolescents. Furthermore, over the years, the placebo response in adult studies has increased, according to a report in the *Journal of the American Medical Association* by Walsh and colleagues in 2002.[1] So adult antidepressant response is not the success story it used to be either.) It is unlikely there is just one reason for this, and we still do not have the answers. It took until 1997 before Emslie and colleagues[2] in Texas broke the curse of equivocal antidepressant response and demonstrated that fluoxetine was more effective than placebo. However, judging by the paucity of really robust findings in many of the industry-sponsored trials with sufficient power to demonstrate a treatment effect, the curse is not fully demolished, and the reasons for either poor treatment response or high placebo response are still not clear.

So, what has happened? What history has borne out is that unhappy children are a heterogeneous group. There are multiple contributors to their symptoms and dysfunction. A magic bullet or two (pill or therapy) may still be in the wings, but we haven't found them yet. What do we do in the meantime?

What we do is to compile a masterful set of contributions like those found in this volume that tackle the subject of treating childhood depression from multiple perspectives. Because depression in young people has been identified as a condition warranting attention, a number of conceptual frameworks have been developed from which empirical treatments have emerged. The chapters included in this comprehensive volume provide the background, the evidence base as it currently stands, and practical suggestions of how to implement each treatment approach. They also address depression in special populations like physically ill children and developmentally disabled children. The contributors are international experts in the field who provide the added advantage of a global perspective on early-onset depression.

It is quite surprising, given the interest in mood disorders in children and adolescents, that there really are no recent volumes on treating depression in young people written for clinicians. Many volumes are available to the lay public. And there are books on childhood depression and on treating adults. This book, however, not only provides a thorough grounding for clinicians of all sorts who treat young people, it does so in a user-friendly way. There are summary points at the start of the chapter, and tables, charts, and lists of useful websites help further synthesize the information.

The editors of this volume have obviously responded to an important need. Dr. Rey, like many who do and have done research in mood disorders, got interested in the field of childhood mood disorders when *DSM-III* criteria allowed the condition to be separated from the myriad of conditions that had "masked" depression previously. Dr. Birmaher could be said to be one of Dr. Joaquim (Kim) Puig-Antich's professional offspring. Dr. Puig-Antich was one of the clinical investigators who helped focus attention on this important area in the 1970s and 1980s. Together they have brought us a state-of-the-art compendium.

I wish I could say we were on the threshold of breaking developments in the treatment of depression in youth. As it stands, *Treating Child and Adolescent Depression* will remain an extremely important source of information for many years to come.

REFERENCES

1. Walsh BT, Seidman SN, Sysko R. Placebo response in studies of major depression: variable, substantial, and growing. *JAMA*. 2002;287:1840–1847.
2. Emslie GJ, Rush AJ, Weinberg WA, et al. Double-blind placebo-controlled study of fluoxetine in depressed children and adolescents. *Arch Gen Psychiatry*. 1997;54:1031–1037.

Gabrielle A. Carlson, MD
Professor of Psychiatry and Pediatrics
Director, Child and Adolescent Psychiatry
Stony Brook University School of Medicine

"They are not useful for my practice" is a frequent complaint put to us by primary care practitioners and mental health professionals when referring to books on the treatment of pediatric depression, the bread and butter of many practices. The chapters on the treatment of depression in widely used general pediatric psychiatry textbooks are usually not detailed enough. Most books focusing on youth depression either summarize the evidence of effectiveness in a scholarly way without dealing with the practical aspects of management (the "how to") or describe one type of treatment (e.g., cognitive behavior therapy, pharmacologic) with little or no attention given to other therapeutic options. Neither meets practitioners' needs. This need has been accentuated by recent controversies surrounding the treatment of depression (e.g., Food and Drug Administration's black box warnings), which have confused and caused uncertainty among clinicians and patients alike.

The book seeks to fill this gap by making evidence-based, up-to-date information on the treatment of child and adolescent depression available but also offering practical advice on the implementation of a wide range of interventions in a variety of clinical situations (e.g., when depression does not respond, when depression is comorbid with other disorders) and when treatment is delivered in particular settings, such as primary care, pediatric medical wards, or cross-culturally. Taking into account the current international literature, the focus of this book is in giving as much practical advice as possible on how to deal with common and uncommon clinical circumstances that arise during treatment, such as when patients are noncompliant, become homicidal or suicidal, develop side effects, or when there is family discord. To that end, most chapters include resources for patients, families, and practitioners, as well as information sheets, rating scales, and other potentially useful aids—most in the public domain, thus able to be used, reproduced, or handed out at no cost.

The first section of the book (three chapters) describes general aspects of depressive illnesses, etiology, and assessment of depressed youth. The second section (17 chapters) discusses practical management, covering topics as diverse as treatment resistance; engaging, involving, educating, and supporting patients, families, and schools; how to use a variety of treatments (pharmacologic, interpersonal psychotherapy, family therapy, complimentary and alternative medicine, etc,); preventing and dealing with side effects and with crisis in the course of treatment; and managing depression in primary care settings. The third section (four chapters) deals with the problems of treating pediatric depression in special groups: the chronically ill, the developmentally disabled, those from culturally diverse backgrounds, and international views and practices.

Interpretation of the data and clinical practice often varies between centers, states in the United States, and between countries. Much can be learned from this diversity of traditions, views, and experience. To that end, we have strived to give the content an international perspective in the language used, in the topics covered, and by engaging contributors from all parts of the world. The aim was that clinicians from Amsterdam, Bangkok, Nairobi, or New York could easily follow the text, ethically adapt the information to the local circumstances, and offer the best possible treatment to their young patients and their families no matter where they are.

We see this volume as a work in progress. Thus we would appreciate readers' comments, advice, and suggestions, which can be sent to jmrey@bigpond.net.au.

Joseph M. Rey
Boris Birmaher

Ava T. Albrecht, M.D.
Clinical Assistant Professor of Child
and Adolescent Psychiatry
Department of Child and Adolescent Psychiatry
New York University School of Medicine;
Associate Director
Adolescent Day Hospital
Bellevue Hospital Center
New York, New York

Joan R. Asarnow, Ph.D.
Professor of Psychiatry and Biobehavioral
Sciences
University of California, Los Angeles (UCLA)
Los Angeles, California

David A. Brent, M.D.
Professor of Psychiatry, Pediatrics, and
Epidemiology
Endowed Chair in Suicide Studies
School of Medicine
University of Pittsburgh;
Academic Chief
Child and Adolescent Psychiatry
Western Psychiatric Institute and Clinic
Pittsburgh, Pennsylvania

John V. Campo, M.D.
Professor of Psychiatry
The Ohio State University;
Chief
Child and Adolescent Psychiatry
Nationwide Children's Hospital and OSU-Harding
Hospital
Columbus, Ohio

Carlo G. Carandang, M.D.
Assistant Professor of Psychiatry
Dalhousie University;
Staff Psychiatrist
Mental Health and Addictions Program
IWK Health Centre
Halifax, Nova Scotia, Canada

Amy H. Cheung, M.D., M.Sc., FRCP (C)
Assistant Professor
Department of Psychiatry
University of Toronto;
Staff Psychiatrist
Division of Youth Psychiatry
Sunnybrook Health Sciences Centre,
Toronto, Canada

Angela W. Chiu, M.A.
Department of Psychology
University of California, Los Angeles (UCLA)
Los Angeles, California

Kathleen F. Clougherty, M.S.W.
Instructor in Clinical Psychiatric Social Work
(in Psychiatry)
Department of Child Psychiatry
Columbia University
New York, New York

Paul Croarkin, D.O.
Assistant Professor of Psychiatry
University of Texas Southwestern Medical Center;
Child and Adolescent Psychiatry
Children's Medical Center
Dallas, Texas

Rasim Somer Diler, M.D.
Assistant Professor of Psychiatry
University of Pittsburgh School of Medicine;
Medical Director
Inpatient Child and Adolescent Bipolar Services
Western Psychiatric Institute and Clinic
Pittsburgh, Pennsylvania

Graham J. Emslie, M.D.
Professor of Psychiatry
University of Texas Southwestern Medical Center;
Chief of Service
Child and Adolescent Psychiatry
Children's Medical Center
Dallas, Texas

Judy Garber, Ph.D.
Professor of Psychology and Human
  Development
Vanderbilt University
Nashville, Tennessee

Neera Ghaziuddin, M.D., MRCPsych (UK)
Associate Professor of Psychiatry
University of Michigan
Ann Arbor, Michigan

**Benjamin I. Goldstein, M.D.,
Ph.D., FRCPC**
Assistant Professor
University of Pittsburgh School of Medicine;
Psychiatrist
Child and Adolescent Bipolar Services
Western Psychiatric Institute and Clinic
Pittsburgh, Pennsylvania

Ian M. Goodyer, M.D., FMed.Sci.
Professor of Child and Adolescent Psychiatry
Section of Developmental Psychiatry
University of Cambridge & Cambridgeshire
  & Peterborough NHS Foundation Trust
Cambridge, United Kingdom

Michael Gordon, M.D., FRANZCP
Honorary Lecturer
Department of Psychological Medicine
Monash University;
Deputy Director
Department of Child Psychiatry
Southern Health (Monash Medical Centre)
Melbourne, Australia

Philip L. Hazell, Ph.D., FRANZCP
Conjoint Professor of Child and Adolescent
  Psychiatry
Concord Clinical School
University of Sydney;
Director
Infant, Child and Adolescent Mental Health
Sydney South West Area Health Service
Sydney, Australia

Maryann O. Hetrick, Ph.D.
Assistant Instructor
University of Texas Southwestern Medical Center
Dallas, Texas

Carroll W. Hughes, Ph.D.
Professor of Psychiatry
University of Texas Southwestern Medical Center
Children's Medical Center
Dallas, Texas

F. Neslihan Inal-Emiroglu, M.D.
Assistant Professor of Child and Adolescent
  Psychiatry
Dokuz Eylul University Medical School
Narlidere, Izmir, Turkey

**Raphael G. Kelvin, MRCPsych.,
DCH, DRCOG**
Associate Lecturer
Section of Developmental Psychiatry,
  Cambridge University;
Consultant in Child and Adolescent
  Psychiatry
Cambridge Child and Adolescent Mental
  Health Service
Cambridgeshire and Peterborough NHS
  Foundation Trust
Cambridge, United Kingdom

Stanley Kutcher, M.D., FRCPC
Sun Life Financial Chair in Adolescent Mental
  Health and Director WHOCollaborating Center
Dalhousie University
IWK Health Centre
Halifax, Nova Scotia, Canada

David A. Langer, M.A.
Department of Psychology
University of California, Los Angeles (UCLA)
Los Angeles, California

Andrés Martin, M.D., M.P.H.
Professor of Child Psychiatry and Psychiatry
Yale Child Study Center;
Medical Director
Children's Psychiatric Inpatient Service
Yale-New Haven Children's Hospital
New Haven, Connecticut

Taryn L. Mayes, M.S.
Faculty Associate
Department of Psychiatry
University of Texas Southwestern Medical Center;
Child and Adolescent Psychiatry
Children's Medical Center
Dallas, Texas

Elizabeth McCauley, Ph.D., ABPP
Professor of Psychiatry and Behavioral
  Sciences
University of Washington;
Associate Director of Child and Adolescent
  Psychiatry
Seattle Children's Hospital and Regional Medical
  Center
Seattle, Washington

Ainslie McDougall, M.Sc.
Research Assistant to Sun Life Financial
Chair in Adolescent Mental Health
Department of Psychiatry
IWK Health Centre
Halifax, Nova Scotia, Canada

Glenn A. Melvin, Ph.D.
Lecturer
Centre for Developmental Psychiatry
  & Psychology
Monash University
Melbourne, Australia

**Sally N. Merry, MB, ChB,
FRANZCP, M.D.**
Senior Lecturer in Psychological Medicine
University of Auckland
Auckland, New Zealand

Laura Mufson, Ph.D.
Associate Professor of Clinical Psychology
  in Psychiatry
Columbia University College of Physicians
  and Surgeons;
Director
Department of Clinical Psychology
New York State Psychiatric Institute
New York, New York

**Andrea Murphy, BSc.Pharm., ACPR,
Pharm.D.**
Assistant Professor
School of Nursing
Dalhousie University;
Research Associate
IWK Health Centre
Halifax, Nova Scotia, Canada

Robert Ortiz-Aguayo, M.D.
Assistant Professor of Psychiatry and Pediatrics
Associate Director Residency Training
University of Pittsburgh Western Psychiatric
  Institute and Clinic of UPMC Presbyterian-
  Shadyside Children's Hospital
Pittsburgh, Pennsylvania

Daniel J. Pilowsky, M.D., M.P.H.
Assistant Professor of Clinical Epidemiology
  and Clinical Psychiatry
Columbia University;
Staff Psychiatrist
New York State Psychiatric Institute
New York, New York

Andres J. Pumariega, M.D.
Professor of Psychiatry
Temple University School of Medicine
Philadelphia, Pennsylvania;
Chair
Department of Psychiatry
The Reading Hospital and Medical Center
Reading, Pennsylvania

Rachel Z. Ritvo, M.D.
Assistant Clinical Professor
Department of Psychiatry and Behavioral
  Sciences
George Washington University
Washington, DC

Kenneth M. Rogers, M.D.
Assistant Professor of Psychiatry
University of Maryland-Baltimore;
Director, Child and Adolescent Psychiatry
  Residency Program
University of Maryland Medical Center
Baltimore, Maryland

Eugenio M. Rothe, M.D.
Associate Professor
Robert Stempel School of Public Health
Florida International University
Miami, Florida

Kirti Saxena, M.D.
Assistant Professor
Division of Child/Adolescent Psychiatry
University of Texas Southwestern Medical
  Center;
Associate Director of Child/Adolescent Psychiatry
  Outpatient Clinic
Children's Medical Center
Dallas, Texas

Karen A. Shoum, M.A.
Doctoral Candidate
Department of Counseling and Clinical
  Psychology
Teachers College
Columbia University
New York, New York

Rongrong Tao, M.D., Ph.D.
Assistant Professor of Psychiatry
University of Texas Southwestern Medical Center;
Child and Adolescent Psychiatry
Children's Medical Center
Dallas, Texas

Bruce J. Tonge, M.D., FRANZCP
Professor and Head of Psychological Medicine
Monash University
Melbourne, Australia;
Head
Centre for Developmental Psychiatry
Monash Medical Centre, Clayton
Victoria, Australia

Helena Verdeli, Ph.D.
Assistant Professor of Clinical Psychology
   in Education
Department of Counseling and Clinical
   Psychology
Teachers College
Columbia University
New York, New York

Garry Walter, Ph.D., FRANZCP
Professor of Child and Adolescent Psychiatry
University of Sydney
Sydney, Australia;
Area Clinical Director
Child and Adolescent Mental Health Services
Northern Sydney Central Coast Health
New South Wales, Australia

Paul O. Wilkinson, M.D.
Clinical Lecturer
Section of Developmental Psychiatry
University of Cambridge;
Locum Consultant
Child and Adolescent Psychiatry
Cambridgeshire and Peterborough NHS
   Foundation Trust
Cambridge, United Kingdom

Leonard Woods, L.C.S.W.
Psychiatric Social Worker IV
Western Psychiatric Institute and Clinic
University of Pittsburgh Medical Center
Pittsburgh, Pennsylvania

Rachel A. Zuckerbrot, M.D.
Assistant Professor of Clinical Psychiatry
Division of Child and Adolescent Psychiatry
Columbia University
New York State Psychiatric Institute
New York, New York

Acknowledgments

We thank the contributors very much; they generously agreed to share their wisdom, knowledge, and clinical experience. We are grateful to our respective families who have endured our spending endless hours in front of the computer; this work would not have been possible without their understanding. We also thank our mentors, teachers, colleagues, and patients and their families who guided us and shared our struggles; together we worked through successes and failures to become better clinicians.

Contents

Foreword v
Preface vii
List of Contributors ix
Acknowledgments xiii

SECTION I General Aspects of Depression

1   Depression in Children and Adolescents 3
JOSEPH M. REY AND PHILIP L. HAZELL

2   Depression: Causes and Risk Factors 17
DANIEL J. PILOWSKY

3   Clinical Assessment of Children and Adolescents With Depression 23
CARLO G. CARANDANG AND ANDRÉS MARTIN

SECTION II Practical Management

4   Introduction to Treating Depression in Children and Adolescents 43
JOSEPH M. REY AND BORIS BIRMAHER

5   Engaging, Involving, Educating, and Supporting Patients,
Families, and Schools During Treatment 54
SALLY N. MERRY AND ELIZABETH MCCAULEY

6   How to Use Medication to Manage Depression .69
GRAHAM J. EMSLIE, RONGRONG TAO, PAUL CROARKIN,
AND TARYN L. MAYES

7   Using Other Biologic Treatments: Electroconvulsive Therapy,
Transcranial Magnetic Stimulation, Vagus Nerve Stimulation,
and Light Therapy 87
GARRY WALTER AND NEERA GHAZIUDDIN

8   How to Use Cognitive Behavior Therapy for Youth
Depression: A Guide to Implementation 100
DAVID A. LANGER, ANGELA W. CHIU, AND JOAN R. ASARNOW

9   How to Use Interpersonal Psychotherapy for
Depressed Adolescents (IPT-A) 114
LAURA MUFSON, HELENA VERDELI, KATHLEEN F. CLOUGHERTY,
AND KAREN A. SHOUM

10   Using Family Therapy 128
LEONARD WOODS

11   Dynamic Psychotherapy for the Treatment of Depression in Youth 140
RACHEL Z. RITVO

12   How to Use Complementary and Alternative Medicine Treatments 151
JOSEPH M. REY

13   Managing Acute Depressive Episodes: Putting It Together in Practice 162
RAPHAEL G. KELVIN, PAUL O. WILKINSON, AND IAN M. GOODYER

14   Preventing, Detecting, and Managing Side Effects of Medications 174
STANLEY KUTCHER, AINSLIE MCDOUGALL, AND ANDREA MURPHY

15   Managing Crises and Emergencies in the Course of Treatment 194
AVA T. ALBRECHT

16   Treatment-Resistant Depression 209
BORIS BIRMAHER AND DAVID A. BRENT

17   Managing Young People With Depression
and Comorbid Conditions 220
MARYANN O. HETRICK, KIRTI SAXENA, AND CARROLL W. HUGHES

18   Managing Adolescents With Comorbid Depression
and Substance Abuse 237
BENJAMIN I. GOLDSTEIN

19   Managing Adolescent Depression in Primary Care 253
AMY H. CHEUNG AND RACHEL A. ZUCKERBROT

20   Prevention of Depression and Early Intervention
With Subclinical Depression 274
JUDY GARBER

SECTION **III** **Particular Issues About Treatment in Specific Groups**

21   Treating Depression in Children and Adolescents
With Chronic Physical Illness 295
ROBERTO ORTIZ-AGUAYO AND JOHN V. CAMPO

22   Treating Depression in the Developmentally Disabled:
Intellectual Disability and Pervasive Developmental Disorders 310
BRUCE J. TONGE, MICHAEL GORDON, AND GLENN A. MELVIN

23   Depression in Immigrant and Minority Children and Youth 321
ANDRES J. PUMARIEGA, EUGENIO M. ROTHE, AND KENNETH M. ROGERS

24   Childhood Depression: International Views
and Treatment Practices 332
F. NESLIHAN INAL-EMIROGLU AND RASIM SOMER DILER

Index 341

General Aspects of Depression

Depression in Children and Adolescents

JOSEPH M. REY AND PHILIP L. HAZELL

KEY POINTS

- Depression is one of the most common psychological disorders in children and adolescents, and as such it needs to be diagnosed and treated not only by specialists but also in primary care settings.
- Often depressive illnesses are chronic, recurrent, and incapacitating, more similar to asthma than pneumonia. This is often overlooked.
- When they grow up, depressed youth are more likely to never marry, be more impaired socially and occupationally, have a poorer quality of life and greater medical and psychiatric morbidity, suffer more depressive episodes, and are more likely to commit suicide than those without depression.
- Diagnosis is complex because depression is a normal human experience, can be a symptom in a variety of physical and psychological disorders, a syndrome, or an illness. Diagnosis requires careful examination of symptoms and impairment, and exclusion of conditions that mimic depression.
- Although not always possible, it is helpful to know which subtype of depression is afflicting a child because of its implications for treatment and prognosis.
- Medical conditions, medications, and substances of abuse can cause symptoms that are similar to depression.
- Depression often co-occurs with other mental disorders. As a result it can be overlooked, particularly when comorbid with attention deficit hyperactivity disorder (ADHD) and disruptive behavior disorders because parents and teachers focus on the annoying behaviors of the child and overlook unhappiness and depressed mood.

Introduction   *Sarah, a thin 11-year-old, is brought to the family physician by her mother. Sarah has been unhappy, saying that life is not worth living, refusing to go to school, and complaining of stomach pains and headache. This problem has become worse over several weeks.*

The challenge of understanding how depression in young people develops, is diagnosed, and treated often begins with presentations like Sarah's. This process is complex because unhappiness is a normal human experience; periods of sadness are a common response to everyday events such as changing school, teasing, the breakup of relationships, parental illness, or exam pressures. Because the word *depression* can mean a symptom in a variety of psychological disorders, a syndrome, or an illness, it is used here to denote an illness, clinical depression, which includes major depressive disorder (MDD) and dysthymia. Thus clinicians need to determine whether Sarah's symptoms fulfill criteria for a psychiatric disorder (e.g., major depression), their relationship to biologic, psychologic, social, and cultural aspects of development, impact on her daily life and adjustment (e.g., on progress at school), connection with family functioning, whether treatment is required, and which treatment is most appropriate. Sarah did not seek help herself but was brought to the physician by her mother, who thought the time was right to seek assistance. This is because many children do not understand they are unwell (e.g., may blame family, school, or friends for their feelings) or are unable to express in words their subjective experiences, or they are frightened and do not want to be evaluated by a clinician. Sarah's need for help was defined by another person, and the clinician should therefore explore what the problem is from the mother's perspective.

A recent World Economic Forum in Davos, Switzerland, discussed depression among other weighty topics. The forum was told that according to the World Health Organization (WHO), depressive illness was the leading cause of disability worldwide in terms of number of people afflicted, and it is forecast to become worse by the year 2020.[1] The fact that a psychiatric illness was discussed at all in such a forum is in itself telling. Besides disability, the cost of treatment is also large, particularly because depression is often a lifelong problem. Also, depression increases the risk of medical illness, academic, work, social, and family problems, and it is the major cause of suicide in youth.[2] As described later in this chapter, depression is one of the most common disorders afflicting not only adults but also the young, and an even greater number of children live with an adult who suffers from the condition.

Little is known about the public's perceptions of depression in the young. However, American people seem to believe childhood depression is a more serious illness than adult depression and in need of formal, even involuntary, treatment.[3] They also perceive depressed youth as potentially violent, probably as a result of the publicity surrounding the tragic Columbine High School events and similar incidents elsewhere.[3] This shows not only that depression in the young is recognized as a serious illness but also that it regrettably carries considerable stigma (e.g., sufferers are perceived as weak, potentially dangerous). By contrast, evidence indicates that depression in the young is often not detected or treated. For example, 66% of depressed adolescents identified in an epidemiologic study had not used any treatment services.[4] However, when they did, they almost always used more than one service (e.g., school counseling, medical, mental health). Of the adolescents who had consulted a physician, all had attended counseling services, and almost all had used mental health services. Only 3% had taken antidepressant medication. This situation might be improving because of education campaigns targeting health professionals and the community at large.

There are suggestions that depression is becoming more common with successive generations and presenting at a younger age.[5] It is also likely that most people who ever suffer from depression will have experienced their first episode before 20 years of age. Childhood depression is therefore too common to be the exclusive domain of specialist services. Just as primary care physicians treat many adults with mild to moderate depressive illness, they may increasingly provide a similar service to children and adolescents; to do so will require gaining knowledge and skills in this area.

DEFINITION

Depression is an episodic or chronic disorder characterized by persistent and pervasive sadness or unhappiness, loss of enjoyment of everyday activities, irritability, boredom, and associated symptoms such as negative thinking, lack of energy, difficulty concentrating, and appetite and sleep disturbance. To have a depressive disorder, the individual's functioning must also be impaired. Depression exists in a continuum, although manifestations may vary according to age, gender, and cultural background. The various subtypes are identified on the basis of symptom severity, pervasiveness, functional impairment, or the presence or absence of manic episodes.

HISTORICAL NOTE

Depression has existed in all recorded historical times. For example, King Saul is depicted as depressed and committing suicide in the Old Testament. Robert Burton in his book *Anatomy of Melancholy* (1621) described not only the symptoms of depression but also explored its psychological and social causes (such as poverty, fear, and solitude). The German psychiatrist Emil Kraepelin (1856–1926) identified "manic depression" (bipolar disorder) as a separate condition. Thus depression in adults is an illness known for a long time and for which new treatments such as psychotherapy, electroconvulsive therapy, and antidepressant drugs were gradually introduced during the 20th century. Yet this was not the case for children.

Psychoanalytic theories mostly posited that depression was the result of superego-driven introjection of aggressive impulses.[6] These theories also assumed that children did not have a well-developed superego and thus could not introject aggression and experience depression. Because psychoanalysis dominated the thinking about depression in the first half of the 20th century, childhood depression was ignored until the 1960s when new currents of thought gathered momentum. For example, according to the proponents of the "masked depression" theory, children can be depressed but express this differently from adults, as conduct problems or physical complaints: "depressive equivalents."[6] Although the concept of masked depression was heavily criticized and subsequently abandoned, the debate rekindled interest on childhood depression, also because many clinicians had noted that children in their practices often showed depressive phenomena. By the 1970s researchers began to accept that childhood depression did exist, and the focus moved on to defining its characteristics.

When the third edition of the *Diagnostic and Statistical Manual of Mental Disorders* of the American Psychiatric Association (*DSM-III*) was published in 1980, many experts already acknowledged that childhood depression shared the essential clinical features of adult depression. The issue was whether children also displayed developmentally specific symptoms, such as somatic complaints, negativism, or aggressiveness, which are not characteristic of the adult syndrome. The following edition, *DSM-IV*, states the core symptoms are the same for children, adolescents, and adults, but it acknowledges the pattern may vary with age, so much so that "irritable mood" in children is accepted as a diagnostic equivalent of depressed mood. The WHO's *International Classification of Diseases,* 10th edition (*ICD-10*) recognizes a similar disorder.

The concept of dysthymic disorder or dysthymia was introduced in *DSM-III* to denote a less severe, less pervasive but more chronic form of depression that often starts during childhood. This diagnosis has been retained with similar characteristics in both *DSM-IV* and *ICD-10,* although questions remain about whether dysthymia is a separate condition.[7]

An update of the classification systems (*DSM-V* and *ICD-11*) is under way, but drastic changes are unlikely. Yet arguments about the existence of specific subtypes (e.g., melancholia), dimensional versus categorical approaches, and the overlap with anxiety disorders (suggesting the existence of one single condition) remain.[8] It has been argued also that major depression can be accurately diagnosed using only three out of five psychological symptoms (depressed mood, lack of interest, worthlessness, poor concentration, and thoughts of death, a subset of the nine symptoms currently used).[9] This has the advantage of being easier to remember. The search now is for objective biologic markers that may help identify the various subtypes of depression earlier and more reliably.

Media stories about a rapid rise in the prescription of antidepressant drugs, unmet expectations regarding their effectiveness, and concerns relating to their safety, particularly about suicidal behavior (see Chapters 6 and 14) have caused anxiety among clinicians, parents, and ill young people. This led some to question again the validity of youth depression, resulting in the reemergence of idiosyncratic or discredited theories, denial of its very existence (e.g., depression in the young is just medicalization of the unhappiness experienced by today's affluent children), trivialization of the illness or stigmatization (e.g., a weakness of character),[10] and a drop in diagnosis and prescription of antidepressants.[11]

EPIDEMIOLOGY

Prevalence estimates for current or recent MDD or dysthymia from selected community surveys of children and adolescents using *DSM-IV* criteria range from 0.9% to 3.4% (Table 1.1). Rates can vary depending on the population, the period considered, informant, and criteria used for diagnosis. The cumulative prevalence (accumulation of new cases in previously unaffected individuals, also known as lifetime prevalence) is much higher. For example, by the age of 16 years, 12% of girls and 7% of boys would have had a depressive disorder at some stage in their lives, according to a study conducted in North Carolina.[12] Prevalence of dysthymic disorder is less well known, but studies suggest a point prevalence ranging from 0.6% to 1.7% in children and 1.6% to 8.0% in adolescents.[5] A further 5% to 10% of young persons have been estimated to exhibit subsyndromal depression (or "minor depression"). Youth with minor depression show considerable impairment, an increased risk of suicide, and of developing major depression.[13]

Earlier epidemiologic studies using *DSM-III-R* criteria produced similar results. For example, Lewinsohn et al.[14] reported a point prevalence for major depression among high school students in

TABLE 1.1 PREVALENCE (%) OF *DSM-IV* DEPRESSIVE DISORDERS (MAJOR DEPRESSION, DYSTHYMIA) ACCORDING TO LARGE EPIDEMIOLOGIC STUDIES OF CHILDREN AND ADOLESCENTS

Population	Children	Adolescents	Females	Males	Overall
1,420 children from North Carolina, 9–13 yr, at first assessment[12(a)]	0.9	3.1	2.8	1.6	2.2
10,438 British children, 5–15 yr[19(b)]	0.4	2.5	1.0	0.9	0.9
3,171 Australian children, 6–17 yr[20(c)]			2.8	3.2	3.0
1,886 children, 4–17 yr, from Puerto Rico[21(d)]			5.2	0.3	3.4
1,107 girls, 12–17 yr, from Sudan[22(b)]			4.4		

[a]Three-month prevalence. [b]Point prevalence. [c]One-year prevalence. [d]Six-month prevalence.

the Unite States of 2.6% (males, 1.7%; females, 3.4%) and 0.5% for dysthymia (males, 0.5%; females, 0.6%). Lifetime prevalence was much higher: 18.5% for major depression and 3.2% for dysthymia.

The ratio of depression in males and females is similar among children but becomes about twice as common among females during adolescence[15] (see Chapter 2). Clinical impressions suggest rates of depression may be especially high in particular groups such as developmentally disabled or indigenous children (e.g., Native Americans, Eskimos, and Australian Aborigines) (see Chapters 21, 22, and 23). An American survey reported that prevalence of depression among attendees of a pediatric primary care service was no greater than that found in the general population.[16] However, the prevalence of depression is substantially higher among patients who suffer from chronic medical conditions (see Chapter 21).

AGE OF ONSET AND COURSE

Depression that begins prior to puberty may be different from depression that begins in adolescence or adult life, or at least more heterogeneous. Also, clinical presentation in children can be different from adolescents (see Chapter 3). Depressed adolescents are more likely to show hopelessness and helplessness, lack of energy or tiredness, hypersomnia, weight loss, substance abuse, delusions, and suicidal ideation and attempts compared with children. Conversely, children are likely to show irritability, hallucinations, comorbid separation anxiety, and ADHD more often.[5] It is during adolescence that depression becomes more common in girls than boys, suggesting the neurobiologic changes underpinning gender differentiation during this period may also be linked to the causation of depression. Whereas younger children respond less predictably to pharmacologic treatments, older adolescents respond to antidepressant drugs in a manner more similar to adults,[17,18] again suggesting that the neurobiologic subtract mediating depression is established or modified during adolescence. The influence of genes on the expression of depression in adolescents is similar to that in adults, whereas in children environmental factors seem to play a more important role. Although much of the depression occurring in adolescence is new-onset disorder, a significant minority of teenagers have already experienced problems in their prepubertal years; for some this is depression, and for others it is an anxiety disorder, ADHD, or conduct problems.[23] Given the overlap of these conditions with depression, clinicians who are treating young people for other psychiatric disorders should, over time, be on the lookout for the emergence of depressive symptoms.

Similar to adults, MDD in youth follows a relapsing course (for definitions of recurrence, relapse, etc., see Table 4.1). An episode of depression in clinically referred groups lasts 7 to 9 months on average, but it is shorter in nonreferred community samples.[13] That is, MDD is a spontaneously remitting illness, which may go some way in explaining the high placebo-response rates in treatment trials. However, there is a 40% probability of recurrence within 2 years, increasing to up to 70% after 5 years. The likelihood of further episodes in adulthood is about 60% to 70%.[5] Thus MDD should optimally be conceptualized as a chronic condition with remissions and recurrences, more similar to asthma or epilepsy than to pneumonia. This has important but often ignored implications for management, which should seek not only to reduce the duration of the depressive episode and lessen its consequences but also to prevent recurrences. The rate of switching to hypomania in young people with depression also seems higher than in adults, with some researchers claiming rates as high as 40%.[13]

Although age at onset does not seem to define separate depressive subgroups, earlier onset is associated with multiple indicators of greater illness burden in adulthood across a wide range of domains, such as never being married, more impaired social and occupational function, poorer quality of life, greater medical and psychiatric comorbidity, more lifetime depressive episodes and suicide attempts, and greater symptom severity.[24] However, predictors of recovery, relapse, and recurrence appear to be similar to those in adult-onset depression. Greater severity, chronicity, recurrences, comorbidity, hopelessness, negative cognitive style, family problems, low socioeconomic status, and exposure to abuse or family conflict are associated with poorer outcome.[13] Risk factors are discussed further in Chapter 2.

CLINICAL PICTURE

Depression affects children in most aspects of their lives, from mood to attitude and behavior, from thinking to body functioning. Table 1.2 lists depressive symptoms and their presentation in the young. In all cases symptoms must be evaluated in the context of the child's developmental stage (e.g., need for sleep, weight changes related to normal growth) and cultural background. Specific populations, such as developmentally disabled or deaf children, may require interpreting symptoms and behavior in the context of their disability and capacity to express unhappiness and distress (see Chapter 22).

TABLE 1.2 CHARACTERISTICS OF DEPRESSIVE SYMPTOMS AS SEEN IN CHILDREN AND ADOLESCENTS

Symptom	Commentary
CORE SYMPTOMS	
Depressed or irritable mood most of the day, nearly every day, as indicated by subjective report or observation made by others	• The mood is often irritable rather than depressed, particularly in children. • Children may not be able to articulate their feelings well. • Adults may overlook the symptom, especially in the presence of comorbid problems. • Irritability can manifest as physical fighting.
Markedly diminished interest or pleasure in all, or almost all, activities most of the day, nearly every day	• It can present as chronic boredom. • A discriminating symptom that can be confused with oppositionality (where the child sullenly refuses to participate in activities). • Some teenagers drop out of structured activities, not because they are depressed, but because their interest has shifted to socializing, or to solitary activities such as computer games. • This can manifest as withdrawal and social isolation. • In comparison with adults, marked anhedonia is rare in youth.
ASSOCIATED SYMPTOMS	
Fatigue or loss of energy nearly every day	• Clinicians must judge whether this symptom may be better explained by intercurrent medical illness (e.g., chronic fatigue syndrome, anemia, viral illness), lack of sleep, or substance use. • Symptoms that seem to be in excess of the level of physical morbidity may still raise the possibility of depression.
Feeling worthless or excessive or inappropriate guilt, nearly every day	• Most young people experience transient crises of confidence. To be significant, these feelings need to be enduring. • Excessive guilt is uncommon but is a discriminating symptom in young people. • Occasionally, these symptoms can be of delusional intensity.

(continued)

TABLE 1.2 CHARACTERISTICS OF DEPRESSIVE SYMPTOMS AS SEEN IN CHILDREN AND ADOLESCENTS (CONTINUED)

Symptom	Commentary
Recurrent thoughts of death, recurrent suicidal ideation, a suicide attempt, or a specific plan for committing suicide	• This does not include fear of dying. • Suicidal thoughts or attempts must always raise the possibility of depression. • Such ideas need to be differentiated from hurtful or manipulative statements made in anger but independent of low mood. Distinguishing them can be difficult in practice. Because depressed youth often have low frustration tolerance, they can become angry and suicidal very easily. • Self-injurious behaviors (e.g., wrist slashing) are very common among adolescents. • More common with increasing age.
Diminished ability to think or concentrate or indecisiveness nearly every day	• This problem usually comes to light because of a decline in academic performance. • In the presence of preexisting problems with attention or concentration, there needs to be a clear increase in the symptom within the context of the depressive episode.
Psychomotor agitation or retardation observable by others and present nearly every day	• In children, this can present as tantrums (also manifestation or irritability). • In the presence of preexisting hyperactivity, there needs to be a clear increase in the symptom within the context of the depressive episode.
Insomnia or hypersomnia nearly every day	• Many teenagers show a normative need for more sleep, plus a tendency to stay up late and to sleep late. • A change in the sleep-wake pattern (for example, sleeping in and refusing to go to school) in the context of sadness or irritability may be a symptom of depression.
Significant weight loss when not dieting or weight gain, or decrease or increase in appetite nearly every day	• In children, consider failure to make expected weight gains. • Teenagers sometimes appear to have lost weight when in fact they have had a growth spurt. • Change in appetite may be confused with food fads. • Craving for food and increased appetite are also common.
OTHER SYMPTOMS OR SIGNS	
Loss of confidence or self-esteem	• As children are easily disheartened by failure and disappointment, the symptom is of clinical significance only if it occurs in conjunction with low mood or irritability.
Frequent unexplained somatic complaints: feeling sick, headaches, stomachaches	• Clinicians must judge whether the symptom may be better explained by intercurrent medical illness or other psychiatric disorders (e.g., anxiety). • Symptoms that seem to be in excess of the level of physical morbidity may still raise the possibility of depression.
Anxiety, phobias, school refusal	• If present premorbidly, have become more severe in the context of the depressive illness. • More common among prepubertal children.
Hopelessness and helplessness	• In excess of the child's circumstances.
Lack of reactivity	• Affect lifts only temporarily in response to pleasant experiences. In repose, the young person still looks depressed.
Hallucinations or delusions	• In psychotic depression. • Usually auditory hallucinations in children; delusions more common in adolescents.

Adapted from Hazell P. Depression. In: David T, ed. *Recent Advances in Paediatrics—21*. London: Royal Society of Medicine; 2004:217–229.

MOOD SYMPTOMS

The core feature of a depressive episode is either a depressed or irritable mood, or loss of interest and enjoyment in all or nearly all activities and pastimes (anhedonia). These symptoms must be pervasive (present for most of the day) and persistent (nearly every day for at least 2 weeks). In practice, children and adolescents often present with behavioral or physical complaints that may obscure the essential features and make detection and diagnosis more difficult. Chronic feelings of worry and boredom are common.

COGNITIVE SYMPTOMS

Cognitive changes are characteristic (depressive thinking) and important because of their implications for treatment. The cognition of depressed youngsters becomes distorted and negative under the influence of their depressed mood, which colors the way they perceive themselves and the world. As a result, they devalue themselves, ignore positive experiences, and focus instead on negative events (e.g., not having receiving a phone call from a friend or an invitation to a party), which are interpreted in a pessimistic, exaggerated, or catastrophic manner ("No one likes me."), resulting in feelings of worthlessness ("I am a failure, a loser."), and creates a vicious cycle that leads to helplessness and hopelessness.

MOTIVATIONAL SYMPTOMS

Difficulty concentrating and making decisions, apathy, and lack of energy and motivation are common. They may retreat to their room and spend inordinate amounts of time lying in bed. These symptoms can result in a deterioration of school performance, withdrawal from sport and social activities, and are often the first manifestation of the illness.

SOMATIC OR NEUROVEGETATIVE SYMPTOMS

Somatic symptoms include poor, restless sleep, appetite changes (overeating and gaining weight or losing appetite and weight), tiredness, and vague or unexplained aches and pains. However, the classic neurovegetative features of *melancholic* depression seen in adults (psychomotor slowing, marked flattening of affect) are uncommon among the young, whose affect usually remains outwardly reactive to their environment, particularly to peers. That is, although they may appear to an observer that they respond and brighten up in that context (e.g., playing basketball with peers), they subjectively report still feeling unhappy ("I have to put on a brave face;" "They play with me because they are sorry for me.").

DIAGNOSIS

Categoric, qualitative diagnoses are the norm in psychiatric taxonomies for a variety of practical reasons. For example, physicians are trained to deal and are more comfortable with an illness/nonillness model; this approach is also more helpful to decide who needs to be treated or not and is usually required by insurers for reimbursement. Yet practitioners need to know there are other approaches (e.g., dimensional or quantitative) and that the boundary between depression and nondepression (e.g., four versus five symptoms, MDD versus subsyndromal depression) is not as clear cut in practice as diagnostic systems seem to convey.[8]

Diagnosis is usually made according to one of the two main classification systems, the *Diagnostic and Statistical Manual of Mental Disorders*, 4th edition *(DSM-IV)*, mostly used in North America and in treatment and research studies, or the *International Classification of Diseases*, 10th edition *(ICD-10)*, often used in European and Asian countries. Although both taxonomies differ in minor aspects (e.g., in the way they define severity; the terms used—*DSM-IV* uses "major depressive episode/disorder," whereas *ICD-10* uses "depressive episode/disorder"), they are quite similar, and this book generally refers to the *DSM-IV* system. Figure 1.1 presents a brief algorithm for the diagnosis of major depression.

It is important to ascertain if the current problems represent a change from the child's previous level of functioning or character. For example, depression should be considered in the differential

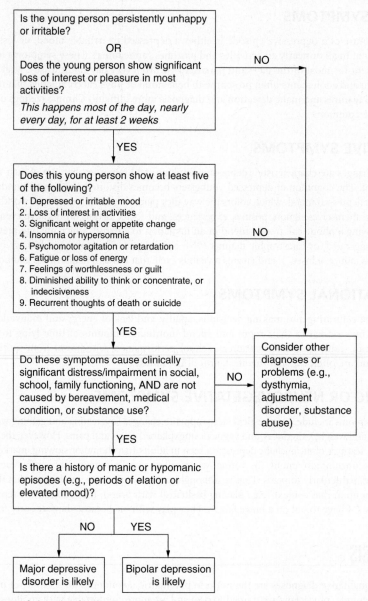

■ Figure 1.1 Brief algorithm for the diagnosis of major depression in young people.

diagnosis of a 14-year-old boy with a 6-month history of oppositional and conduct symptoms and no previous behavior problems. Similarly, depression may account for the recent academic failure of a 15-year-old girl who had previously topped her class (for further discussion of practical aspects of diagnosis, see Chapter 3).

RELIABILITY

Agreement between clinicians making diagnoses of MDD in clinic settings is only moderate (e.g., *kappa* = 0.5 to 0.6) but not very different from the reliability of most emotional disorders.[25] Factors that influence agreement include the informants used, the type of sample (clinic, community), practitioners' experience, presence of comorbid diagnoses, and whether clinicians have undergone training to ensure similar knowledge and frames of reference. Supplementing clinical evaluations with rating scales or structured diagnostic interviews enhances agreement. The reliability of a diagnosis of dysthymic disorder is lower.

INFORMANT

Much evidence shows that parents and teachers underestimate depressive feelings in the young. Additionally, reports and questionnaire data from different informants often disagree. This does not necessarily imply untruthfulness; it often reflects observers' difficulty interpreting children's emotions and behavior, and their limited knowledge of the child (e.g., teachers observe the young person's behavior and emotions in the classroom but not at home or in social situations). For example, in an epidemiologic survey of 1,340 adolescents 13 to 17 years of age, 72% of the 64 adolescents who reported clinically significant depression were not perceived as depressed by their parents. Conversely, 67% of the 55 adolescents reported as depressed by parents did not report clinically significant depression themselves.[4] Hence it is essential to interview the child, often on several occasions, to obtain an accurate picture of how the young person is feeling. The key clinical skill of integrating information from several sources is often difficult in this context, but, contrary to what happens with other conditions such as conduct disorder or ADHD, clinicians should usually give more weight to young persons' reports when diagnosing depression, although information from parents and teachers should also be sought and considered. Chapter 3 offers suggestions on how to integrate data from several informants in everyday practice.

SEVERITY

As with most medical conditions, evaluating the severity of a depressive episode is important because treatment guidelines use severity as a yardstick to indicate what type of treatment should be administered[2,13] and to estimate the risk-to-benefit ratio. Severity is also a key feature to bear in mind when interpreting or applying the results of treatment studies. Results obtained in mildly depressed patients may not necessarily pertain to more disturbed populations. For example, most randomized controlled treatment trials have excluded suicidal participants, whereas suicidal thoughts and attempts are very common in depressed young people in clinic settings.

Table 3.3 presents the rating of severity of depressive episodes according to the *DSM-IV*. *ICD-10* uses a list of ten symptoms and divides depression into nondepressed (fewer than four symptoms), mild (four symptoms), moderate (five or six symptoms), and severe (seven or more symptoms with or without psychotic features). The National Institute for Clinical Excellence (NICE) in the United Kingdom differentiates mild depression, moderate to severe depression, and severe depression with psychotic features. The NICE guideline acknowledges the limitation of categorizing severity of depressive illnesses by symptom count alone.[2] Given the inadequate definitions of severity, not backed by empirical evidence, assessment of severity is largely based on clinical consensus and on the skills and experience of the clinician. Apart from depressive symptoms and impairment, other factors, particularly risk to self or others, also impinge on deciding which treatment setting is more appropriate and are indicators of severity. For example, an adolescent with high suicide risk may require hospitalization, whereas another with an otherwise similarly severe depression but with low risk of suicide may not.

SUBTYPES OF DEPRESSION

Over the years researchers have hypothesized the existence of many subtypes of depression (e.g., primary and secondary, endogenous and reactive, neurotic and psychotic) based on etiologic speculation, often without convincing empirical data or clinical usefulness. Some of these concepts are still popular in a number of countries or settings. This notwithstanding, subtyping depressive illness is relevant because different types of depression have implications for treatment and prognosis. For example, seasonal mood disorder may specifically respond to light therapy, a double depression (dysthymia plus major depression) would be an indicator of poorer prognosis, and treatment of bipolar depression (or bipolar disorder I or II: depressed episode) is different from that of unipolar depression.

TABLE 1.3 SOME SUBTYPES OF DEPRESSION RELEVANT TO CLINICAL PRACTICE

Unipolar depression	Major depression when there is no history of a manic, mixed, or hypomanic episode.
Bipolar depression	Major depression when there is history of at least one (not drug-induced) manic hypomanic, or mixed episode. This is equivalent in *DSM-IV* to bipolar I—depressed (if the episode was manic or mixed) or bipolar II—depressed (if the episode was hypomanic).
Psychotic depression	When, in the absence of other psychotic disorder, the young person displays hallucinations or delusions in addition to symptoms of major depression.
Melancholic depression, major depression with melancholic features, or melancholia	When episodes are characterized by prominent neurovegetative changes such as weight loss, psychomotor retardation, marked sleep disturbance, diurnal mood variation, and lack of reactivity.
Dysthymic disorder or dysthymia	When there is a chronically depressed mood for at least 1 year but not severe enough to qualify for a diagnosis of major depression. Symptom-free intervals last <2 months and there is an absence of manic, hypomanic, or mixed episodes.
Double depression	When a major depressive episode occurs in a young person already suffering from dysthymia.
Seasonal depression (major depression with seasonal pattern, seasonal affective disorder)	When the beginning and remission of major depression follow a pattern (for at least 2 years) related to specific times of the year, usually onset during fall or winter and remission in spring. It should be differentiated from depression triggered by school stress because both usually coincide with the school calendar.
Mood disorder not otherwise specified (NOS)	When young people present with significant mood symptoms and impairment but do not clearly meet criteria for a specific mood disorder, often because of mixed presentations (e.g., depressive and manic symptoms).
Adjustment disorder with depressed mood	When clinically significant depressive symptoms (unhappiness, tearfulness, hopelessness) or impairment occur within 3 months of identifiable stressors and do not meet criteria for major depression or bereavement. It is expected that symptoms will disappear within 6 months once stressors have ceased.
Minor depression, subsyndromal depression, subclinical depression	When a depressive episode falls short of meeting the full criteria for major depression (e.g., one core symptom, and one to three associated symptoms, and very mild disability). This term is mostly used in prevention studies and interventions.

Table 1.3 summarizes the most widely used subtypes of depression. Other subtypes include depression arising from medical illness or substance use (listed in Table 1.4), catatonic depression, postpsychotic depression, and premenstrual dysphoric disorder. The last condition, not yet formally included in *DSM-IV*, is characterized by incapacitating depressed mood, anxiety, and lability that are linked with the menstrual cycle, most notably during the week preceding menstruation.

COMORBIDITY

This section introduces the general issues associated with comorbidity, which are dealt with further in Chapters 3 and 17. Comorbidity refers to the simultaneous occurrence of two or more distinct conditions in the one individual. This is a common and complex issue across all child and adolescent mental disorders that has considerable theoretical and practical implications—for example, for treatment—and is still not resolved satisfactorily. Reflecting this uncertainty, the *DSM-IV* and *ICD-10* systems deal differently with comorbidity. *DSM-IV* prescribes that, with few exceptions, if the young person meets concurrent criteria for two, three, or more disorders (e.g., MDD, ADHD, and oppositional

TABLE 1.4 COMMON MEDICAL CONDITIONS THAT CAN PRESENT WITH SYMPTOMS MIMICKING DEPRESSION IN CHILDREN AND ADOLESCENTS[a]

Medication Induced	Substance Induced	Infections	Neurologic	Endocrine	Other
Accutane	Alcohol	Acquired	Epilepsy	Addison disease	Anemia
Anticonvulsants	Amphetamines	immunodeficiency	Migraine	Cushing disease	Chronic
(e.g., valproate)	Cocaine	syndrome (AIDS)	Radiation	Diabetes	fatigue
Antihypertensives	Marijuana	Encephalitis	therapy	Hypopituitarism	syndrome
(e.g., clonidine,	Opiates	Infectious	Traumatic	Premenstrual	Chronic renal
ß-blockers)	Solvent or petrol	mononucleosis	brain	dysphoric	failure
Benzodiazepines	sniffing	Influenza	injury	disorder	Electrolyte
Cimetidine				Thyroid	abnormalities
Corticosteroids				disorders	Irritable
Oral contraceptives					bowel
Stimulants (e.g.,					syndrome
amphetamines,					Malignancies
methylphenidate)					Malnutrition
					Wilson disease

[a]Modified from Weller EB, Weller RA, Rowan AB, et al. Depressive disorders in children and adolescents. In: M. Lewis, ed. *Child and Adolescent Psychiatry: A Comprehensive Textbook.* Philadelphia, PA: Lippincott Williams & Wilkins; 2002:773.

defiant disorder), each of the conditions should be diagnosed, as long as the symptoms of one disorder are not accounted for by the other condition. For example, if a child meets criteria for oppositional defiant disorder (ODD) and if irritability is better accounted for by the ODD, this symptom is not considered for major depression. The problem is that some investigators do not follow this rule because it requires a degree of inference, thus reducing reliability. This is one of the reasons for the high rate of comorbidity in many research studies. In this line, of the children with any *DSM-IV* diagnosis in an epidemiologic study, 22% had two, 5% three, and 2% four concurrent diagnoses.[19] On the contrary, *ICD-10* stipulates that some of the combinations observed represent distinct disorders and should receive only one diagnosis. That is, *ICD-10* assumes that symptoms of several conditions appearing simultaneously are more likely to be the manifestation of a single disorder with an atypical presentation than of two or more separate conditions. A youth meeting criteria for major depression and conduct disorder would be diagnosed as suffering from "depressive conduct disorder," according to *ICD-10,* and with both MDD and conduct disorder, according to *DSM-IV.* Comorbidity becomes of particular theoretical interest when the observed frequency of co-occurrence is greater than the frequency expected by chance alone. This would suggest the presence of one condition increases the risk of suffering from the other, often true with physical illnesses (e.g., diabetes and heart disease).

Data from community surveys suggest that depression comorbid with other disorders is the norm rather than the exception in children and adolescents, even more so in clinic settings. This is because the likelihood of referral of such a child is a function of the combined likelihood of referral for each disorder separately, a phenomenon known as the Berkson effect. These children also show greater impairment than children with a single diagnosis. Comorbidity is often associated with worse adult outcomes. For example, childhood MDD comorbid with conduct disorder or substance abuse is associated with a higher likelihood of severe or violent offending by age 24 than when major depression, conduct disorder, or substance abuse occur alone.[26]

The more frequent psychiatric disorders comorbid with depression include anxiety disorders, conduct problems, ADHD, obsessive compulsive disorder, and learning difficulties. An epidemiologic study[12] showed that in a 3-month period, 28% of the young people diagnosed with a depressive disorder also had an anxiety disorder, 7% ADHD, 3% conduct disorder, 3% oppositional defiant disorder, and 1% substance use disorder. The practical implication is that establishing whether a child shows symptoms of one condition (e.g., major depression) is only a first step in the evaluation; clinicians ought to inquire for symptoms of other conditions as well.

The link between depression and anxiety (both described as *emotional* or *internalizing* disorders) is well known because depressive and anxiety symptoms often coexist, and individuals frequently experience depressive and anxiety episodes at different times in their lives. Suffering from a depressive episode not only increases the risk of further depressive episodes (homotypic continuity) but also of anxiety disorders (heterotypic continuity).[8,12,27]

Depression is frequently comorbid with posttraumatic stress disorder.[28] Adolescents in particular are vulnerable to depression and suicidality in the year following a traumatic event. Mechanisms include so-called survivor guilt that others died or were severely injured, complicated bereavement, problems in carrying out tasks of daily living owing to impaired concentration or to intrusive memories, and distress arising from chronic anxiety symptoms. Other psychiatric complications of traumatic stress that may interact with depression include panic disorder, other anxiety disorders, disruptive behaviors, dissociative disorder, and substance misuse.[28]

DEPRESSION AND PERSONALITY DISORDER

Personality traits become progressively ingrained during adolescence and early adulthood. Borderline personality styles are of particular relevance to depression because affected individuals are dysphoric and extremely sensitive to rejection. Their fears of abandonment can be accompanied by intense but usually brief episodes of sadness, anger, or irritability, which sometimes culminate in episodes of self-harm. Both a depressive disorder and borderline personality traits or disorder can coexist. Depression, on the one hand, can be misdiagnosed when adolescents with dramatic personality styles present with sadness, irritability, and self-loathing; on the other hand, a depressive episode can exaggerate otherwise normal personality traits, suggesting that a personality disorder exists when that might not be the case. In the latter situation, the symptoms of personality disorder would remit once the individual has recovered from the depressive episode. Diagnosis of personality disorder should be provisional in a depressed adolescent and made on the basis of symptoms and functioning outside of the depressive episode. Perfectionistic and obsessional traits are also seen in adolescents with depression, but given their high prevalence in the community they may actually be underrepresented in clinical populations.[29]

DEPRESSION AND SUICIDAL BEHAVIOR

Suicide is one of the leading causes of death in adolescents in the United States and worldwide. For each completed suicide in the young, there are about 100 reported suicide attempts. Suicidal thoughts are common among the young; about one in six girls 12 to 16 years of age reports having them in the previous 6 months (one in ten for boys), but rates in clinic samples are much higher. Although suicide is the result of complex interactions in which individual and psychosocial factors as well as mental health problems play a role, considerable evidence indicates that depression is the strongest risk factor. About 60% of depressed young people report having thought about suicide, and 30% actually attempt suicide. The risk increases if there have been suicides in the family, if the young person has attempted suicide previously, and if there are other comorbid psychiatric disorders (e.g., substance abuse), impulsivity, aggression, access to lethal means (e.g., firearms), exposure to negative events (e.g., disciplinary crises, physical or sexual abuse), among others.[13] Suicidal behaviors and risk need to be carefully evaluated in every depressed young person (see also Chapters 3 and 15).

THE BURDEN OF CHILDHOOD DEPRESSION

It was estimated that in 2001 adult depression caused the third largest burden of disease in high-income countries—measured in disability-adjusted life years—just behind ischemic heart disease and cerebrovascular disease.[30] The burden of illness comprises direct, indirect, and intangible costs. Direct costs include medical (e.g., outpatient, inpatient, and pharmaceutical expenses) and nonmedical costs such as transport and social services. Indirect costs comprise productivity loss due to absences from the workplace or reduced productivity caused by morbidity and premature death. Intangible costs result from the diminished quality of life of the sufferer and their families. There are still few studies of the cost of depression in adults with methodologies of varying quality, but estimates suggest that depression poses a considerable burden.[31] For example, a study in Sweden showed that costs of depression had increased from a total of €1.7 billion in 1997 to €3.5 billion in 2005. The main reason for the increase was growing indirect costs (e.g., sick leave and early retirement); direct costs had been relatively stable.[32]

Few data on the economic burden of depression in childhood are currently available.[33] However, assuming a large continuity into adulthood of the disorder, burden is likely to be very substantial in most areas, including mortality.[2,32,34] For example, one study estimated that a randomly selected

21-year-old woman with early-onset major depressive disorder in 1995 could expect future annual earnings that were 12% to 18% lower than those of a randomly selected 21-year-old woman whose onset of major depressive disorder occurred after age 21 or without major depression.[35] Data on burden of depression are important and will probably highlight the cost effectiveness of prevention, early detection, and treatment, and they will underscore the potential key role of primary care service providers in this endeavor.

RESOURCES FOR PRACTITIONERS

References 2, 5, and 8.

Athealth.com: A provider of mental health information and services for mental health practitioners and patients: http://www.athealth.com/index.html

Texas Department of State Health Services: Mental Health Programs Initiatives, Children's Medication Algorithm Project: http://www.dshs.state.tx.us/mhprograms/CMAPmddED.shtm

Most of the websites listed for patients and families also provide information for practitioners.

RESOURCES FOR PATIENTS AND FAMILIES

A self-help website based in the United Kingdom for adolescents (mostly) and parents with good information and aids: http://www.ru-ok.com/index.html

Depression in Children and Adolescents, NIMH: http://www.nimh.nih.gov/health/topics/depression/depression-in-children-and-adolescents.shtml

Depression Center at HealthyPlace.com has considerable information on depression for both practitioners and sufferers: http://www.healthyplace.com/communities/depression/ index.asp

NYU Child Study Center: http://www.aboutourkids.org/families/disorders_treatments/az_disorder_guide/depressive_disorders

Mood Disorders Society of Canada: http://www.mooddisorderscanada.ca/depression/ index.htm#

Depression Alliance: A site from the United Kingdom supporting people with depression: http://www.depressionalliance.org/index.html

Beyondblue: An Australian site with information, resources, and support for sufferers: http://www.beyondblue.org.au/index.aspx?

Black Dog Institute: http://www.blackdoginstitute.org.au/index.cfm

Reach Out! A web-based service that inspires young people to help themselves through tough times: http://www.reachout.com.au/home.asp

Graham P, Hughes C. *So Young, So Sad, So Listen.* 2nd ed. London: The Royal College of Psychiatrists; 2005 (Paperback; 56 pp.).

REFERENCES

1. Murray CJL, Lopez AD. Alternate projections of mortality and disability by cause 1990–2020: global burden of disease study. *Lancet.* 1997;349:1498–1504.
2. National Institute for Health and Clinical Excellence. *Depression in Children and Young People: Identification and Management in Primary, Community and Secondary Care.* National Clinical Practice Guideline No. 28. Leicester, UK: The British Psychological Society; 2005. Available at http://www.nice.org.uk/nicemedia/pdf/cg028fullguideline.pdf
3. Perry BL, Pescosolido BA, Martin JK, et al. Comparison of public attributions, attitudes, and stigma in regard to depression among children and adults. *Psychiatr Serv.* 2007;58:632–635.
4. Rey JM, Sawyer MG, Clark JJ, et al. Depression among Australian adolescents. *Med J Aust.* 2001;175:19–23.
5. Birmaher B, Ryan ND, Williamson DE, et al. Childhood and adolescent depression: a review of the past 10 years. Part I. *J Am Acad Child Adolesc Psychiatry.* 1996;35:1427–1439.
6. Carlson G, Garber J. Developmental issues in the classification of depression in children. In: Rutter M, Izard CE, Read PB, eds. *Depression in Young People: Developmental and Clinical Perspectives.* New York: Guilford Press; 1986:399–434.
7. Goodman SH, Schwab-Stone M, Lahey BB, et al. Major depression and dysthymia in children and adolescents: discriminant validity and differential consequences in a community sample. *J Am Acad Child Adolesc Psychiatry.* 2000;39:761–770.
8. Cole J, McGuffin P, Farmer AE. The classification of depression: are we still confused? *Br J Psychiatry.* 2008;192:83–85.

9. Andrews G, Slade T, Sunderland M, et al. Issues for DSM-V: simplifying DSM-IV to enhance utility: the case of major depressive disorder. *Am J Psychiatry.* 2007;164:1784–1785.

10. Timimi S. Rethinking childhood depression. *BMJ.* 2004;329:1394–1396.

11. Olfson M, Marcus SC, Druss BG. Effects of Food and Drug Administration warnings on antidepressant use in a national sample. *Arch Gen Psychiatry.* 2008;65:94–101.

12. Costello EJ, Mustillo S, Erkanli A, et al. Prevalence and development of psychiatric disorders in childhood and adolescence. *Arch Gen Psychiatry.* 2003;60:837–844.

13. Birmaher B, Brent D, AACAP Work Group on Quality Issues, et al. Practice parameter for the assessment and treatment of children and adolescents with depressive disorders. *J Am Acad Child Adolesc Psychiatry.* 2007;46: 1503–1526. Available at: http://www.aacap.org/galleries/PracticeParameters/InPress_2007_Depressivedisorders. pdf

14. Lewinsohn PM, Hops H, Roberts RE, et al. Adolescent psychopathology: I. Prevalence and incidence of depression and other DSM-III-R disorders in high school students. *J Abnorm Psychol.* 1993;102:133–144.

15. Hankin BL, Abramson LY, Moffitt TE, et al. Development of depression from preadolescence to young adulthood: emerging gender differences in a 10-year longitudinal study. *J Abnorm Psychol.* 1998;107:128–140.

16. Costello EJ, Costello AJ, Edelbrock C, et al. Psychiatric disorders in pediatric primary care: prevalence and risk factors. *Arch Gen Psychiatry.* 1988;45:1107–1116.

17. Hazell P, O'Connell D, Heathcote D, et al. Tricyclic drugs for depression in children and adolescents. *Cochrane Database Syst Rev.* 2002;2:CD002317.

18. Bridge JA, Iyengar S, Salary CB, et al. Clinical response and risk for reported suicidal ideation and suicide attempts in pediatric antidepressant treatment: a meta-analysis of randomized controlled trials. *JAMA.* 2007;297:1683–1696.

19. Ford T, Goodman R, Meltzer H. The British Child and Adolescent Mental Health Survey 1999: the prevalence of DSM-IV disorders. *J Am Acad Child Adolesc Psychiatry.* 2003;42:1203–1211.

20. Sawyer M, Arney F, Baghurst P, et al. The mental health of young people in Australia: key findings from the child and adolescent component of the national survey of mental health and well-being. *Aust N Z J Psychiatry.* 2001;35:806–814.

21. Canino G, Shrout PE, Rubio-Stipec M, et al. The DSM-IV rates of child and adolescent disorders in Puerto Rico. Prevalence, correlates, service use, and the effects of impairment. *Arch Gen Psychiatry.* 2004;61:85–93.

22. Shaaban KMA, Baashar TA. A community study of depression in adolescent girls: prevalence and its relation to age. *Med Principles Pract.* 2003;12:256–259.

23. Carlson GA. The challenge of diagnosing depression in childhood and adolescence. *J Affect Disord.* 2000;61:3–8.

24. Zisook S, Lesser I, Stewart JW, et al. Effect of age at onset on the course of major depressive disorder. *Am J Psychiatry.* 2007;164:1539–1546.

25. Rey JM, Plapp JM, Stewart GW. Reliability of psychiatric diagnosis in referred adolescents. *J Child Psychol Psychiatry.* 1989;30:879–888.

26. Copeland WE, Miller-Johnson S, Keeler G, et al. Childhood psychiatric disorders and young adult crime: a prospective, population-based study. *Am J Psychiatry.* 2007;164:1668–1675.

27. Fergusson DM, Horwood LJ, Boden JM. Structure of internalizing symptoms in early adulthood. *Br J Psychiatry.* 2006;189:540–546.

28. Perrin S, Smith P, Yule W. The assessment and treatment of post-traumatic stress disorder in children and adolescents. *J Child Psychol Psychiatry.* 2000;41:277–289.

29. Parker G, Roy K. Adolescent depression: a review. *Aust N Z J Psychiatry.* 2001;35:572–580.

30. Lopez AD, Mathers CD, Ezzati M, et al. Global and regional burden of disease and risk factors, 2001: systematic analysis of population health data. *Lancet.* 2006;367:1747–1757.

31. Luppa M, Heinrich S, Angermeyer MC, et al. Cost-of-illness studies of depression. A systematic review. *J Affect Disord.* 2007;98:29–43.

32. Sobocki P, Lekander I, Borgstrom F, et al. The economic burden of depression in Sweden from 1997 to 2005. *Eur Psychiatry.* 2007;22:146–152.

33. Lynch FL, Clarke GN. Estimating the economic burden of depression in children and adolescents. *Am J Prevent Med.* 2006;31(suppl 1):S143–S151.

34. Weissman MM, Wolk S, Goldstein RB, et al. Depressed adolescents grown up. *JAMA.* 1999;281:1707–1713.

35. Berndt ER, Koran LM, Finkelstein SN, et al. Lost human capital from early-onset chronic depression. *Am J Psychiatry.* 2000;157:940–947.

Depression: Causes and Risk Factors

DANIEL J. PILOWSKY

KEY POINTS

- Depression in youth is likely the result of a complex set of interactions between biologic vulnerabilities and environmental influences.
- Before puberty, depression is relatively rare and equally prevalent in males and females. Starting with puberty, the incidence (new cases) of depression increases markedly, and female depression becomes more prevalent than depression in males.
- Biologic vulnerabilities may result from the child's genetic endowment and from prenatal factors.
- Environmental influences may be proximal (e.g., the child's family) or distal (school and neighborhood characteristics).
- Parental depression is the most consistently replicated risk factor for depression in the offspring.
- Stressful life events—especially loss events—may increase the risk for depression. This risk may be augmented when children process loss events (or other stressful life events) using negative attributions.
- Parental rejection may create a depression diathesis, especially when other risk factors are present.
- Distal influences, that is, the social environment that includes neighborhood and schools, may increase or decrease the risk.

Introduction   *Depression is likely to be multidetermined, and therefore it is unlikely that a single cause or risk factor will explain its development. When examining the multiple risk factors involved, the task is no longer teasing out genetic from environmental factors but understanding how they relate to each other. However, understanding the interplay between genes and environments, including the prenatal environment, is in its early stages. Risk factors for depression should be considered at several levels, including individual, familial, and social, as they interact in complex causal webs. Nevertheless, they are presented separately in this chapter to facilitate their understanding.*

Risk factors may be fixed (e.g., gender) or subject to change (e.g., maladaptive cognitions). The latter are potential targets of preventive interventions.

INDIVIDUAL RISK FACTORS

GENETIC

Genetic factors clearly increase the risk for depression.[1] Even though numerous estimates of heritability have been published, usually based on twin studies, the specific genetic pathways are still being studied. Until recently, behavioral geneticists estimated that genetic factors accounted for about 40% of the variance in both males and females, with most of the remaining variance explained by individuals' unique environment.[2] One the main findings in recent twin studies is that hereditability for depression is greater in females than in males.[3] For example, a large study of Swedish twins revealed that hereditability was 29% and 42% in males and females, respectively.[4] Another recent finding is that at least some genetic pathways include genes that may interact with a variety of childhood stressful life events, especially with maltreatment.[5,6] These interactions have so far been limited to the serotonin transporter gene, but others may emerge as more knowledge is gained. From a clinical viewpoint, the implication is that the same event (e.g., maltreatment in childhood) may have a large depressogenic impact on one adolescent and little on another.

GENDER

Major depression is relatively rare before puberty and equally distributed between boys and girls or slightly more prevalent in boys. Two changes occur with puberty. First, major depression becomes more frequent in both genders. Second, major depression and depressive symptoms become two to three times more prevalent in girls than in boys, as is the case in adulthood.

Multiple explanations have been proposed for this phenomenon, including genetic, hormonal, and social theories.[3] Even though there might be genetic differences, the evidence is not conclusive.[7] Recurrent estrogen withdrawal, beginning with puberty, may interfere with one of the functions of estrogens (i.e., the neutralization of corticoids released during stress), thus increasing the risk of stress-related depressive episodes.[8] Among the many psychosocial factors proposed to explain the higher prevalence of adolescent depression in girls, theories that posit dissimilar affiliative needs have received a lot of attention. Even though both genders seek friends, girls are more likely to become emotionally invested in a friendship network and to have a higher turnover of close friends than boys. Thus girls are more exposed to disappointments in their relationships, and these disappointments may increase the risk for depression in adolescence.[3,9]

STRESSFUL LIFE EVENTS

An extensive literature suggests that stressful life events often precede the onset of depressive episodes.[10–12] It is noteworthy, however, that such events precede other psychiatric disorders as well.[13] Some events seem to precipitate depressive episodes, whereas others may create a vulnerability to depression. Child maltreatment may operate both ways. Sexual abuse in childhood may increase the risk for depression, anxiety, eating disorders, and self-injurious behaviors in adolescence[14,15] and create a vulnerability for adult depression.[16–18] Child maltreatment, including physical and sexual abuse, is one of the childhood events most consistently associated with higher rates of depression and anxiety in adolescence and adulthood.[14,19] Losses, such as a death in the family or loss of a close friend, seem to precipitate depressive episodes, and this association has some specificity; that is, losses are more likely to be associated with depression than with other disorders.[13]

ATTACHMENTS AND EARLY CHILDHOOD

Abundant evidence indicates that the quality of early attachments contributes to later depressive and anxious symptoms.[20] Early emotional deprivation, which may result from disrupted attachments, may increase the responsiveness of the hypothalamic-pituitary-adrenal axis, thus altering responses to later stress.[21–23] Clinical evidence also shows that disrupted attachments may be associated with severe early deprivation.[24]

COGNITIVE STYLES

Cognitive theories of depression suggest that individuals who have negative beliefs about themselves or about the world perceive stressors—such as stressful life events and their consequences—negatively. This pessimistic outlook may in turn increase the risk of depression in these individuals.[25] Empirical evidence from longitudinal studies shows that negative cognitions and a negative explanatory style predict depressive symptoms, and the association is stronger in older children and adolescents.[26–28] Overall, the evidence that negative cognitions increase the risk for depression in youth is solid. What is not clear, however, is whether these cognitions are an early manifestation of clinical depression or a causal factor. Additionally, if negative cognitions are indeed a causal factor, the question of why certain children develop negative cognitions remains unanswered.

ANXIETY IN CHILDHOOD

Anxiety disorders are the most common co-occurring conditions among youth with depression.[25] Furthermore, anxiety disorders often precede the onset of depression, which has been observed in high-risk family studies as well as in clinical samples. Typically, anxiety disorders in school-age children are followed by major depression in adolescence.[29–31] Interpreting the meaning of the sequence, from anxiety to later depression, is complex. Anxiety in childhood and depression in adolescence could be sequential manifestations of a single disorder (heterotypic continuity), and anxiety disorders, and perhaps symptoms, may indeed be a risk factor for major depression. Disruptive behavior disorders may also precede the onset of depression.[32,33] Peer rejection, academic failure, and social isolation may increase the risk of depression in these children.[34]

FAMILIAL RISK FACTORS

PARENTAL DEPRESSION

Parental depression is one of the most consistently replicated risk factors for depression in childhood and adolescence,[25,35–37] and the increased risk is likely to be influenced by both genetic and environmental factors. Compared to offspring of nondepressed parents, children of depressed parents are about three to four times more likely to develop a mood disorder. Even at 5 years of age, children of depressed mothers exhibited increased peer conflict and aggression in a well-designed study.[38] Children of depressed mothers are also at increased risk for other disorders. Weissman et al., using data from a three-generation study, described a typical developmental sequence among children of depressed mothers; it consists of an increased prevalence of behavioral and anxiety disorders in school-age children, depression and substance use in adolescents, and depression and substance abuse in the early adult years.[35,39] Fortunately, the impact of maternal depression may be at least partially reversible. A study assessed mothers and children while the mothers were depressed and 3 months after the initiation of treatment of maternal depression. There was an overall decrease (11%) in rates of diagnoses in children of mothers whose depression remitted, compared with an 8% increase in rates of diagnoses in children of mothers who remained depressed.[40]

Parental depression is associated with a higher risk of major depression in their offspring—eightfold for childhood onset and fivefold for early-adult onset—but not with major depression of adolescent-onset.[41] The incidence of major depression increases markedly in adolescence, especially in girls, regardless of parental depression status.[42] Different causal pathways may be associated with offspring depression in childhood, adolescence, and adulthood. Recent evidence of a negative impact of paternal depression on young children has generated interest in widening research to include depressed fathers.[43]

Although many studies of children of depressed parents have been conducted, little is known about psychopathology among parents of depressed children. A study of parents of clinically depressed children found that major depression was the most common disorder in parents of both sexes, but it was more prevalent in mothers. Substance abuse and antisocial pathology was more prevalent in fathers.[44] A more recent study screened 117 mothers seeking treatment for their depressed children, and it found that 17% screened positive for panic disorder, 17% for generalized anxiety disorder, and 14% for major depression. Few screened positive for alcohol (2%), drug use (1%), or abuse.[45]

PARENTAL RELATIONSHIPS, PARENTING, AND FAMILY FUNCTIONING

Parental depression is associated with marital and family discord,[46] and these factors are associated with depression in the offspring.[47] Some evidence also indicates that marital discord may be associated with other offspring disorders.[48,49] One limitation of this literature is that these factors may have a different impact on children from families with and without a depressed parent. In families with a depressed parent, the impact of parental depression may overshadow the impact of most other risk factors. For example, Pilowsky et al. reported that affectionless control, a type of parenting characterized by lack of affection and a controlling parenting style, was associated with a fivefold increase in the risk for major depression in children of nondepressed parents but was not associated with a significantly increased risk among children of depressed parents.[47] Thus it is important to consider separately the impact of familial risk factors in children of depressed parents and in unselected clinical and community samples.

A meta-analysis revealed that parenting accounted for almost 8% of the variance in childhood depression, compared with <6% of the variance in child externalizing problems and <4% of the variance in childhood anxiety.[50] Parental rejection and parental control were found to be consistently associated with depression in the offspring, the former more so than the latter. Parental hostility toward the child, a subdimension of the parental rejection construct, was most strongly associated with childhood depression.[50]

Parenting can be defined as the practices used to rear a child. This includes, among others, providing nurture, protection, love, and guidance. Studies have often found two factors underlying different types of parenting. These are called care and control (resulting in four types of parenting according to whether there is high or low levels of care and control—for example, affectionless-controlling, caring-non controlling) or demandingness and responsiveness, which also result in four parenting styles (indulgent, authoritarian, authoritative, and uninvolved).

Among the many familial risk factors studied, marital discord deserves special attention because of the consistent evidence of its contribution to increased risk for depression in the offspring and for other psychiatric symptoms and disorders.[51,52] Marital conflict and parenting are closely related because marital conflict may lead to maladaptive parenting.[53]

INTERPERSONAL AND PSYCHOANALYTIC THEORIES

Garber[25] suggests two significant links between interpersonal vulnerability and depression. First, there are attachment and parenting deficits in families with a depressed parent. Second, depressed adolescents themselves have interpersonal difficulties including poorer communication and problem-solving skills. Additionally, they are less assertive than nondepressed children. Although interpersonal difficulties may increase the risk for adolescent depression, depression itself may lead to interpersonal difficulties, such as the lack of assertiveness typically seen in depressed adolescents.

Contemporary psychoanalytic theories of depression in adolescence often view attachment deficits as a vulnerability factor. Some evidence indicates that deficits in attachment are associated with subsequent depression,[54] but attachment deficits have also been linked to other disorders.[55] The development of new instruments for measuring attachment in children may contribute to more empirical research in this area.[56] Additionally, some psychodynamically oriented theorists focus on external and internal losses as precipitants of depressive episodes in adolescence.[57] External losses may include the death of a parent or relative (see "Stressful Life Events" earlier). Internal losses may include the loss of the internalized parental images of childhood or the loss of the capacity for the free imaginative play characteristic of childhood.[57]

SOCIAL RISK FACTORS

Children do not only depend on their caregivers for achieving and maintaining psychological well-being. Their well-being also depends on the resources offered by schools and neighborhoods. High-quality schools and after-school programs, parks, recreational facilities, and freedom from violence—a set of factors often grouped under the conceptual umbrella of "social capital"—may increase or decrease the risk for depression.[58] Recent research suggests that neighborhood characteristics, such as percentage of households living in poverty in a given neighborhood, social control (i.e., whether there is an expectation that somebody will intervene in certain situations, such as a child skipping school), and social cohesion (i.e., a perceived willingness of neighbors to help each other), impact on children's mental health. More specifically, neighborhood characteristics explain a substantial proportion of the variance in children's internalizing scores, a reflection of depressive and anxiety-related symptoms.[59]

REFERENCES

1. Thapar A, Rice F. Twin studies in pediatric depression. *Child Adolesc Psychiatr Clin N Am*. 2006;15:869–881.
2. Thapar A, McGuffin P. Genetic influences on life events in childhood. *Psychol Med*. 1996;26:813–820.
3. Goldberg D. The aetiology of depression. *Psychol Med*. 2006;36:1341–1347.
4. Kendler KS, Gatz M, Gardner CO, et al. A Swedish national twin study of lifetime major depression. *Am J Psychiatry*. 2006;163:109–114.
5. Caspi A, Sugden K, Moffitt TE, et al. Influence of life stress on depression: moderation by a polymorphism in the 5-HTT gene. *Science*. 2003;301:386–389.
6. Kaufman J, Yang B-Z, Douglas-Palumberi H, et al. Social supports and serotonin transporter gene moderate depression in maltreated children. *Proc Natl Acad Sci U S A*. 2004;101:17316–17321.
7. Staley JK, Sanacora G, Tamagnan G, et al. Sex differences in diencephalon serotonin transporter availability in major depression. *Biol Psychiatry*. 2006;59:40–47.
8. Seeman MV. Psychopathology in women and men: focus on female hormones. *Am J Psychiatry*. 1997;154:1641–1647.
9. Goodyer IM, Herbert J, Tamplin A, et al. Recent life events, cortisol, dehydroepiandrosterone and the onset of major depression in high-risk adolescents. *Br J Psychiatry*. 2000;177:499–504.
10. Hammen C, Ellicott A, Gitlin M, et al. Sociotropy/autonomy and vulnerability to specific life events in patients with unipolar depression and bipolar disorders. *J Abnorm Psychol*. 1989;98:154–160.
11. Brown GW, Harris T. Social origins of depression: a reply. *Psychol Med*. 1978;8:577–588.
12. Hammen C, Davila J, Brown G, et al. Psychiatric history and stress: predictors of severity of unipolar depression. *J Abnorm Psychol*. 1992;101:45–52.
13. Tiet QQ, Bird HR, Hoven CW, et al. Relationship between specific adverse life events and psychiatric disorders. *J Abnorm Child Psychol*. 2001;29:153–164.
14. Mullen PE, Martin JL, Anderson JC, et al. The effect of child sexual abuse on social, interpersonal and sexual function in adult life. *Br J Psychiatry*. 1994;165:35–47.
15. Swanston HY, Plunkett AM, O'Toole BI, et al. Nine years after child sexual abuse. *Child Abuse Negl*. 2003;27:967–984.
16. Mullen PE, Martin JL, Anderson JC, et al. The long-term impact of the physical, emotional, and sexual abuse of children: a community study. *Child Abuse Negl*. 1996;20:7–21.
17. Bifulco A, Moran PM, Baines R, et al. Exploring psychological abuse in childhood: II. Association with other abuse and adult clinical depression. *Bull Menninger Clin*. 2002;66:241–258.
18. Kendler KS, Kuhn JW, Prescott CA. Childhood sexual abuse, stressful life events and risk for major depression in women. *Psychol Med*. 2004;34:1475–1482.
19. Swanston HY, Tebbutt JS, O'Toole BI, et al. Sexually abused children 5 years after presentation: a case-control study. *Pediatrics*. 1997;100:600–608.
20. Field TM. Early interactions between infants and their postpartum depressed mothers. *Infant Behav Dev*. 2002;25:25–29.
21. Gunnar MR. Stress effects on the developing brain. In: Romer D, Walker EF, eds. *Adolescent Psychopathology and the Developing Brain: Integrating Brain and Prevention Science*. New York: Oxford University Press; 2007:127–147.
22. Heim C, Meinlschmidt G, Nemeroff CB. Neurobiology of early-life stress. *Psychiatric Ann*. 2003;33:18–26.
23. Heim C, Nemeroff CB. The impact of early adverse experiences on brain systems involved in the pathophysiology of anxiety and affective disorders. *Biol Psychiatry*. 1999;46:1509–1522.
24. Rutter ML, Kreppner JM, O'Connor TG. Specificity and heterogeneity in children's responses to profound institutional privation. *Br J Psychiatry*. 2001;179:97–103.
25. Garber J. Depression in children and adolescents: linking risk research and prevention. *Am J Prevent Med*. 2006;31:S104–S125.
26. Weisz JR, Southam-Gerow MA, McCarty CA. Control-related beliefs and depressive symptoms in clinic-referred children and adolescents: developmental differences and model specificity. *J Abnorm Psychol*. 2001;110:97–109.
27. Abela JR. The hopelessness theory of depression: a test of the diathesis-stress and causal mediation components in third and seventh grade children. *J Abnorm Child Psychol*. 2001;29:241–254.
28. Abela JR, Aydin C, Auerbach RP. Operationalizing the "vulnerability" and "stress" components of the hopelessness theory of depression: a multi-wave longitudinal study. *Behav Res Ther*. 2006;44:1565–1583.
29. Avenevoli S, Stolar M, Li J, et al. Comorbidity of depression in children and adolescents: models and evidence from a prospective high-risk family study. *Biol Psychiatry*. 2001;49:1071–1081.
30. Merikangas KR, Zhang H, Avenevoli S, et al. Longitudinal trajectories of depression and anxiety in a prospective community study. *Arch Gen Psychiatry*. 2003;60:993–1000.

31. Cole DA, Peeke LG, Martin JM, et al. A longitudinal look at the relation between depression and anxiety in children and adolescents. *J Consulting Clin Psychol.* 1998;66:451–460.

32. Lahey BB, Loeber R, Burke J, et al. Waxing and waning in concert: dynamic comorbidity of conduct disorder with other disruptive and emotional problems over 7 years among clinic-referred boys. *J Abnorm Psychol.* 2002;111:556–567.

33. Mick E, Biederman J, Santangelo S, et al. The influence of gender in the familial association between ADHD and major depression. *J Nerv Ment Dis.* 2003;191:699–705.

34. Keiley MK, Lofthouse N, Bates JE, et al. Differential risks of covarying and pure components in mother and teacher reports of externalizing and internalizing behavior across ages 5 to 14. *J Abnorm Child Psychol.* 2003;31:267–283.

35. Weissman MM, Wickramaratne P, Nomura Y, et al. Offspring of depressed parents: 20 years later. *Am J Psychiatry.* 2006;163:1001–1008.

36. Hammen C, Adrian C, Gordon D, et al. Children of depressed mothers: maternal strain and symptom predictors of dysfunction. *J Abnorm Psychol.* 1987;96:190–198.

37. Weissman MM, Wickramaratne P, Nomura Y, et al. Families at high and low risk for depression: a 3-generation study. *Arch Gen Psychiatry.* 2005;62:29–36.

38. Hipwell AE, Murray L, Ducournau P, et al. The effects of maternal depression and parental conflict on children's peer play. *Child Care Health Dev.* 2005;31:11–23.

39. Weissman MM, Gammon GD, John K, et al. Children of depressed parents. Increased psychopathology and early onset of major depression. *Arch Gen Psychiatry.* 1987;44:847–853.

40. Weissman MM, Pilowsky DJ, Wickramaratne PJ, et al. Remissions in maternal depression and child psychopathology: a STAR*D-child report. *JAMA.* 2006;295:1389–1398.

41. Weissman MM, Wickramaratne P. Age of onset and familial risk in major depression. *Arch Gen Psychiatry.* 2000;57:513–514.

42. Wickramaratne PJ, Weissman MM. Onset of psychopathology in offspring by developmental phase and parental depression. *J Am Acad Child Adolesc Psychiatry.* 1998;37:933–942.

43. Ramchandani P, Stein A, Evans J, et al. Paternal depression in the postnatal period and child development: a prospective population study. *Lancet.* 2005;365:2201–2205.

44. Mitchell J, McCauley E, Burke P, et al. Psychopathology in parents of depressed children and adolescents. *J Am Acad Child Adolesc Psychiatry.* 1989;28:352–357.

45. Ferro T, Verdeli H, Pierre F, et al. Screening for depression in mothers bringing their offspring for evaluation or treatment of depression. *Am J Psychiatry.* 2000;157:375–379.

46. Keitner GI, Miller IW. Family functioning and major depression: an overview. *Am J Psychiatry.* 1990;147:1128–1137.

47. Pilowsky DJ, Wickramaratne P, Nomura Y, et al. Family discord, parental depression, and psychopathology in offspring: 20-year follow-up. *J Am Acad Child Adolesc Psychiatry.* 2006;45:452–460.

48. Du Rocher Schudlich TD, Cummings EM. Parental dysphoria and children's internalizing symptoms: marital conflict styles as mediators of risk. *Child Dev.* 2003;74:1663–1681.

49. Burke L. The impact of maternal depression on familial relationships. *Int Rev Psychiatry.* 2003;15:243–255.

50. McLeod BD, Weisz JR, Wood JJ. Examining the association between parenting and childhood depression: a meta-analysis. *Clin Psychol Rev.* 2007;27:986–1003.

51. Cummings EM, Keller PS, Davies PT. Towards a family process model of maternal and paternal depressive symptoms: exploring multiple relations with child and family functioning. *J Child Psychol Psychiatry.* 2005;46:479–489.

52. Davies PT, Cummings E. Marital conflict and child adjustment: an emotional security hypothesis. *Psychol Bull.* 1994;116: 387–411.

53. Schoppe-Sullivan SJ, Schermerhorn AC, Cummings E. Marital conflict and children's adjustment: evaluation of the parenting process model. *J Marriage Fam.* 2007;69:1118–1134.

54. Lancaster G, Rollinson L, Hill J. The measurement of a major childhood risk for depression: comparison of the Parental Bonding Instrument (PBI) 'Parental Care' and the Childhood Experience of Care and Abuse (CECA) 'Parental Neglect.' *J Affective Dis.* 2007;101:263–267.

55. Allen JP, Porter M, McFarland C, et al. The relation of attachment security to adolescents' paternal and peer relationships, depression, and externalizing behavior. *Child Dev.* 2007;78:1222–1239.

56. Target M, Fonagy P, Shmueli-Goetz Y. Attachment representations in school-age children: the development of the child attachment interview (CAI). *J Child Psychother.* 2003;29:171–186.

57. Zaslow S. Depressed adolescents. In: O'Brien JD, Pilowsky DJ, Lewis OW, eds. *Psychotherapies with Children and Adolescents: Adapting the Psychodynamic Process.* Washington, DC: American Psychiatric Association; 1992:209–230.

58. Fitzpatrick KM, Piko BF, Wright DR, et al. Depressive symptomatology, exposure to violence, and the role of social capital among African American adolescents. *Am J Orthopsychiatry.* 2005;75:262–274.

59. Xue Y, Leventhal T, Brooks-Gunn J, et al. Neighborhood residence and mental health problems of 5- to 11-year-olds. *Arch Gen Psychiatry.* 2005;62:554–563.

Clinical Assessment of Children and Adolescents With Depression

CARLO G. CARANDANG AND ANDRÉS MARTIN

KEY POINTS

- Although the core symptoms of depression are similar across the life span, developmental differences exist and should be taken into account in the assessment.
- With increasing age, there generally is an increase in melancholic symptoms, delusions, and suicidal ideation and attempts. In contrast, younger children tend to have more separation anxiety, behavior problems, temper tantrums, and hallucinations.
- Direct interviews with children and adolescents are critical because parents and teachers may not be aware of the youth's depressive symptoms.
- Discrepant information between parents and their children should be solved in a cordial and non-judgmental way.
- Assessment of suicidal and homicidal ideation and behaviors is mandatory.
- The interview process and screening questions used by research interviews, such as the Schedule for Affective Disorders and Schizophrenia for School Age Children, Present and Lifetime Version (KSADS-PL), can be useful.
- Detection and diagnosis can be enhanced by using parent and child self-report measures.

Introduction

The preceding chapters focused on the phenomenology, etiology, course, and prognosis of children and adolescents with depression. This chapter presents a practical approach to evaluating young persons for depression. As such, we focus on the "how to" rather than on the "what is" of pediatric depression. Much of what we do as clinicians is not exclusively informed by evidence or hard data. In the end, unless a connection is made with our young patients and their families and unless we master the process of assessing pediatric depression, no amount of evidence will be applied to its fullest.

The goals of assessment are to (1) establish if the patient suffers from psychiatric disorders and, if so, which ones, (2) elicit the factors that may have caused or contributed to the initiation of these problems and to their persistence (genetic, developmental, familiar, social), (3) evaluate patients' normal level of functioning and the extent this has been impaired by the illness, (4) identify areas of strength as well as potential supports within the family and the wider social environment, and (5) build trust and rapport. It is assumed that you are familiar with a psychiatric evaluation and aware that the interview is the main tool in assessing patients, based not only on what patients and families disclose but also by observing their behavior and interactions—with the clinician, family members, toys, and others.

Assessment of a child or adolescent differs from that of an adult in several respects. Whereas most adults seek help on their own behalf, children rarely do so. As a result, parents or caregivers are often the primary source of information. Greater emphasis is placed on corroborative history from teachers or other persons who know the patient. Also, the developmental level of the child has to be taken into account when considering symptoms and functioning. However, it is similar to assessing adults in that it requires clinicians to obtain a detailed history, to conduct a mental status examination (and a physical examination when necessary), to integrate all the data in a formulation, diagnosis, and differential diagnosis, to convey this information back to patients and family, and to negotiate a plan for treatment.

Assessment of young persons typically requires more time than adults (2 to 5 hours). Briefer assessment is undertaken in an emergency, but this is usually followed by more extensive evaluation at a later point. Dealing with families also requires specific skills and techniques, which are described in Chapter 10.

As discussed in Chapter 1, two classification systems are used for diagnosis: the *Diagnostic and Statistical Manual of Mental Disorders,* 4th edition (*DSM-IV*),[1] and the World Health Organization's *International Classification of Diseases,* 10th edition (*ICD-10*).[2] We refer to the *DSM-IV* in this chapter, in line with the rest of the book. The focus is on the *DSM-IV* depressive disorders, which include major depressive disorder and dysthymic disorder. The word *youth* and *young person* are used to refer to both children and adolescents. The word *depression* is used to refer to both major depressive disorder and dysthymia.

GENERAL RECOMMENDATIONS ABOUT ASSESSMENT

The initial evaluation involves obtaining data from multiple sources, which include the youth, parents, and teachers. This comprises interviews with the youth alone (and, if indicated, the parents alone) and interviews with both the youth and parents.

Confidentiality should be discussed at the onset. This includes explaining that information will be kept confidential unless the patient's life or other persons' lives are at risk. The role of clinicians as mandated reporters of abuse (in most countries) should also be explained. Because child protection is paramount, disclosures of abuse to the clinician from the child or others need to be shared with the local child protection agency. Sensitive issues such as substance abuse, sexual activity, and pregnancy would not warrant breaking confidentiality unless there are special circumstances; it is better to encourage the youth to share this information with the parents. In the United States (according to the Health Insurance Portability and Accountability Act), it should be explained that the government has the right to access patients' medical records. Youth and parental consent to contact other informants (e.g., teachers) should also be obtained.

CONDUCTING THE ASSESSMENT INTERVIEW

The youth interview is critical because parents and teachers tend to underreport depressive symptoms.[3] Clinicians differ in their view about how this should be achieved; some prefer seeing adolescents first and then together with the parents—or parents alone, if one expects too much conflict. For children, the opposite is often preferred: to see the child together with parents or parents alone first, and then interviewing the child alone. Children are less likely to answer questions reliably about mood, time concepts, comparing themselves to their peers, and questions that require the child to use judgment.[4] Interviewing the parent first allows the eliciting of relevant information and the time course of symptoms, which can be used later when interviewing the child.[5] For example, the interviewer can start by stating that parents have described periods when the child looks sad or angry, and asking the child to describe the feelings during these times, or having the child point to a face on a chart with a variety of expressions/emotions. This can help children with chronological data (e.g., "your parents said you have been sad since the New Year" rather than "tell me about your moods over the last 2 months."). Questions need to be simple (e.g., dealing with one concrete issue at a time: "Have you been feeling so bad that you have been crying often in the last few days?"), not long or complicated (e.g., several issues in one question: "Have you been feeling sad, having problems sleeping, or not concentrating at school?"). Avoid leading questions (more likely to draw "yes" answers and more false positives) and vague, open-ended questions (more likely to draw "I don't know" answers and more false negatives).

Many adolescents prefer to be interviewed alone first. Adolescents value their privacy and independence and are more likely to share information if they know it will be kept confidential.

Clinicians should outline the parameters by which they will share information with the parents, which mainly includes safety issues, such as suicidal and homicidal thoughts. The youth should also be made aware that disclosures of abuse will result in a call to local child protective services. Contrary to popular views, asking about suicide will not induce or trigger the youth to commit suicide. Young persons are often relieved when a caring clinician asks about their suicidal thoughts.

Gaining the trust of depressed young persons is often a challenge; however, without trust, valid information is less likely to be obtained. Apathy ("sure, whatever") and withdrawal (no eye contact, no talking) are common responses. Starting with favorite hobbies or pleasurable topics is often helpful to get the young person talking. Finding a common interest between clinician and young person is even better, with care not to overdo it.

Parents can be interviewed alone if sensitive information needs to be discussed. The interview with the parents should focus on the patient's depressive and other symptoms, antecedent triggers, school and social functioning, and family history. Opening a "Pandora's box" is not the goal of an initial assessment.

After the interviews with the patient and family, if the case is difficult or complex, it may be helpful to debrief with a colleague. It is useful to spend some time processing the information, considering the differential diagnoses and treatment, and scoring rating scales. Once a provisional diagnosis and treatment plan are formulated, the clinician can debrief the patient and parents. Psychoeducation is often the focus at this stage because the family usually has questions regarding diagnoses, prognosis, and treatment.

RECONCILING CONFLICTING DATA AMONG PARENT, YOUTH, AND OTHER SOURCES

Many instances arise when youth give opposite information to their parents. Further inconsistencies can come from other sources, such as teachers, friends, and medical records. Basically the clinician needs to meet together with the child and parent(s) and in a nonjudgmental way resolve discrepancies. Clinicians can also use either the "best-estimate diagnoses" or the "or" rule to reconcile differences.

The *best estimate diagnosis* is the process by which clinicians synthesize all available data, resolve discrepancies between data sources, and use their clinical judgment to arrive at the final diagnosis.[6] Using guidelines to resolve discrepancies between data sources results in good to excellent test-retest reliability. These include the following:[7]

- Data from direct interviews are given more weight than to other reports.
- When data are limited regarding family history, positive reports receive greater weight than negative reports.
- Regardless of source, positive reports of symptoms in excess of the minimum requirements to meet diagnostic criteria receive more weight than positive reports of symptoms that barely meet criteria.
- Symptoms supported by more convincing examples should be given more weight than those supported by vague or ambiguous examples.
- Data from informants with greater contact with the patient are given more weight than from those with less contact.

Another method to resolve discrepancies is the "or" rule, where a symptom is counted toward the criteria if either the parent or youth endorses the symptom. The "or" rule maximizes sensitivity at the cost of specificity[8] and may be useful in cases in which young persons minimize symptoms. However, this method may result in an increase in the number of comorbid diagnoses.

DETECTING DEPRESSION IN CHILDREN AND ADOLESCENTS

Detecting depression can be difficult because depressed youth are often dismissed as having problems related to bad behavior, or their behavior is attributed to a "phase" of development such as adolescent angst. Table 3.1 outlines common presentations.

TABLE 3.1 PRESENTATIONS AND CIRCUMSTANCES THAT SHOULD RAISE SUSPICIONS OF MAJOR DEPRESSION

Symptoms	• Sustained negative mood change: irritability, sadness • Changes in sleep patterns or appetite • Drop in energy • Complaints of boredom • Suicidal ideation; thoughts of death • Excessive somatic complaints (especially children) • Low self-esteem (especially adolescents) • Behavioral symptoms (irritability, anger, noncompliance, temper tantrums in children)
Consequences of depression	• Drop in school performance • Relationship problems, family conflict • Drug abuse
Other circumstances	• Family history of depression • Victim of bullying, abuse

Sustained Negative Mood Change

One of the key factors is duration: The mood problem (irritability, sadness, anhedonia) lasts most of the day (e.g., more than half the time awake) and for most days of the week, with a minimum duration of 2 weeks (in practice, many clinicians and researchers prefer a longer duration, e.g., 4 weeks). Children often have trouble verbalizing their own feelings or deny feelings of sadness or irritability. The clinician should then rely on other informants and on observable behaviors (e.g., tearfulness) to complete the assessment.

Suicidality

Many youth who show suicidal behavior suffer from depression. Suicide is the leading *preventable* cause of death in young persons 15 to 24 years of age in the developed world. Many completed suicides are related to psychiatric illness, particularly mood disorders associated with impulsivity, history of abuse, and substance use[9] (see also Chapter 15).

Excessive Somatic Complaints

Frequent visits to the school nurse or the pediatrician because of somatic complaints that are in excess of what is to be expected with a particular medical illness may be a telltale sign of depression. Children and developmentally delayed youths with depression often present with excessive somatic complaints. This may also be secondary to anxiety that often accompanies depression.

Behavior Problems

Severe, recurrent temper tantrums above and beyond what would be expected for the developmental stage can be a manifestation of depression in children and adolescents. Conduct problems and oppositional behavior can also be a sign of depression. A marked and persistent change of behavior in a child or adolescent when there was no disruptive conduct previously should raise a red flag for depression.

Drop in School Performance

Depression affects young persons' ability to focus on schoolwork and the motivation to complete it. Problems with sleep-wake cycle associated with depression may contribute to youth missing classes or, in severe cases, stopping school attendance altogether. Some eventually drop out of school. Thus it is important to follow-up depressed youth who are *in school* and those who have *dropped out of school.*

Relationship Problems, Family Conflict

Problems with peers and family can both trigger or be the result of a depressive episode (see Chapters 2 and 10).

Drug Abuse

Young persons with depression often resort to drugs to feel better. Substance use greatly increases the risk for suicide; all substance-abusing adolescents should be screened for depression (see also Chapter 18).

Family History of Depression

The offspring of depressed parents are at increased risk of depression (see Chapter 2). Thus a positive family history should raise suspicions that the youth may have this disorder. However, offspring of depressed parents are also at risk of developing other disorders such as anxiety and attention deficit hyperactivity disorder (ADHD).

Being Bullied or Abused

Bullying and physical, emotional, or sexual abuse can trigger or exacerbate a depressive episode.

ASSESSING DEPRESSIVE EPISODES AND DIAGNOSING DEPRESSIVE DISORDERS

Mnemonics, such as SIGECAPS, are helpful to remember the *DSM-IV* criteria for mood disorders. Table 3.2 lists what each letter of the mnemonic stands for and examples of developmentally-appropriate questions to elucidate each symptom.[10]

To meet *DSM-IV* criteria for a major depressive episode, at least five out of the nine symptoms should have been present for at least 2 weeks; one of the symptoms being either depressed mood or anhedonia (loss of interest or pleasure). Except for depressed mood, the other criteria for a major depressive episode are contained in the mnemonic SIGECAPS.

It is important to assess the current (or most recent) depressive episode as well as prior depressive episodes, and to evaluate their severity (Table 3.3). This is important because treatment for a single episode differs from that of recurrent depression, and treatment for mild to moderate depression is different from severe depression. Mood charts (see Resources for Families section) can be helpful to map out depressive episodes, illustrating frequency or number of episodes, triggers, duration, and severity.

Episodicity is a critical characteristic of subjects with mood disorders, although a minority may have chronic symptoms (see Chapter 1). However, a common error is to make a diagnosis of "major depressive episode." The correct diagnosis is "major depressive disorder," single or recurrent episode, and mild, moderate, or severe.

Dysthymic disorder is diagnosed using the same mnemonic for depression, except that the last two criteria (psychomotor agitation/retardation and suicidality) are not used (Table 3.4).

For dysthymia, the child or adolescent shows depressed mood or irritability for most of the day, more days than not, and for 1 year at least. In addition, the young person ought to have at least two of the symptoms in Table 3.4. It is also required not to have been without depressive symptoms for >2 months at a time and not to have had a major depressive episode during that year. The following is a case vignette of dysthymic disorder in an adolescent:

> David is a 15-year-old boy in grade 9. He lives with his parents and younger sister. David has been failing school over the past year. He exhibits much anger at school and at home most days of the week. He often becomes angry at school because he does not want to deal with people, and he has received multiple in-school suspensions. He feels "crummy" about himself and that he is not getting enough credit for the effort he is putting to complete his schoolwork. He is not able to concentrate, and this frustrates him even further as he claims he tries to complete the work. He has difficulty falling asleep and is fatigued throughout the day. He denies suicidal ideation, feelings of guilt or hopelessness, reports good appetite, and still enjoys hanging out with his friends and playing his guitar. Besides school, his other problem is his relationship with his father, who tells David what to do, is very short and punitive, especially about school problems.

TABLE 3.2 MNEMONIC FOR MAJOR DEPRESSIVE EPISODE IN ADDITION TO DEPRESSED MOOD (SIGECAPS)

Symptom/Mnemonic	Stands for:	Selected Screening Questions from the KSADS[a]
Depressed mood	• Depressed mood	• Have you ever felt sad, blue, down, or empty? • Did you feel like crying? When was that? Do you feel (___) now? • Was there ever another time you felt (___)?
S	• **S**leep In**S**omnia	• Do you have trouble sleeping? How long does it take you to fall asleep? • Do you wake up in the middle of the night? How many times? • How long does it take you to fall back asleep? Are you waking up earlier than you had to? Do you feel rested upon awakening?
	• Hyper**S**omnia	• Are you sleeping longer than usual? • Do you go back to sleep after you wake up in the morning?
I	• **I**rritability	• Was there ever a time when you got annoyed, irritated, or cranky at little things? • Did you ever have a time when you lost your temper a lot? When was that? Are you like that now? Was there ever another time you felt (___)? • What kinds of things made you (___)?
	• Poor self-**I**mage (low self-esteem)	• How do you feel about yourself? Do you like yourself? Why? or Why not? • Do you think of yourself as pretty or ugly? • Do you think of yourself as bright or stupid? • Do you like your personality, or do you wish it were different? • How often do you feel this way about yourself?
	• Lack of **I**nterest in pleasurable activities (anhedonia), apathy, low motivation, or boredom	• What are the things you do for fun? Enjoy? • Has there ever been a time you felt bored a lot of the time? When? Do you feel bored a lot now? Was there another time you felt bored a lot? • Did you look forward to doing the things you used to enjoy? • Did you have as much fun doing them as you used to before you began feeling (sad, etc.)? • If less fun, did you enjoy them a little less? Much less? Not at all?
G	• Feelings of **G**uilt	• When people say or do things that are good, they usually feel good, and when they say or do something bad, they feel bad about it. Do you feel bad about anything you have done? What is it? How often do you think about it? When did you do that? • What does it mean if I said I feel guilty about something? How much of the time do you feel like this?
	• Feelings of hopelessness	• What do you think is going to happen to you? Do you think you are going to get better? Any better? Do you think we can help you? How? • What do you want to do (to be) when you grow up? Do you think you'll make it? Why not? Have you given up on life?
E	• Loss of **E**nergy • Fatigue	• Have you been feeling tired? How often? • When did you start feeling so tired? Was it after you started feeling (___)? Do you take naps because you feel tired? How much?

(continued)

TABLE 3.2 MNEMONIC FOR MAJOR DEPRESSIVE EPISODE IN ADDITION TO DEPRESSED MOOD (SIGECAPS) (CONTINUED)

Symptom/Mnemonic	Stands for:	Selected Screening Questions from the KSADS[a]
		• Do you have to rest? Do your limbs feel heavy? Is it very hard to get going? To move your legs? Do you feel like this all the time?
C	• Poor **C**oncentration • Indecisiveness	• Do you know what it means to concentrate? Sometimes children have a lot of trouble concentrating. For instance, they have to read a page from a book and can't keep their mind on it, so it takes much longer to do it or they just can't do it, can't pay attention. • Have you been having this kind of trouble? When did it begin? • Is your thinking slowed down? If you push yourself very hard can you concentrate? Does it take longer to do your homework? When you try to concentrate on something, does your mind drift off to other thoughts? Can you pay attention in school?
A	• Decrease or increase in **A**ppetite or weight • Failure to make expected weight gains in children	• How is your appetite? Do you feel hungry often? • Are you eating more or less than before? • Have you lost any weight since you started feeling sad? How do you know? • Have you gained any weight since you started feeling sad? How do you know?
P	• **P**sychomotor agitation or	• Since you've felt sad, are there times when you can't sit still, or you have to keep moving and can't stop? Do you walk up and down?
	• **P**sychomotor retardation	• Since you started feeling (sad) have you noticed that you can't move as fast as before? Have you found it hard to start talking? • Has your speech slowed down? Do you talk a lot less than before?
S	• **S**uicidal ideation, plan, or attempt	• Sometimes children who get upset or feel bad think about dying or even killing themselves. Have you ever had such thoughts? How would you do it? Did you have a plan? Have you actually tried to kill yourself? • When? What did you do? Any other things? Did you really want to die? • Did you ask for any help after you did it?
	• Thoughts of death	• Sometimes children who get upset or feel bad, wish they were dead or feel they'd be better off dead. Have you ever had these types of thoughts? When? Do you feel that way now? Was there ever another time you felt that way?
	• **S**elf-harm behaviors	• Did you ever try to hurt yourself? Have you ever burned yourself with matches/candles? Or scratched yourself with needles/a knife? Your nails? Or put hot pennies on your skin? Anything else? Why did you do it? How often? Do you have many accidents? What kind? How often? • Some kids do these types of things because they want to kill themselves, and other kids do them because it makes them feel a little better afterwards. Why do you do these things?

[a]Reproduced from the Schedule for Affective Disorders and Schizophrenia for School Age Children, Present and Lifetime Version (KSADS-PL),[10] with permission from Dr. J. Kaufman. SIGECAPS was developed by Carey Gross (cited in S. Nassir Ghaemi, *Mood Disorders: A Practical Guide,* Lippincott Williams & Wilkins, 2003, page 11)

TABLE 3.3 RATING SEVERITY OF DEPRESSIVE EPISODE[1]

Mild	• Few, if any, symptoms in excess of those required to make the diagnosis • Minor impairment of functioning
Moderate	• Symptoms and functional impairment between "mild" and "severe"
Severe without psychotic features	• Several symptoms in excess of those required to make the diagnosis • Severe impairment of functioning
Severe with psychotic features	• Delusions or hallucinations also present
In partial remission	• Currently has some depressive symptoms without meeting full criteria for a depressive episode, • Or no longer has any depressive symptoms for less than 2 months
In full remission	• No depressive symptoms for the past 2 months

DEVELOPMENTAL DIFFERENCES IN THE CLINICAL PRESENTATION OF DEPRESSION

Children and adolescents with depression have an overall clinical presentation that is similar to adults; discrepancies can be attributed to age and developmental level.[11–15] Some studies,[11–14] but not all,[16] have reported that depressed children have more somatic complaints, psychomotor agitation, anxiety symptoms, behavior problems, ADHD-like symptoms, hallucinations, and depressed affect, whereas adolescents presented with more melancholic symptoms (e.g. anhedonia, guilt, early morning wakening, weight loss), delusions, suicidal behaviors, and substance abuse. The following is a case vignette of a depressed child:

Joel is a 9-year-old boy who lives with his mother and younger sister. He presents to his family doctor with excessive stomach pains. On further interview, Joel has been very moody, irritable, and extremely defiant with his mother. His stomach pains worsen at school, resulting in frequent visits to the school nurse. Joel often worries that something dire will happen to his mother, and he has missed many days of school over the past several months, frequently calling his mother to pick him up. His teacher is concerned because Joel is usually a good student and is not having the good grades he had achieved previously. He hardly sleeps due to the stomach pain and is not hungry. After his parents' divorce last year, he rarely sees his father and has recently started talking about dying.

The following case illustrates an adolescent with depression:

Chantal is a 16-year-old girl, entering grade 11. She lives at home with her mother, father, and younger brother. She is anxious, self-conscious, and gets average grades in school. At the beginning of the school year her performance deteriorated and she complained of being unable to focus in class. She began experimenting with cannabis, stating it helped her to relax. Her parents noticed increasing irritability at home and with friends. She refused to follow her parents' rules, despite having been compliant in the past, and she became openly defiant and disrespectful. She was observed making negative comments about herself. She also reported chronic tiredness. A few months later, she became tearful, spent most of her time in her room, and did not want to go out with her friends. She was eating more, mainly junk food, gaining 15 pounds in 4 months. She had trouble sleeping, felt exhausted, and "dragging her feet" throughout the day.

TABLE 3.4 MNEMONIC FOR DYSTHYMIC EPISODE

- **S**leep
- **I**rritability
- **G**uilt
- **E**nergy
- **C**oncentration
- **A**ppetite

DIFFERENTIAL DIAGNOSIS

Because several disorders can present with similar symptoms (see Table 17.1), it is important to clarify which disorder best accounts for the symptoms. Differential diagnosis for depression includes bipolar depression, adjustment disorder with depressed mood, bereavement, posttraumatic stress disorder (PTSD), oppositional defiant disorder (ODD), ADHD, pervasive developmental disorder, and mood disorder related to a general medical condition (including substance-induced depression) (see also Chapter 1).

BIPOLAR DISORDER

Bipolar disorder should always be ruled out because a first episode of depression can be the initial mood episode of both bipolar disorder and unipolar depression. Family history of bipolar disorder, psychotic symptoms, and medication-induced mania may be telltale signs of bipolar disorder.[15] When treating a young person with depression, it is important for the clinician to monitor longitudinally the occurrence of manic or hypomanic symptoms, which may signal the emergence of a bipolar disorder.

To meet the *DSV-IV* criteria for a manic episode, a young person needs to exhibit persistent mood elevation or irritable mood for at least 1 week and also meet criteria for at least three of the following symptoms (or four if the mood is irritable) as contained in the mnemonic DIGFAST (Table 3.5). The following is a vignette of a preadolescent who presents initially with a depressive episode but subsequently develops a manic episode:

> Amy is 12 years old. For the past 3 months she felt sad almost every day, crying often and for no reason. Her appetite decreased and she lost about 7 pounds. She also had trouble falling asleep, waking up several times at night. She felt tired and with no energy during the day. Although she had said that life was not worth living, she did not have a suicidal plan. Amy stopped calling friends, playing piano and guitar, which she used to enjoy, and did not talk much with her parents. Over the next few days Amy seemed to be feeling better. She started to call her friends and appeared to have more energy. She became more talkative and resumed playing piano and guitar. Her parents noticed that she began to giggle a lot, which was unusual for Amy. On a Friday night she called her friends to come over to play a game. Throughout the game Amy giggled uncontrollably and began telling jokes, put socks on her ears and danced around. Because her friends did not look amused, Amy angrily told them to leave. Her parents were awakened at 2 AM on Saturday by Amy playing piano and singing out loud. She explained she was practicing to be the best musician ever, and wanted to go on tour with her music. She said that these and other thoughts raced through her head. Parents had trouble following her because she was talking very fast and giggling. The following Monday parents received a call from school saying that Amy was laughing uncontrollably in class and acting childish, and she was sent home where she was closely watched by her parents. After a week, Amy began to slowly unwind, becoming increasingly depressed and withdrawn, much like before.

TABLE 3.5 MNEMONIC FOR MANIC EPISODE

Distractibility	• Inability to filter out unimportant external stimuli
Insomnia	• Decreased need for sleep
Grandiosity	• Inflated self-worth
Flight of ideas	• Racing thoughts
Activity	• Increase in goal-directed **A**ctivities
Speech	• Pressured **S**peech
Thoughtlessness	• Highly reckless behaviors without regard for severe consequences • Hypersexuality, spending sprees

Developed by William Falk (cited in S. Nassir Ghaemi, *Mood Disorders: A Practical Guide*, Lippincott Williams & Wilkins, 2003, page 13).

ADJUSTMENT DISORDER WITH DEPRESSED MOOD

In adjustment disorder, depressive symptoms (sadness, tearfulness, hopelessness) appear after the occurrence of an identifiable stressor and do not meet criteria for a major depressive episode. According to the *DSM-IV*, the symptoms should occur within 3 months of the onset of the stressor(s), and must not last >6 months after the offset of the stressor(s). Here is a case vignette of adjustment disorder with depressed mood:

> Nicky is a 16-year-old girl who lives with her mother and had been attending grade 9. Over the past 2 months, Nicky exhibited depressive symptoms, characterized by tearfulness and disrupted sleep patterns. Nicky and her mother were evicted from their apartment 4 months ago and spent several weeks at a homeless shelter. They have since found an apartment to rent, but Nicky is now worried that her mother will kick her out of the house because Nicky recently turned 16, and her mother had been making comments that Nicky should find a job because she has to take care of herself eventually. Nicky and her mother fought constantly; at times they did not have money to buy food. Nicky dropped out of school because her home life was too stressful to even worry about schoolwork. She denies suicidal ideations. She spends most of her day isolated in her room.

BEREAVEMENT

Young persons can present with depressive symptoms immediately after the death of a loved one. The symptoms may include sadness and associated symptoms of poor appetite, insomnia, and lack of concentration. If the symptoms last >2 months, or are particularly severe (e.g., psychotic, high suicidality) or incapacitating, then major depressive disorder should be considered.

POSTTRAUMATIC STRESS DISORDER

PTSD shares symptoms with and can mimic depression. Symptoms of depression (with the overlapping PTSD symptom in parentheses) are anhedonia (numbing of responsiveness), social isolation (detachment from others), hopelessness (sense of foreshortened future), disrupted sleep patterns (increased arousal), irritability (increased arousal), and difficulty concentrating (increased arousal). Consider depression if the patient also has suicidality. Consider PTSD if there has been abuse or if the patient reexperiences the traumatic event, which in children can manifest as repetitive play with expression of the trauma. However, the co-occurrence of PTSD and major depression is frequent.

ODD, ADHD, AND PERVASIVE DEVELOPMENTAL DISORDER

Depressed youth may be more prone to oppositional and defiant behaviors as a consequence of irritability, and temper tantrums may be a manifestation of depressed mood. However, in depression, the behavioral problems usually start after the onset of depressive symptoms. Additionally, behavioral problems in a depressed youth without a comorbid behavior disorder are less severe than those of youths with a behavior disorder alone or comorbid depression and behavior disorder. Behavior problems are also more chronic in youths with a behavioral disorder alone or with comorbid depression and behavior disorder.[17] Regarding autistic spectrum disorders, depressive-like symptoms can appear to overlap with symptoms of autism, such as lack of social reciprocity, failure to develop peer relationships, and poor eye contact.

MOOD DISORDER DUE TO GENERAL MEDICAL CONDITION

Many medical conditions can mimic depression (see Table 1.4 in Chapter 1). As such, it is important for nonphysicians, such as psychologists, to have a close working relationship with a physician, so a referral can be made to rule out medical conditions presenting with depressive symptoms. A complete physical examination is required only if there is suspicion of a medical problem or signs of a medical illness.

To rule out medication-induced depression, a thorough evaluation of current and previous medications should be obtained, with special attention to the onset and offset of symptoms in relation to medication changes. Medications such as corticosteroids, contraceptives, and isotretinoin are associated with depressive symptomatology, and the last one with suicidal behaviors.[15]

To exclude substance-induced depression, a thorough substance use history is needed (see Chapter 18). A urine toxicology screen can help identify substances not discussed during the interviews or when doubts linger.

Infectious diseases such as mononucleosis and neurologic disorders such as migraine and traumatic brain injury (TBI) should be ruled out. Laboratory investigations should be ordered as indicated, such as a Monospot test for mononucleosis, an electroencephalogram for epilepsy, and magnetic resonance imaging for TBI. If cognitive deficits and executive functioning are a concern with someone with TBI or a history of concussions, then a referral for neuropsychological testing may be considered.

Endocrine illnesses such as thyroid disorders and diabetes should also be excluded and laboratory investigations sought as indicated: serum free thyroxine and thyroid-stimulating hormone for thyroid disorders; serum glycosylated hemoglobin, fasting glucose levels, and urinalysis for diabetes. Other conditions to consider include anemia, electrolyte abnormalities, and malnutrition.

RATING SCALES AND STRUCTURED DIAGNOSTIC INTERVIEWS

Rating scales are an important part of assessment by providing efficient detection and measurement of depressive symptoms and other relevant domains. Rating scales are not designed to substitute for the clinical interview—the gold standard—and clinicians should not blindly use them based on their popularity or widespread use, but rather because of the scale's psychometric properties.[18]

Structured diagnostic interviews are frequently used in research settings to improve reliability. Diagnostic interviews range from unstructured (such as the clinical interview) to semistructured (e.g., Schedule for Affective Disorders and Schizophrenia for School Age Children, Present and Lifetime Version, KSADS-PL)[10] to fully structured (e.g., Diagnostic Interview Schedule for Children Version-IV, DISC-IV).[19] Semistructured interviews require much time and training, whereas fully structured interviews require minimal training. In adults, the combination of diagnostic interviews and self-report scales is the state of the art for evidence-based assessment of depression.[20] A similar recommendation has been made for children.[8]

RATING SCALES FOR DEPRESSION

We focus on scales in the public domain and other selected scales based on psychometric properties and usefulness (Table 3.6). A comprehensive review can be found elsewhere.[21]

The CED-D (Center for Epidemiological Studies Depression Scale) was designed for adults but has been validated for adolescents, and it has good psychometric properties in adolescents. The CES-DC (Center for Epidemiological Studies Depression Scale for Children) was designed for youth 6 to 17 years of age. It has poor reliability and validity in children but better in adolescents.[22] Neither the CES-D nor the CES-DC are suitable for children, but both may be useful in adolescents.[21] The Depression Self-Rating Scale (DSRS) uses a very simple language—therefore suitable for children[23]—and has been validated in both community and clinical settings.[24–26] However, its ability to discriminate depression from other disorders is in question. Should this be answered, the DSRS has potential for widespread use.[21]

The remaining scales discussed are copyrighted. The Children's Depression Rating Scale-Revised (CDRS-R) is clinician rated and requires integrating information from parent, child, and clinical observations.[27] The CDRS-R has good interrater reliability and is sensitive to medication effects. As such, it is widely used in treatment studies. The CDRS-R has a special niche because it incorporates both the clinician's interview and other sources of information.[21] The Beck Depression Inventory (BDI) is a self-report very widely used in adolescents.[28] The BDI is brief, available in several languages, and has a version for use in primary care, the BDI-PC. The BDI has good psychometric properties and is especially good at discriminating depressed adolescent outpatients from nondepressed adolescents. However, no parent version is available. In addition, its ability to measure severity in adolescents is suspect. Nonetheless, the BDI has a large database from diverse samples, which helps

TABLE 3.6 SELECTED SCALES TO RATE DEPRESSIVE SYMPTOMS

Scale	Rater (Target Group)	Comments
CDRS-R: Children's Depression Rating Scale-Revised[27]	Clinician (Children, adolescents)	• Widely used as outcome measure in treatment studies • Requires integrating information from parent, child, and clinical observation • Good interrater reliability • Sensitive to medication effects
BDI: Beck Depression Inventory[28]	Self (Adolescents)	• Brief; very widely used in adolescents • Good psychometric properties; especially good for discriminating depressed outpatients from nondepressed • Available in several languages • No parent version; one version for use in primary care: BDI-PC • Not good for measuring severity of depressive episode
CES-D/CES-DC: Center for Epidemiologic Studies-Depression Scale[39]	Self, parent (Children, adolescents)	• Brief • Free of charge; public domain • May be useful for screening but has limited usefulness in clinic settings • Discriminant validity problematic • There is a less-well-researched parent version • Not very useful for children
CDI: Children's Depression Inventory[29]	Self (Children, adolescents)	• Very widely used • Good psychometric properties but not very specific • No parent version • Available in several languages • Discriminate validity is poor, particularly in children • Validity of younger children's self-report arguable • Not very appropriate for adolescents
RADS/RCDS: Reynolds Adolescent/ Child Depression Scales[30,31]	Self, parent (Adolescents, children)	• Widely used, mostly in school samples • Good psychometric properties • Available in several languages • Decreased ability to detect treatment effects compared to other scales • Good for non-clinical samples and may be one of the best screening tools
MFQ: Mood and Feelings Questionnaire[32]	Self, parent, teacher (Children, adolescents)	• Good screening instrument in community • Good clinical instrument • Good psychometric properties • Short and long versions for children and parents • Free for clinical or research use, with permission • Can be downloaded at http://devepi.mc.duke.edu/MFQ.html
DSRS: Depression Self-Rating Scale[23]	Self (Children, adolescents)	• Suitability to children; very simple language • Free of charge; public domain • Ability to discriminate from other disorders is suspect; more studies needed • Potential for widespread use
KADS: Kutcher Adolescent Depression Scale[36]	Self (Adolescents)	• May be useful in non-clinical and clinical settings for adolescents • Brief versions available • New; more validation studies needed • Free of charge for clinical work; other uses require permission

define its usefulness for a range of applications.[21] The Children's Depression Inventory (CDI) is a very widely used self-report available in several languages.[29] However, the CDI has several drawbacks: It has no parent version, is not very appropriate for adolescents, discriminant validity is poor (particularly in children), and the validity of younger children's self-report is questionable.[21] The Reynolds Adolescent/Child Depression Scales (RADS/RCDS) are self-report and parent-reported scales.[30,31] The RADS/RCDS are widely used, mostly in school samples, and available in several languages. They have good psychometric properties and have been tested in diverse samples. The RADS is one of the best screening tools[21] but less helpful in the clinical context because it has difficulty detecting treatment effects. The Mood and Feelings Questionnaire (MFQ) has multiple reporters, including self (MFQ-C), parent (MFQ-P), and teacher.[32] The MFQ is a good screening instrument in the community and useful in clinic settings.[33,34] The MFQ-C and MFQ-P have good psychometric properties, especially when used in combination, and they are able to identify depression in youths with diverse demographic and clinical characteristics.[34] Short and long versions are available. The Kutcher Adolescent Depression Scale (KADS) is self-rated and may be useful in nonclinical and clinical settings; initial studies suggest good psychometric properties.[35,36] Short versions of the KADS are also available and have potential as screening tools.

STRUCTURED DIAGNOSTIC INTERVIEWS

As summarized in Table 3.7, we focus on two widely used interviews, the Schedule for Affective Disorders and Schizophrenia for School Age Children, Present and Lifetime Version (KSADS-PL)[10] and the Diagnostic Interview Schedule for Children Version-IV (DISC-IV).[19]

The KSADS-PL[10] is semistructured, has several modules, is widely used in treatment research, and has good psychometric properties. The module for affective disorders can be used separately. Among the diagnostic interviews, the KSADS-PL has the best test-retest reliability for mood and anxiety disorders.[37] However, it is time consuming and requires considerable training. It also requires interviewing the child, parents, and, if possible, obtaining information from the school. Discrepancies between sources of information are resolved by the clinician, as mentioned earlier in this chapter regarding reconciling disagreements between informants.

The DISC-IV[19] is highly structured, modular, and can be administered via computer. It is useful in epidemiologic research, and the module for mood disorders can be used separately. However, the

TABLE 3.7 SELECTED STRUCTURED DIAGNOSTIC INTERVIEWS

Scale	Rater (Target Group)	Comments
K-SADS-PL: Schedule for Affective Disorders and Schizophrenia for School Age Children, Present and Lifetime Version[10]	Clinician (Children, adolescents)	• Widely used in treatment research • Good psychometric properties • Excellent test-retest reliability, especially for affective disorders • Semistructured; time consuming • Requires interviewing the child, parents, and, if possible, obtaining information from school; discrepancies between sources of information need to be determined by the clinician • Requires training • Module for affective disorders can be used separately • Free of charge • http://www.wpic.pitt.edu/ksads/default.htm
DISC-IV: Diagnostic Interview Schedule for Children Version-IV[19]	Lay interviewers (Children, adolescents)	• Highly structured • Time consuming and monotonous • Module for mood disorders can be used separately • Useful in epidemiologic research • Requires some training, minimized with computer-assisted administration

interrater reliability does not approach that of the other instruments. Substantial diagnostic disagreement has been found between DISC-IV diagnoses and clinician diagnoses, with kappa values ranging from −0.04 for anxiety disorders, to 0.11 for mood disorders, to 0.22 for ADHD.[38] The DISC-IV is time consuming and can be monotonous. Although administering the DISC-IV requires some training, this is minimized with computer-assisted administration.

SCALES FOR MULTIPLE SYMPTOM DOMAINS AND SCREENING PURPOSES

Table 3.8 lists scales that can be employed as screening instruments that measure multiple symptom domains. The Strengths and Difficulties Questionnaire (SDQ) is a self-, parent-, and teacher-report scale.[40,41] It is very brief (fits in one page) and is free of charge for noncommercial purposes. High SDQ scores—upper 10% in a community sample—were associated with increased psychiatric risk. The SDQ has high specificity (high proportion of true negatives) but low sensitivity (lower proportion of true positives),[42] which is acceptable for a screening instrument.

The Achenbach System of Empirically Based Assessment (ASEBA) is a self-, parent-, and teacher-report scale.[43] The questionnaires are long (100+ items), yet it is very widely used in research and clinic settings. The ASEBA identifies several "narrow-band" syndromes, including anxiety-depression. It has low specificity.

ASSESSMENT OF FUNCTIONING

Table 3.9 lists selected scales to assess functioning (a comprehensive review can be found elsewhere[44]). The Children's Global Assessment Scale (CGAS) is a clinician-rated instrument that produces a global rating of functioning based on Axis V of the *DSM-IV*.[45] The CGAS is widely used in treatment studies because it is sensitive to treatment effects and has good psychometrics.[44,46] Although the CGAS is easy to score, it requires time to gather data from several sources to do the rating. The Clinical Global Impression Scale (CGI) is also clinician rated and produces a global score.[47] It is fast, easy to score, and includes severity and improvement scales. The CGI is widely used in treatment studies as a primary or secondary outcome measure. The Health of the Nation Outcome Scales for Children and Adolescents (HoNOSCA) are clinician rated and a semistructured

TABLE 3.8 SELECTED SCALES TO RATE MULTIPLE SYMPTOM DOMAINS IN CHILDREN AND ADOLESCENTS THAT CAN BE USED FOR SCREENING PURPOSES

Scale	Rater (Target Group)	Comments
SDQ: Strengths and Difficulties Questionnaire[40,41]	Self, parent, teacher (Children, adolescents)	• Very brief: 25 items divided among 5 scales, all on one page • Strongly correlated with the longer Child Behavior Check List (see ASEBA) and with comparable ability to discriminate between community and clinic status • High specificity; good psychometrics as a screening instrument • Free for noncommercial purposes • Used worldwide • Translations available in most languages at http://www.sdqinfo.com/
ASEBA: Achenbach System of Empirically Based Assessment[43]	Self, parent, teacher	• Long questionnaires (>100 items) • Several "narrow-band" syndromes, including anxiety-depression • Low specificity • Very widely used in research and clinic settings • Translations available in most languages at http://www.aseba.org/index.html

TABLE 3.9 SELECTED SCALES TO RATE IMPROVEMENT, PSYCHOSOCIAL FUNCTIONING/ IMPAIRMENT, AND QUALITY OF LIFE

Scale	Rater (Target Group)	Comments
CGAS: Children's Global Assessment Scale[45]	Clinician (Children, adolescents)	• Global ratings of functioning based on Axis 5 of *DSM-IV* • Widely used in treatment studies • Sensitive to treatment effects • Good psychometrics • Free of charge
CGI: Clinical Global Impressions Scale[47]	Clinician (Children, adolescents)	• Severity and improvement scales • Global ratings; fast and easy • Widely used in treatment studies as primary or secondary outcome measure • Free of charge; public domain
HoNOSCA: Health of the Nation Outcome Scales for Children and Adolescents[48]	Clinician (Children, adolescents)	• Rates the global burden of psychiatric problems during the past month • Semistructured interview of parent and youth • Self-report and parent report also developed • Widely used in Europe and Australia • Good psychometrics but questions about reliability • Free of charge
PQ-LES-Q: Pediatric Quality of Life Enjoyment and Satisfaction Questionnaire[50]	Self (Children, adolescents)	• Good psychometric properties • Used in some recent treatment studies for pediatric depression • New; need more validation studies in community samples • Free of charge for noncommercial uses
SAICA: Social Adjustment Inventory for Children and Adolescents[51]	Clinician (Children, adolescents)	• Limited psychometric data • Long; at least 30 minutes needed • Not widely used • Minimizes clinician judgment by being respondent based • No training required • Free of charge

interview of parent and youth.[48] The HoNOSCA rates the global burden of psychiatric problems during the past month; it is widely used in Europe and Australasia. It has good psychometric properties, but reliability is still in question.[49] The Pediatric Quality of Life Enjoyment and Satisfaction Questionnaire (PQ-LES-Q) is a self-report, has good psychometric properties, and has been used in treatment studies for pediatric depression. It measures dimensions not accounted for by the commonly used global assessment scales.[50] Although showing promise, the PQ-LES-Q is a new scale and requires more validation studies, especially in community samples. The Social Adjustment Inventory for Children and Adolescents (SAICA) is clinician rated and measures multiple domains of social functioning.[51] It has limited psychometric data and is long (it takes at least 30 minutes),[44] which may explain why it is not widely used. Nonetheless, the SAICA has some advantages: It is free, minimizes clinician's judgment by being respondent based, and does not require training.

OTHER ASSESSMENT ISSUES

COMORBIDITY

When assessing a depressed youth, comorbid psychiatric disorders should be considered and are frequently uncovered. The most common are anxiety disorders, disruptive behavior disorders, and substance abuse.[15] Comorbid medical illnesses are not uncommon. Further discussion on the diagnosis and treatment of depression comorbid with other disorders can be found in Chapter 17.

TREATMENT HISTORY

An assessment of prior treatments is essential; this includes medication and psychotherapy. The types of treatment, their duration, drug dosages, side effects, adherence to treatment, and whether patients responded or depression had remitted should be ascertained.

PARENTAL PSYCHOPATHOLOGY

Another important part of the assessment is to ascertain sensitively and discreetly the level of parental psychopathology, if any—particularly parental depression, which is associated with longer time to recovery, more severe symptoms, more recurrences, earlier onset, and more psychosocial impairment in depressed youth.[52–54] Parental psychopathology can be assessed with rating scales appropriate for adults, and it can be done concurrently with the assessment of their children.

REFERRAL TO A CHILD PSYCHIATRIST

Unfortunately, referral to a child psychiatrist in most parts of the world is largely determined by resource issues, given the undersupply (see Chapter 24). Referrals should be made for complex cases, such as severe depression, treatment-resistant depression, depression with comorbidities, psychotic depression, bipolar depression, suicidal or homicidal thoughts, and so on. The ideal child psychiatric assessment may be performed by a multidisciplinary team including, in addition to a child psychiatrist, psychologists, social workers, occupational therapists, and pediatricians.

Important as a multidisciplinary and team-based approach can be, it is essential for someone to remain the hub of the treatment, as a main person for the patient to connect and feel comfortable with, as well as to coordinate the various approaches and to ensure things do not fall through the cracks. Involving others should not be a default clinical position but a proactive and carefully thought through decision. Although a multidisciplinary team is preferable, a child psychiatrist or any competent clinician should be able to evaluate a child or adolescent in all these domains.

WHERE TO TREAT THE YOUTH WITH DEPRESSION

The decision where to treat a depressed youth depends on multiple factors, such as severity of depressive episode, presence of suicidal ideation, psychotic symptoms, degree of functioning, and psychosocial environment. The least restrictive setting should always be considered. However, the following should be red flags to think about inpatient hospitalization: severe suicidal ideation, significant plan or actual suicidal attempt; homicidal ideation; severe depressive symptoms; poor adherence to treatment; poor response despite appropriate treatment; severe agitation or psychotic symptoms; substance abuse; chaotic environment for a child or adolescent who is not responding to treatment or at risk for suicide, substance abuse, is being abused or at high risk for abuse.

RESOURCES FOR PRACTITIONERS

Birmaher B, Brent D, AACAP Work Group on Quality Issues. Practice parameter for the assessment and treatment of children and adolescents with depressive disorders. *J Am Acad Child Adolesc Psychiatry.* 2007;46:1503–1526.

Abela J, Hankin B, eds. *Handbook of Depression in Children and Adolescents.* New York: Guilford Press; 2007.

Zalsman G, Brent DA eds. Depression. *Child Adolesc Psychiatr Clin N Am.* 2006;15(4):827–1088.

Shaffer D, Waslick BD, eds. *The Many Faces of Depression in Children and Adolescents.* Washington, DC: American Psychiatric Publishing; 2002.

NICE: Depression in children and young people: identification and management in primary, community and secondary care, available at http://www.nice.org.uk/guidance/CG28

A comprehensive list of screening tools and rating scales and description is available at http://www.massgeneral.org/schoolpsychiatry/screeningtools_table.asp and http://www.adelaide.edu.au/library/guide/med/menthealth/scales.html#P

RESOURCES FOR PATIENTS AND FAMILIES

Example of a mood chart: http://www.psychiatry24x7.com/bgdisplay.jhtml?itemname= mooddiary
Naparstek N. *Is Your Child Depressed? Answers to Your Toughest Questions.* New York: McGraw-Hill; 2006.

REFERENCES

1. American Psychiatric Association. *Diagnostic and Statistical Manual of Mental Disorders.* 4th ed. Washington, DC: American Psychiatric Association; 1994.
2. World Health Organization. *International Statistical Classification of Diseases and Health Related Problems (the) ICD-10.* 2nd ed. Geneva: World Health Organization; 2004.
3. Jensen PS, Rubio-Stipec M, Canino G, et al. Parent and child contributions to diagnosis of mental disorder: are both informants always necessary? *J Am Acad Child Adolesc Psychiatr.* 1999;38:1569–1579.
4. Granero R, Ezpeleta L, Domenech JM, et al. Characteristics of the subject and interview influencing the test-retest reliability of the Diagnostic Interview for Children and Adolescents—Revised. *J Child Psychol Psychiatry.* 1998;39:963–972.
5. Ryan ND. Diagnosing pediatric depression. *Biol Psychiatry.* 2001;49:1050–1054.
6. Leckman JF, Sholomskas D, Thompson WD, et al. Best estimate of lifetime psychiatric diagnosis: a methodological study. *Arch Gen Psychiatry.* 1982;39:879–883.
7. Klein DN, Ouimette PC, Kelly HS, et al. Test-retest reliability of team consensus best-estimate diagnoses of Axis I and II disorders in a family study. *Am J Psychiatry.* 1994;151:1043–1047.
8. Klein DN, Dougherty LR, Olino TM. Toward guidelines for evidence-based assessment of depression in children and adolescents. *J Clin Child Adolesc Psychol.* 2005;34:412–432.
9. Conwell Y, Duberstein PR, Cox C, et al. Relationships of age and Axis I diagnoses in victims of completed suicide: a psychological autopsy study. *Am J Psychiatry.* 1996;153:1001–1008.
10. Kaufman J, Birmaher B, Brent D, et al. Schedule for affective disorders and schizophrenia for school-age children-present and lifetime version (K-SADS-PL): initial reliability and validity data. *J Am Acad Child Adolesc Psychiatry.* 1997;36:980–988.
11. Ryan ND, Puig-Antich J, Ambrosini P, et al. The clinical picture of major depression in children and adolescents. *Arch Gen Psychiatry.* 1987;44:854–861.
12. Carlson GA, Kashani JH. Phenomenology of major depression from childhood through adulthood: analysis of three studies. *Am J Psychiatry.* 1988;145:1222–1225.
13. Yorbik O, Birmaher B, Axelson D, et al. Clinical characteristics of depressive symptoms in children and adolescents with major depressive disorder. *J Clin Psychiatry.* 2004;65:1654–1659.
14. Ginicola MM. Children's unique experience of depression: using a developmental approach to predict variation in symptomatology. *Child Adolesc Psychiatry Ment Health.* 2007;1:9.
15. Birmaher B, Brent D, AACAP Work Group on Quality Issues. Practice parameter for the assessment and treatment of children and adolescents with depressive disorders. *J Am Academy Child Adolesc Psychiatry.* 2007;46:1503–1526.
16. Kovacs M, Paulauskas SL. Developmental stage and the expression of depressive disorders in children: an empirical analysis. In: Ciccheti D, Schneider-Rosen K, eds. *Childhood Depression.* San Francisco: Jossey-Bass; 1984:59–80.
17. Carlson GA, Cantwell DP. Unmasking masked depression in children and adolescents. *Am J Psychiatry.* 1980;137:445–449.
18. Myers K, Winters NC. Ten-year review of rating scales. I: Overview of scale functioning, psychometric properties, and selection. *J Am Acad Child Adolesc Psychiatry.* 2002;41:114–122.
19. Shaffer D, Fisher P, Lucas CP, et al. NIMH Diagnostic Interview Schedule for Children Version IV (NIMH DISC-IV): Description, differences from previous versions, and reliability of some common diagnoses. *J Am Acad Child Adolesc Psychiatry.* 2000;39:28–38.
20. Joiner TE, Walker RL, Pettit JW, et al. Evidence-based assessment of depression in adults. *Psychol Assess.* 2005;17:267–277.
21. Myers K, Winters NC. Ten-year review of rating scales. II: Scales for internalizing disorders. *J Am Acad Child Adolesc Psychiatry.* 2002;41:634–659.
22. Fendrich M, Weissman MM, Warner V. Screening for depressive disorder in children and adolescents: validating the center for epidemiologic studies depression scale for children. *Am J Epidemiol.* 1990;131:538–551.
23. Birleson P. The validity of depressive disorder in childhood and the development of a self-rating scale: a research report. *J Child Psychol Psychiatry.* 1981;22:73–88.
24. Ivarsson T, Lidberg A, Gillberg C. The Birleson Depression Self-Rating Scale (DSRS). Clinical evaluation in an adolescent inpatient population. *J Affect Disord.* 1994;32:115–125.
25. Ivarsson T, Gillberg C. Depressive symptoms in Swedish adolescents: normative data using the Birleson Depression Self-Rating Scale (DSRS). *J Affect Disord.* 1997;42:59–68.
26. Denda K, Kako Y, Kitagawa N, et al. Assessment of depressive symptoms in Japanese school children and adolescents using the Birleson Depression Self-Rating Scale. *Int J Psychiatry Med.* 2006;36:231–241.

27. Poznanski EO, Mokros HB. *Children's Depression Rating Scale, Revised (CDRS-R)*. Los Angeles, Calif: Western Psychological Services; 1996.

28. Beck AT, Steer RA. *Beck Depression Inventory (BDI) Manual*. 2nd ed. San Antonio, Tex: Psychological Corporation; 1993.

29. Kovacs M. *Children's Depression Inventory Manual*. North Tonawanda, NY: Multi-Health Systems; 1992.

30. Reynolds WM. *RCDS, Reynolds Child Depression Scale*. Odessa, Fla: Psychological Assessment Resources; 1989.

31. Reynolds WM. *RADS, Reynolds Adolescent Depression Scale*. Odessa, Fla: Psychological Assessment Resources; 1987.

32. Angold A, Costello EJ, Messer SC, et al. The development of a short questionnaire for use in epidemiological studies of depression in children and adolescents. *Int J Meth Psychiatr Res*. 1995;5:237–249.

33. Thapar A, McGuffin P. Validity of the shortened mood and feelings questionnaire in a community sample of children and adolescents: a preliminary research note. *Psychiatry Res*. 1998;81:259–268.

34. Daviss WB, Birmaher B, Melhem NA, et al. Criterion validity of the mood and feelings questionnaire for depressive episodes in clinic and non-clinic subjects. *J Child Psychol Psychiatry*. 2006;47:927–934.

35. LeBlanc JC, Almudevar A, Brooks SJ, et al. Screening for adolescent depression: comparison of the Kutcher adolescent depression scale with the Beck Depression Inventory. *J Child Adolesc Psychopharmacol*. 2002; 12:113–126.

36. Brooks SJ, Krulewicz SP, Kutcher S. The Kutcher Adolescent Depression Scale: assessment of its evaluative properties over the course of an 8-week pediatric pharmacotherapy trial. *J Child Adolesc Psychopharmacol*. 2003;13:337–349.

37. Renou S, Hergueta T, Flament M, et al. Entretiens diagnostiques structurés en psychiatrie de l'enfant et de l'adolescent. *Encephale*. 2004;30:122–134.

38. Lewczyk CM, Garland AF, Hurlburt MS, et al. Comparing DISC-IV and clinician diagnoses among youths receiving public mental health services. *J Am Acad Child Adolesc Psychiatry*. 2003;42:349–356.

39. Roberts RE, Lewinsohn PM, Seeley JR. Screening for adolescent depression: a comparison of depression scales. *J Am Acad Child Adolesc Psychiatry*. 1991;30:58–66.

40. Goodman R, Scott S. Comparing the strengths and difficulties questionnaire and the child behavior checklist: Is small beautiful? *J Abnorm Child Psychol*. 1999;27:17–24.

41. Bourdon KH, Goodman R, Rae DS, et al. The strengths and difficulties questionnaire: U.S. normative data and psychometric properties. *J Am Acad Child Adolesc Psychiatry*. 2005;44:557–564.

42. Goodman R. Psychometric properties of the strengths and difficulties questionnaire. *J Am Acad Child Adolesc Psychiatry*. 2001;40:1337–1345.

43. Achenbach TM, Rescorla LA. *Manual for the ASEBA School-Age Forms & Profiles*. Burlington: University of Vermont; 2001.

44. Winters NC, Collett BR, Myers KM. Ten-year review of rating scales, VII: Scales assessing functional impairment. *J Am Acad Child Adolesc Psychiatry*. 2005;44:309–338.

45. Bird HR, Yager TJ, Staghezza B, et al. Impairment in the epidemiological measurement of childhood psychopathology in the community. *J Am Acad Child Adolesc Psychiatry*. 1990;29:796–803.

46. Shaffer D, Gould MS, Brasic J, et al. A Children's Global Assessment Scale (CGAS). *Arch Gen Psychiatry*. 1983;40:1228–1231.

47. Guy W. *ECDEU Assessment Manual for Psychopharmacology*. 2nd ed. Washington, DC: U.S. Department of Health, Education, and Welfare, Public Health Service, Alcohol, Drug Abuse, and Mental Health Administration, National Institute of Mental Health, Psychopharmacology Research Branch, Division of Extramural Research Programs; 1976.

48. Gowers SG, Harrington RC, Whitton A, et al. Brief scale for measuring the outcomes of emotional and behavioural disorders in children. Health of the Nation Outcome Scales for Children and Adolescents (HoNOSCA). *Br J Psychiatry*. 1999;174:413–416.

49. Harnett PH, Loxton NJ, Sadler T, et al. The health of the nation outcome scales for children and adolescents in an adolescent in-patient sample. *Aust N Z J Psychiatry*. 2005;39:129–135.

50. Endicott J, Nee J, Yang R, et al. Pediatric Quality of Life Enjoyment and Satisfaction Questionnaire (PQ-LES-Q): reliability and validity. *J Am Acad Child Adolesc Psychiatry*. 2006;45:401–407.

51. John K, Gammon GD, Prusoff BA, et al. The Social Adjustment Inventory for Children and Adolescents (SAICA): testing of a new semistructured interview. *J Am Acad Child Adolesc Psychiatry*. 1987;26:898–911.

52. Warner V, Weissman MM, Fendrich M, et al. The course of major depression in the offspring of depressed parents. Incidence, recurrence, and recovery. *Arch Gen Psychiatry*. 1992;49:795–801.

53. Lieb R, Isensee B, Höfler M, et al. Parental major depression and the risk of depression and other mental disorders in offspring: a prospective-longitudinal community study. *Arch Gen Psychiatry*. 2002;59:365–374.

54. Lewinsohn PM, Olino TM, Klein DN. Psychosocial impairment in offspring of depressed parents. *Psychol Med*. 2005;35:1493–1503.

Practical Management

Introduction to Treating Depression in Children and Adolescents

JOSEPH M. REY AND BORIS BIRMAHER

KEY POINTS

- There is a need to train frontline providers to recognize and manage depressive illnesses and to educate them in scientifically proven treatments.
- To understand the research literature fully, it is useful to be familiar with the meaning of technical terms such as *response, remission, relapse, number needed to treat or harm, augmentation treatment,* and *treatment resistance.*
- Not causing harm or ensuring that benefits of treatment outweigh the risks is the first principle of bioethics.
- Informing patients and parents about the benefits and risks of interventions is at the core of ethical practice. Without that, informed consent is not possible.
- Not obtaining children's assent or cooperation often leads to adherence problems and can scuttle the best laid treatment plans.
- Off-label prescribing poses an extra burden on practitioners who need to be particularly careful explaining what off-label implies, its potential risks and benefits.
- Prescribing a psychotropic drug can in itself have an important psychological impact.
- Research on the placebo effect, large in major depression, highlights the importance of a good therapeutic relationship for better outcomes.
- Supportive management is probably a better option than watchful waiting and likely to be more acceptable to clinicians and parents.
- Prescribing antidepressants implies an obligation in the prescriber to monitor side effects and response adequately.
- Patients treated with antidepressants are often undertreated (e.g., remain at a low dose for too long or continue on an ineffective medication with only partial improvement) or not treated for long enough.
- Apart from preventing relapse and recurrence, an important function of continuation treatment is to achieve further improvement among partial responders.
- According to controlled trial data, clinicians can expect that up to 42% of depressed youth who initially respond will relapse or have a recurrence between 12 and 36 weeks in spite of adequate treatment.
- Ignoring family psychopathology may result in nonresponse to treatment, crises, and relapse or recurrence of the illness. This may require referring parents for treatment in their own right.

Introduction   *"The burden of suffering experienced by children with mental health needs and their families has created a health crisis in this country. Growing numbers of children are suffering needlessly because their emotional, behavioral, and developmental needs are not being met"*[1] *(p. 1). The U.S. Surgeon's General report on children's mental health begins with these words, which can rightly be applied to the situation in most countries and in particular to depressive illness. To remediate this state of affairs in the United States, one of the goals for the future agreed on was to train frontline* *providers to recognize and manage mental health issues, and educate them in sci-entifically proven treatments[1] (p. 8)—goals relevant for most countries. These wor-thy aspirations were outlined in 2000; almost 10 years later we learn that there is still much room for improvement. For example, in spite of—probably unrealistic—recommendations by the U.S. Food and Drug Administration (FDA) that depressed children and adolescents should be seen often at the beginning of treatment, only 5% had the recommended number of visits.[2] Chapters 1, 19, and 24 highlight that there are not enough trained professionals, physicians and nonphysicians, to meet the treatment needs of depressed youth worldwide. In the United States, two thirds of the prescriptions of antidepressants for depressed youth between 1998 and 2005 were written by nonpsychiatrists,[2] stressing the importance of improving the knowl-edge and skills of primary care professionals (see Chapter 19).*

DEFINITIONS

Table 4.1 summarizes the definitions of *response, partial response, remission, relapse, recurrence, phases of treatment*, as well as terms used to describe various types or aspects of treatment relevant to everyday practice. These concepts are often referred to in the chapters that follow and in research reports; practitioners need to be familiar with their meaning to interpret research data correctly.

TABLE 4.1 DEFINITION OF TERMS OFTEN USED IN THE TREATMENT OF MAJOR DEPRESSION

Outcome[a]

Response	After onset of treatment, if the patient shows no symptoms or a significant reduction in depressive symptoms for at least 2 weeks.
Partial response	The youth no longer fulfills criteria for MDD, but clinically relevant depressive symptoms or some functional impairment remain.
Sustained response	When patient is very much improved or very improved in at least two assessments conducted 6 weeks apart.
Remission	When there has been a period of >2 weeks but <2 months with no or very mild depressive symptoms and no or minimal functional impairment.
Recovery	Absence of significant symptoms of depression (e.g., no more than one or two mild symptoms) for >2 months and no functional impairment.
Relapse	When symptoms and impairment meeting criteria for a major depressive episode reappear during a period of remission (i.e., <2 months after symptoms subsided).
Recurrence	When symptoms and impairment severe enough to meet criteria for a major depressive episode return during a period of recovery (i.e., >2 months after symptoms subsided). This can be considered a new episode of the illness.
Treatment resistance	There is no wide agreement about a definition of resistance to treatment. Chapter 16 proposes that a patient should be deemed treatment-resistant when symptoms meeting criteria for MDD and functional impairment persist after 8 to 12 weeks of optimal treatment (pharmacological, CBT, or IPT) and a further 8 to 12 weeks of an alternative antidepressant or augmentation therapy with other medication or evidence-based psychotherapy.
Number needed to treat (NNT)	The number of individuals who need to be treated to prevent one additional case or bad outcome (i.e., resolution of a depressive episode). Data from RCTs are required to compute NNT, which is equal to one divided by the rate or response in the control group minus the rate of response in the treatment group (this is also called "absolute risk reduction"). For example, the TADS study[25] reported that 71% of participants treated with fluoxetine plus CBT were much or very much improved; the result for placebo was 35%. In this case NNT $= 1/(0.35-0.71) = 2.7$. That is, three patients (it is customary to round to the next whole number) will need to be treated with fluoxetine combined with CBT for one patient to show much or very much improvement. The lower the NNT, the more effective the intervention.

(continued)

TABLE 4.1 DEFINITION OF TERMS OFTEN USED IN THE TREATMENT OF MAJOR DEPRESSION (CONTINUED)

Outcome[a]

Number needed to harm (NNH)	NNH indicates how many patients need to be exposed to a risk factor (e.g., medication) to cause harm in one patient who would not have been harmed otherwise. NNH is calculated similarly to NNT with the difference that NNH refers to an unwanted effect; it also requires data from RCTs. NNH is the inverse of attributable risk (that is, the rate of an unwanted effect in those taking placebo minus the rate in those treated with the medication). NNH equals one divided by the rate in nonexposed minus rate in exposed. For example, the same TADS study[25] reported that 11.9% of participants treated with fluoxetine alone had reported some harm-related event, compared with 5.4% for placebo. In this case NNH = $1/(0.119-0.054) = 15.4$. That is, 15 depressed patients will need to be treated with fluoxetine for one patient to suffer a harm-related event attributed to the medication. In the case of NNH, the higher the number, the safer the intervention.

Phases of Treatment[a]

Acute	The initial phase of treatment, which aims to achieve response and ultimately remission. It usually last 6 to 12 weeks.
Continuation	Once response or remission is achieved, treatment (pharmacologic, booster sessions of psychosocial treatments) is continued in all depressed youths to consolidate the gains of the acute phase, further symptom reduction, and to avoid relapses. This phase usually lasts 3 to 9 months.
Maintenance	After a patient has recovered, maintenance treatment (pharmacologic, booster sessions of psychosocial treatments) is used to prevent recurrences in patients with a recurring or chronic disorder. Duration varies, but it can be indefinite.

Types of Treatment

First line	Appropriately safe treatments whose efficacy is supported by several, consistent RCTs, such as fluoxetine (Chapter 6), CBT (Chapter 8), and IPT (Chapter 9).
Second line	Treatments whose effectiveness has not been demonstrated by RCTs (e.g., escitalopram, dynamic psychotherapy) or have greater risks or side effects than first-line treatments (e.g., ECT). Second-line treatments are justified when first-line treatments have been ineffective or could not be tolerated (Chapters 6 and 16).
Optimization	Increasing the medication or psychotherapy to a maximum tolerable dose or lengthening the duration of treatment. This is the first strategy that should be considered to improve response (Chapters 6 and 16).
Switching	Changing one treatment, which has been ineffective or not tolerated, for another. Switching can be from psychotherapy to medication, from medication to psychotherapy, from one type of psychotherapy to another, and from one medication to another. In the case of medication, switching usually requires stopping or cross-tapering (reducing gradually one drug while the other is progressively introduced) (Chapter16).
Augmentation	When two or more treatments that target the same symptoms or illness are combined to achieve synergy of action and a better response (Chapter 6). Both psychological (e.g., CBT) and pharmacologic (e.g., fluoxetine) treatments can be combined to improve outcome. Different classes of drugs can also be combined to augment response (e.g., an SSRI and lithium). The main risk of augmentation is increasing side effects (Chapters 6 and 14) and cost.
Adjunct treatments	Adjunctive agents generally target specific symptoms (e.g., sleep, agitation) with the expectation that once the depression improves, the adjunct treatment will no longer be required. For example, trazodone and mirtazapine are often used as adjunct and transient treatments for insomnia. The main risk of using adjunctive treatments is increasing side effects (Chapters 6 and 14) and cost..

(continued)

TABLE 4.1 DEFINITION OF TERMS OFTEN USED IN THE TREATMENT OF MAJOR DEPRESSION (CONTINUED)

Types of Treatment	
Off-label	When medications are prescribed for indications or in patient groups (e.g., children, elderly) other than those approved by the regulatory bodies. Regrettably, most drugs are not formally licensed for use in children, resulting in much off-label prescription in pediatric patients (Chapter 6). Because regulatory bodies (such as the FDA in the United States, EMEA for the European Union) may approve specific medications or not, what is considered off-label prescription can vary from country to country. Off-label use, although legal, places added responsibilities on the prescriber.
Generic drugs	Generic medications are drugs produced and distributed after the patent protection (20 years for pharmaceuticals) afforded to the original developer has expired (e.g., fluoxetine). Generics are assumed to have identical properties to the original brand but usually are substantially cheaper.

[a]Modified from the American Academy of Child and Adolescent Psychiatry Practice Parameters for the Assessment and Treatment of Children and Adolescents with Depressive Disorder.[18]
CBT, cognitive behavior therapy; ECT, electroconvulsive therapy; EMEA, European Medicines Agency; FDA, Food and Drug Administration; IPT, interpersonal psychotherapy; MDD, major depressive disorder; RCTs, randomized controlled trials; SSRI, selective serotonin reuptake inhibitor; TADS, Treatment for Adolescents with Depression Study.

ETHICAL ISSUES

The chapters that follow largely focus on "what to do" when treating pediatric depression. However, it is also important to highlight the ethical aspects of treatment and what to avoid. The key issues of confidentiality and safety are not discussed here because they are dealt with in most chapters of the book applied to the specific topics.

"PRIMUN NON NOCERE"

Not causing harm or, at the very least, ensuring that benefits of treatment far outweigh the risks, is one of the principles of bioethics (*nonmaleficence*—the duty not to inflict harm).[3] That is, to recommend a treatment, the chances of helping patients with it should be higher than the probability of harming them; in other words, the risk/benefit ratio should be favorable.

Clinicians often use too narrow a gauge to appraise benefit versus risk. The potential gains from an intervention must be considered not only against the direct unwanted effects (e.g., akathisia, suicidal thoughts) but also against the financial and emotional cost, stigma, and inconvenience of treatment. Some of these costs are relevant to psychosocial treatments such as cognitive behavior therapy (CBT), interpersonal psychotherapy (IPT), dynamic, and family therapies, in which unwanted effects are often ignored when in fact the financial and time demands of treatment (e.g., missing time at work for parents, missing school or activities for children) can cause stress, particularly in already stretched families, and may undermine the sometimes marginal benefits of treatment. This can be a problem also in specialist services in which small parcels of the treatment plan are farmed out to various members of the multidisciplinary team, all needing a share of patients' and families' time for investigative and therapeutic input (discussed also in Chapter 5). When weighing the risks, the wider implications of not treating the depressive episode need to be considered also. Apart from the ongoing suffering and distress, these include potential deleterious outcomes such as suicide, school failure, and substance use.

Errors or poor judgment in delivering treatment are not the only ways in which we may harm our patients. This can happen in other, more subtle forms, such as through inadequate assessment, by neglecting to involve the child or family actively, haphazard and ad hoc decisions, not tailoring treatment to the needs and circumstances of the individual patient, and by impatience resulting in unnecessary changes to treatment, to name a few. Clinical experience, patient complaints, and malpractice suits repeatedly show that many flawed treatment decisions stem from an inadequate assessment resulting in misdiagnosis, lack of awareness of comorbid conditions, or ignorance of concurrent or previous treatments or side effects. As highlighted in Chapter 3 and other parts of the book, a good initial evaluation is the basis for sound treatment planning.

INFORMED CONSENT

"We were not told"—that selective serotonin reuptake inhibitors (SSRIs) may increase the risk for suicidal behavior—was the main complaint voiced by angry parents whose children they believed had committed suicide as a result of treatment with SSRIs during hearings by the Food and Drug Administration, which subsequently resulted in "black box" warnings.[4] Probably parents were not told because at that time clinicians did not know themselves, and this matter is still unresolved,[5–7] although "it is much more likely that suicidal behavior leads to treatment than that treatment leads to suicidal behavior"[8] (see also Chapters 6 and 14). Telling patients and parents about the benefits and risks of interventions is at the core of ethical practice. Without that, they will be able to only give "uninformed" consent.

Information must be provided in a way patients and parents can understand (in their own language in the case of non-English speakers or other minorities—as highlighted in Chapter 23), and it should include benefits and risks of alternative interventions. Data from randomized controlled trials (RCTs) allow computation of the benefits and risks of treatments in a practical and easy-to-understand way. Number needed to treat and number needed to harm (Table 4.1) can thus be obtained and discussed with families to assist them in making decisions. For example, a recent meta-analysis[9] based on data from 13 trials and 2,910 participants concluded that 10 depressed youth need to be treated with an SSRI for one patient to overcome a major depressive episode, and 112 need to be treated for one patient to suffer harm, to develop suicidal thoughts. Although data of this kind about pharmacologic interventions are growing, much less is known about unwanted effects of psychosocial treatments, a topic that has received scant attention.

Providing families with information to research the existing treatments using some of the many resources currently available is also helpful, even though some of the information may be biased or misleading, particularly on the Internet. Resources for patients and families are listed at the end of most chapters here; their inclusion does not mean that the authors, editors, or publisher endorsed its content.

Not giving adequate information or not obtaining informed consent undermines *autonomy*,[3] which refers to individuals' right to make decisions about themselves and their own health care. In most countries, children <14 years cannot give consent; they are not considered by law to be autonomous individuals; parents have the capacity to give consent on their behalf. The status of those between 14 and 16 years of age is less clear, and their capacity to consent varies between jurisdictions and depending on the specific treatment (e.g. electroconvulsive therapy). Informed consent in the case of incarcerated or mentally retarded youth and state wards poses particular challenges and is open to abuse by institutions and caregivers. In any case, clinicians have the duty to ensure that children are safe, respect their wishes whenever possible, and, if appropriate, seek their *assent*.

Assent means (1) helping children gain a developmentally appropriate understanding of the nature of their illness, (2) explaining what they can expect (good and bad) with the treatment, (3) evaluating patients' understanding of the situation, including whether they are being inappropriately pressured, and (4) seeking an expression of the patients' willingness to accept the treatment.[10] Not obtaining children's assent or cooperation often leads to adherence problems and can scuttle the best laid treatment plans.

OFF-LABEL PRESCRIBING

Chapters 6 and 14 deal with some of the issues with off-label prescribing. The reality is that many medications, psychotropic and nonpsychotropic, are not formally approved for use in young people. Considering only approved drugs would substantially reduce clinicians' options to treat most pediatric disorders including depression, particularly treatment-resistant or severe cases. Further, practitioners are confronted with the fact that evidence for many treatments is lacking (although lack of evidence does not necessarily mean lack of effectiveness), and a large percentage of patients do not present with single, clear-cut disorders but with complex, mixed clinical pictures in which treatment can become symptom driven (e.g., aggression) rather than disorder specific. Nevertheless, prescribing off-label drugs poses an extra burden and potential liability on practitioners, who need to be particularly careful in explaining what off-label means, and the potential benefits and risks without instilling false hope or excessive fear,[3] so that a meaningful informed consent is obtained. Assessing the risk/benefit ratio in off-label treatments is problematic and has been subject to manipulation.[11]

Not all off-label prescribing is the same: Some older medications may not be formally approved for children but their use is widely sanctioned by experience and consensus, whereas off-label use of newly introduced drugs could be considered quasi-experimental and would require extra precautions. Note that psychosocial treatments do not undergo the same licensing processes as medication (licensing is not required); thus the off-label concept does not apply to them.

OTHER ISSUES INFLUENCING TREATMENT

STIGMA

Many patients, particularly older children, adolescents, and people from some minority groups (see Chapter 23), see mental health treatment—and a psychiatric diagnosis—as stigmatizing.[12] It is relevant that depression is often perceived as a more serious illness, for example when compared with ADHD.[13] Youth worry that family members, peers, and others in their social network may think they are "mad" or dangerous, become apprehensive about being marginalized, and feel embarrassed or ashamed.

Clinicians, out of familiarity with the task of prescribing, may not realize that the mere act of prescribing a psychotropic drug can have a huge psychological impact on children and parents.[3] Young people often attribute magical properties or powers to medication, such as taking over one's mind, making those who take it do what they don't want, or behave like zombies. Having to take medication conspicuously (e.g., during school hours) can be embarrassing and exposes children to ridicule or bullying, thus the importance of thoughtful scheduling of doses. Exploring these anxieties when prescribing, often not done unless specifically raised by the family, can minimize hazards, reduce anxiety, improve adherence, and increase satisfaction with treatment.

TIME PRESSURES

Concern about the need to spend so much time dealing with the matters described—not directly related to evaluation and treatment of the illness itself but critical to its success—is a common response when reading what is required for competent, ethical management. Practitioners often feel these issues are all well and good but do not apply to the real world because such time demands are rarely acknowledged by funding agencies, service managers, health insurance companies, or even patients and their parents. Pressures are exacerbated by the higher cost this entails and a worldwide shortage of trained professionals. As a result, clinicians are often pressured to cut corners, see more patients in ever shorter periods, and achieve results quickly, leading to a feeling that theory is largely irrelevant to practice. Although acknowledging these tensions, one can struggle to achieve appropriate standards and use one's considerable prestige and influence to challenge these pressures and to educate patients.

PLACEBO RESPONSE: NUISANCE OR OPPORTUNITY?

One of the most puzzling aspects of the treatment of depression is the high rate of placebo response, estimated at about 50% in RCTs examining the pharmacologic treatment of MDD in youth.[9] Similar results have been reported in adults and, if anything, placebo response seems to be on the increase.[14] Although placebo response is considered a nuisance in treatment trials, it has been proposed that, if harnessed, it could create therapeutic opportunities.[15]

The placebo effect can be separated into the patient's response to (1) observation and assessment, (2) the administration of the placebo, and (3) the patient–practitioner interaction.[16,17] A trial involving patients with irritable bowel syndrome has shown that a combination of placebo with an augmented patient–practitioner interaction produced a clinically significant improvement above a nonenhanced patient–practitioner interaction and waiting list in a dose-response manner.[17] Although it is unclear whether these results can be extended to the treatment of depression, they highlight the importance of investing time and effort developing a good therapeutic relationship. Many chapters in the book emphasize that building trust and rapport with young patients is a key aspect of successful treatment. This research provides empirical support for this recommendation.

GOALS OF TREATMENT

The aims of treatment are to reduce to a minimum the symptoms, impairment, and duration of the depressive episode, as well as prevent its recurrence. The last is particularly important, given that pediatric depression is often a recurring condition (see Chapter 1). Clinicians ought to aim high, to achieve full remission of symptoms and a return to premorbid levels of functioning. Anything less is a suboptimal outcome because persistence of depressive symptoms increases the likelihood of poor psychosocial outcomes, suicide, and other problems (e.g., substance abuse), as well as relapse and recurrence.[18] Yet RCTs often use their own definitions of response, usually a reduction of symptoms below a predetermined cutoff, without taking into account the length of time patients have been with minimal or no symptoms; this makes generalizing the results of RCTs to everyday practice difficult, a problem compounded by selective reporting of RCTs.[19] Very few studies examine sustained response or recovery.[20,21]

WHEN TO TREAT

WATCHFUL WAITING

Watchful waiting is an approach to managing illnesses in which time is allowed to pass before further treatment is considered.[22] Watchful waiting is often used in conditions with a high likelihood of self-resolution or where the risks of treatment may outweigh the benefits (e.g., benign prostate cancer). A key component of watchful waiting is the use of an explicit protocol to ensure a timely transition to another form of management, if necessary. The United Kingdom's National Institute for Health and Clinical Excellence (NICE) guidelines introduced watchful waiting as a strategy "for children and young people with diagnosed mild depression who do not want an intervention or who, in the opinion of the healthcare professional, may recover with no intervention, a further assessment should be arranged, normally within 2 weeks."[23] Given that a proportion of depressed children and adolescents recover spontaneously or with minimal treatment, watchful waiting should not be ignored when depression and risk for harm are not severe. According to the NICE guidelines, other treatment options should be offered if after 4 weeks of watchful waiting, symptoms do not improve.

SUPPORTIVE MANAGEMENT

In a similar vein, the American Academy of Child and Adolescent Psychiatry (AACAP) practice parameter states that instead of medication "it is reasonable, in a patient with a mild or brief depression, mild psychosocial impairment, and the absence of clinically significant suicidality or psychosis, to begin treatment with education, support, and case management related to environmental stressors in the family and school. It is expected to observe response after 4 to 6 weeks of supportive therapy."[18] That is, education, support, and case management—*supportive management*—is a valid treatment option. Although little researched, supportive management is widely used in practice for the treatment of depressed youth and is not very different from *specialized treatment as usual* (described in Chapter 13) and *active monitoring* (described in Chapter 19). Supportive management is probably a better option than watchful waiting and likely to be more acceptable to clinicians and parents. Its importance is also highlighted by the data on placebo response.[17]

INITIATING MEDICATION

There is some disagreement among practitioners about when to start medication. Although the advice provided in this book is largely consistent, small disagreements in the recommendations in different chapters can be explained by different interpretations of the evidence or actual lack of empirical data. For example, Chapter 6 highlights that the "NICE guidelines for pediatric depression do not recommend antidepressant treatment in this age group until after specific psychotherapy has failed (and then only during ongoing psychotherapy). This stance is not supported by empirical data and in fact it may be unethical to delay medication treatment for six to eight weeks in severely depressed adolescents." Yet the NICE position—currently under review—has been adopted by many clinicians to a greater or lesser extent, particularly outside the United States. The European Union guidelines are similar to those of NICE (e.g., fluoxetine should be used *only after* the patient has failed to respond after four to six sessions of psychological treatment).[24] Inconsistencies are compounded by the fact that definitions of severity of depression are poorly operationalized and not very helpful for everyday clinical practice (see Chapters 1 and 3).

The AACAP practice parameter states that, although moderate depression may respond to CBT or IPT alone, more severe depressive episodes generally require treatment with antidepressants.[18] In the absence of complicating factors such as patient or parent refusal, most clinicians would find it difficult to justify waiting 4 to 6 weeks before starting medication in a severely depressed youth. This does not mean, however, that in many cases (particularly in primary care settings) it will be wise to wait 1 or 2 weeks, assuming that safety issues are adequately dealt with. This time allows for one or two additional consultations and a better assessment of the child, building rapport, providing education, and permits a superior evaluation of the true severity of the symptoms and impairment, which are often exaggerated by the emotions surrounding the crisis (e.g., a suicide attempt) that often leads to referral or presentation. Knee-jerk changes in treatment in response to crises and ad hoc management plans are counterproductive (see Chapters 13 and 15).

MONITORING TREATMENT

The AACAP practice parameter states:

> "The FDA recommends that depressed youths should be seen every week for the first 4 weeks and biweekly thereafter, although it is not always possible to schedule weekly face-to-face appointments. In this case, evaluations should be briefly carried out by telephone, but it is important to emphasize that there are no data to suggest that the monitoring schedule proposed by the FDA or telephone calls have any impact on the risk of suicide.[18]"

Although the FDA requirement of initial weekly follow-up might be unrealistic, as suggested by the low adherence to this recommendation in practice,[2] it is clear that prescribing antidepressants implies an obligation on the part of the prescriber to monitor side effects and response adequately.

HOW HARD SHOULD WE TREAT?

UNDERTREATMENT

"Patients treated with antidepressants are often under-treated (e.g. remain at a low dose for too long or continue on an ineffective medication with only partial improvement)" (see Chapter 6). Undertreatment—not enough medication or not for long enough—is a common error in clinical practice, true also for pediatric depression. Chapter 16 stresses that optimizing treatment is one of the first steps when managing depressed youth who do not improve.

The length of treatment is also important. There is growing data showing that up to 12 weeks of antidepressant treatment may be required to achieve response or recovery (see Chapter 16) and that recurrence after ceasing medication is common. Longitudinal studies of clinical and community samples show that recurrence of depression is as high as 20% to 60% by 1 to 2 years after remission and up to 70% after 5 years.[18]

Figure 4.1 shows response rates from 12 to 36 weeks in the Treatment for Adolescents with Depression Study (TADS).[21,25] Many adolescents with major depression who had not responded during the acute treatment phase (12 weeks) did respond during continuation treatment (weeks 12 to 36).[25] Figure 4.1 also illustrates the added benefit of continuing treatment for at least 24 weeks, irrespective of the type of treatment. Although participants treated with the combination of fluoxetine and CBT or fluoxetine alone responded earlier and more often, response rates for the three treatments converged after 18 weeks. About 20% failed to respond at 36 weeks, also irrespective of the type of treatment.

The 12-week results of TADS are tempered by the fact that "combination treatment had the highest rate of symptomatic remission, but even in that condition, the rate of remission was only 37%. Fully half of those subjects termed responders, a common endpoint in clinical trials, still had significant

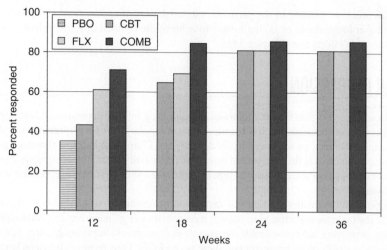

■ **Figure 4.1** Response rates according to type and duration of treatment based on the Treatment for Adolescents with Depression Study (12 week data from reference 25; 18–36 week data from reference 21). CBT, cognitive behavior therapy; COMB, combined fluoxetine and cognitive behavior therapy; FLX, fluoxetine; PBO, placebo.

residual symptoms."[20] The proportion of participants who recovered fully by 36 weeks has not yet been published but is likely to be substantially lower than the rates for response. In the TADS,[21] 95 of the 242 participants (39%) were considered not to have a *sustained response* at 12 weeks of treatment. The majority (74%) of these achieved either definite or possible sustained response by week 36 (80% with combined CBT and fluoxetine, 62% with fluoxetine, 77% with CBT; differences not statistically significant). These results and other studies[26] suggest that an important function of continuation treatment (with medication or psychotherapy) may be to achieve further improvement among partial responders; it remains to be seen whether this applies to remission as well as to response.[20]

RELAPSE AND RECURRENCE

In a study by Emslie and his colleagues,[27] 102 patients with major depression 7 to 18 years of age whose depression had responded or remitted after 12 weeks of treatment with fluoxetine were randomly allocated to continuation treatment with fluoxetine or placebo for a further 24 weeks. Relapse rates by week 24 were high in both groups but almost twice as common (69% versus 42%) and earlier in the placebo versus the fluoxetine group. Most relapses occurred during the first 12 weeks of continuation treatment, particularly in participants with residual depressive symptoms.

Of the 147 patients who had achieved sustained response by week 12 in the TADS,[21] 15% did not maintain their sustained response, with rates differing according to treatment modality (12% for combined CBT and fluoxetine group, 26% for fluoxetine, 3% for CBT; significantly lower for CBT than for fluoxetine). Put together, these data show that clinicians can expect that up to 42% of depressed youth who initially respond will relapse or have a recurrence between 12 and 36 weeks *in spite of adequate treatment*.

OPTIMAL DOSAGE

How quickly should optimal dosage be achieved? RCTs are constrained by the time available to reach the optimal dose, because extending the trial duration becomes prohibitively expensive, and by the narrow range of patients included. Yet increasing the dose rapidly to achieve optimal dosage quickly may result in more unwanted effects and dropouts. Also, optimal dose might vary substantially according to the patient, for example if the child has a comorbid physical illness (see Chapter 21) or a pervasive developmental disorder (see Chapter 22). Clinicians in everyday practice do not usually need to reach the optimal dose as quickly as in RCTs, as far as optimal dosage is achieved. With some exceptions (e.g., when depression is very severe or the risk is high), the goal should be to adapt treatment as much as possible to the particular circumstances of each patient and family. This may mean starting at lower doses or taking longer to achieve the optimal dose, to enhance compliance and minimize side effects (see Chapter 14).

BIPOLAR DEPRESSION

Many of the chapters emphasize the importance of detecting bipolar depression. Identifying bipolar depression is difficult because the first manifestation of bipolar disorder is often a major depressive episode during childhood or adolescence. As described in Chapters 3 and 6, a thorough assessment looking for specific clues is the best way to minimize the risk of missing this diagnosis. Primary care practitioners who suspect the existence of bipolar depression should, if possible, consult with a pediatric psychiatrist.

A description of the treatment of bipolar depression is outside the scope of this book, and readers interested in the topic are encouraged to consult recent reviews (e.g., reference 28). Although a diagnosis of bipolar depression has considerable therapeutic and prognostic implications, very limited empirical evidence is available on its treatment and there are no RCTs. Thus recommendations largely rely on extrapolation of adult data to children, always fraught with dangers. The most important aspect to keep in mind is that antidepressants should be used with caution when bipolar depression is suspected.

Many clinicians believe that antidepressants may trigger or worsen manic symptoms, but this has neither been confirmed nor ruled out in RCTs in either adults or children, and there are no RCTs showing that antidepressants are effective, even when combined with mood stabilizers.[29,30] A further problem in youth is that similarities between "behavioral activation," a side effect of SSRIs, and mania or hypomania make it difficult to detect emergent manic symptoms in clinical practice. Martin et al.[31] examined this problem in a sample of 87,920 patients 5 to 29 years of age followed for a median of 41 weeks. They reported that overall, 6% of patients became manic and that patient age and antidepressant class each contributed to the risk of conversion. The conversion rate among antidepressant-treated patients (7.7%) was threefold that among nonexposed ones (2.5%). Risk was highest for tricyclic antidepressants (odds ratio, 3.9) and in the younger age group (10- to 14-year-olds).

PARENTS AND THE WIDER CONTEXT

The AACAP practice parameter[18] acknowledges that it is virtually impossible to treat a depressed child or adolescent successfully without the close involvement of parents, and each phase of treatment should include family and school whenever possible. Family and school involvement are an integral part of *supportive management*[18] and *specialized treatment as usual* (see Chapter 13).

Chapter 2 highlights the growing body of evidence about the role that parental psychopathology, particularly maternal depression and family conflict, plays in the causation and maintenance of depression in youth. The impact on a depressed child of untreated parental psychopathology cannot be ignored because research shows that reduction or remission of parental depressive symptoms is related to a reduction in child symptoms.[32] Further, parental psychiatric disorder and family conflict are often found in cases in which depressed youth fail to respond to treatment and may trigger crises during treatment, as described in Chapters 15 and 16. The implication is that clinicians need to consider if parental disorder such as depression exists and, if so, how this thorny issue can be dealt with. Several chapters (e.g., Chapter 10), provide guidance on how to approach this matter constructively and how to refer the parent or parents for treatment on their own right without alienating them or undermining the child's management.

REFERENCES

1. U.S. Public Health Service. *Report of the Surgeon General's Conference on Children's Mental Health: A National Action Agenda.* Washington, DC: Department of Health and Human Services; 2000.
2. Morrato EH, Libby AM, Orton HD, et al. Frequency of provider contact after FDA advisory on risk of pediatric suicidality with SSRIs. *Am J Psychiatry.* 2008;165:42–50.

3. Dell ML, Vaughan BS, Kratochvil CJ. Ethics and the prescription pad. *Child Adolesc Psychiatr Clin N Am.* 2008;17:93–111.
4. Moynihan R. FDA advisory panel calls for suicide warnings over new antidepressants. *Br Med J.* 2004;328:303.
5. Birmaher B, Brent D, AACAP Work Group on Quality Issues. Practice parameter for the assessment and treatment of children and adolescents with depressive disorders. *J Am Acad Child Adolesc Psychiatry.* 2007;46:1503–1526.
6. Rey JM, Martin A. SSRIs and suicidality in juveniles: review of the evidence and implications for clinical practice. *Child Adolesc Psychiatr Clin N Am.* 2006;15:221–237.
7. Katz LY, Kozyrskyj AL, Prior HJ, et al. Effect of regulatory warnings on antidepressant prescription rates, use of health services and outcomes among children, adolescents and young adults. *Can Med Assoc J.* 2008; 178:1005–1011.
8. Brent D. Antidepressants and suicidal behavior: cause or cure? *Am J Psychiatry.* 2007;164:989–991.
9. Bridge JA, Iyengar S, Salary CB, et al. Clinical response and risk for reported suicidal ideation and suicide attempts in pediatric antidepressant treatment: a meta-analysis of randomized controlled trials. *JAMA* 2007; 297:1683–1696.
10. Committee on Bioethics of the American Academy of Pediatrics. Informed consent, parental permission, and assent in pediatric practice. *Pediatrics.* 1995;95:314–317.
11. Psaty BM, Ray W. FDA guidance on off-label promotion and the state of the literature from sponsors. *JAMA.* 2008;299:1949–1951.
12. Perry BL, Pescosolido BA, Martin JK, et al. Comparison of public attributions, attitudes, and stigma in regard to depression among children and adults. *Psychiatr Serv.* 2007;58:632–635.
13. Pescosolido B, Jensen P, Martin J, et al. Public knowledge and assessment of child mental health problems: findings from the National Stigma Study-Children. *J Am Acad Child Adolesc Psychiatry.* 2008;47:339–349.
14. Walsh BT, Seidman SN, Sysko R. Placebo response in studies of major depression: variable, substantial, and growing. *JAMA.* 2002;287:1840–1847.
15. Andrews G. Placebo response in depression: bane of research, boon to therapy. *Br J Psychiatry.* 2001;178: 192–194.
16. Kaptchuk TJ. Powerful placebo: the dark side of the randomized controlled trial. *Lancet.* 1998;351:1722–1725.
17. Kaptchuk TJ, Kelley JM, Conboy LA, et al. Components of placebo effect: randomised controlled trial in patients with irritable bowel syndrome. *Br Med J.* 2008;336:999–1003.
18. Birmaher B, Brent D, AACAP Work Group on Quality Issues. Practice parameter for the assessment and treatment of children and adolescents with depressive disorders. *J Am Acad Child Adolesc Psychiatry.* 2007;46:1503–1526.
19. Turner EH, Matthews AM, Linardatos E, et al. Selective publication of antidepressant trials and its influence on apparent efficacy. *N Engl J Med.* 2008;358:252–260.
20. Brent D. Glad for what TADS adds, but many TADS grads still sad. *J Am Acad Child Adolesc Psychiatry.* 2006;45:1461–1464.
21. Rohde P, Silva SG, Tonel ST, et al. Achievement and maintenance of sustained response during the Treatment for Adolescents with Depression Study continuation and maintenance therapy. *Arch Gen Psychiatry.* 2008;65:447–455.
22. http://en.wikipedia.org/wiki/Watchful_waiting
23. National Institute for Health and Clinical Excellence. *Depression in Children and Young People: Identification and Management in Primary, Community and Secondary Care.* National Clinical Practice Guideline No. 28. Leicester, UK: The British Psychological Society; 2005.
24. Eaton L. European agency approves use of fluoxetine for children and teens. *Br Med J.* 2006;332:1407.
25. Treatment for Adolescents with Depression Study (TADS) Team. Fluoxetine, cognitive-behavioral therapy, and their combination for adolescents with depression *JAMA.* 2004;292:807–820.
26. Clarke GN, Rohde P, Lewinsohn PM, et al. Cognitive-behavioral treatment of adolescent depression: efficacy of acute group treatment and booster sessions. *J Am Acad Child Adolesc Psychiatry.* 1999;38:272–279.
27. Emslie GJ, Kennard BD, Mayes TL, et al. Fluoxetine versus placebo in preventing relapse of major depression in children and adolescents. *Am J Psychiatry.* 2008;165:459–467.
28. Smarty S, Findling RL. Psychopharmacology of pediatric bipolar disorder: a review. *Psychopharmacology.* 2007;191:39–54.
29. Goldberg JF, Perlis RH, Nassir Ghaemi S, et al. Adjunctive antidepressant use and symptomatic recovery among bipolar depressed patients with concomitant manic symptoms: findings from the STEP-BD. *Am J Psychiatry.* 2007;164:1348–1355.
30. Sachs GS, Nierenberg AA, Calabrese JR, et al. Effectiveness of adjunctive antidepressant treatment for bipolar depression. *N Engl J Med.* 2007;356:1711–1722.
31. Martin A, Young C, Leckman JF, et al. Age effects on antidepressant-induced manic conversion. *Arch Pediatr Adolesc Med.* 2004;158:773–780.
32. Gunlicks ML, Weissman MM. Change in child psychopathology with improvement in parental depression: a systematic review. *J Am Acad Child Adolesc Psychiatry.* 2008;47:379–389.

Engaging, Involving, Educating, and Supporting Patients, Families, and Schools During Treatment

SALLY N. MERRY AND ELIZABETH MCCAULEY

KEY POINTS

- Engagement strategies must take into account the youth's developmental level, the setting where depression presents, and family, ethnic, and cultural issues and beliefs.
- It is hard for parents to ask for help, particularly if they did not recognize the problem and teachers or health professionals raised the issue or if adolescents sought help of their own accord.
- With children, it is important to engage the parents while making the child feel included. With adolescents, it is important to engage the adolescent while making the family members feel included.
- Involving young persons in decisions about treatment at all stages of management increases adherence.
- Providing parents, youth, and teachers with information about depression and its management is best done both verbally and by giving written resources.
- The impact on a family of living with a depressed child can be considerable. Interacting with a miserable or irritable young person is wearisome, particularly if other family members are struggling with their own problems.
- Parents may need guidance to differentiate between normal teenagers' ups and downs and a depressive disorder and the part they may play lessening or exacerbating symptoms.
- Parents should be given clear instructions about what to do if they are worried about their child's illness, including contact numbers of the treating clinician, crisis teams, or emergency services. They also need to know what to do if there has been an episode of self-harm.
- Engaging with schools can take several forms, including community-based therapists providing education and consultation, policy consultation to promote a positive school climate, school-based screening programs, and actual delivery of mental health services.
- School personnel need education to identify the signs and symptoms of depression, suicide risk, understand when and how to talk with a young person who seems in despair, and how to facilitate getting help.
- Schools should have procedures to deal with concerns about depressed students and those at risk of harming themselves or others.
- Working in specialist mental health services poses particular challenges in engaging young people. Care is often provided by a multidisciplinary team, and the severity and complexity of disorders are higher and require more of the family's time.

Introduction

All health care professionals face the task of engaging children, adolescents, and families in treatment for depression. As highlighted in earlier chapters, depression in the young is common and costly to the community. Despite this, 50% to 75% of children and adolescents with clinically significant depression are untreated.[1] In most countries the capacity of specialist mental health services is limited; schools and primary health care services have an important role in the detection and early management of pediatric depression. The process of engagement depends on who identifies the problem, on the developmental level of the child or adolescent, and on the setting. Stigma around mental health problems may be a barrier to accessing help and developing a good relationship with clinicians trying to provide care. There are particular challenges in engaging young persons and their families who do not recognize there is a depressive disorder, or in situations where depression coexists with a physical illness. In some settings, such as schools, adolescents may seek help but may be reluctant to have their parents involved. For optimal delivery of care for depressive disorders, children and their immediate family should all be involved in the care plan. In this chapter "parent" is used to mean parents, guardians, and care-givers; "child," "youth," and "young people" are used to mean both children and adolescents unless specified otherwise.

ENGAGING AND SUPPORTING CHILDREN AND ADOLESCENTS

The way in which youth and their families may be engaged in the assessment and treatment process depends on their developmental level. Evaluation is described in detail in Chapter 3.

CHILDREN

In clinical practice, children are seldom seen without a parent, and depression often arises within the context of family or social difficulties (see Chapter 2). Clinicians therefore have the task of engaging with both the child and family members. It is important to have strategies to ensure the child is included in all stages of the assessment process and involved in the management plan. Communication with the child depends on the child's developmental level and his or her verbal and cognitive ability. The language and approach must be appropriate to the child's age (e.g., toys or drawings in younger children). Time available varies from setting to setting, so techniques need to be tailored to the child and the situation. Here are some tips that often facilitate engagement:

- Start engagement at the first contact—greet the child specifically.
- Early in the consultation talk to the child about things they are interested in (e.g., friends, siblings, activities, school, pets, birthdays).
- Ensure the child is brought into the conversation regularly during the interview.
- Translate information for the child in an age appropriate style. Check that children understand what you are talking about.
- Ask children if they have questions.

ADOLESCENTS

Adolescence is a time when young people move from dependence on parents to independent functioning. This stage is accompanied by a greater affinity for peers and an increase in novelty seeking and risk taking. Cognitively, adolescents move to increased abstract thought, although brain development, and accompanying judgment, is not complete until the mid-20s. Adolescents and those around them have to adjust to rapid developmental changes with negotiations over levels of independence that typically continue throughout adolescence.

To support the need for independence and to establish a working relationship, it is important to spend time alone with the adolescent. This allows for a more accurate monitoring of mood and of risk behaviors that may be associated with mood disorders, such as substance abuse, suicidal thoughts and behaviors, and sexual activities. Parents should also be given time alone with the therapist and be kept informed of progress.

There are strategies that can be used to engage depressed adolescents and their families. Adolescents report that they appreciate it if clinicians take an interest in them, rather than just in their problems. The HEADDS interview (mnemonic for *H*ome, *E*ducation/employment/eating, *A*ctivities, *D*iet, *D*rugs/cigarettes/alcohol, *S*exuality/suicidality/depression/safety)[2,3] (see Appendix 5.1) provides a good framework for assessing the psychosocial situation of adolescents and supports the

TABLE 5.1 MOTIVATIONAL INTERVIEWING STRATEGIES

Avoid argument
   Confrontation is counterproductive
   The adolescent's recognition of need to change is a most powerful agent

Express empathy
   Builds trust
   Ambivalence is expected; acknowledging it leads to change

Support self-efficacy
   Hope, reinforce all efforts towards change, increase accountability

Roll with resistance
   Points of resistance are critical to understanding barriers to change
   Resistance when not reinforced is diminished
   Leads to more exploration of the adolescent's perspective

Develop discrepancy
   "Motivation for change occurs when people perceive a discrepancy between where they are and where they want to be."

Adapted from Miller WR, Rollnick S. *Motivational Interviewing: Preparing People for Change.* 2nd ed. New York: Guilford Press; 2002.

development of rapport. Motivational interviewing[4] offers another useful set of techniques to engage adolescents and their parents and to enhance willingness to consider changing maladaptive behaviors (Table 5.1). In this approach the aim is to build on the adolescent's own reasons (e.g., plans, desires) for making a change. Strategies include the use of open-ended questions and responses that affirm adolescents' thoughts and feelings by reflecting their ideas back to them. For example, "If I am following you correctly, it sounds like you are feeling pretty overwhelmed by school right now." Summary statements can also be used, such as "Just to review what we talked about today, it sounds like you are feeling pretty stressed out but are willing to try getting to bed earlier over the next couple of weeks to see if that is helpful."

As with other physical and mental health problems, a depressive disorder may impede the development of independence and sap self-confidence. Having a "mental illness" has a potentially negative influence on the adolescent's sense of identity. A number of challenges are raised for parents as well. They may become more protective and may have a sense of guilt and responsibility; alternatively, parents can become rejecting, critical, and punitive, particularly if depression manifests itself with irritability, noncompliance, and rejection of family values. These responses may impact on the relationship with the therapist. Labeling the problem as "depression" or "depressive illness" allows the adolescent and the family to distinguish between the person and the problem. Externalizing the difficulty has the advantage that adolescents, parents, and therapist can join forces and work together to find strategies to deal with the difficulties.

Providing adolescents with information about the causes and treatment of depression allows them to participate in decisions about management. Knowing that depressive disorder is common and strategies are available to deal with it is helpful. Adolescents may find it easier to talk about stress management or motivational problems than depression as an illness. Fact sheets and websites can be used to supplement information given by clinicians. (see Resources for Patients, Families, and Teachers at the end of the chapter.)

Giving adolescents details about interventions, *choice* about the preferred treatment, and discussing with them and their families how family members might be involved promotes a sense of efficacy. The process of "shared decision making" improves outcome in the management of depression.[5] This should then be followed by including adolescents in active monitoring of their progress (e.g., through the use of rating scales) and discussing with them options at all stages of therapy. Here are some tips to facilitate engagement with adolescents (see also Chapter 3):

- Greet the adolescent specifically.
- Be friendly.
- Give adolescents and families some time separately with you.
- Explain confidentiality and its limits clearly during the first interview.

- Make sure you use language that is developmentally appropriate.
- Start by taking an interest in the adolescent generally, not just in their problems (ask about school, hobbies, and friends).
- Develop the treatment plan jointly with the adolescent.
- Give choice where possible.
- Don't try to be what you are not (e.g., "cool"—if you are not).
- Avoid medical jargon.
- Talk about their strengths, not only about difficulties.

TALKING ABOUT SUICIDE AND SELF-HARM

The risk of suicide must be monitored in all young persons who are treated for depression, particularly in those who are on antidepressant medications (see Chapter 14). Because of the evidence that media coverage of suicide acts can increase the risk of completed suicide, there has been concern that raising the issue of suicidal ideation and behavior in a clinical context may increase risk. In fact, clear evidence indicates that asking about suicidal ideation and behavior in this context does not increase risk.[6]

Managing risk while maintaining a good relationship with the young person can be challenging, and it is best done collaboratively with the youth. Asking about the context of the risk, and asking the young person what precipitated the thoughts or actions is helpful. It is also worth asking about times when the young person had thought about self-harm or suicide but had not acted on it. Finding out the strategies they have used themselves can be applied to support the youth's sense of their own strengths, and to prompt discussion about other methods that could be used to reduce self-destructive behavior. It may be helpful to develop an action plan that the young people can use if they feel their risk has increased. This could include things the youth could do and supportive people the young person could approach. Involving families in managing risk is discussed later.

USING TECHNOLOGY TO ENHANCE ENGAGEMENT

Young people use mobile phones and the Internet extensively to communicate with each other, and there is increasing interest in their clinical applications. Clinicians can take advantage of text messaging or e-mail to remind about appointments, give prompts about tasks set in therapy sessions, and get quick progress reports from the young person, among others. Using technology for these purposes is in its infancy but is bound to have a multitude of applications and to become more important.

ENGAGING AND SUPPORTING FAMILIES

Engagement and response to treatment are substantially predicted by family factors. There are high rates of psychopathology (e.g., maternal depression, paternal alcohol abuse) in families of depressed children and adolescents and also high rates of family conflict[7] (see Chapter 2). Addressing these factors has the potential to improve the overall situation of the depressed child, strengthen engagement, and prevent recurrences.[8] The way in which families are involved depends on the developmental stage of the child and on the setting in which the presentation occurs. Parents may bring the child for assessment and treatment without telling the child of their concerns. Depression may be uncovered in the context of a consultation for another disorder. In primary care settings, for example, most depressed young persons present with somatic symptoms.[9] Adolescents may access care on their own and may or may not want to involve parents. Differing approaches are clearly needed for these differing scenarios.

Parents and other family members have a valuable contribution to make. They can be engaged as active partners by asking to provide information on the young person's symptoms, monitor progress (e.g., by completing rating scales or questionnaires), support therapeutic interventions, and help the child to watch for signs of relapse. Support for parents to help them address unresolved conflict in the family or negative approaches to therapy by one or more family members may also be critical for a positive outcome (see Chapter 10).

A number of options are available to consider if parents do not recognize depression or the need for treatment. In schools, youth clinics, and where the young person is able to give informed consent, it may be possible to provide care for the youth without involving the parents. This limits therapeutic options, particularly where family discord is an issue, but it gives the young person access to support and care. In other settings, for example where there are fees for services, it may be difficult to provide care without involving the parents. Contacting the parents in a nonconfrontational way, talking to them about concerns about their child, and exploring their own perceptions of the situation may help forge an alliance and may resolve the situation. If this is not the case, it is important to be clear about the consequences of not addressing the problem. If parents remain unconvinced, the risk to the child must be weighed. If there is serious risk of harm or depression is severe, it may be necessary to inform the relevant child protection services; in extreme cases, involuntary treatment may be required.

Where parents want their child—or more often teenager—to have treatment and the child does not want it, it is useful to start by seeing the adolescent alone to find out their perceptions of the situation and to discuss with them the concerns of those around. Sometimes adolescents have a plan to address the problem and it may be worth supporting this, trying to get their agreement to review success or otherwise with their parents or the therapist. After discussing the situation, adolescents may be prepared to attend a couple of appointments, to see the therapist elsewhere, or to attend a different facility. Alternatively, it may be possible to coach parents to provide support.

With pre-pubertal children, parents are in a particularly good position to help, which should include monitoring diet, exercise, and sleep—encouraging sensible behaviors in these areas—helping resolve immediate stressors like bullying at school, reducing family conflict (e.g., by refusing to fight with the child, by keeping disagreements between themselves out of the family arena), and by spending positive time with the child. This could include playing a favorite game, reading stories, or taking them on outings.

Many teenagers report they would like to spend more time with their parents, and teenagers who are depressed need support. Direct questions such as "How do you feel?" or "How was your day?" often lead to noncommittal answers, but teenagers, like most of us, like people to take an interest in them. This may be best accomplished less directly (e.g., by parents offering a drink and a snack and sitting and having one themselves). Chatting about general things often provides an opening to the teenager to talk about what is troubling them.

CHILDREN IN OUT-OF-HOME SITUATIONS

Involvement of parents in situations where the youth is a ward of the state or is in foster care is a complex issue. The extent and type of involvement by the parents should be decided depending on the individual situation, keeping in mind that the welfare of the young person is paramount, and the child's views should be taken into consideration in any decisions. The first priority is to ensure the young person is not at risk of harm, particularly if there is a history of abuse. If contact with one or both parents is very distressing for the child, or if contact puts the young person at risk, then involvement of the parents may be limited. These decisions should not rest on the shoulders of the therapist alone but involve liaison with child protection services, the wider family group where possible, and at times the juvenile justice system. In some countries such as New Zealand, provision is made for "family group conferences," which afford a forum for family members and professionals from the health, child protection, education, and justice systems to work together and find solutions. It is helpful to have a specific person to provide support for the child and argue the case for them, either formally—through a "counsel for the child"—or informally.

COMMUNICATION

It is hard for parents to ask for help. It is even more difficult when they have not recognized that there is a problem and the issue is raised by a teacher, health professional, or where an adolescent has sought help of their own accord. As a rule of thumb, with children it is important to engage the parents while making the child feel included. With adolescents it is important to engage the adolescent while making the family members feel included. Greeting all family members specifically, setting up clear expectations at the beginning of a consultation, providing separate time for children and their parents, and checking with parents about their own well-being (being careful not to imply that parents are the target of treatment) are all strategies that can be used to make family members feel valued and supported. Adherence to a management plan is unlikely unless all involved think the plan is a good one. It is therefore important to reach agreement with the young person and their parents about the best way forward. Where there is disagreement, it is critical to try and resolve this. Even in cases when adolescents are seen on their own, it is advisable to see one or both parents from time to time (if at all possible with the knowledge and permission of the patient), it is advisable to see one or both parents from time to time. This can take just a few minutes at the beginning or end of the consultation, with or without the adolescent present. The aim is to keep parents informed, facilitate communication, clarify issues, and to validate adolescents' reports—not always realistic or truthful.

EDUCATION

Although parents report that receiving information about depression is helpful, adding a formal parent psychoeducation package to existing treatment has not yet resulted in improved outcomes.[10–12] This may be related to high dropout rates because of the demands of the packages and to the practical difficulties of attending a regular program while running a home, getting to work, and dealing with a depressed child. However, ensuring that parents are informed about depression, treatment options, and involving them in decisions about management is part of good and ethical practice.[13]

Depression often recurs, so that ongoing monitoring of mood, recognition of early signs of recurrence, and ensuring access to help early in the course of the illness are important roles for family members. The relationship between depression and bipolar disorder should also be highlighted. Developing jointly with the young person and key family members a list of early warning signs of depression and mania and an action plan are ways of minimizing this risk.

Providing parents and youth with information about depression and its natural history and management is best done both verbally and by giving written resources. It is unrealistic to expect people to remember all the information discussed, particularly if they are worried or stressed. Providing fact sheets or details about reliable websites gives them a resource to refer back to. Making a note in the medical record of the information provided gives some protection against complaints that parents (and young people) were not told what to do about a number of different scenarios.

SUPPORT

The impact on a family of living with a depressed child can be considerable. Interacting with a miserable or irritable young person is wearisome, particularly if other family members are struggling with their own problems or psychopathology. Thus screening for difficulties in parents and siblings and ensuring their access to help is important.[8,13] Given the high rate of depression in parents of depressed children, it may we worth having self-help resources on hand.

Parents may respond to a depressed child by becoming overprotective. This is not likely to be helpful because it will increase the child's sense of helplessness and failure. Parents can be warned specifically about this possibility (perhaps by discussing the issue in the third person (e.g., "Some parents find they feel really protective when their child is depressed, but this may make the depression worse because it makes the child feel helpless."). The potential negative effects of being overprotective and the advantages of encouraging children to do things for themselves to increase their sense of efficacy can be discussed with the parents. They should be given practical advice about how much to expect from the child. Giving parents an outline of cognitive strategies such as problem solving, activity scheduling, and so on, allows them to contribute to the child's recovery and helps them avoid encouraging the child to take on the role of an invalid. For example, children should in most cases continue to attend school despite their depression. A reduced workload, perhaps with less homework, may be negotiated, and the child can be encouraged to complete the work set. Parents could help depressed children break tasks down into small parts, reward effort, and help children realize that tackling small tasks may lead to improved mood, as it often does.

Some parents become critical and rejecting of the child and will not make allowances for the depression. The risk for this is particularly high when children are irritable. In this case parents should be informed about the nature of depression and its effects, and of the negative consequence of fighting with depressed children or continually criticizing them. Parents may need guidance to differentiate between normal teenagers' ups and downs and a depressive disorder and to recognize the part they may play in exacerbating or lessening things. This can be less confronting if put in the third person (e.g., "Some parents find it really hard not to snap back if their child is being very irritable. It is worth watching out for this as we know that having arguments with parents or feeling criticized by parents makes things worse. Some parents find they have to leave the room or bite their tongue to try and keep the peace. Is this a problem for you? Have you found any good ways of dealing with this?"). Clinicians ought to acknowledge the difficulties and stresses parents often face, particularly if depression is comorbid with other conditions, as it often is (see Chapter 17). Suggesting ways in which they can get time for themselves to decrease overall stress, encouraging them not to voice criticism of the young person, and identifying and avoiding triggers that may precipitate arguments may be helpful.

MANAGING RISK

How to deal with crises and emergencies (suicidal and homicidal behavior, running away, etc.) is discussed in detail in Chapter 15. Suffice to say here that families need information about the risk of self-harm or suicide. Parents are usually wary of raising the issue of self-harm with their child, thus depriving the young person of potential support. They can be reassured that asking about suicidal thoughts is likely to be helpful, not harmful. Parents should be told to take talk of suicide or self-harm seriously. Warning signs that parents should watch for include the following:

- Threats of suicide or self-harm
- Talking about or writing about death or suicide
- Saying things like "I'd be better off dead," "Nobody cares," "There is no way out of this"
- Engaging in reckless behavior or having a lot of accidents
- Suicide plans

If parents are concerned they should be encouraged to:

- Stay calm;
- Ask children directly if they are thinking of suicide/self-harm;
- Be supportive and nonjudgmental;
- Reassure the child that it is possible to get help;
- Supervise the child;
- Remove anything children might use to harm themselves (pills, guns, knives, etc.); and
- Help children access appropriate help (family doctor, child and adolescent mental health service or specialist, crisis team).

Parents should be given clear instructions about what to do if they are worried, including the contact numbers of the treating clinician, crisis teams, or emergency services. Parents also need to know what to do if there has been an episode of self-harm or a suicide attempt (e.g., to ensure that urgent care for the child is provided, including what emergency services should be called or in which circumstances the child should be taken to the emergency room and where). Parents should also be clear about the role of the treating clinician and whether or not to call the clinician in an emergency. Once appropriate care has been provided and the child is safe, parents will need an opportunity to talk about what has happened, their worries, guilt, and anger.

SOCIAL AND CULTURAL CONTEXT

The extent to which children are seen on their own and the extent to which parents are involved need to be tailored to the particular family and take into account cultural norms. The cultural context influences how depression presents and is perceived, as well as engagement strategies. Ethnic and racial groups vary in their beliefs about mental illness and the acceptability of discussing and addressing these issues. Treating depression in immigrants and minority groups is discussed in detail in Chapter 23. However, it is worth emphasizing that children and adolescents from immigrant families face the stress of trying to fit into a new culture; parents often adhere to more traditional values and frequently hold negative attitudes regarding mental health issues. Those in fringe and marginalized groups are also at greater risk of depression,[14] and sensitivity to the demands of each family's situation is necessary. This includes gay, lesbian, bisexual, and transgendered youth.

Families from indigenous communities in some colonized countries have high rates of mental health problems in general, and of depression in particular.[15–17] The effects of loss of land, of traditional social structures, and of language are thought to play an important part in the development of depressive disorder.[18] Therapy perceived to come from the colonizing culture may be regarded as inappropriate, unhelpful, and out of touch with traditions and cultural norms that are held dear. It is impossible for every clinician to be "expert" in multiple cultures; in many cases it is best to help the young person and family find a care provider who has cultural expertise or involving someone in a multidisciplinary team with skills dealing with that particular group (see Chapters 23 and 24). If that is not possible, it is helpful if clinicians are not afraid to admit their limited knowledge and seek input from the patient and family about their culture. Often this allows professionals to get a clearer sense of the beliefs and values central in each case. Simple statements like "I'm going to need your help to understand the beliefs and attitudes of your school (or family, community) and how that affects you" can be used.

WORKING WITH SCHOOLS

Schools are key partners in the promotion of positive mental health and the provision of mental health services for depressed youth. Academic achievement, feeling connected to the school, and supportive relationships with peers reduce the risk for depression; academic, and learning problems, peer harassment, and isolation increase the risk.[19,20] There is a growing recognition of the association between positive mental health and academic achievement.[21] Depression can undermine school performance and attendance and lead to decreased involvement with peers and school activities. School personnel, like primary care providers, are in a good position to identify children and adolescents at risk and face growing expectations about the management of the mental health needs of their students. In the United States, for example, school districts offer a variety of health services, including school-based health centers that provide medical and mental health care on site, with the number of these centers growing from 120 in 1988 to nearly 1,400 across 45 states by 2001.[21–24] These programs improve academic performance[21] and emotional health,[25] and they reduce mental health and emergency room visits and hospitalizations.[22,23]

Engaging with schools in the mental health care of children can take a variety of forms, including community-based therapists providing education and consultation about management of depressed young people, policy consultation aimed at promoting a positive school climate, school-based screening programs to identify youth at risk, and actual delivery of mental health services. Table 5.2 summarizes some of the areas in which mental health service providers can work with or within schools. At all points, it is critical that school personnel are actively engaged as part of the

---

TABLE 5.2 WORKING WITH OR WITHIN SCHOOLS TO MANAGE DEPRESSED STUDENTS

- Promotion of a positive school culture
- Development of a no-bullying climate
- Education of staff and faculty:
  - Signs and symptoms of depression
  - Signs and symptoms of common co-occurring anxiety, conduct, attention deficit hyperactivity, substance abuse, and learning problems
- Education of staff and faculty regarding communication skills:
  - Validation of feelings
  - Problem-solving skills
  - Conflict resolution
- Prevention strategies:
  - Antibullying programs
  - Programs to address specific needs:
    - Help with homework
    - Activities to increase positive social engagement
    - Conflict-resolution programs

prevention or treatment team and that mental health care providers know what school resources are available because these can contribute to an optimal treatment program. Many schools have homework centers, tutors, and social activities that can be used to address specific learning and social difficulties, thus expanding the scope of intervention.

COMMUNICATION

It is critical for the care provider, even if school based, to elicit input from teachers and other school personnel about the young person's ability to function at school. Potential contact people include school counselors, vice-principals, core teachers, and school nurses. It may be useful to ask the core teacher to complete a questionnaire such as the Teacher Report Form[26] because this provides information on social, academic, and behavioral domains (see Chapter 3 for other scales and questionnaires). Because permission has to be obtained from parents and child before a teacher is approached, agreement about how and what to communicate to the teacher must be established. Sending a brief cover letter asking for input because the youth is involved in an evaluation "of growth and development" may suffice. However, many parents and youth are comfortable with a more detailed exchange, especially when they realize it may be in the youth's best interest for the teacher to understand they are struggling with depression, which may be contributing to difficulties completing assignments or getting to class. Failure to communicate with school means that strategies employed at school can be at odds with the objectives of the mental health treatment program.

EDUCATION

Teachers and school personnel may need education so they can identify the signs and symptoms of depression and manic switch, assess suicide risk, understand when and how to talk with a young person who seems in despair—using validation of feelings coupled with identification of effective coping strategies—and how to facilitate getting additional help for that youth. Reminding school personnel that depression frequently presents in the form of somatic complaints, particularly in younger children, is critical. It is also important to help teachers recognize that symptoms of depression, such as anhedonia and irritable mood, can be easily misinterpreted as negative attitude and lack of effort, and to help them understand that problems such as attention deficit disorder and depression can occur together. School personnel also benefit from understanding the central role stressful life events can play in triggering a depressive episode.[27] They are in a good position to monitor the responses of youth exposed to various stressors in the community or at home. Education for school personnel may also include information on emotional development with particular attention to the developmental challenges of adolescence.[28] This includes acknowledging the increased moodiness that comes with puberty and the normal adolescent interest in risk taking and questioning authority.

School personnel also play a role in communicating concerns to parents but may benefit from learning how best to discuss mental health issues, especially when dealing with families from varied cultural and ethnic backgrounds. In these situations, focusing on the positive attributes of the young person, concerns about stress management, and positive school involvement can be an effective way to begin a conversation with parents. Finally, it is important to provide information on evidence-based treatment so school personnel can direct students and parents toward optimal care.

There are many ways of providing education for school personnel on these topics. Principals often welcome brief presentations with a focus on practical solutions and concrete strategies as part of their teacher training, in-service days, or parent-teacher nights. Many schools have newsletters or electronic communication systems that welcome brief pieces on topics of interest like recognizing the signs of depression, what to do if a teen talks about suicide, and so on. Many materials are available at no cost via the Internet. They are user friendly and provide how-to ideas about talking with youth about depression, suicide, cutting, and so on (see section on resources at the end of the chapter). It is also important to intervene in times of national or community crises such as when there is a shooting or a youth suicide in a school. These unfortunate events provide an avenue for education about how to identify risk, talk with teens in distress, and communicate risk to parents via teachers and parent forums. Schools may need assistance to develop their protocols about how to respond to youth at risk.

MANAGING RISK

Because schools have heightened concern about students who may be at risk of harming themselves or others, it is necessary to include education about how to identify and manage youth along the continuum of depression and risk. Although teachers cannot be expected to manage major mental health problems, we can encourage them to take an active role by appropriately noting or asking about feelings of depression or thoughts of self-harm in their students. Reassure teachers that questions such as "You seem a bit down these days, I worry that you are feeling depressed" or "I noticed your essays are very focused on death and want to make sure you are not thinking about harming yourself" can be asked without increasing the risk of self-harm.[6] In these instances, teachers need to know that validating the youth's feelings and connecting them with the school counselor, nurse, parent, or therapist is an effective and sufficient intervention.

Many times schools want assurance that a youth who has attempted suicide or engaged in threatening behavior is "safe" to return to school. In these instances it is necessary to complete an evaluation of the child as soon as possible and then to work with the school, adolescent, and parents to get the youth reintegrated into school as soon as clinically indicated. Because no absolute assurances can be given, with youth and parents' permission, communicate the general outline of the treatment plan and what school personnel should watch for and should do if concerning signs crop up. Identifying a person in the school with whom the youth is comfortable who can check on the youth and receive concerns from teachers and staff is helpful. This person and appropriate school personnel need to know who to contact if concerns arise. Only when the treatment team is willing to step up to these responsibilities will the school staff feel comfortable in having the child back.

Nowadays schools, particularly in the United States, are even more concerned about disturbed youth's potential to harm others. It is important to inform them that in spite of the horrific nature of school-based shootings, homicides in schools remain rare in the United States, with <1% of all youth homicides occurring in schools.[29] That said, it is critical to encourage teachers and school staff to take indicators of this type of risk seriously, and to express their concern to youth who make threatening statements in their writings, artwork, or behavior, as well as connecting those youth with the school counselor, nurse, or administrator assigned to handle these issues. In cases of significant risk of harm to self or other, teachers should be directed to actually walk with the youth to the office of the appropriate staff member and, with the youth present, calmly state their worry and the reason behind it, allowing the youth opportunity to explain their feelings and behaviors. Calling caring and respectful attention to worrisome behavior without drawing conclusions lets students know that the people around them are paying attention to them, care about them, and want to make sure they are safe.

Although schoolwide mental health screening programs are beyond the scope of this chapter, brief screening tools with good psychometric properties are available free of charge (see Chapter 3) and can be useful for school counselors or nurses. These questionnaires can also be used to educate students about signs and symptoms of depression and to put into perspective how they are feeling and how distressed they are. For young people with mild depression, teachers and school counselors can be encouraged to use "active monitoring" as a first-line intervention.[30]

If screening tools are used, a referral system must be in place so school personnel know what to do if a student needs evaluation or treatment. A recent universal school-based mental health screening with sixth-grade students found that 15% reported feeling distressed; follow-up assessments revealed that only 13% of these "distressed" youth were in need of a mental health referral, and the majority were in need of academic assistance or support within the school.[31]

COORDINATING CARE

When a young person has persistent or severe depression, or there are concerns about safely, schools need a system for communicating their concerns to the young people and parents and for facilitating access to appropriate care. Unless schools have on-site mental health services, they need to establish procedures and collaborative relationships with mental health agencies in their communities to ensure timely access to service. In turn, care providers can work with the local schools to establish these procedures. For instance, working with depressed young people in the community may highlight a need for a broader school effort to promote emotional health among students. This could take the form of advocating for a schoolwide antibullying program[32–34] or providing guidelines for policies and procedures to manage suicidal students.

ENGAGING PATIENTS AND FAMILIES IN SPECIALIST MENTAL HEALTH SERVICES

Working in specialist mental health services poses particular challenges in engaging young people. The severity and complexity of disorders are higher, usually requiring longer consultations, and it is expected that children and their families will attend often and longer. Engagement strategies developed for dialectical behavioral therapy (DBT)[35] can be useful, particularly when working with adolescents. These include outlining a recommended approach, then stepping back and asking the reluctant adolescent or family to think carefully about their ability to commit themselves to the treatment, and clear delineation of the rules and expectations of the therapy—requiring active, not passive engagement.

In specialist services there will be a greater proportion of young people who have not responded to treatment, which is not always effective.[36] Clinicians need to maintain hope and support when symptoms persist. Do not underestimate the importance of helping young people maximize function in the face of ongoing symptoms and supporting them in confronting these issues. Similarly, families need support and should be encouraged to attend to their own needs as well as to those of their child.

It is particularly disappointing when the therapy provided by "experts" is ineffective or only partially effective. Patients and relatives may become angry and health professionals defensive, which is unhelpful. Rather than showing unrealistic optimism, acknowledge the limitations of current treatments, empathize with the young person and family, and express regret over the limitations of current interventions. It is hard to keep seeing young people and families when treatment is not helpful. However, staying the distance and providing a place where it is possible to talk about these difficulties is an important role for clinicians.

In specialist services, care is often provided by a multidisciplinary team; seeing a number of different people can be bewildering. It is helpful to have a key worker who provides ongoing care, clear information about the roles of other team members (a written outline with names, contact numbers, and roles is useful), and ensuring that all members of the team consistently give the same information.

Compulsory detention and treatment is almost inevitably distressing and may result in a lack of trust in mental health professionals and disengagement. Inform the youth and family about the legal process, give explanations for the actions taken, and provide them with information about their rights. Once the young person has improved, it is worth taking time to discuss their feelings about the actions taken, acknowledge distress from the process, and develop a plan to avoid the need for compulsory assessment and treatment in the future.

RESOURCES FOR PATIENTS, FAMILIES, AND TEACHERS

Matthew Johnstone, *I Had a Black Dog* (Pan Macmillan Australia, 2005). This short book describes depression and what helps in cartoon format. It is an excellent introduction to depression for patients and families and should appeal to a wide range of people.

T. Wigney, K. Eyers, G. Parker, eds., *Journeys with the Black Dog* (Allen and Unwin, 2007). This book contains firsthand accounts from people who have suffered from depression.

These are some websites that provide information on depression specifically for young people: http://www.kidshealth.org/, http://www.thelowdown.co.nz/, http://www.ybblue.com.au/, and http://www.sortoutstress.co.uk/

RESOURCES FOR PROFESSIONALS

Evidence-based treatment for children and adolescents; Society of Clinical Child and Adolescent Psychology: http://sccap.tamu.edu/EST/; http://www.clinicalchildpsychology.org

GLAD-PC: Toolkit http://www.glad-pc.org/documents/GLAD-PCToolkit.pdf

REFERENCES

1. Emslie GJ. Improving outcome in pediatric depression. *Am J Psychiatry.* 2008;165:1–3.
2. Goldenring JM, Cohen E. Getting into adolescent heads. *Contemp Pediatr.* 1988;5:75–90.
3. Goldenring JM, Rosen D. Getting into adolescent heads: an essential update. *Contemp Pediatr.* 2004; 21:64–90.
4. Miller WR, Rollnick S. *Motivational Interviewing: Preparing People for Change.* 2nd ed. New York: Guilford Press; 2002.
5. Clever SL, Ford DE, Rubenstein LV, et al. Primary care patients' involvement in decision-making is associated with improvement in depression. *Med Care.* 2006;44:398–405.
6. Gould MS, Marrocco FA, Kleinman M, et al. Evaluating iatrogenic risk of youth suicide screening programs. *JAMA.* 2005;293:1635–1643.
7. Garber J. Depression and the family. In: Hudson JL, Rapee RM, eds. *Psychopathology and the Family.* San Diego: Elsevier; 2005:386.
8. Gunlicks ML, Weissman MM. Change in child psychopathology with improvement in parental depression: a systematic review. *J Am Acad Child Adolesc Psychiatry.* 2008;47:379–389.
9. Martinez R, Reynolds S, Howe A. Factors that influence the detection of psychological problems in adolescents attending general practices. *Br J Gen Pract.* 2006;56:594–599.
10. Clarke GN, Hawkins W, Murphy M, et al. School-based primary prevention of depressive symptomatology in adolescents: findings from two studies. *J Adolesc Res.* 1993;8:183–204.
11. Clarke GN. Prevention of depression in at-risk sample of adolescents. In: Essau CA, Petermann F, eds. *Depressive Disorders in Children and Adolescents: Epidemiology, Risk Factors and Treatment.* Northvale, NJ: Jason Aronson Press; 1999:341–360.
12. Fristad MA, Goldberg-Arnold JS, Gavazzi SM. Multi-family psychoeducation groups in the treatment of children with mood disorders. *J Marital Fam Ther.* 2003;29:491–504.
13. Birmaher B, Brent D, AACAP Work Group on Quality Issues. Practice parameter for the assessment and treatment of children and adolescents with depressive disorders. *J Am Acad Child Adolesc Psychiatry.* 2007; 46:1503–1526.
14. Hegna K, Wichstrom L. Suicide attempts among Norwegian gay, lesbian and bisexual youths: general and specific risk factors. *Acta Sociol.* 2007;50:21–37.
15. Durie M. Mental health and Maori development. *Aust N Z J Psychiatry.* 1999;35:5–12.
16. Baxter JJ, Kokaua J, Wells JE, et al. Ethnic comparisons of the 12 month prevalence of mental disorders and treatment contact in Te Rau Hinengaro: The New Zealand Mental Health Survey. *Aust N Z J Psychiatry.* 2006;40:905–913.
17. Hunter E. Disadvantage and discontent: a review of issues relevant to the mental health of rural and remote indigenous Australians. *Aust J Rural Health.* 2007;15:88–93.
18. Brown R. Australian indigenous mental health. *Aust N Z J Ment Health Nurs.* 2001;10:33–41.
19. Eccles JS, Lord SE, Roeser RW, et al. The association of school transitions in early adolescence with developmental trajectories through high school. In: Schulenberg J, Maggs JL, Hurrelmann K, eds. *Health Risks and Developmental Transitions During Adolescence.* New York: Cambridge University Press; 1997:283–320.
20. Goodyer IM, Wright C, Altham P. Recent achievements and adversities in anxious and depressed school age children. *J Child Psychol Psychiatry.* 1990;31:1063–1077.
21. Geierstanger SP, Amaral G, Mansour M, et al. School-based health centers and academic performance: research, challenges, and recommendations. *J Sch Health.* 2004;74:347–352.
22. Santelli J, Kouzis A, Newcomer S. School-based health centers and adolescent use of primary and hospital care. *J Adolesc Health.* 1996;19:267–275.
23. Anglin T, Naylor KE, Kaplan DW. Comprehensive school-based health care: high school students' use of medical, mental health, and substance abuse services. *Pediatrics.* 1996;97:318–331.
24. Clark D, Clasen C, Stolfi A, et al. Parent knowledge and opinions of school health services in an urban public school system. *J Sch Health.* 2002;72:18–22.
25. Gall G, Pagano ME, Desmond SM, et al. Utility of psychosocial screening at a school-based health center. *J Sch Health.* 2000;70:292–298.
26. Achenbach TM. *Manual of the Teacher's Report Form and 1991 profile.* Burlington: University of Vermont, Department of Psychiatry; 1991.
27. National Institute for Health and Clinical Excellence. *Depression in Children and Young People: Identification and Management in Primary, Community and Secondary Care.* National Clinical Practice Guideline No. 28. Leicester, UK: The British Psychological Society; 2005.
28. Steinberg L, Dahl R, Keating D, et al. The study of developmental psychopathology in adolescence: integrating affective neuroscience with the study of context. In: Cicchetti D, ed. *Handbook of Developmental Psychopathology.* New York: John Wiley; 2004.
29. Centers for Disease Control and Prevention. School-associated student homicides: United States, 1992–2006. *Mor Mortal Wkly Rep.* 2008;57:33–36. Available at http://www.cdc.gov/mmwr/preview/mmwrhtml/mm5702a1.htm

30. Cheung AH, Zuckerbrot RA, Jensen PS, et al. Guidelines for adolescent depression in primary care (GLAD-PC): II. Treatment and ongoing management. *Pediatrics.* 2007;120:e1313–1326.

31. Vander-Stoep A, McCauley E, Thompson KA, et al. Universal emotional health screening at the middle school transition. *J Emotion Behav Dis.* 2005;13:213–223.

32. Department for Education and Skills. *Bullying: Don't Suffer in Silence—An Anti-bullying Pack for Schools.* London: Department for Education and Skills (DfES) Publications; 2002.

33. Espelage DL, Swearer SM. *Bullying in American Schools: A Social-Ecological Perspective on Prevention and Intervention.* Mahwah, NJ: Erlbaum; 2004.

34. Hawker DS, Boulton MJ. Twenty years' research on peer victimization and psychosocial maladjustment: a meta-analytic review of cross-sectional studies. *J Child Psychol Psychiatry.* 2000;41:441–455.

35. Miller AL, Rathus JH, Linehan MM. *Dialectical Behavior Therapy with Suicidal Adolescents.* New York: Guilford Press; 2007:346.

36. Jensen P. After TADS, can we measure up, catch up and ante up? *J Am Acad Child Adolesc Psychiatry.* 2006;45:1456–1460.

HEADDS Psychosocial Interview for Adolescents[a]

HEADDS can be tailored to the situation. A comprehensive set of questions is given below. The assessment can be done briefly using the first questions in each domain.

Home
- Take an interest in who lives in the home, what the relationships are like, and what people do together.
- Ask about what parents do for a living, and how much time they spend at home.
- Find out if the young person has ever lived away from home (to uncover history of running away/incarceration). Does the young person feel safe at home?

Education/Employment
- Ask about the school: Is it enjoyable, are there any problems?
- Ask which class the young person is in and the number of schools in the past 3 to 4 years.
- Ask about favorite subjects and subjects where there are problems. Find out about the relationship with teachers and if there are particularly supportive teachers.
- Ask about grades and compare with previous grades. Check whether there have been problems in school with peers? Teachers? Bullying? Cyberbullying? What happened?
- Find out about current or past employment. Hours per week? Problems with employers/employees?

Activities
- Ask how the young person likes to spend free time. Where? With whom?
- Ask what things they do with friends for fun. What about with the family?
- Ask about sports, clubs, projects, religious groups.
- Find out if there is a closest friend or group of friends. What's that relationship like?

Diet
- Find out about the diet, the number of meals in the day. and about snacks.

- Ask about body image and attempts to lose or gain weight. (Pursue a more detailed history of eating-disordered behavior as needed.)

Drugs, cigarettes, alcohol
- Ask about experimentation with different drugs like alcohol, tobacco, cannabis.
- Ask about use at school, among friends or family members. Amount, frequency, patterns of use. How were/are drugs obtained?
- Has the use ever gotten the young person into trouble with friends, in school, at home, with the law? Have they ever done anything they regretted afterward when they were using?
- Have they ever been in a car with an intoxicated driver? What could they do to avoid that situation in the future? Is there someone they could call who would come and get them?
- Have they ever been in drug treatment? Any family members ever been in drug treatment?

Sexuality
- Explain that many young people experiment with their sexuality these days, and ask about sexual experiences.
- Ask if they have been attracted to anyone. To guys, girls, or both?
- Ask if there have been any romantic relationships and whether that involved having sex.
- Find out about sexual experiences. Were they with males, females, or both? Were they wanted? Unpleasant? Confusing?
- Have they ever had an infection from having sex? Any pregnancy?
- Find out about contraception.
- Ask about sexual abuse.

Suicidality/Depression
- Ask what the young person does when stressed.
- Ask, "Have you ever experienced a *low mood* or felt *really down* for more than a few hours at a time?"
- "Did it ever last more than a few days?"
- "Did it affect your ability to do things?" If yes, go on to screen for other depressive symptoms.
- Did it ever affect sleep? Appetite? Ability to enjoy things? Behavior with others (make you irritable or moody)?

- Have you ever felt hopeless? Helpless?
- Did your feelings ever make you want to hurt or kill yourself? Did you ever come up with a plan? Did you ever carry out a plan? What happened? How are you doing now?
- Does your family have a history of mental health problems?

Safety
- Topics to include in conversation: domestic violence, relationship violence, drug use, need for barrier contraceptive use, gun availability, and seat-belt use.

[a]Adapted from Goldenring JM, Cohen E. Getting into adolescent heads. *Contemp Pediatr.* 1988;5:75–90, and Goldenring JM, Rosen D. Getting into adolescent heads: an essential update. *Contemp Pediatr.* 2004;21:64–90.

How to Use Medication to Manage Depression

GRAHAM J. EMSLIE, RONGRONG TAO,
PAUL CROARKIN, AND TARYN L. MAYES

KEY POINTS

- In treating depression, medications can target depressive symptoms, augument partial response, or treat associated symptoms.
- Fluoxetine, citalopram, and sertraline are recommended for the initial treatment of depression, with fluoxetine having the strongest evidence.
- Given the high rate of comorbidity, initiating antidepressant medication is based on the judgment that the depression is primary (meaning it is the most disabling or not a consequence of another disorder).
- Response or nonresponse or adverse effects of treatment during a previous episode will influence the choice of medication for the current episode. Also, patients' previous experience with medication will influence adherence.
- Prior to initiating treatment with antidepressants, patients must be screened for suicidal behavior. Suicidality should be monitored carefully during treatment.
- It is important to monitor changes in depressive symptoms using standardized forms such as the Quick Inventory of Depressive Symptoms (QIDS) rather than global judgment.
- Patients are often undertreated (e.g., remain at a low dose for too long or continue on an ineffective medication with only partial improvement). An adequate trial may last up to 12 weeks because of decisions to increase the dose or initial difficulties with tolerance. A review of the treatment plan is essential if patients continue to have symptoms after 3 months of treatment.
- An alternative selective serotonin reuptake inhibitor (SSRI) is recommended as the second line of treatment (fluoxetine, citalopram, sertraline, escitalopram, or paroxetine—in adolescents only).
- Although to date none of the non-SSRI drugs have been shown to be effective in acute treatment, this would not preclude use of these medications (e.g., venlafaxine, bupropion, mirtazapine, or duloxetine). At this time, these agents are generally recommended in patients who have failed to respond to adequate SSRI treatments.
- Information to guide augmenting strategies in treating children and adolescents is very limited, and recommendations are generally based on adult data. Medications for augmentation include lithium, triiodothyronine (T3), bupropion, atypical antipsychotics, buspirone, and psychostimulants.

Introduction

Like many advances in medicine, discovery of antidepressants occurred serendipitously when, in 1954, Bloch and colleagues reported improved mood in patients treated with iproniazid for tuberculosis.[1] Kuhn also reported decreased depressed mood with imipramine, which was being studied as a tranquilizer.[2] Subsequently, monoamine oxidase inhibitors (MAOIs) and tricyclics (TCAs) began to be used as antidepressants.

In 1973, Weinberg and colleagues presented data on diagnosis of depression in a cohort of 72 children with learning difficulties in the *Journal of Pediatrics*.[3] In the article, he also described treatment of 19 children with antidepressants. The editor felt compelled to add, "the Editor feels it is necessary to stress extreme caution (1) in identifying any child as having a depressive illness, and (2) in prescribing any medication for such a disorder." The editor also recommended future research directions for pediatric depression, including randomized, placebo-controlled trials.[3]

Over the next 20 years, research into antidepressant treatment for pediatric depression increased, but only about 250 children were involved in randomized controlled trials (RCTs) worldwide during that period. The inability to demonstrate efficacy of TCAs in pediatric populations suggested that extrapolating from adult data was problematic, so additional studies specific to children and adolescents with depression were needed. The first positive trial of fluoxetine in children and adolescents (8 to 18 years of age) with MDD was funded by the National Institute of Mental Health (NIMH).[4] In 1997, the FDA Modernization Act made it mandatory that all new compounds with potential use in the pediatric age group be studied in children and adolescents. Furthermore, the act encouraged pediatric research on medications approved for adults that were also being used in children and adolescents.[5] This was followed by the Best Pharmaceuticals for Children Act in 2002, which established a process for studying medications in pediatric populations to improve clinical trial investigations (e.g., clinical study design, weight of evidence, ethical and labeling issues, etc.). However, even with these acts, there were problems with new pediatric data, including lack of research infrastructure and methodologic flaws in study design, and design of optimal trials was still undetermined. Regardless of these limitations, these studies have provided substantial information in the use of antidepressants in the pediatric population, with over a 200% increase in children and adolescents enrolled in RCTs in the past 10 years. Increasing data on both pharmalogic and non-pharmalogic treatments resulted in guidelines for treating depression in the pediatric population that parallel adult depression treatment.[6–8] Contrary to these guidelines, the recommendation in European countries has been not to use antidepressants in children and adolescents except for their approved indication (only obsessive compulsive disorder) or in conjunction with psychotherapy following nonresponse to psychotherapy alone.[9–10]

The increased pediatric data also suggested that treatment of antidepressants caused increased suicidality (suicidal behavior and ideation), with 4% of subjects on active treatment and 2% of subjects on placebo reporting increased suicidality. There were no completed suicides in any of these trials.[11] These findings resulted in an advisory from the Food and Drug Administration (FDA) and "black box" warnings for all antidepressants. A recent meta-analysis on antidepressant RCTs in children and adolescents, in contrast, reported that benefits outweigh risks in SSRIs and novel antidepressants.[12]

Based on the available empirical data, antidepressants continue to be an effective treatment for pediatric depression, and SSRIs are considered the first-line medication for this population.[6–8] In this chapter, we review rational approaches to medication management in children and adolescents with depression. Specifically, we discuss (1) general management issues, (2) acute medication management (including dosing, pharmacokinetics, and safety), (3) use of adjunctive and augmenting agents, and (4) continuation and maintenance treatment.

GENERAL MANAGEMENT

General issues to consider prior to initiating medication treatment include diagnosis, previous treatments, safety assessment, measurement of outcomes, and psychoeducation.

DIAGNOSIS

Diagnosis is based on an interview with the child and parent separately (as well as other available sources, such as teachers) to establish the presence of a current MDD episode (see Chapter 3). Currently, information on medication management is only available for MDD; however, clinicians often extrapolate from MDD data and adult data to consider medication treatment for dysthymic disorder and depressive disorder not otherwise specified. As part of the diagnostic evaluation, assessment of comorbid conditions is important. Given the high rate of comorbidity, initiating antidepressant medication is based on the judgment that the depression is primary (in this context, meaning it is the most disabling or *not* a consequence of another disorder).

Because depression is an episodic disorder, assessment includes past history of the illness, as well as the phase of current treatment (if applicable). Treatment for depression involves three phases: acute, continuation, and maintenance (see Table 4.1 for definitions). *Acute treatment* refers to initial treatment designed to achieve *response* (significant reduction in depressive symptoms) and ultimately *remission* (minimal or no symptoms). The goal of treatment is remission, although most RCTs include response as the primary aim. *Continuation treatment* follows acute treatment, with the goal of preventing *relapse* of symptoms of the treated episode and consolidating symptom improvement for a longer duration (*recovery*). Continuation treatment generally lasts 4 to 9 months following remission. Maintenance treatment, which lasts 1 to 3 years, is aimed at preventing new episodes, or *recurrences*, of depression in participants who have recovered from their index episode.[13–15]

PREVIOUS TREATMENT

Consideration of treatment history addresses three areas: current episode, past episodes, and non-pharmacologic interventions. In evaluating patients who have already had treatment for this episode, clinicians must consider whether previous medication trials have been optimal. This involves assessing the dose administered, duration of treatment, and compliance. The Antidepressant Treatment History Form is an instrument that quantifies the adequacy of prior treatments with antidepressants. This has been used extensively in adults; however, few guidelines are available for child and adolescent patients.[16] Obviously, response or nonresponse or adverse effects of treatment during a previous episode will influence medication choice for the current episode. Also, patients' previous experience with medication will influence adherence.

Assessment of the quality and quantity of specific psychotherapy is a consideration prior to initiating medication. Specific psychotherapies such as cognitive behavioral therapy (CBT) and interpersonal therapy (IPT) significantly reduce depression when compared with control groups (reviewed in Chapters 8 and 9). Most guidelines suggest using either a specific therapy or medication for youth who do not respond to nonspecific interventions;[6,7] however, the National Institute for Health and Clinical Excellence (NICE) guidelines for pediatric depression do not recommend antidepressant treatment in this age group until after specific psychotherapy has failed (and then only during ongoing psychotherapy).[10] This stance is not supported by empirical data, and in fact it may be unethical to delay medication treatment for 6 to 8 weeks in severely depressed adolescents.

The current evidence suggests that options include integration of medication and psychotherapy, sequencing of treatment, or combination treatment. A trial of psychotherapy could precede a medication trial (as recommended by the NICE guidelines) or follow response to medication.[17–22] Alternatively, both medication and psychotherapy could be initiated together. Data from the Treatment for Adolescents with Depression Study (TADS) trial suggest some advantage of combined treatment;[23] however, combination treatment following a brief psychosocial intervention was not superior to medication alone in a second study.[24] Two smaller studies also failed to demonstrate greater efficacy with combination treatment over monotherapy in reducing depression.[25–26] Sequencing of treatment can be considered depending on patient preference, severity of depression, or availability of treatments.

SAFETY ASSESSMENT

Prior to initiating medication treatments, two important areas need to be addressed: history of suicidal behavior and family psychiatric history. In the general population, studies have found that up to 5% of 14- to 18-year-olds report having suicidal thoughts.[27] Another study reports that as many as 19% of teenagers (15 to 19 years of age) in the general population have suicidal ideation, and nearly 9% make an actual suicide attempt over a 12-month period.[28] The rates of suicidal thinking and suicide attempts are even more frequent in youth receiving care for depression. In all, 35% to 50% of them have made, or will make, a suicide attempt.[29–30] Thus assessment of suicidal thinking and behaviors (including examination of suicidal behavior versus nonsuicidal self-injurious behavior) prior to initiating treatment, as well as ongoing assessment throughout treatment, is important.[31] Managing suicidal behavior during treatment is discussed in Chapter 15. In addition, the

FDA also recommended monitoring for symptoms of anxiety, agitation, panic attacks, insomnia, irritability, hostility (aggressiveness), impulsivity, akathisia (psychomotor restlessness), hypomania, and mania because these symptoms have been reported in adult and pediatric patients being treated with antidepressants.

Family history of suicides and of bipolar disorder is also important to assess. Although family history of bipolar disorder would not preclude antidepressant treatment, it would indicate that antidepressant medication should be initiated cautiously.

MEASUREMENT OF OUTCOMES

The goal of depression treatment is full remission of symptoms[15] and restoration of functioning, not simply response to treatment. Implementation of evidence-based guidelines improves outcome in adults[32] and children.[33] However, even when following guidelines, clinicians frequently underdose or change treatment too quickly, vary substantially in visit frequency, and vary in how they assess outcome.[34] Often, global judgment is used instead of specific symptom assessment, even though global judgment is less accurate.[35] Severity of depression and functioning need to be assessed at baseline and throughout treatment using standardized measures. This process of measurement-based care was used successfully in real-world clinic settings in the 2006 NIMH-funded adult Sequenced Treatment Alternatives to Relieve Depression (STAR*D) trial.[36]

In assessing depression severity in children and adolescents, several instruments are available, including clinician-rated, self-report, and parent report. One option is the Quick Inventory of Depressive Symptoms,[37] which has a clinician, parent, and child rating, assesses all nine criteria of depressive symptoms, and correlates with the CDRS-R.[38] A recent review provides details about various rating scales for depression in the pediatric age group;[39] their characteristics and usefulness are also described in Chapter 3.

PSYCHOEDUCATION

As noted earlier, parents and families participate in treatment decisions. As such, they need to have sufficient information about the benefits and risks of medication treatment (as well as other treatment interventions) (see Chapter 4). A parent medication guide endorsed by the American Psychiatric Association and the American Academy of Child and Adolescent Psychiatry is an excellent resource for parents (see Resources for Patients and Families). This guide includes information about depression, treatment interventions, and risks associated with antidepressant treatment, including an explanation of the "black box" warning and the concerns about suicidality with antidepressants. Although such a handout is helpful, it is equally important to review the information with families verbally, allowing adequate time to answer all their questions.

MEDICATION TREATMENT STRATEGIES

Medications for depression are used for a variety of reasons: to treat depressive symptoms, to augment in partial response, and to treat associated symptoms. Empirical evidence of medications used to treat these problems is provided later. In addition, the pharmacologic aspects of these treatments are detailed. Table 6.1 provides practical implications of the pharmacologic aspects of medications that are considered when choosing an antidepressant.

ACUTE TREATMENT

Figure 6.1 shows the updated algorithm developed for the Texas Childhood Medication Algorithm Project (CMAP) for depression.[8] It is important to understand that these recommendations are a guide—not a mandate—to clinicians and are based on a synthesis of available data. Clinicians are free to deviate but, ideally, would have a good clinical reason (e.g., previous family member response, side-effect profile, opinion related to a specific profile of the patient, etc.). Data on which medications work for which patients is not yet available, and therefore clinical judgment for individual patients is critically important.

TABLE 6.1 PRACTICAL IMPLICATIONS OF PHARMACOLOGICAL ASPECTS OF TREATMENT

Term	Meaning	Practical implications When Choosing an Antidepressant
Half-life	Indicates the time it takes from administration of a drug for the plasma concentration to halve through metabolism and elimination.	Drugs with a short half-life (such as paroxetine) need to be taken more often (e.g., several times a day) than those with a long half-life (e.g., fluoxetine) to achieve steady therapeutic plasma concentrations. Drugs with a short half-life are more likely to cause withdrawal or discontinuation symptoms if doses are missed.
Time to steady state	The time required from first dose of a drug to reach a point at which the amount of drug going into the body is equivalent to the amount cleared. Peak and trough levels are consistent at this point. This period is 4 or 5 half-lives. This time applies to any dosage change or discontinuation of the drug as well.	Drugs with a longer time to steady state require more time to reach stable plasma levels. This could result in more time required for therapeutic effects. Some side effects may be more problematic during transitions to steady state. Drugs with longer time to steady state (e.g., fluoxetine) require greater washout periods if switching to alternative agents.
Volume of distribution	The volume in which an amount of drug would be uniformly distributed in the body. Antidepressants generally have large volumes of distribution.	Drugs with a higher volume of distribution have greater extravascular than intravascular concentrations. This can lead to longer half-lives and durations of action. Volume of distribution is influenced by many physiologic factors, such as body size, cardiac and renal functioning, amount of adipose tissue and extracellular water (which fluctuates throughout human development).
Cytochrome P450 enzyme inhibited (see also Chapter 14)	Cytochromes are heme-containing enzymes located in the intestines and liver that metabolize drugs, toxins, steroids, lipids, and fatty acids. Cytochrome enzymes are involved in phase I metabolism of psychotropic medications. Drugs can hinder (inhibition) or activate (induction) the functioning of a cytochrome enzyme.	Drugs that induce or inhibit cytochrome enzymes can cause significant drug–drug interactions. Inhibitors can lead to unexpected increases in the plasma level of other concurrent medications metabolized by the enzyme. Inducers of an enzyme can lead to unexpected decreases in the plasma level of another drug that is cleared by the enzyme. Children with medical comorbidities or complex medical treatment may benefit from a medication with minimal cytochrome effects (e.g., citalopram).
Kinetics	Pharmacokinetics refers to how the body impacts the concentration and distribution of a drug over time. Linear (first-order) kinetics refers to drugs that have a proportional elimination from the bloodstream. The amount eliminated is related to the concentration in the bloodstream. Nonlinear (zero-order) kinetics refers to situations in which the body's elimination process is saturated. Hence a defined amount of drug is removed over time, regardless of blood levels.	Drugs with linear kinetics (e.g., citalopram, sertraline, bupropion) have more predictable blood concentrations after dosing changes. Drugs with nonlinear kinetics (e.g., paroxetine) have more unpredictable blood concentrations after dosing changes. This should be considered when titrating antidepressants in children and adolescents.

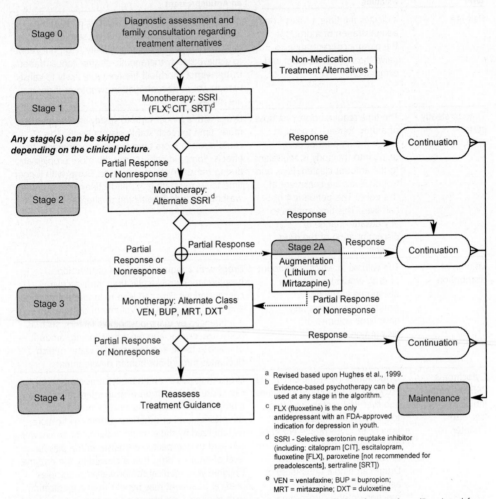

■ **Figure 6.1 Texas Childhood Medication Algorithm Project (CMAP) for depression.** (Reprinted from Hughes CW, Emslie GJ, Crismon ML, et al. Texas Children's Medication Algorithm Project: update from Texas Consensus Conference Panel on Medication Treatment of Childhood Major Depressive Disorder. *J Am Acad Child Adolesc Psychiatry.* 2007;46:667–686, with permission from the Texas Department of State Health Services.)

Stage 1

Based on results of published and unpublished trials, recommendations were to initiate treatment with one of three SSRIs: fluoxetine, citalopram, or sertraline, each having at least one positive RCT, with the strongest evidence for fluoxetine. Either there is inadequate data to warrant a recommendation for other SSRIs (e.g., escitalopram) or reasons to limit their use (e.g., paroxetine). Table 6.2 lists the pharmacokinetic and efficacy data for SSRIs in pediatric populations. Generally, adolescents showed greater drug/placebo differences than children in all SSRIs, with the exception of fluoxetine.[12,40]

Fluoxetine has three positive RCTs,[4,23,41] two of which were government funded.[4,23] It is not clear whether the positive trials with fluoxetine are caused by methodological differences from other antidepressant trials or to the pharmacokinetic profile.[42] Fluoxetine is generally initiated at 10 mg, with an increase to 20 mg following 1 week, provided the patient is tolerating the medication. Based on the two fluoxetine trials that included prepubertal children, 20 mg appears to be a sufficient dose for

TABLE 6.2 EFFICACY, PHARMACODYNAMICS, AND PHARMACOKINETICS OF SSRIs

Medication	Level of Evidence	Half-Life	Time to Steady State	Volume of Distribution	Cytochrome P450 Enzyme Inhibited	Kinetics
Fluoxetine	A*	4–6 days	>4 wk	20–45 L/kg	1A2 (weak) 2B6 (moderate) 2C9 (moderate) 3A4 (moderate) 2C19 (potent) 2D6 (potent)	Nonlinear
Citalopram	A	20 hr	6–10 days	14–16 L/kg	2D6 (weak)	Linear
Sertraline	A	26 hr	5–7 days	20 L/kg	1A2 (weak) 3A4 (moderate) 2B6 (moderate) 2D6 (moderate at low doses, potent at high doses)	Linear
Escitalopram	B	27–32 hr	7 days	15 L/kg	2D6 (weak)	Linear
Paroxetine	B	21 hr	7–14 days	3–12 L/kg	1A2 (weak) 2C9 (weak) 2C19 (weak) 3A4 (moderate) 2B6 (potent) 2D6 (potent)	Nonlinear

Level of Evidence:
A: At least one positive double-blind, randomized, controlled trial (A* signifies at least two positive double-blind, randomized, controlled trials).
B: Positive prospective open-label trials but no positive RCT.

the younger age group. In adolescents, however, dose may need to be increased to 30 to 40 mg if they are not adequately responding to 20 mg.[23,40] In a study of 29 children and adolescents (9 to 17 years of age) who had not responded to 9 weeks of treatment with fluoxetine, participants were randomized to continue on 20 mg (n = 20) or increase to 40 to 60 mg (n = 14; 40 mg for 4 weeks with the option to increase to 60 mg in the event of inadequate response to 40 mg). At the conclusion of this study phase, 10 patients (71%) on 40 to 60 mg/day were responders (≥30% reduction on the CDRS-R), compared with 5 patients (36%) on 20 mg/day ($p = 0.128$).[43] Although the study was too small to detect statistical significance, there appears to be potential benefit in increasing the dose in youth who are not responding to the target dose. It is rare for patients <18 years to require doses beyond 40 mg.

Citalopram has one positive[44] and one negative trial,[45] and it has limited cytochrome P450 inhibition. Like fluoxetine, the initial citalopram dose is 10 mg, and then increased to 20 mg after 1 week. Dose may be increased to 30 to 40 mg if there is inadequate response after 4 to 6 weeks of treatment, although there are currently no studies evaluating dose-related response in the pediatric age group.

Sertraline demonstrated efficacy in two combined trials,[46] and moderate interaction in P450 enzymes. Dosing for sertraline begins at 25 mg for 1 week. Following 1 week, dose is increased to 50 mg for a week, followed by 100 mg (the target dose is 100 mg). Youth with inadequate improvement following 4 to 6 weeks of treatment at 100 mg may be increased to 150 to 200 mg/day. Table 6.3 lists the formulations and dosing for SSRIs.

During the initial stage of treatment, visits are more frequent. The FDA recommended weekly visits for 4 weeks, followed by biweekly visits for 1 month, and again after a total of 3 months of treatment. Although it is not clear if this recommendation has changed clinical practice,[47–48] it does support the need for frequent monitoring early in treatment to assess improvement, adjust dose, and monitor for worsening of depression or emergence of adverse events, such as suicidal behaviors or mania.

Patients treated with antidepressants are often undertreated (e.g., remain at a low dose for too long or continue on an ineffective medication with only partial improvement). Therefore, as noted earlier,

TABLE 6.3 SSRI FORMULATIONS AND DOSING[a]

Medication	Formulations	Initial Dose	Target Dose	Maximum Dose
Citalopram	*Tablet:* 10 mg, 20 mg, 40 mg *Solution:* 10 mg/5 mL	10 mg	20–40 mg	60 mg
Escitalopram	*Tablet:* 5 mg, 10 mg, 20 mg *Solution:* 5 mg/5 mL	5–10 mg	10–20 mg	30 mg
Fluoxetine	*Capsule:* 10 mg, 20 mg, 40 mg *Tablet:* 10 mg *Solution:* 20 mg/5 mL	10 mg	20–40 mg	60 mg
Paroxetine	*Tablet:* 10 mg, 20 mg, 30 mg, 40 mg *Tablet CR:* 12.5 mg, 25 mg, 37.5 mg *Suspension:* 10 mg/5 mL	10 mg	20–40 mg	50 mg
Sertraline	*Tablet:* 25 mg, 50 mg, 100 mg *Solution:* 20 mg/mL	12.5–25 mg	50–150 mg	200 mg

[a]These drugs, formulations, and doses refer to the United States at the time of writing and may be different or not be available in other countries.

clinicians are encouraged to monitor response to the medication systematically, with the goal of treatment being remission of symptoms. An adequate trial of medication may last up to 12 weeks because of decisions to increase the dose or initial difficulties with tolerance. However, for patients continuing to have significant symptoms after 3 months of treatment, a change in the treatment plan is needed.

Stage 2

Once it is clear that a patient requires a different antidepressant, the second line of treatment is an alternate SSRI. Any of the first-line treatments may be used (fluoxetine, citalopram, or sertraline), or escitalopram or paroxetine (adolescents only) may be used as a second-line treatment. Escitalopram has one RCT in children and adolescents, which was not positive. However, in the adolescent subgroup, escitalopram led to significantly improved CDRS-R scores compared with placebo ($p = .047$).[49] A second adolescent trial has been completed, and results are pending. The pharmacokinetics of escitalopram is similar to that of citalopram, although the half-life of escitalopram is slightly longer (see Table 6.2). Because escitalopram is the active (S)-enantiomer of citalopram and twice as potent as citalopram with respect to serotonin inhibition,[50] dosing is lower for escitalopram. Initial dose is 5 to 10 mg/day, with the target dose of 10 to 20 mg for children and adolescents. Youth should not generally exceed 30 mg/day of escitalopram.

Paroxetine has been studied in three RCTs of pediatric MDD. One adolescent trial demonstrated positive efficacy on some outcomes,[51] but a second adolescent trial was negative.[52] The only paroxetine trial to include both children and adolescents was also negative and led to higher dropout rates in children, suggesting it may not be well tolerated in the younger age group.[53] Dosing of paroxetine in this study may have been too high for children. Pharmacokinetic studies of paroxetine in children and adolescents demonstrate nonlinear kinetics (see Table 6.1). Half-lives in children and adolescents are generally shorter than those reported in adults. However, there is wide variability in half-lives, peak blood levels, and blood concentrations that may relate to cytochrome P450 2D6 phenotypes. Blood levels at 10 mg/day were stable in one small sample of children and adolescents. At higher dosages, children are likely to have greater systemic exposure than adolescents.[54] Because of concerns about tolerance in children, paroxetine is recommended only for adolescents (≥12 years). Target dose for adolescents is 20 to 40 mg/day, with a maximum dose of 50 mg/day.

Stage 3

For patients who have failed to respond to this second medication trial, prior to initiating the next medication, it is essential to conduct a major reassessment to (1) determine if the initial diagnosis was correct, (2) evaluate whether there are ongoing or unrecognized comorbid disorders (e.g., substance abuse), and (3) assess the adequacy of psychosocial interventions. It is also possible that

TABLE 6.4 EFFICACY, PHARMACODYNAMICS, AND PHARMACOKINETICS OF NON-SSRIs

Medication	Level of Evidence	Half-Life	Time to Steady State	Volume of Distribution	Cytochrome P450 Enzyme Inhibited	Kinetics
Bupropion	B	Biphasic: 1.5 hr 14 hr	8 days	27–60 L/kg	2D6 (potent)	Linear
Bupropion SR	B	21 hr	8 days	27–60 L/kg	2D6 (potent)	Linear
Duloxetine	C	12.5 hr	3 days	27.7 L/kg	1A2 (potent) 2D6 (potent)	Linear
Mirtazapine	B	20–40 hr	4 days	4.8 L/kg	No known inhibition substrate for: 1A2, 2D6, 3A4	Linear
Venlafaxine XR	B	10.3 hr	3 days	Unknown	2D6 (weak) 3A4 (weak)	Linear

Level of Evidence:
A: At least one positive double-blind, randomized, controlled trial.
B: Positive prospective open-label trials but no positive RCT.
C: Retrospective chart reviews and case reports.

intervening psychosocial difficulties or unrecognized parental psychopathology may be contributing to nonresponse. If these issues have been adequately addressed, then the recommendation for stage 3 is a non-SSRI, such as venlafaxine, bupropion, mirtazapine, or duloxetine. Although to date no non-SSRI has been shown to be effective in acute treatment of pediatric depression,[55,56] this would not preclude use of these medications in patients who have failed to respond to SSRI treatments. Table 6.4 lists the efficacy and pharmacokinetic information for non-SSRIs.

Venlafaxine has been examined in three RCTs of children and adolescents with MDD. Two of these studies, both sponsored by Wyeth-Ayerst, showed no difference between venlafaxine and placebo. However, when the two studies were combined, the adolescent subgroup showed a significant difference between drug and placebo on the CDRS-R change score (−24.4 versus −19.9, respectively; $p = 0.02$), suggesting that adolescents may show more response to venlafaxine treatment than younger children.[56] Another study[57] also showed no difference between venlafaxine and placebo but was underpowered (n = 40). In the safety analyses conducted by the FDA, venlafaxine was the only antidepressant to have significantly more suicide-related adverse events than placebo, which was primarily because of increased suicidal ideation.[11] Initial dosing for venlafaxine is 75 mg daily for immediate release and 37.5 to 75 mg for extended release, with a dose increase of 75 mg/day every 4 to 7 days. Maximum doses are 225 to 300 mg (see Table 6.5).

Two multicenter trials of children and adolescents (7 to 17 years of age) with MDD were conducted to compare mirtazapine (15 to 45 mg/day) and placebo for 8 weeks of treatment. There were no significant differences on any of the outcome variables in either study, which may have been because of a high placebo response rate in both studies.[55] For example, in the first study, 59.8%

TABLE 6.5 NON-SSRI FORMULATIONS AND DOSING[a]

Medication	Formulations	Initial Dose	Target Dose	Maximum Dose
Bupropion Bupropion SR	*Tablet:* 75 mg, 100 mg *Tablet ER:* 100 mg, 150 mg, 200 mg	100 mg	300 mg	300 mg
Bupropion XL	*Tablet ER:* 150 mg, 300 mg	150 mg	450 mg	450 mg
Duloxetine	*Capsule:* 20 mg, 30 mg, 60 mg	20 mg bid	40–60 mg	60 mg
Mirtazapine	*Tablet:* 15 mg, 30 mg, 45 mg *Tablet Dissolve:* 15 mg, 30 mg, 45 mg	7.5–15 mg	15–45 mg	45 mg
Venlafaxine XR	*Capsule:* 37.5 mg, 75 mg, 150 mg	37.5 mg	150–225 mg	300 mg

[a]These drugs, formulations, and doses refer to the United States at the time of writing and may be different or not be available in other countries.

responded to mirtazapine (based on CGI-I ≤2) compared to 56.8% on placebo; in the second study, mirtazapine had a response rate of 53.7%, compared to 41.5% for placebo. Initial doses are 7.5 mg to 15 mg given at bedtime, increasing by 15 mg every 1 to 2 weeks to a maximum dose of 45 mg given once daily (Table 6.5). At low doses, the histamine antagonism of mirtazapine is more prominent and may lead to sedation and increased appetite.

There are currently no RCTs of bupropion for MDD in children and adolescents, although one study compared bupropion and placebo in youth with comorbid ADHD and depression (n = 24). By the end of 8 weeks of treatment, 21 subjects (88%) were responders (CGI-I ≤2, at least "much improved") in depression, 15 (63%) in ADHD, and 14 (58%) in both disorders.[58] Despite lack of available data, bupropion prescriptions are on the rise since the FDA black box warning, probably in part because of lack of data—and therefore no data on increased suicidality for this population.[59] The extended-release preparation is given once daily at 150 mg. After 4 to 7 days, this can be increased to 300 mg daily. It is important to give single daily doses early in the day to avoid insomnia or agitation at bedtime.

Duloxetine was released in 2004; because of its relatively recent availability, there are currently no pediatric depression trials. Two case reports have suggested that duloxetine may improve experience of pain and depressive symptoms in three adolescent females with chronic or severe pain and depressive symptoms.[60–61] Dosing for children and adolescents is not yet well defined, but adult dosing recommendations suggest initiating duloxetine at 40 mg/day in two divided doses, with a target dose of 40 to 60 mg/day.

Although an alternate SSRI is currently considered the second-line treatment, with non-SSRIs as third-line treatments, there are limited data available on treatment-resistant depression in youth (discussed in detail in Chapter 16). In the Sequential Treatment Alternatives to Relieve Depression (STAR-D) study, 727 adults who failed a trial of citalopram were randomized to a second monotherapy antidepressant: sertraline (n = 238), bupropion SR (n = 239), or venlafaxine XR (n = 250). All three medication groups showed similar rates of response and remission, with approximately one out of every four participants reaching remission with the second-line medication.[62] Thus, in adults, similar outcomes were found whether they used a second SSRI or an alternative medication.

ALTERNATIVE MEDICATION TREATMENT OPTIONS

Other antidepressants (fluvoxamine, nefazodone, TCAs, and MAOIs) may be used for youth who do not respond to SSRIs or non-SSRIs, although currently no empirical data support their use. Fluvoxamine is a SSRI approved for the treatment of pediatric obsessive compulsive disorder (OCD); however, it is not indicated for adult depression and therefore not widely used clinically for this disorder in the United States (in adults or children). Nefazodone has shown some efficacy in adolescents with MDD.[63] In 2003, the sale of brand-name nefazodone (Serzone) was discontinued in many countries because of the possibility of hepatic damage (leading to death or requiring a liver transplant in some cases) related to its use. In May 2004, Serzone was withdrawn from the market in the United States. Generic preparations are still available. However, nefazodone carries a black box warning regarding the risk of life-threatening hepatic failure, so it is not generally used for children and adolescents. TCAs are not usually included in treatment guidelines for pediatric MDD because of lack of efficacy and increased rates of adverse events.[64] In the paroxetine trial by Keller and colleagues, imipramine was used as an active comparator; 31.5% of subjects on imipramine withdrew because of adverse events, compared to 9.7% and 6.9% on paroxetine and placebo, respectively.[51] Finally, use of MAOIs has been limited in the pediatric age group owing to difficulties managing the diet. However, a transdermal selegiline patch, which has reportedly fewer side effects and contraindications, has recently been marketed, and it may be an alternative treatment for pediatric patients, particularly those who do not respond to SSRIs and other novel antidepressants.

SAFETY

In addition to efficacy, it is important to monitor for side effects to improve compliance in children and adolescents taking antidepressants (see Chapter 14). Although there is great individual variability, common side effects of SSRIs include headaches, nausea, vomiting, diarrhea, dizziness, bruxism, somnolence, vivid dreams, fluctuations in appetite, weight loss, weight gain, tremors, akathisia, rashes, and increased sweating. Some of these side effects resolve over time. The literature also suggests that SSRIs can increase the risk of bleeding.[65] Sexual side effects, such as erectile dysfunction, diminished libido, and anorgasmia, may also occur. Mirtazapine, nefazodone, and bupropion do not have sexual side effects.

Discontinuation symptoms may occur with abrupt changes in dosages, which is more common in antidepressants with short half-lives. SSRIs and novel antidepressants (such as mirtazapine, nefazodone, and bupropion) have a higher margin of safety in overdoses compared to MAOIs and TCAs. However, patients have died with large ingestions.[66]

SSRIs and other atypical antidepressants should not be taken with any of the MAOIs because these combinations may lead to confusion, high blood pressure, tremor, hyperactivity, and death. In addition, concurrent tryptophan can cause headaches, nausea, sweating, and dizziness when taken with an SSRI. Coadministration of these antidepressants with tramadol hydrochloride can cause seizures, although this is rare. Patients taking Pimozide, an antipsychotic medication, should not take SSRIs. Bupropion should not be given to patients with eating disorders or those who have epilepsy or are at high risk for seizures. Because of potential changes in blood pressure and heart rate, blood pressure must be monitored closely in patients taking venlafaxine or duloxetine.

TCAs have anticholinergic side effects such as dry mouth, blurred vision, and constipation. Weight gain often occurs with long-term use. Cardiovascular effects include tachycardia, hypertension, arrhythmias, and conduction blocks, and children may be more susceptible. Other adverse effects include rashes, blood dyscrasias, sweating, and hepatoxicity.[67–68]

MAOIs have multiple common side effects and serious safety concerns. These include hepatotoxicity, orthostatic hypotension, weight gain, dizziness, fatigue, sexual side effects, fatigue, headaches, sexual side effects, urinary hesitancy, and disrupted sleep. Patients can develop a hypertensive crisis if tyramine is ingested. Life-threatening drug–drug interactions can occur with sympathomimetics, meperidine, other narcotics, and other serotonergic agents.[69]

Suicidal ideation and behaviors are common symptoms of depression. For example, in the TADS trial, 29.2% of adolescents reported significant suicidal ideation at baseline.[70] The FDA also recommended monitoring for "associated symptoms," including anxiety, agitation, panic, insomnia, irritability, hostility, impulsivity, akathisia, hypomania, and mania. Thus patients receiving antidepressant treatment should be monitored for such psychiatric symptoms (including suicidality), and health care providers should adjust treatment interventions as needed (e.g., reduce dose or discontinue the medication). Clearly, the recent controversies have highlighted the need to assess antidepressant-specific adverse events before and during treatment.

During antidepressant treatment, one potential concern is behavioral activation or switching from depression to mania or hypomania. However, limited data are available on the prevalence of such activation with antidepressant treatment in the pediatric population. As noted by Goodman and colleagues, one of the difficulties in identifying manic switching or activation is that clinicians and researchers use a variety of terms to describe these adverse events (e.g., mania, hypomania, agitation, akathisia, activation, etc.).[71] Despite the limited data, some youth may exhibit such activation. Pediatric patients who have a family history of bipolar disorder warrant close monitoring during antidepressant treatment because manic/hypomanic switching may be predicted by a positive family history.[72]

AUGMENTING, ADJUNCTIVE, AND ALTERNATIVE TREATMENTS

Medications used for augmentation include lithium, triiodothyronine (T3), bupropion, atypical antipsychotics, buspirone, and psychostimulants. Table 6.6 lists the formulations and dosing information for these medications. These issues are discussed in Chapter 16, too; see also Table 4.1 for definitions.

LITHIUM

Lithium is the most studied augmenting agent in adult depression, with at least 11 RCT augmentation studies, two double-blind, drug–drug comparison trials, and 15 open trials. Overall, both the controlled and open-label studies indicated efficacy of lithium augmenting TCAs;[73] however, the

TABLE 6.6 FORMULATIONS AND DOSING[a] FOR AUGMENTING AGENTS

Medication	Formulations	Initial Dose	Target Augmentation Daily Dose	Maximum Daily Dose
Lithium	*Lithium Carbonate Capsule:* 150 mg, 300 mg, 600 mg *Lithobid Tablet:* 300 mg *Eskalith Tablet:* 450 mg *Lithium Citrate Elixir:* 300 mg/5 mL	150–300 mg daily	600–1200 mg daily (BID to TID)	Adjust to serum level of 0.6 to 1.1 mEq/L
Liothyronine sodium (T3)	*Tablet:* 0.005 mg, 0.025 mg, 0.05 mg	25 µg	25–50 µg	50 µg
Bupropion	*IR Tablet:* 75 mg, 100 mg *SR Tablet:* 100 mg, 150 mg *XL Tablet:* 150 mg, 300 mg	75–100 mg	150 mg	300 mg
Buspirone	*Tablet:* 5 mg, 7.5 mg, 10 mg, 15 mg	5–10 mg	20–30 mg	60 mg
ATYPICAL ANTIPSYCHOTICS				
Clozapine	*Tablet:* 25 mg, 100 mg	25 mg daily	50–100 mg daily	400 mg
Risperidone	*Tablet:* 0.25 mg, 0.5 mg, 1 mg, 2 mg, 3 mg, 4 mg *Elixir:* 1 mg/mL Oral disintegrating tablet: 0.5 mg, 1 mg, 2 mg, 3 mg, 4 mg *Injectable depot preparation*	0.25 to 0.5 mg daily	2–3 mg daily	4–6 mg
Olanzapine	*Tablet:* 2.5 mg, 5 mg, 7.5 mg, 10 mg, 15 mg, 20 mg *Oral disintegrating tablet:* 5 mg, 10 mg, 15 mg, 20 mg *Injectable preparation*	2.5 to 5 mg daily	5–10 mg daily	20 mg
Quetiapine	*Tablet:* 25 mg, 50 mg, 100 mg, 200 mg, 300 mg, 400 mg	25–50 mg daily	200–300 mg daily	600–800 mg
Ziprasidone	*Capsule:* 20 mg, 40 mg, 60 mg, 80 mg *Injectable preparation*	20–40 mg daily	120 mg daily	160 mg
Aripiprazole	*Tablet:* 1 mg, 2 mg, 5 mg, 10 mg, 15 mg, 20 mg, 30 mg *Solution:* 1 mg/mL	1–5 mg daily	5–10 mg daily	20 mg

[a]These drugs, formulations, and doses refer to the United States at the time of writing and may be different or not be available in other countries.

benefit of lithium is less evident with newer antidepressants.[74] The majority of the 11 placebo-controlled studies included patients resistant to TCA treatment, and only two studies included SSRI treatment-resistant patients. Controlled studies are needed for newer antidepressants before concluding that lithium is less effective as an augmenting agent to newer antidepressants.

No controlled studies of lithium augmentation have been done in pediatric populations. Two small open studies indicated the efficacy of lithium as an augmenting agent in pediatric patients who did not have adequate response to TCA treatment. The dose of lithium ranged from 600 mg to 1200 mg per day. Hand tremor, dizziness, nausea, dry mouth, fatigue, and polyuria were the most frequently reported side effects, but they were not considered to be related to the serum lithium level. No patient discontinued the treatment owing to the side effects of lithium. The assessment of lithium augmentation in these two studies was relatively short (e.g., 3 to 6 weeks).[75–76]

The current recommendation for lithium augmentation would be initially to augment at low doses (i.e., 150 to 300 mg for 2 to 3 weeks) and, if not effective, consider dosing to achieve therapeutic serum levels (0.8 to 1.0 mg/kg).

TRIIODOTHYROXINE (T3)

Triiodothyronine (T3) is the second most studied augmenting agent in adult depression. The results, however, are mixed. Although three of the four RCTs indicate efficacy, one study was negative and resulted in a negative pooled analyses of all four studies.[77,78] However, neither controlled nor open-label studies have been done in the pediatric population. Augmentation dosing is generally 25 to 50 µg/day.

BUPROPION

Sustained-release bupropion is used in the United States as an augmenting agent in the pediatric population, although currently no data are available on the effectiveness of this strategy. Sustained-release bupropion is an effective augmenting agent in adults who have experienced inadequate improvement with a SSRI.[36,79] Generally, a trial of low-dose augmentation would be made before going to full dose.

ATYPICAL ANTIPSYCHOTICS

Empirical evidence has started to emerge for augmenting with atypical antipsychotics in depressed adults with partial response. Papakostas and colleagues recently completed a meta-analysis of 10 RCTs that used atypical antipsychotics (olanzapine, risperidone, quetiapine) as augmenting agents for 1,500 mostly SSRI treatment-resistant depressed adults. They found a pooled remission rate of 47.4% for atypicals and 22.3% for placebo. Discontinuation rate owing to adverse effects were higher in the atypical group than the placebo group.[80]

Recently, a double-blind placebo-controlled study of aripiprazole also found efficacy in depressed adults who did not have adequate response to 8 weeks of SSRI treatment.[81] No controlled trials are available in pediatric depression. A chart review of 10 cases demonstrated efficacy and limited side effects (sedation and an average of about 5 pounds weight gain) of adding quetiapine to treat depressed adolescents who failed at least one 8-week adequate trial of an SSRI.[82]

OTHER AUGMENTING STRATEGIES

Other strategies have included addition of buspirone and psychostimulants. It is important to recognize that these are strategies to improve symptoms of depression, not specifically to treat comorbid anxiety or ADHD. No data are available on these combinations.

ADJUNCTIVE AGENTS

The distinction between augmenting response (i.e., some synergy of medications to provide a more complete response) and adjunctive treatments is important, although at times the distinction is not always clearly evident. Adjunctive agents would generally target specific symptoms (e.g., sleep, agitation), with the expectation that once the depression is improved, the additional treatment would no longer be needed and would be discontinued. Alternatively, augmenting agents resulting in remission would generally be continued as long as the primary treatment was needed. That is, what gets you well is what keeps you well. An example would be the use of atypical antipsychotics. If an atypical was used after partial response to a SSRI to augment the treatment, it would be continued as long as the SSRI was used. If, however, an atypical was initiated (along with treatment for depression) because of agitation, when the depression and agitation improved, consideration would be made to discontinue the atypical with the assumption that the agitation was a symptom or result of the depressive episode.

Insomnia is a frequent symptom of depression, and use of adjunctive hypnotics is common in adults. A study by Fava and colleagues[83] in 2006 noted that subjects treated with an SSRI and a hypnotic showed more improvement than SSRI and placebo on symptoms of depression after excluding the sleep item. Sleep difficulties are also among the most common residual symptom in adolescents who respond to treatment.[84] However, there is minimal to no efficacy or safety data on the use of hypnotics in children and adolescents, and there are concerns, particularly in children, that paradoxical effects may occur. Therefore, there are currently no clear recommendations about the use of hypnotics in this age group. The most commonly prescribed sleeping aids in the pediatric age group appear to be over-the-counter medications.[85] Clearly, more research is needed.

ALTERNATIVE TREATMENTS

Pediatric patients use alternative or complementary medicine frequently. A recent Canadian study found that 50% of children in general pediatric clinics use some form of alternative treatment.[86] The evidence of efficacy, however, is scarce. St. John's wort, omega-3 fatty acid, and S-adenosyl methionine are among the most studied herbal/natural remedies for adult depression. These treatments are discussed in Chapter 12.

CONTINUATION AND MAINTENANCE TREATMENT

Based on adult research, most guidelines and algorithms recommend continued treatment with the successful antidepressant for 6 to 9 months following response.[6–8] One small pilot study of children and adolescents with depression also demonstrated that continued treatment with fluoxetine prevented relapse and delayed time to relapse.[87] Emslie and colleagues[88] have recently completed the first large continuation trial in pediatric depression. Of 102 participants randomized to fluoxetine (n = 50) or placebo (n = 52) following response to 12 weeks of open treatment with fluoxetine, 42.0% (n = 21) relapsed on fluoxetine compared to 69.2% (n = 36) on placebo (p = 0.005). Time to relapse was significantly shorter in the placebo-treated group, further demonstrating the need for continued treatment for 6 to 9 months following initial treatment response. To date, maintenance studies have not yet been reported in pediatric depression, although guidelines recommend maintenance treatment (1 to 2 years) for youth with risk factors for recurrence (e.g., multiple episodes, chronic depression, etc.).

DISCONTINUATION

After a successful continuation or maintenance treatment, antidepressants can typically be discontinued. Usually, it is prudent to taper antidepressant medications slowly to avoid untoward effects, particularly when using medications with short half-lives. For example, TCAs can produce cholinergic rebound if stopped too quickly. Rapid cessation of venlafaxine, fluvoxamine, sertraline, citalopram, escitalopram, and paroxetine can all cause a discontinuation or withdrawal syndrome. This may consist of flulike symptoms, dizziness, anxiety, mood lability, agitation, lethargy, paraesthesia, nausea, vivid dreams, insomnia, abdominal pain, and fatigue. These symptoms are often misinterpreted as an exacerbation of depression.

Discontinuation symptoms can occur within 1 to 2 days of stopping medication or up to 1 to 2 weeks later. This condition is usually self-limited and resolves in 3 to 4 weeks. In some cases, particularly with MAOIs, it can become more serious. Fluoxetine can generally be discontinued rapidly because it has a long half-life and is thought to "auto-taper." A randomized clinical trial in adults comparing fluoxetine discontinuation to interruption of sertraline or paroxetine therapy indicated that abrupt withdrawal of paroxetine and, to a lesser extent, sertraline was more likely to provoke unpleasant symptoms than fluoxetine discontinuation.[89] If withdrawal symptoms occur, the antidepressant can be reintroduced and tapered more gradually. There are no definitive studies regarding children and adolescents. In general, TCA dosages can be decreased by 25 mg every 3 to 4 days. Clinicians can taper SSRIs and MAOIs over 2 to 3 weeks in most cases.[90] Patients and families should be educated about the possibility of discontinuation symptoms prior to tapering antidepressants. Because depression is often a lifelong illness, further education should focus on recognizing symptoms of recurrence and when to seek future treatment.

CONCLUSIONS

It is frequently difficult to move beyond the controversies and natural reluctance to prescribe antidepressants to children and adolescents. Yet, used rationally and systematically, medication management is an essential component of treatment for moderate to severe depression in this age group.

Rational and systematic medication management is based on accurate diagnosis, development of a therapeutic alliance, and concomitant management of stressors associated with depression and sequelae of the illness. If antidepressants are used, then choice of treatment is rational (i.e., one step at a time) and uses evidence-based treatments. Measurement of illness severity and side effect burden throughout treatment is essential.

RESOURCES FOR PRACTITIONERS

References 8, 10, 12, 52, 67, and 89.

American Academy of Child and Adolescent Psychiatry. Practice Parameter for the Assessment and Treatment of Children and Adolescents with Depressive Disorders. Reference 6 and http://www.aacap.org/galleries/PracticeParameters/InPress_2007_DepressiveDisorders.pdf

Texas Children's Medication Algorithm Project: http://www.dshs.state.tx.us/mhprograms/mddpage.shtm

SAMHSA's National Mental Health Information Center (NMHIC). Child, Adolescent & Family: http://mentalhealth.samhsa.gov/cmhs/ChildrensCampaign/default.asp

RESOURCES FOR PATIENTS AND FAMILIES

A parent medication guide endorsed by many medical societies and associations can be found at http://www.parentsmedguide.org/parentsmedguide.pdf

Antidepressants for children: Explore the pros and cons at http://www.mayoclinic.com/health/antidepressants/MH00059

National Institute of Mental Health (NIMH): Antidepressant Medications for Children and Adolescents: Information for Parent and Caregivers. http://www.nimh.nih.gov/health/topics/child-and-adolescent-mental-health/antidepressant-medications-for-children-and-adolescents-information-for-parents-and-caregivers.shtml

REFERENCES

1. Bloch RG, Doonief AS, Buchberg AS, et al. The clinical effect of isoniazid and iproniazid in the treatment of pulmonary tuberculosis. *Ann Intern Med.* 1954;40:881–900.
2. Kuhn R. The treatment of depressive states with G 22355 (imipramine hydrochloride). *Am J Psychiatry.* 1958;115:459–464.
3. Weinberg WA, Rutman J, Sullivan L, et al. Depression in children referred to an educational diagnostic center: diagnosis and treatment. Preliminary report. *J Pediatr.* 1973;83:1065–1072.
4. Emslie GJ, Rush AJ, Weinberg WA, et al. Double-blind placebo controlled study of fluoxetine in depressed children and adolescents. *Arch Gen Psychiatry.* 1997;54:1031–1037.
5. FDA. *FDA Modernization Act of 1997.* Available at: http://www.fda.gov/cber/genadmin/fdamod97.pdf
6. American Academy of Child and Adolescent Psychiatry. Practice parameter for the assessment and treatment of children and adolescents with depressive disorders. *J Am Acad Child Adolesc Psychiatry.* 2007;46: 1503–1526.
7. Cheung AH, Zuckerbrot RA, Jensen PS, et al. Guidelines for adolescent depression in primary care (GLAD-PC): Part II. Treatment and ongoing management. *Pediatrics.* 2007;120:e1313–1326.
8. Hughes CW, Emslie GJ, Crismon ML, et al. Texas Children's Medication Algorithm Project: update from Texas Consensus Conference Panel on Medication Treatment of Childhood Major Depressive Disorder. *J Am Acad Child Adolesc Psychiatry.* 2007;46:667–686.
9. European Medicines Agency. April 2005. European Medicines Agency Press Release, European Medicines Agency finalizes review of antidepressants in children and adolescents. Available at: www.emea.eu.int/pdfs/human/press/pr/12891805en.pdf
10. National Institute for Health and Clinical Excellence (NICE). Depression in children and young people: identification and management in primary, community and secondary care. September 2005. Available at: http://www.nice.org.uk/guidance/index.jsp?action=byID&o=10970
11. Hammad TA, Laughren T, Racoosin J. Suicidality in pediatric patients treated with antidepressant drugs. *Arch Gen Psychiatry.* 2006;63:332–339.
12. Bridge JA, Iyengar S, Salary CB, et al. Clinical response and risk for reported suicidal ideation and suicide attempts in pediatric antidepressant treatment: a meta-analysis of randomized controlled trials. *JAMA.* 2007;297:1683–1696.
13. Depression Guideline Panel. *Depression in Primary Care: Vol. 1. Detection and Diagnosis.* Clinical Practice Guideline, No. 5. Rockville, Md: U.S. Department of Health and Human Services, Public Health Service, Agency for Health Care Policy and Research. AHCPR Publication No. 93-0550, 1993.

14. Frank E, Prien RF, Jarrett RB, et al. Conceptualization and rationale for consensus definitions of terms in major depressive disorder. Remission, recovery, relapse, and recurrence. *Arch Gen Psychiatry.* 1991;48:851–855.

15. Rush AJ, Kraemer HC, Sackeim HS, et al. Report by the ACNP Task Force on response and remission in major depressive disorder. *Neuropsychopharmacology.* 2006;31:1841–1853.

16. Sackeim HA. The definition and meaning of treatment-resistant depression. *J Clin Psychiatry.* 2001;62 (suppl 16):10–17.

17. Bockting C, Schene A, Spinhoven P, et al. Preventing relapse/recurrence in recurrent depression with cognitive therapy: a randomized controlled trial. *J Consult Clin Psychol.* 2005;73:647–657.

18. Fava GA, Grandi S, Zielezny M, et al. Cognitive behavioral treatment of residual symptoms in primary major depressive disorder. *Am J Psychiatry.* 1994;151:1295–1299.

19. Fava G, Fabbri S, Sonino N. Residual symptoms in depression: an emerging therapeutic target. *Prog Neuropsychopharmacol Biol Psychiatry.* 2002;26:1019–1027.

20. Paykel ES, Scott J, Teasdale JD, et al. Prevention of relapse in residual depression by cognitive therapy: a controlled trial. *Arch Gen Psychiatry.* 1999;56:829–835.

21. Perlis R, Nierenberg A, Alpert J, et al. The effects of adding cognitive therapy to fluoxetine dose increase on risk of relapse and residual depressive symptoms in continuation treatment of major depressive disorder. *J Clin Psychopharmacol.* 2002;22:474–480.

22. Teasdale JD, Segal ZV, Williams JM, et al. Prevention of relapse/recurrence in major depression by mindfulness-based cognitive therapy. *J Consult Clin Psychol.* 2000;68:615–623.

23. Treatment for Adolescents with Depression Study (TADS) team. Fluoxetine, cognitive-behavioral therapy, and their combination for adolescents with depression. *JAMA.* 2004;292:807–820.

24. Goodyer I, Dubicka B, Wilkinson P, et al. Selective serotonin reuptake inhibitors (SSRIs) and routine specialist care with and without cognitive behaviour therapy in adolescents with major depression: randomised controlled trial. *BMJ.* 2007;335:142.

25. Clarke G, Debar L, Lynch F, et al. A randomized effectiveness trial of brief cognitive-behavioral therapy for depressed adolescents receiving antidepressant medication. *J Am Acad Child Adolesc Psychiatry.* 2005;44: 888–898.

26. Melvin GA, Tonge BJ, King NJ, et al. A comparison of cognitive-behavioral therapy, sertraline, and their combination for adolescent depression. *J Am Acad Child Adolesc Psychiatry.* 2006;45:1151–1161.

27. King RA, Schwab-Stone M, Flisher AJ, et al. Psychosocial and risk behavior correlates of youth suicide attempts and suicidal ideation. *J Am Acad Child Adolesc Psychiatry.* 2001;40:837–846.

28. Grunbaum JA, Kann L, Kinchen SA, et al. Youth risk behavior surveillance—United States, 2001. *J Sch Health.* 2002;72:313–328.

29. Fombonne E, Wostear G, Cooper V, et al. The Maudsley long-term follow-up of child and adolescent depression. 2. Suicidality, criminality and social dysfunction in adulthood. *Br J Psychiatry.* 2001;179:218–223.

30. Kovacs M, Goldston D, Gatsonis C. Suicidal behaviors and childhood-onset depressive disorders: a longitudinal investigation. *J Am Acad Child Adolesc Psychiatry.* 1993;32:8–20.

31. Posner K, Oquendo MA, Gould M, et al. Columbia Classification Algorithm of Suicide Assessment (C-CASA): classification of suicidal events in the FDA's pediatric suicidal risk analysis of antidepressants. *Am J Psychiatry.* 2007;164:1035–1043.

32. Dennehy EB, Suppes T, Rush AJ, et al. Does provider adherence to a treatment guideline change clinical outcomes for patients with bipolar disorder? Results from the Texas Medication Algorithm Project. *Psychol Med.* 2005;35:1695–1706.

33. Emslie GJ, Hughes CW, Crismon ML, et al. A feasibility study of the childhood depression medication algorithm: the Texas Children's Medication Algorithm Project (CMAP). *J Am Acad Child Adolesc Psychiatry.* 2004;43:519–527.

34. Trivedi MH, Rush AJ, Gaynes BN, et al. Maximizing the adequacy of medication treatment in controlled trials and clinical practice: STAR*D measurement-based care. *Neuropsychopharmacology.* 2007;32:2479–2489.

35. Biggs MM, Shores-Wilson K, Rush AJ, et al. A comparison of alternative assessments of depressive symptom severity: a pilot study. *Psychiat Res.* 2000;96:269–279.

36. Trivedi MH, Fava M, Wisniewski SR, et al. Medication augmentation after the failure of SSRIs for depression. *N Engl J Med.* 2006;354:1243–1252.

37. Rush AJ, Trivedi MH, Ibrahim HM, et al. The 16-item Quick Inventory of Depressive Symptomatology (QIDS) Clinician Rating (QIDS-C) and Self-Report (QIDS-SR): a psychometric evaluation in patients with chronic major depression. *Biol Psychiatry.* 2003;54:573–583.

38. Moore HK, Hughes CW, Mundt JC, et al. A pilot study of an electronic, adolescent version of the quick inventory of depressive symptomatology. *J Clin Psychiatry.* 2007;68:1436–1440.

39. Myers K, Winters NC. Ten-year review of rating scales. II: Scales for internalizing disorders. *J Am Acad Child Adolesc Psychiatry.* 2002;41:634–659.

40. Mayes TL, Tao R, Rintelmann JW, et al. Do children and adolescents have differential response rates in placebo-controlled trials of fluoxetine? *CNS Spectrum.* 2007;12:147–154.

41. Emslie GJ, Heiligenstein JH, Wagner KD, et al. Fluoxetine for acute treatment of depression in children and adolescents: a placebo-controlled, randomized clinical trial. *J Am Acad Child Adolesc Psychiatry*. 2002;41: 1205–1215.

42. Emslie GJ, Ryan ND, Wagner KD. Major depressive disorder in children and adolescents: clinical trial design and antidepressant efficacy. *J Clin Psychiatry*. 2005;66(suppl 7):14–20.

43. Heiligenstein JH, Hoog SL, Wagner KD, et al. Fluoxetine 40–60 mg versus fluoxetine 20 mg in the treatment of children and adolescents with a less-than-complete response to nine-week treatment with fluoxetine 10–20 mg: a pilot study. *J Child Adolesc Psychopharmacol*. 2006;16:207–217.

44. Wagner KD, Robb AS, Findling RL, et al. A randomized, placebo-controlled trial of citalopram for the treatment of major depression in children and adolescents. *Am J Psychiatry*. 2004;161:1079–1083.

45. von Knorring AL, Olsson GI, Thomsen PH, et al. A randomized, double-blind, placebo-controlled study of citalopram in adolescents with major depressive disorder. *J Clin Psychopharmacol*. 2006;26:311–315.

46. Wagner KD, Ambrosini P, Rynn M, et al. Efficacy of sertraline in the treatment of children and adolescents with major depressive disorder: two randomized controlled trials. *JAMA*. 2003;290:1033–1041.

47. Morrato EH, Libby AM, Orton HD, et al. Frequency of provider contact after FDA advisory on risk of pediatric suicidality with SSRIs. *Am J Psychiatry*. 2008;165:42–50.

48. Emslie GJ. Improving outcome in pediatric depression. *Am J Psychiatry*. 2008;165:1–3.

49. Wagner KD, Jonas J, Findling RL, et al. A double-blind, randomized, placebo-controlled trial of escitalopram in the treatment of pediatric depression. *J Am Acad Child Adolesc Psychiatry*. 2006;45:280–288.

50. Rao N. The clinical pharmacokinetics of escitalopram. *Clin Pharmacokinet*. 2007;46:281–290.

51. Keller MB, Ryan ND, Strober M, et al. Efficacy of paroxetine in the treatment of adolescent major depression: a randomized, controlled trial. *J Am Acad Child Adolesc Psychiatry*. 2001;40:762–772.

52. Berard R, Fong R, Carpenter DJ, et al. An international, multicenter, placebo-controlled trial of paroxetine in adolescents with major depressive disorder. *J Child Adolesc Psychopharmacol*. 2006;16:59–75.

53. Emslie GJ, Wagner KD, Kutcher S, et al. Paroxetine treatment in children and adolescents with major depressive disorder: a randomized, multicenter, double-blind, placebo-controlled trial. *J Am Acad Child Adolesc Psychiatry*. 2006;45:709–719.

54. Findling RL, Nucci G, Piergies AA, et al. Multiple dose pharmacokinetics of paroxetine in children and adolescents with major depressive disorder or obsessive-compulsive disorder. *Neuropsychopharmacology*. 2006; 31:1274–1285.

55. Cheung AH, Emslie GJ, Mayes TL. Review of the efficacy and safety of antidepressants in youth. *J Child Psychol Psychiatry*. 2005;46:735–754.

56. Emslie GJ, Findling RL, Yeung PP, et al. Efficacy and safety of venlafaxine ER in the treatment of pediatric major depressive disorder. *J Am Acad Child Adolesc Psychiatry*. 2007;46:479–488.

57. Mandoki MW, Tapia MR, Tapia MA, et al. Venlafaxine in the treatment of children and adolescents with major depression. *Psychopharmacol Bull*. 1997;33:149–154.

58. Daviss WB, Bentivoglio P, Racusin R, et al. Bupropion sustained release in adolescents with comorbid attention-deficit/hyperactivity disorder and depression. *J Am Acad Child Adolesc Psychiatry*. 2001;40:307–314.

59. Nemeroff CB, Kalali A, Keller MB. Impact of publicity concerning pediatric suicidality data on physician practice patterns in the United States. *Arch Gen Psychiatry*. 2007;64:466–472.

60. Desarkar P, Das A, Sinha VK. Duloxetine for childhood depression with pain and dissociative symptoms. *Eur Child Adolesc Psychiatry*. 2006;15:496–499.

61. Meighen KG. Duloxetine treatment of pediatric chronic pain and co-morbid major depressive disorder. *J Child Adolesc Psychopharmacology*. 2007;17:121–127.

62. Rush AJ, Trivedi MH, Wisniewski SR, et al. Bupropion-SR, sertraline, or venlafaxine-XR after failure of SSRIs for depression. *N Engl J Med*. 2006;354:1231–1242.

63. Emslie GJ, Findling RL, Rynn MA, et al. Efficacy and safety of nefazodone in the treatment of adolescents with major depressive disorder. *J Child Adolesc Psychopharmacol*. 2002;12:299.

64. Hazell P, O'Connell D, Heathcote D, et al. Tricyclic drugs for depression in children and adolescents. *Cochrane Database Syst Rev*. 2002;(2):CD002317.

65. Turner MS, May DB, Arthur RR, et al. Clinical impact of selective serotonin reuptake inhibitors therapy with bleeding risks. *J Intern Med*. 2007;261:205–213.

66. Oström M, Eriksson A, Thorson J, et al. Fatal overdose with citalopram. *Lancet*. 1996;348:339–340.

67. Nelson JC. Tricyclic and tetracyclic drugs. In: Schatzberg AF, Nemeroff CB, eds. *The American Psychiatric Publishing Textbook of Psychopharmacology*. Washington, DC: American Psychiatric Publishing; 2004.

68. Wilens TE, Biederman J, Baldessarini RJ, et al. Cardiovascular effects of therapeutic doses of tricyclic antidepressants in children and adolescents. *J Am Acad Child Adolesc Psychiatry*. 1996;35:1491–1501.

69. Yamada M, Yasuhara H. Clinical pharmacology of MAO inhibitors: safety and future. *Neuro Toxicology*. 2004;25:215–221.

70. Emslie GJ, Kratochvil CJ, Vitiello B, et al. Treatment for adolescents with depression study (TADS): safety results. *J Am Acad Child Adolesc Psychiatry*. 2006;45:1440–1455.

71. Goodman WK, Murphy TK, Storch EA. Risk of adverse behavioral effects with pediatric use of antidepressants. *Psychopharmacology.* 2007;191:87–96.

72. Craney JL, Geller B. A prepubertal and early adolescent bipolar disorder-I phenotype: review of phenomenology and longitudinal course. *Bipolar Dis.* 2003;5:243–256.

73. Bschor T, Bauer M. Efficacy and mechanisms of action of lithium augmentation in refractory major depression. *Curr Pharm Des.* 2006;12:2985–2992.

74. Carvalho AF, Cavalcante JL, Castelo MS, et al. Augmentation strategies for treatment-resistant depression: a literature review. *J Clin Pharmacol Ther.* 2007;32:415–428.

75. Ryan ND, Meyer V, Dachille S, et al. Lithium antidepressant augmentation in TCA-refractory depression in adolescents. *J Am Acad Child Adolesc Psychiatry.*1988;27:371–376.

76. Strober M, Freeman R, Rigali J, et al. The pharmacotherapy of depressive illness in adolescence: II. Effects of lithium augmentation in nonresponders to imipramine. *J Am Acad Child Adolesc Psychiatry.* 1992; 31:16–20.

77. Aronson R, Offman H, Joffe R, et al. Triiodothyronine augmentation in treatment of refractory depression. *Arch Gen Psychiatry.* 1996;53:842–848.

78. Abraham G, Milev R, Stuart Lawson J. T3 augmentation of SSRI resistant depression. *J Affect Dis.* 2006;91: 211–215.

79. Fava M, Rush AJ, Thase ME, et al. 15 years of clinical experience with bupropion HCl: from bupropion to bupropion SR to bupropion XL. *Prim Care Companion J Clin Psychiatry.* 2005;7:106–113.

80. Papakostas GI, Shelton RC, Smith J, et al. Augmentation of antidepressants with atypical antipsychotic medications for treatment-resistant major depressive disorder: a meta-analysis. *J Clin Psychiatry.* 2007;68: 826–831.

81. Berman RM, Marcus RN, Swanink R, et al. The efficacy and safety of aripiprazole as adjunctive therapy in major depressive disorder: a multicenter, randomized, double-blind, placebo-controlled study. *J Clin Psychiatry.* 2007;68:843–853.

82. Pathak S, Johns ES, Kowatch RA. Adjunctive quetiapine for treatment-resistant adolescent major depressive disorder: a case series. *J Child Adolesc Psychopharmacol.* 2005;15:696–702.

83. Fava M, McCall WV, Krystal A, et al. Eszopiclone co-administered with fluoxetine in patients with insomnia coexisting with major depressive disorder. *Biol Psychiatry.* 2006;59:1052–1060.

84. Kennard B, Silva S, Vitiello B, et al. Remission and residual symptoms after acute treatment of adolescents with major depressive disorder. *J Am Acad Child Adolesc Psychiatry.* 2006;45:1404–1411.

85. Owens JA, Babcock D, Blumer J, et al. The use of pharmacotherapy in the treatment of pediatric insomnia in primary care: rational approaches. A consensus meeting summary. *J Clin Sleep Med.* 2005;1:49–59.

86. Jean D, Cyr C. Use of complementary and alternative medicine in a general pediatric clinic. *Pediatrics.* 2007;120:e138–141.

87. Emslie GJ, Heiligenstein JH, Hoog SL, et al. Fluoxetine treatment for prevention of relapse of depression in children and adolescents: a double-blind, placebo-controlled study. *J Am Acad Child Adolesc Psychiatry.* 2004;43:1397–1405.

88. Emslie GJ, Kennard BD, Mayes TL, et al. Fluoxetine vs. placebo to prevent relapse of MDD in children and adolescents. *Am J Psychiatry.* 2008;165:459–467.

89. Rosenbaum JF, Fava M, Hoog SL, et al. Selective serotonin reuptake inhibitor discontinuation syndrome: a randomized clinical trial. *Biol Psychiatry.* 1998;44:77–87.

90. Lader M. Pharmacotherapy of mood disorders and treatment discontinuation. *Drugs.* 2007;67:1657–1663.

DISCLOSURES

Graham Emslie receives research support from the National Institute of Mental Health, Eli Lilly, Organon, Shire, Somerset, Forest Laboratories, and Biobehavioral Diagnostics Inc. He is a consultant for Forest Laboratories, Inc., Eli Lilly, GlaxoSmithKline, Wyeth-Ayerst, Shire, and Biobehavioral Diagnostics Inc. and is on the Speaker's Bureau for McNeil. Paul Croarkin, Rongrong Tao, and Taryn Mayes report no competing interests.

Using Other Biologic Treatments: Electroconvulsive Therapy, Transcranial Magnetic Stimulation, Vagus Nerve Stimulation, and Light Therapy

GARRY WALTER AND NEERA GHAZIUDDIN

KEY POINTS

- Electroconvulsive therapy (ECT), transcranial magnetic stimulation (TMS), vagus nerve stimulation (VNS), and light therapy are treatments quite different from each other in nature and scope.
- The use of VNS and TMS in young persons should at this point be deemed experimental and for cases that are severe and have not responded to any other type of treatment.
- Light therapy is considered one of the first-line treatments for patients with seasonal affective disorder (SAD).
- Although these treatments may prove beneficial for young people with depression, many patients and families are apprehensive about their use (with the possible exception of light therapy). These are some of the key questions for clinicians to consider:
  ○ Is the diagnosis for which the treatment is to be given accurate, thus justifying use of the treatment?
  ○ Have adequate trials of pharmacotherapy and psychotherapy been undertaken? (This question is less relevant for SAD and light therapy.)
  ○ Have the potential benefits and risks of treatment been clearly conveyed to young patients and parents prior to commencement? (This is particularly important, because the evidence base for these treatments is often not strong.)
  ○ How should these treatments be integrated with other treatments (e.g., medication, psychotherapy) while being used and after cessation?
- Clinicians need to be familiar with the local legal requirements for the administration of ECT, which vary widely between jurisdictions. For example, after a parent or a guardian has consented, some U.S. states require that several child and adolescent psychiatrists concur about the need for ECT before it is administered.
- Because of the strong, often extreme, emotions this treatment can generate, the decision about the need for ECT should not be made lightly and informed consent processes must be carefully followed.
- Neuropsychological assessment should be completed prior to ECT (unless the patient is too ill or disorganized), on completion of the course, and 3 to 6 months later to evaluate potential cognitive deficits.
- Side effects of ECT are typically mild and transient. These may include short-term memory disturbance, headache, muscle and joint pain, drowsiness, post-ECT confusion, nausea, and disinhibition.

Introduction

Although pharmacotherapy (Chapter 6) is the most commonly employed biologic treatment for depression in young people, a range of other biologic therapies have been used or show potential. This chapter focuses on electroconvulsive therapy (ECT)—because of the much larger number of studies and longer history of use when compared with the other treatments described—but we also briefly consider transcranial magnetic stimulation (TMS), vagus nerve stimulation (VNS), and light therapy. This chapter should also be read in conjunction with Chapter 16 on treatment-resistant depression. Table 7.1 summarizes the evidence for effectiveness, taking into account not only the scarce data from treatment studies in adolescents but also by extrapolating information from adult studies.

TABLE 7.1 SUMMARY OF NONPHARMACOLOGIC BIOLOGIC TREATMENTS FOR DEPRESSION IN ADOLESCENTS

Treatment	Earliest Published Report as Psychiatric Treatment in Young Persons	Controlled Study(ies)	Quality of Overall Evidence	Strength of Recommendation	Comments
ECT	1942[1]	No	**	✓✓	Relatively large number of published reports; limited data in preadolescents; controlled trials unlikely to be conducted.
TMS	2001[2]	No[a]	*	✓	Few studies, but early results promising.
VNS	No studies	No	No studies	✓	Experimental treatment. No studies in young people with psychiatric illness.
Light therapy	1986[3]	Yes	*	✓✓	Data limited, but includes controlled trial reporting positive results.

ECT, electroconvulsive therapy; TMS, transcranial magnetic stimulation; VNS, vagus nerve stimulation.
***Multiple high-quality scientific studies with homogeneous results; **At least one relevant high-quality study or multiple adequate studies; *Expert opinion, case studies, or standard of care.
✓✓Useful and effective; ✓✓Weight of evidence/opinion is in favor; ✓Usefulness not established.
[a]The reports by Walter et al.[2] and Loo et al.[4] include data extracted from controlled studies and data from the first two subjects in a controlled trial, respectively.

ELECTROCONVULSIVE THERAPY

ECT, one of the oldest treatments in psychiatry, entails the production of a brief passage of current through the brain via electrodes placed on the scalp, resulting in a generalized seizure. Its use in young people was first described in the early 1940s by Heuyer and colleagues,[1,5] who concluded that ECT is a safe procedure and often effective in children and adolescents with melancholia. Soon after, however, the use of ECT in the young appeared to decline, probably owing to apprehension about potential (but unproved) harmful effects and the advent of psychotropic drugs.[6] Negative perceptions have contributed to ECT being outlawed for children and adolescents in several U.S. states. Adolescents today constitute about 1% of all patients treated with ECT.

EFFECTIVENESS AND INDICATIONS

Several reports over the past 20 years[6–10] have suggested that ECT is effective for the treatment of unipolar and bipolar disorders in adolescents. However, it is noteworthy that, to date, there has not been a single randomized controlled trial (RCT) in this age group. A comprehensive review of ECT in children and adolescents, published in 1997,[6] examined 60 reports and emphasized that the overall quality of studies was poor. It warrants digressing to note that ECT may also be effective in the treatment of adolescents with schizoaffective disorder, schizophrenia, other psychotic disorders, catatonia, and neuroleptic malignant syndrome.

The response rate to ECT among adolescents is 60% to 80% for mood disorders (and somewhat lower for psychoses),[6] based on case series. Given this situation, it is necessary to extrapolate data from adult research, which has produced similar results, although adolescents may not necessarily respond in the same way as adults. ECT is the most effective treatment available for adult patients with severe depression, producing significant or complete symptom remission in >70%. Data from 90 RCTs[11] in adults with depressive illness of varying severity suggest the following:

- Real ECT (that is, where an electric current is applied) is more effective in the short term than sham ECT (when no electric current is applied).
- Stimulus parameters have an influence on efficacy.
- Bilateral ECT is more effective than unilateral ECT.
- Raising the electrical stimulus above the individual's seizure threshold increases the efficacy of unilateral ECT at the expense of increased cognitive impairment.
- In trials comparing ECT with pharmacotherapy, ECT produced greater benefit than the use of certain antidepressants (although the trials were of variable quality).
- The combination of ECT with pharmacotherapy was not superior to ECT alone.

Comorbid psychiatric disorders, including personality disorder, are not a reason to deny ECT, although response may be less consistent in such patients. For example, in one study,[12] there was a 27% response rate in adolescents with both major depression and personality disorder, compared with a 71% response rate in adolescents with major depression alone. Response rates and indications for ECT are similar in adolescents and adults.[13,14]

In general, after successful ECT, individuals must continue pharmacologic or another sort of treatment to maintain the improvement. Although ECT is often highly effective for the treatment of an index episode of depression, the long-term outcome is variable. For instance, following ECT treatment, patients may remain symptom free for an extended period of time but may experience recurrence and, in the longer term, they may not differ significantly from psychiatric controls in areas of social or school functioning. Taieb et al.[15] examined a small group of adolescents with psychotic depression or bipolar disorder over 5 years and found that school functioning was more likely to be associated with illness severity than type of treatment received.

The American Academy of Child and Adolescent Psychiatry[16] suggests that ECT may be considered for a child or adolescent who suffers from a severe psychiatric disorder (unipolar or bipolar mood disorder, or other condition), who may be resistant to or unable to tolerate conventional treatment and/or whose safety is compromised when waiting for response from such treatment (e.g., the patient is not eating or drinking or is acutely suicidal). The United Kingdom's National Institute of Clinical Excellence (NICE) recommends that ECT should only be considered for adolescents with very severe depression and either life-threatening symptoms (such as suicidal behavior) or intractable and severe symptoms that have not responded to other treatments.[17]

ECT is rarely used in prepubertal children, as noted earlier, and NICE does not recommend using ECT for children <12 years. However, encouraging results have been observed in this age group when ECT has been used for serious and/or refractory disorders. For instance, Russell et al.[18] described a prepubertal child who was successfully treated with ECT for severe depression and catatonic features. Esmaili and Malek[19] described a 6-year-old girl with similar clinical features and outcome.

SIDE EFFECTS

Side effects of ECT are typically mild and transient and not dissimilar to those reported for adult patients. These may include headache, muscle and joint pain, drowsiness, post-ECT confusion, nausea, memory complaints, and disinhibition.[6,12] Disturbance of short-term memory is a well-known side effect of ECT, with greater disturbance of impersonal than autobiographical memories.[20] Advances in treatment technique over the past decade have enabled a reduction of adverse cognitive effects of ECT. Nearly all ECT devices currently used deliver a lower current, brief-pulse electrical stimulation, compared with the earlier machines that had sine wave output. With a brief-pulse electrical wave, a therapeutic seizure may be induced with as little as a third the electrical power of the older method, thereby reducing the potential for confusion and memory disturbance.

Cognitive Effects

To date, only two studies have focused on the cognitive effects of ECT in adolescents. The first, by Cohen et al.,[21] compared 10 adolescents with severe mood disorders treated, on average, 3.5 years earlier, with controls. All patients, except one who was mildly hypomanic, were in remission at the time of follow-up assessment. Objective tests did not reveal significant group differences for short-term memory, attention, new learning, and objective memory scores. It was also found that poorer cognitive performance was significantly associated with greater psychopathology. The second study, of 16 adolescents treated with ECT, was by Ghaziuddin et al.[22] Complete recovery of cognitive functions with return to pre-ECT functioning was noted at the second post-ECT testing (8.5 ± 4.9 months after the last treatment). A large body of evidence in adult patients shows that memory loss, anterograde, and, more commonly, retrograde, can occur.[20] Usually these improve after a few weeks and months, but some amnesia can persist for longer.

Prolonged Seizures

Prolonged seizures (>180 seconds) during treatment and, rarely, spontaneous seizures after full recovery from anesthesia have been reported. Guttmacher and Cretella[23] described prolonged seizures in two of their four patients, and Moise and Petrides[8] in 3 of 13 patients. The exact cause of these seizures or their clinical relevance is not fully understood at this time. However, lower-seizure threshold among adolescent patients is a likely contributing factor.

Structural Abnormalities

Fears that ECT may cause gross structural brain pathology have not been supported by decades of methodologically sound research in both humans and animals.[24] Nevertheless, at present there are no data specific for children or adolescents regarding the effect of ECT on brain structure.

Death

The literature on ECT use in young people has reported only one fatality, a 16-year-old girl with neuroleptic malignant syndrome (NMS) who died 10 days after her last ECT.[25] However, this outcome was possibly related to continued administration of a neuroleptic medication, despite her NMS, rather than ECT per se. Adult data show death rates of about 1 per 25,000 treatments, which is similar to the death rate of general anesthesia.

LEGISLATION

The use of ECT has been legislated in many jurisdictions, particularly when administered involuntarily to patients unable to give informed consent and to juveniles, but legislation varies considerably. For example, California prohibits the use of ECT for children <12 years. Minors between 12 and 15 years of age may only receive ECT if, in addition to the other provisions authorizing ECT, the circumstances are life threatening and the unanimous opinion of three child psychiatrists appointed by the mental health commissioner is in favor of ECT. In Texas, amendments to the legislation in 1993 resulted in the prohibition of ECT in patients <16 years. In France, Iceland, Latvia, the Netherlands, Norway, Portugal, Romania, Spain, and Turkey, only the written consent of the nearest relative or the legally appointed guardian is required. ECT is prohibited in some cantons in Switzerland, but patients can travel to different cantons to receive treatment.

ATTITUDES TOWARD ELECTROCONVULSIVE THERAPY

Studies of persons who received ECT as adolescents and their parents[26–28] suggest that the majority had very positive views about the treatment. For example, young patients would have it again if required, they would recommend it to others, and they rate the underlying illness, for which ECT was given, worse than the treatment. Such positive attitudes are reassuring for would-be recipients of the treatment, and they help offset negative views about the treatment in the wider community.

PRACTICAL ASPECTS OF TREATMENT WITH ELECTROCONVULSIVE THERAPY

Assessment

The following requirements[16,29] are suggested for all young people in whom ECT is considered:

1. A comprehensive psychiatric history and psychiatric diagnosis
2. Decisions about the adequacy of previous treatments and "treatment resistance" (see Chapter 16)
3. Complete medical history and physical examination (further investigations, such as blood tests, EEG, brain computed tomography, and magnetic resonance imaging, are dictated by the clinical assessment)
4. Review of concurrent drug use
5. If possible, baseline neuropsychological assessment (the minimum standard recommended by the American Academy of Child and Adolescent Psychiatry[16] is a memory assessment, but a more comprehensive battery may be considered.[29])

There are no absolute medical contraindications to ECT. For example, Ghaziuddin et al.[30] described a successful outcome in an adolescent girl who had a complicated neurologic history. The patient had undergone craniotomy for a brainstem astrocytoma and suffered extensive postsurgical neurologic deficits (third and seventh nerve damage, hemiparesis, and a ventricular-peritoneal shunt for hydrocephalous). Despite her complicated neurologic presentation, she achieved remission with eight treatments. Additionally, patients with comorbid medical conditions who were successfully treated with ECT have been reported.

Informed Consent and Consultation

Because of the strong, often extreme, emotions that ECT can generate, the decision about the need or advisability for the treatment should not be made lightly and informed consent processes should be followed carefully in all age groups, but particularly in minors. In many jurisdictions, parents or legal guardians have the authority to consent to ECT on behalf of their children. At the same time, however, most clinicians recognize the importance of adolescents' assent. Further, both consent and assent should be regarded as a process and not as an event at a single moment in time. For example, adolescents unable to assent at the start of a treatment course may become better able to do so with improvement in their clinical condition. Many specialized services provide written information (see Appendix 7.1), videos, or DVDs depicting the treatment to assist patients and their families in the consent process. Practitioners also need to be aware of the local legislative requirements and adhere to them. This usually calls for the opinion of one or more child psychiatrists.

Procedure

ECT is preferably administered after the adolescent has been hospitalized,[16] although it can also be performed as a day-only procedure. Administering the treatment requires the expertise of a multidisciplinary team, which includes a psychiatrist, anesthesiologist, and nursing staff, and appropriate physical facilities. ECT is administered in a specially designated area or suite.[16,29] In general, concurrent use of medication should be discouraged unless clinically necessary. Some drugs known to interfere with ECT in adults (e.g., benzodiazepines) should be stopped. Treatments are generally administered two or three times per week, and a "course" may include anywhere between 6 and 18 treatments (or occasionally more). Each treatment session is usually completed within an hour, which includes the time necessary for recovery from general anesthesia. There are ongoing debates about the optimal electrode placement (unilateral or bilateral) and how the dose of electricity for the patient should be determined. For more detailed information regarding these and other aspects of the procedure, see references 11, 16, and 29.

FOLLOW-UP

Because ECT is a short-term treatment for an acute illness episode, a recurrence of depression is not uncommon. Hence adolescents treated with ECT must have a careful follow-up treatment plan to enhance the likelihood of improvement being maintained and recurrences prevented. The plan may include pharmacotherapy and psychosocial treatments. Although widely used among adult patients, there are few reports in adolescents regarding "maintenance ECT" treatment—ECT at regular intervals following the course, to prevent relapse.

Although cognitive function should be clinically assessed during the course of ECT, because of the risk of memory impairment, it is recommended that neuropsychological assessment should also be performed on completion of the course and then 3 to 6 months later.

TRANSCRANIAL MAGNETIC STIMULATION

Transcranial magnetic stimulation (TMS) operates on the principle that passing a current through a coil held close to the head produces a magnetic field, which, in turn, induces a current in the brain. In the mid-1980s, TMS began to be used as an investigative tool to assess the integrity of motor pathways. Within a few years, its potential therapeutic application was being studied, particularly in relation to mood disorders. For treatment purposes, a variant of TMS known as repetitive TMS (rTMS), in which magnetic pulses are repeated at intervals of one or more per second, is used. Meta-analyses have reported a modest rate of improvement in adults with depression,[31] although effectiveness appears to have improved in recent trials, which used new paradigms of stimulation.[32]

EFFECTIVENESS

Table 7.1 summarizes the effectiveness of rTMS. As with most psychiatric treatments, the number of studies conducted in adults far exceeds those in children and adolescents. The first report describing rTMS as a psychiatric treatment in young persons[2] ascertained the experience of rTMS researchers through an e-mail listserv. Seven recipients of rTMS, 16 to 18 years of age, were identified. Of these, three had unipolar depression (two of whom improved with rTMS) and one had bipolar disorder, depressive phase (rTMS was ineffective in this patient). In a controlled trial of rTMS in adolescents with major depression, rTMS was found to be effective in the first two patients, each 16 years old, who received active rTMS treatment.[4] The trial is continuing.

To date, Bloch et al.[33] have reported the largest sample. In that open-label study, 9 adolescents with severe resistant depression, 16 to 18 years of age, were treated with rTMS; three of the patients reached the primary outcome measure of >30% reduction in the Children's Depression Rating Scale-Revised.

SIDE EFFECTS

Side effects of rTMS in adults are generally mild and transient. The more common are headache and scalp pain, arising from stimulation of scalp muscles. Gilbert et al.[34] reviewed the side effects in 28 studies that had described TMS in >850 children (collectively including subjects whose ages ranged from infancy to late adolescence and with a variety of conditions, excluding depression). No seizures or other adverse events were found, although it was suggested there may have been inadequate reporting of mild side effects. It is also worth noting that the studies examined by Gilbert were not treatment studies, so the form of TMS was nonrepetitive TMS. One of the seven patients described in Walter et al.[2] reported a headache, and one patient in the series described by Bloch et al.[33] developed a brief hypomanic episode. In the latter patient, hypomania did not recur when rTMS was resumed. Cognitive status in several domains, as measured by a range of psychometric instruments, was not negatively affected by rTMS in the treatment studies of Loo et al.[4] and Bloch et al.[33]

The most serious potential side effect of rTMS is seizure, which has been reported in adults (rarely) but not adolescents. The sonic artifact of rTMS could affect hearing—the reason earplugs are worn for the procedure—but there is no evidence for hearing impairment in children or adolescents.

The tolerability of TMS is supported by findings in a study of attitudes of young recipients regarding the treatment.[35] Thirty-four out of 40 children (healthy or with ADHD), 6 to 13 years of age, who had single-pulse TMS would have it again and ranked TMS as more enjoyable than a long car ride. Attitudes to rTMS among children or adolescents have not been evaluated, but in adult recipients of rTMS the treatment is viewed favorably.[36]

PROCEDURE

Unlike ECT, the rTMS treatment procedure does not entail producing a convulsion and, accordingly, it does not require a general anesthetic or muscle relaxant. The treatment is administered in a designated TMS suite, usually as an outpatient. The optimal characteristics of the stimulus have not been determined for adults, let alone young people, but the favored area of stimulation for all ages is the dorsolateral left prefrontal cortex, and stimulus frequencies in the 5- to 20-Hz range are generally used, with stimulus intensity calculated according to the patient's resting motor threshold.[37] The optimal length of treatment course and frequency of treatment sessions are unknown; in comparison with modern ECT, which is given two to three times weekly, rTMS is sometimes administered daily. A typical treatment session takes about 20 minutes.

There are no absolute contraindications to rTMS, but a thorough medical review, including neurologic assessment and medication history, is required. Neurologic disorders and certain medication may increase the risk of seizure.

It is worth digressing briefly to mention a variety of new experimental techniques, yet to be tested in trials in children, that incorporate magnetic and/or electrical stimulation. These include magnetic seizure therapy (MST), transcranial direct current stimulation (tDCS), and focal electrically administered seizure therapy (FEAST). MST, for example, uses a sufficient dose of TMS, under anesthesia, to produce a focal (treatment) seizure. The rationale is that the seizure will impact those regions of the brain hypothesized to be involved in antidepressant response but will not affect the deeper brain structures believed to mediate the cognitive side effects of ECT.[38]

VAGUS NERVE STIMULATION

Vagus nerve stimulation (VNS) has been successfully used in the treatment of refractory epilepsy in children and adults, and it has been investigated with adults with resistant chronic or recurrent depression, with encouraging results.[39–41] To date, no trials have been conducted for psychiatric disorders in young persons (Table 7.1). The VNS apparatus consists of a small pacemaker-like pulse generator, a flexible bipolar lead, an external programming wand, and programming software. The pulse generator, implanted by a surgeon subcutaneously in the upper left chest, sends intermittent electrical stimulation to the left vagus nerve.[42] The scientific basis for VNS is that the vagus nerve sends sensory information to the nucleus of the solitary tract, which then projects to the forebrain, limbic system, locus ceruleus, raphe nucleus, and other brain regions.[42] The treatment is not without side effects. In the trials of VNS for adult psychiatric disorders, the most common side effects, all transient, were voice alteration, cough, neck pain, and dyspnea. In a recent open-label study of 11 patients, one patient committed suicide and another had recurrence of pulmonary emboli, but these events were thought to be unrelated to the VNS.[43] VNS does not appear to impair cognitive function.[44]

In July 2005, the Food and Drug Administration (FDA) approved VNS for the "adjunctive long-term treatment of chronic or recurrent depression for patients 18 years of age or older who are experiencing a major depressive episode and have not had an adequate response to four or more adequate antidepressant treatments." The approval was not without controversy, and the use of VNS for depression in children and adolescents should at this point be considered experimental.

LIGHT THERAPY

Light therapy (or "phototherapy") is the recommended treatment for people with seasonal affective disorder (SAD), a condition initially described by Rosenthal and colleagues almost 25 years ago as a recurrent depressive illness in which depression develops in fall or winter and subsides in spring or summer.[45] Less is known about the prevalence, characteristics, and optimal treatment of this illness in young people compared with adults. Nevertheless, it has been suggested that SAD may occur in 3% to 4% of school-age children and that the clinical features are similar to those found in adults.[46,47]

EFFECTIVENESS

Table 7.1 summarizes the effectiveness of light therapy. The beneficial effects of phototherapy in young persons with SAD were first reported by Rosenthal et al.[3] and Sonis et al.[48] in small case series (7 cases and 5 cases, respectively). The major study remains that of Swedo et al.,[49] in which 28 children (ages 7 to 17 years) with SAD were randomly assigned to receive active treatment (1 hour of bright-light therapy plus 2 hours of "dawn simulation") or placebo (1 hour of clear goggles plus 5 minutes of low-intensity dawn simulation) for 1 week. The active treatment group fared better. A subsequent study[50] found that yearly treatment with light therapy is effective for managing seasonal recurrences.

It warrants mentioning the results of a recent meta-analysis of light therapy,[51] restricted to patients 18 to 65 years of age. Apart from showing that light therapy reduced symptom severity more than placebo for SAD, it was found that light therapy also reduced symptom severity more than placebo for nonseasonal depression, although not when used as an adjunct to pharmacotherapy. This raises the possibility that light therapy may have a role for nonseasonal depression in young people.

SIDE EFFECTS

Light therapy appears to be safe and well tolerated, including in very young children.[52] If side effects occur, they tend to be mild and transient. Nevertheless, these may include headaches, eyestrain, irritability or anxiety, insomnia, nausea, fatigue, dryness of the eyes, nasal passages, and sinuses, and sunburn. The treatment does not appear to cause damage to the eyes, although patients and families not uncommonly inquire about this. In recent years, companies have been making "blue light" units. It has been suggested that blue light is effective and safe for SAD, but there is less data compared with standard light therapy.

PROCEDURE

Several types of "light boxes" are commercially available (they cost about $250 to $350 US). They are generally portable, and there are both desk/tabletop and freestanding models. Commonly, the young person sits 1 to 3 feet in front of a light unit delivering about 10,000 lux of bright light, initially for about half an hour early in the morning at home. The duration of daily exposure is then gradually increased to an hour over two weeks. It is not necessary to stare at the light box to derive its full benefits; just facing it with one's eyes open is generally sufficient, so a young person can engage in other activities while receiving treatment.[53] The benefits of light therapy are not always immediately apparent. It has been recommended that one should not discontinue light therapy before 2 weeks of correct and consistent use.[53]

RESOURCES FOR PATIENTS AND FAMILIES

Electroconvulsive Therapy

ECT in Scotland: A Guide to Electroconvulsive Therapy: The Latest Evidence. This guide was produced by the Scottish ECT Accreditation Network (SEAN) and designed to give an impartial presentation of the current evidence and advice on ECT for patients, carers, and lay people: http://sean.org.uk/Main/Guide

From the American Psychiatric Association: http://www.psych.org/research/apire/training_fund/clin_res/index.cfm

The Royal Australian and New Zealand College of Psychiatrists "Clinical Memorandum" on ECT is regularly updated and freely available: http://www.ranzcp.org/pdffiles/clinicalmemem/cm12.pdf

Electroconvulsive therapy (ECT): Treating severe depression and mental illness: information from the Mayo Clinic website. http://www.mayoclinic.com/health/electroconvulsive-therapy/MH00022/UPDATEAPP=0

Information about ECT at an Australian site supporting people with depression: http://www.depressionet.com.au/treatments/electro-convulsive-therapy-ect.html

From the SANE Australia website (a charity formed by relatives working for a better life for people affected by mental illness): http://www.sane.org/information/factsheets/electroconvulsive_therapy_(ect).html

There is considerable anti-ECT information on the Internet. Websites with anti-ECT content include: the Citizens Commission on Human Rights (CCHR): http://www.cchr.org/index/5276/6608/ and Mind: http://www.mind.org.uk/Information/Booklets/Making+sense/ECT.htm

A brief history of ECT by R.M.E. Sabbatini, MD, is available at: http://www.cerebromente.org.br/n04/historia/shock_i.htm

Repetitive Transcranial Magnetic Stimulation

From the National Alliance on Mental Illness website: http://www.nami.org/Content/ContentGroups/Helpline1/Transcranial_Magnetic_Stimulation_(rTMS).htm and at the Mayo Clinic website: http://www.mayoclinic.com/health/transcranial-magnetic-stimulation/MH00115

Vagus Nerve Stimulation

Information about VNS is available at http://www.vagusnervestimulation.com and http://www.vnstherapy.com

Light Therapy and Seasonal Affective Disorder

From the American Psychiatric Association: http://www.healthyminds.org/multimedia/LTFSAD fctsheetFinal.pdf

From the Society of Light Treatment and Biological Rhythms: http://www.websciences.org/sltbr

Detailed information about the practical aspects of light therapy is provided in reference 53.

RESOURCES FOR PROFESSIONALS

Walter G, Rey JM, Mitchell P. Practitioner review: ECT in adolescents. *J Child Psychol Psychiatry.* 1999;40:325–334.

The Practice Parameter of the American Academy of Child and Adolescent Psychiatry on electroconvulsive therapy with adolescents is available at: http://www.aacap.org/galleries/PracticeParameters/ECT.pdf

The ECT Handbook, 2nd ed.: The third report of the United Kingdom's Royal College of Psychiatrists' Special Committee on ECT presents the latest clinical guidelines for psychiatrists who prescribe electroconvulsive and practitioners who administer it. It clarifies the place of ECT in contemporary practice and reviews the evidence for its efficacy. It was published in 2005 and is available free of charge at http://www.rcpsych.ac.uk/files/pdfversion/cr128.pdf

ECT On-Line (part of Psychiatry On-Line) has considerable information about ECT research: http://www.priory.co.uk/psych/ectol.htm

The UK's National Institute for Health and Clinical Excellence (NICE) guidance on transcranial magnetic stimulation for severe depression is available at http://www.nice.org.uk/nicemedia/pdf/IPG242GUIDANCE.pdf

REFERENCES

1. Heuyer G, Bour X, Feld M. Electrochoc chez les adolescents. *Ann Med Psychol.* 1942;2:75–84.
2. Walter G, Tormos J, Israel J, et al. TMS in young persons: a review of known cases. *J Child Adolesc Psychopharmacol.* 2001;11:69–76.
3. Rosenthal NE, Carpenter CJ, James CP, et al. Seasonal affective disorder in children and adolescents. *Am J Psychiatry.* 1986;143:356–358.
4. Loo C, McFarquhar T, Walter G. TMS in adolescent depression. *Australas Psychiatry.* 2006;14:81–85.
5. Heuyer G, Bour X, Leroy R. L'electrochoc chez les enfants. *Ann Med Psychol.* 1943;2:402–407.
6. Rey JM, Walter G. Half a century of ECT in young people. *Am J Psychiatry.* 1997;154:595–602.
7. Bertagnoli MW, Borchardt CM. A review of ECT for children and adolescents. *J Am Acad Child Adolesc Psychiatry.* 1990;29:302–307.
8. Moise FN, Petrides G. Electroconvulsive therapy in adolescents. *J Am Acad Child Adolesc Psychiatry.* 1996; 35:312–318.
9. Ghaziuddin N, King CA, Naylor MW, et al. Electroconvulsive treatment in adolescents with pharmacotherapy refractory depression. *J Child Adolesc Psychopharmacol.* 1996;6:259–271.
10. Etain B, Le Heuzey MF, Mouren-Simeoni MC. Electroconvulsive therapy in the adolescent: clinical considerations apropos a series of cases. *Can J Psychiatry.* 2001;46:976–981.
11. National Institute for Health and Clinical Excellence. Guidance on the use of electroconvulsive therapy. Technology Appraisal Guidance 59. London: National Institute for Health and Clinical Excellence; 2003:11–12. Available at: http://www.nice.org.uk/nicemedia/pdf/59ectfullguidance.pdf.

12. Walter G, Rey JM. Has the practice and outcome of ECT in young persons changed? Findings from a whole population study. *J ECT*. 2003;19:84–87.

13. Bloch Y, Levcovitch Y, Bloch AM, et al. Electroconvulsive therapy in adolescents: similarities to and differences from adults. *J Am Acad Child Adolesc Psychiatry*. 2001;40:1332–1336.

14. Stein D, Kurtsman L, Stier S, et al. Electroconvulsive therapy in adolescent and adult psychiatric inpatients: a retrospective chart design. *J Affect Disord*. 2004;82:335–342.

15. Taieb O, Flament MF, Chevret S, et al. Clinical relevance of electroconvulsive therapy (ECT) in adolescents with severe mood disorder: evidence from a follow-up study. *Eur Psychiatry*. 2002;17:206–212.

16. American Academy of Child and Adolescent Psychiatry. Practice Parameter for use of electroconvulsive therapy with adolescents. *J Am Acad Child Adolesc Psychiatry*. 2004;43:1521–1539.

17. National Institute for Health and Clinical Excellence. Depression in children and young people: identification and management in primary, community and secondary care. National Clinical Practice Guideline No. 28. Leicester, UK: The British Psychological Society; 2005:131.

18. Russell PS, Tharyan P, Kumar A, et al. Electroconvulsive therapy in a pre-pubertal child with severe depression. *J Postgrad Med*. 2002;48:290–291.

19. Esmaili T, Malek A. Electroconvulsive therapy in a six-year-old girl suffering from major depressive disorder with catatonic features. *Eur J Psychiatry*. 2007;16:58–60.

20. Lisanby SH, Maddox JH, Prudic J, et al. The effects of electroconvulsive therapy on memory of autobiographical and public events. *Arch Gen Psychiatry*. 2000;77:581–590.

21. Cohen D, Taieb O, Flament M, et al. Absence of cognitive impairment at long-term follow-up in adolescents treated with ECT for severe mood disorders. *Am J Psychiatry*. 2000;157:460–462.

22. Ghaziuddin N, Laughrin D, Giordani B. Cognitive side effects of electroconvulsive therapy in adolescents. *J Child Adolesc Psychopharmacol*. 2001;10:269–276.

23. Guttmacher LB, Cretella H. Electroconvulsive therapy in one child and three adolescents. *J Clin Psychiatry*. 1988;49:20–23.

24. Devanand DP, Dwork AJ, Hutchinson ER, et al. Does ECT alter brain structure? *Am J Psychiatry*. 1994;151:957–970.

25. Kish SJ, Kleinert R, Minauf M, et al. Brain neurotransmitter changes in three patients who had a fatal hyperthermia syndrome. *Am J Psychiatry*. 1990;147:1358–1363.

26. Walter G, Koster M, Rey JM. Electroconvulsive therapy in adolescents: experience, knowledge, and attitudes of recipients. *J Am Acad Child Adolesc Psychiatry*. 1999;38:594–599.

27. Walter G, Koster M, Rey JM. Views about treatment among parents of adolescents who had received ECT. *Psychiatr Serv*. 1999;50:701–702.

28. Taieb O, Flament MF, Corcos M, et al. Electroconvulsive therapy in adolescents with mood disorder: patients' and parents' attitudes. *Psychiatry Res*. 2001;104:183–190.

29. Walter G, Rey JM, Mitchell P. Practitioner Review: ECT in adolescents. *J Child Psychol Psychiatry*. 1999;40:325–334.

30. Ghaziuddin N, DeQuardo JR, Ghaziuddin M, et al. Electroconvulsive treatment in an adolescent treated with craniotomy. *J Child Adolesc Psychopharmacol*. 1999;9:63–69.

31. Loo CK, Mitchell PB. A review of the efficacy of transcranial magnetic stimulation (TMS) treatment for depression, and current and future strategies to optimize efficacy. *J Affect Dis*. 2005;88:255–267.

32. Gross M, Nakamura L, Pascual-Leone A, et al. Has repetitive transcranial magnetic stimulation (rTMS) treatment for depression improved? A systematic review and meta-analysis comparing the recent vs. the earlier rTMS studies. *Acta Psychiatr Scand*. 2007;116:165–173.

33. Bloch Y, Grisaru N, Harel EV, et al. Repetitive transcranial magnetic stimulation in the treatment of depression in adolescents: an open label study. *J ECT*. 2008;24:156–159.

34. Gilbert DL, Garvey MA, Bansal AS, et al. Should TMS research in children be considered minimal risk? *Clin Neurophysiol*. 2004;115:1730–1739.

35. Garvey MA, Kaczynski KJ, Becker DA, et al. Subjective reactions of children to single-pulse TMS. *J Child Neurol*. 2001:16:891–894.

36. Walter G, Martin J, Kirkby K, et al. Transcranial magnetic stimulation: experience, knowledge and attitudes of recipients. *Aust N Z J Psychiatry*. 2001;35:58–61.

37. Stein D, Weizman A, Bloch Y. Electroconvulsive therapy and TMS: can they be considered valid modalities in the treatment of pediatric mood disorders? *Child Adolesc Psychiatr Clin N Am*. 2006;15:1035–1056.

38. Morales OG, Henry ME, Nobler MS, et al. Electroconvulsive therapy and repetitive transcranial magnetic stimulation in children and adolescents: a review and report of two cases of epilepsia partialis continua. *Child Adolesc Psychiatr Clin N Am*. 2005;14:193–210.

39. Rush AJ, George MS, Sackeim HA, et al. Vagus nerve stimulation (VNS) for treatment-resistant depression: a multicenter study. *Biol Psychiatry*. 2000;47:276–286.

40. Sackeim HA, Rush AJ, George MS, et al. Vagus nerve stimulation (VNS) for treatment-resistant depression: efficacy, side effects and predictors of outcome. *Neuropsychopharmacology*. 2001;25:713–728.

41. Marangell LB, Rush AJ, George MS, et al. Vagus nerve stimulation (VNS) for major depressive episodes: one year outcomes. *Biol Psychiatry*. 2002;51:280–287.

42. Martinez JM, Marangell LB, Hollrah L. Vagus nerve stimulation: current use and potential applications in child and adolescent psychiatry. *Child Adolesc Psychiatr Clin N Am*. 2005;14:177–191.

43. Corcoran CD, Thomas P, O'Keane V. Vagus nerve stimulation in chronic treatment-resistant depression: preliminary findings of an open-label study. Br J Psychiatry. 2006;189:282–283.

44. Sackeim HA, Keilp JG, Rush AJ, et al. The effects of vagus nerve stimulation on cognitive performance in patients with treatment-resistant depression. *Neuropsychiatry Neuropsychol Behav Neurol*. 2001;14:53–62.

45. Rosenthal NE, Sack DA, Gillin JC, et al. Seasonal affective disorder: a description of the syndrome and preliminary findings with light therapy. *Arch Gen Psychiatry*. 1984;41:72–80.

46. Carskadon MA, Acebo C. Parental reports of seasonal mood and behavior changes in children. *J Am Acad Child Adolesc Psychiatry*. 1993;32:264–269.

47. Swedo SE, Pleeter JD, Richter DM, et al. Rates of seasonal affective disorder in children and adolescents. *Am J Psychiatry*. 1995;152:1016–1019.

48. Sonis WA, Yellin AM, Garfinkel BD, et al. The antidepressant effect of light in seasonal affective disorder of childhood and adolescence. *Psychopharmacol Bull*. 1987;23:360–363.

49. Swedo SE, Allen AJ, Glod CA, et al. A controlled trial of light therapy for the treatment of pediatric seasonal affective disorder. *J Am Acad Child Adolesc Psychiatry*. 1997;36:816–821.

50. Giedd JN, Swedo SE, Lowe CH, et al. Case series: seasonal affective disorder: a follow-up report. *J Am Acad Child Adolesc Psychiatry*. 1998;37:218–220.

51. Golden R, Gaynes B, Ekstrom RD, et al. The efficacy of light therapy in the treatment of mood disorders: a review and meta-analysis of the evidence. *Am J Psychiatry*. 2005;162:656–662.

52. Saha S, Pariante CM, McArdle TF, et al. Very early onset seasonal affective disorder: a case study. *Eur Child Adolesc Psychiatry*. 2000;9:135–138.

53. Rosenthal NE. *Winter Blues: Everything You Need to Know to Beat Seasonal Affective Disorder*. Rev. ed. New York: Guilford Press; 2006.

Example of Information About ECT for Young Patients and Their Families

What is Electroconvulsive Therapy?

Electroconvulsive therapy (ECT) is a treatment for certain mental disorders that was discovered almost 60 years ago. It is given by a team of specialist doctors and nurses. One of the doctors, an anesthetist, puts the patient to sleep for a short while with an anesthetic. While the patient is asleep, an electric current is applied to the head by another doctor. A brief seizure, which can hardly be noticed because the muscles are relaxed, follows. The patient is then taken to a recovery room and is looked after by trained nurses. The whole procedure takes about 10 minutes. ECT is usually given two or three times weekly. Most patients need 6 to 12 treatments, but a few patients require more.

How does ECT work?

An imbalance of chemicals is thought to cause most mental disorders for which ECT is given. ECT corrects this imbalance, though how it actually does this is not known. A lot of research is currently being done to discover this.

Is ECT an approved treatment?

All major medical and psychiatric organizations, including the American Psychiatric Association, Royal College of Psychiatrists (UK), and Royal Australian and New Zealand College of Psychiatrists, approve the use of ECT and have guidelines for how it should be given.

Why do young people have ECT?

The main reason is severe depression. Young people with this condition may feel unhappy, be unable to enjoy anything, sleep poorly, and feel suicidal. ECT is also sometimes used to treat mania and schizophrenia.

How often is ECT given to young people?

ECT is used more often in adults, but the treatment is occasionally used for young people. About 1% of people who have ECT are teenagers. When used, it is after medication and other treatments have not helped or have caused serious side effects.

How effective is ECT?

More than half of the young people who have ECT improve a great deal or recover fully from their symptoms. This is very good given how unwell the person is just before ECT and the fact that other treatments did not work. ECT does not stop the person becoming unwell again. It is thus important that most people start taking medication again after ECT and be followed-up by their doctor.

How safe is the treatment?

ECT is very safe. The risks are the same as those for an operation needing a brief anesthetic. When thinking about safety, it is also worth keeping in mind the bad effects of other treatments as well as the risks of not treating the condition at all. Suicide, for example, is not rare in people who are severely depressed.

What are the main side effects of ECT?

The side effects of ECT are mild and don't last long. Some people complain of headache after waking from the anesthetic but this is brief and goes away with analgesics. A few people complain of muscle aches for a short while. Some people complain of memory problems. This stops once the treatment has finished.

Does ECT damage the brain?
There is NO evidence to suggest this. Studies of brain structure and function show that ECT does not injure the brain.

Who gives consent for ECT?
The doctor recommending ECT will discuss this treatment with the patient and the patient's family and provide time for them to ask questions about the treatment. If the patient and family choose to go ahead with ECT, the patient will then sign a consent. When patients can't understand what they are told about ECT (usually because of their illness), a panel made up of a doctor, a lawyer, and a patient representative will consider whether ECT treatment should be used.*

Why has ECT had such a bad image?
After ECT was discovered, it was used for all mental disorders. Drug treatments were not around at the time and there were few other treatments. Also, muscle relaxants were not given, resulting in more side effects from the seizure. Movies such as *The Snake Pit* and *One Flew Over the Cuckoo's Nest* gave negative accounts for ECT, and this helped to create a bad image. As practiced these days, ECT is a safe, even lifesaving treatment, used for particular illnesses and according to strict guidelines.

*This is the most common procedure but requirements vary from state to state and from country to country.
Source: Walter G, Rey JM, Mitchell P. Practitioner Review: ECT in adolescents. *Journal of Child Psychology and Psychiatry and Allied Disciplines* 1999;40:325–334. © Copyright 1999. Wiley-Blackwell Publishing Ltd. Reproduced with permission.

How to Use Cognitive Behavior Therapy for Youth Depression: A Guide to Implementation

DAVID A. LANGER, ANGELA W. CHIU, AND JOAN R. ASARNOW

KEY POINTS

- Considerable evidence indicates that cognitive behavior therapy (CBT), alone or in combination with medication, is effective in the acute treatment of major depression in youth.
- Combined treatment (CBT plus medication) appears to be the treatment for youth with moderate to severe depression with the best risk/benefit ratio, although the specific benefits of CBT are less clear with more severe depression.
- The combination of medication and CBT appears to be the best treatment for depressed adolescents who did not respond to an adequate medication trial.
- Efficacy of CBT is likely to be influenced by the characteristics of the specific CBT used, the patient population, clinician's characteristics, and other parameters.
- A CBT program contains three somewhat overlapping phases: conceptualization, skills and application training, and relapse prevention.
- A typical CBT session begins by collaboratively setting an agenda for the session, reviewing homework from the previous week, teaching and practicing the current cognitive-behavioral skill, addressing crises and issues that have arisen in the youth's life over the previous week, helping the youth summarize the skills that have been learned during the session, and allocating practice/homework assignments.
- CBT is often provided weekly. Increasing session frequency is encouraged, particularly at the start of treatment if youth present with severe or chronic symptoms.
- Different CBT approaches vary in the amount of parent involvement. However, at a minimum, most CBT clinicians recommend some family psychoeducation regarding depression and family or parent sessions.
- The first goal of the activity module is to identify links between mood and activities in the youth's life experience, followed by increasing the number of pleasant activities.
- The cognitive module is rooted in the cognitive model of depression that views depressive symptoms as consequences of negative thought patterns. This module helps youth discriminate between "helpful" thoughts and "unhelpful" thoughts, develop strategies for generating more helpful thoughts, and practice using helpful thought patterns in response to potential stressful situations.
- Depressed youth may often behave in ways that push others away. When they argue with family members and friends, they feel worse. The communication and problem-solving modules aim to equip youth with skills to build and maintain healthy relationships.
- Common barriers to CBT can include perceived stigma associated with mental health treatment, immature cognitive skills, crises, and lack of completion of homework.
- Younger patients require more active play-oriented approaches, whereas close family involvement is often less important for adolescents.

Introduction   *Michelle is a 15-year old white girl living with her biological parents and her 12-year old sister. She presented with an acute onset of a depressive episode after her family moved 3 months earlier. Michelle's mother expressed concern about Michelle's school refusal, depressed mood, irritability, sudden loss of interest in extracurricular activities, apathy toward making new friends, and frequent complaints of headaches. In addition, Michelle's academic performance has deteriorated significantly.*

This chapter focuses on the use of CBT with youth like Michelle. CBT is an established treatment for youth depression, supported by substantial evidence documenting efficacy under controlled conditions, and recent data supporting effectiveness under usual practice conditions.[1,2] The general CBT model is based on the assumption that depressive symptoms are associated with an individual's behavioral responses and thought patterns, and changes in behavioral and thought patterns will help the youth feel better and cope more effectively. In this chapter we begin by reviewing the evidence base supporting the value of CBT, followed by a detailed description of how to use CBT with youth like Michelle.

THE EVIDENCE BASE AND PRACTICE PARAMETERS

Current practice parameters for the treatment of youth depression emphasize the value of beginning with a psychosocial treatment and considering medication or combined psychosocial and medication treatments for youth who fail to respond to an initial course of psychosocial treatment or present with severe depression.[2] Emphasis on psychosocial treatment has been strengthened by recent warnings regarding the risk of suicidality with antidepressant medications.[3] In the next section, we review the evidence supporting the efficacy and effectiveness of CBT for youth depression. To parallel the practice parameters, we (1) begin with the efficacy of CBT as a monotherapy, relative to alternative psychosocial treatment strategies, (2) proceed to a review of the data on the efficacy of CBT in combination with medication treatment, and (3) conclude with the evidence on effectiveness under routine practice conditions.

COGNITIVE BEHAVIOR THERAPY AS A MONOTHERAPY

Extant research supports the efficacy of CBT, relative to wait-list, inactive control, and active control conditions. Effect sizes for CBT have varied somewhat. Early meta-analyses reported impressive outcomes, with effect sizes ranging from 1.02 to 1.27,[4,5] far surpassing Cohen's[6] criteria for a large effect, set at 0.80; more recent meta-analyses, which examined a broader group of "treatments with cognitive components," have found a smaller average effect size, 0.35, which is statistically similar to the effects of other psychosocial treatments.[7] Thus, although the overall data support the efficacy of CBT, treatment efficacy is likely to be impacted by the characteristics of the specific CBT, the patient population, clinician characteristics, and other parameters.

COMBINATION THERAPY: CBT COMBINED WITH MEDICATION

Two recent large scale studies have underscored the value of combination treatment, in which youth receive CBT plus medication. First, the multisite Treatment for Adolescents with Depression Study (TADS)[8] randomized moderately to severely depressed adolescents to receive CBT alone, medication alone (fluoxetine), CBT plus medication, or pill placebo. After 12 weeks of acute treatment, medication alone and CBT plus medication outperformed placebo. Although youth receiving CBT alone did not significantly differ from youth in the placebo condition, there was some evidence that combining CBT and medication led to reduced suicidality, enhancing the safety of medication treatment. After 36 weeks of treatment, response rates were identical for CBT alone and fluoxetine alone (81%), with a slight, nonsignificant advantage (86% response rate) continuing for combined treatment.[9]

Thus it appears that combination treatment or medication alone leads to accelerated recovery, but with time, recovery rates look similar for CBT and medication monotherapies. However, it is important to note that there were some moderators of treatment response in the TADS, which should be acknowledged when considering CBT. For instance, in TADS, combined treatment was more beneficial for adolescents with milder presentations of depression, whereas youth with more severe depression responded similarly to the combined treatment and monotherapy with fluoxetine.[10] Additionally, not all studies have shown an advantage for combined CBT plus medication.[11,12] Lastly, because nonresponders were offered additional treatment at the end of the TADS trial, data are not available on longer term outcomes for youth assigned to the placebo condition, leaving open questions regarding whether longer term improvement was owing to the effects of active treatments or to the natural trend toward recovery seen in adolescent depression.

Results of the Treatment of Resistant Depression in Adolescents study (TORDIA)[13] also support the value of combination therapy. This study was the first to examine treatment strategies for youth who failed to respond to an initial trial of antidepressant medication (as opposed to the TADS sample of youth who were excluded if they had demonstrated prior treatment resistance). Results indicated that at the end of 12 weeks of acute treatment, youth receiving combined CBT plus a change in medication were more likely to show an adequate clinical response when compared with youth receiving a change in medication alone. Thus results of the TORDIA study support the value of adding CBT as a second-step treatment for youth who fail to respond to initial medication treatment.

EFFECTIVENESS OF COGNITIVE BEHAVIOR THERAPY UNDER ROUTINE PRACTICE CONDITIONS

The Youth Partners in Care Study (YPIC)[1] examined the effectiveness of a quality improvement intervention aimed at improving access to evidence-based depression treatment (CBT and/or medication) through primary care among youth screened for probable depression. In this study, usual providers in the participating health care organizations were trained in manualized CBT for depression. When given a choice of treatment type, patients and providers chose higher rates of CBT relative to medication.[1] Results indicated that youth in the intervention condition, relative to youth receiving usual care, showed both increased rates of CBT and psychosocial treatment and improved depression outcomes, suggesting that the improved outcomes were associated with the increased rate of psychosocial treatment, primarily CBT.[1] With a more severe sample of youth with major depressive disorder selected for selective serotonin reuptake inhibitor (SSRI) treatment by their primary care providers, Clarke and colleagues found only a weak advantage for combined CBT and medication compared with medication alone.[14] Moreover, a British effectiveness/pragmatic trial found no advantage at 12 to 24 weeks for combined CBT plus SSRI medication versus SSRI medication, with both conditions including usual clinical care and the sample including youth with definite and probable major depression who had failed to respond to a brief initial psychosocial intervention.[11,15] These studies thus underscore the complexity of translating research findings to usual care settings.

SUMMARY OF COGNITIVE BEHAVIOR THERAPY EFFICACY/EFFECTIVENESS

In summary, the bulk of the evidence supports the efficacy of CBT in the acute treatment of depressed youth and that CBT can be delivered under routine practice conditions with beneficial effects. For youth with moderate to severe depression, combined treatment (CBT plus medication) appears to be the treatment with the best risk/benefit ratio. For youth who fail to respond to an initial SSRI trial, the addition of CBT leads to improved outcomes.[13] However, extant effectiveness data suggest that translating these findings to usual care contexts may be complex, raising questions regarding the added value of combined CBT plus medication under more routine practice conditions (e.g., versus controlled treatment trials).[1,11,12,14,15] Although the majority of CBT research has focused on adolescents,[7] CBT is also effective with younger school-age children with depressive symptoms.[16-18] Note, however, that to date no published randomized controlled trials have documented the efficacy of CBT for school-age children with depressive disorders.

PRINCIPLES OF COGNITIVE BEHAVIOR THERAPY

CBT is based on two major assumptions: (1) depressed mood states are associated with an individual's behaviors and thoughts, and (2) changing behavioral and cognitive patterns leads to reductions in depressive symptoms and improved functioning. The model presented in most CBT programs is one in which a youth is exposed to a range of stressors and responds to these stressors with feelings (emotional states), thoughts, and behaviors. Sometimes these feelings, thoughts, and behaviors make the youth feel worse and contribute to downward spirals in which sad/bad feelings lead to unhelpful negative thoughts and behaviors, which lead to worse feelings and even more negative thoughts and behaviors. The goal of treatment is to turn upward these downward depressive spirals. This is done by understanding how one's feelings, thoughts, and behaviors are interconnected and developing strategies for finding more helpful patterns of thinking and behaving, which in turn lead to better feelings. In this chapter, we emphasize our approach for adolescents that is based on the manual of Clarke and colleagues[19] and combines elements of approaches developed originally by Meichenbaum[20] and Seligman, Jaycox, and colleagues.[21] We also describe other approaches, including those for younger children.

CONDUCTING A CBT PROGRAM FOR DEPRESSED YOUTH

PHASES

A CBT program for depressed youth can be viewed as containing three phases: conceptualization, skills and application training, and relapse prevention. The focus of treatment varies over time, with an initial emphasis on conceptualization, followed by a focus on skills training and application practice, and concluding with relapse prevention and termination. However, each component listed here is addressed throughout treatment (e.g., the therapist continues to emphasize the CBT model of depression and relapse prevention is anticipated from the early phase of treatment). Nonspecific factors such as a strong therapeutic relationship and alliance with the youth and family are viewed as necessary conditions for treatment.

Conceptualization

CBT builds on a strong therapeutic relationship and a "collaborative empiricism" through which the clinician adopts the role of "coach." The clinician, youth, and parents (as appropriate) systematically consider and "gather data" to help inform the treatment and develop strategies for coping with depression, changing thoughts and behaviors that contribute to depression. This approach emphasizes the active involvement of the youth in treatment. A successful CBT program for youth depression involves working with the youth to understand the cognitive-behavioral model of depression and how treatment is likely to be beneficial. The youth and clinician "collaborate" to discover the influence of thoughts and behaviors on the youth's mood and the cognitive-behavioral strategies that are most effective for the individual youth.

Skills Training and Application Training

The second major task in CBT is to build the youth's cognitive and behavioral skills for coping with depression and help the youth practice those skills in real-world scenarios. Skills that are polished during the session will not help the youth unless the clinician specifically trains for generalization as each skill is learned (e.g., using practice assignments/homework to be done outside of the session), enlisting the help of parents and others (e.g., friends, teachers) who can help the youth apply his or her skills outside of the therapy session.

Relapse Prevention

As therapeutic work comes to a close, it is important to address the youth and family's strategies to maintain therapeutic gains. The clinician and youth identify potential stressors and develop plans to cope with those stressors. General coping strategies are emphasized because it is not possible to anticipate all possible future stresses. The clinician works with the youth and his or her family to recognize signs of depression early. This way the youth can use his or her coping strategies before the downward spiral of depression has gained momentum and seek treatment early if depressive symptoms begin to escalate. The goal during the relapse prevention phase is to provide the youth and family with strategies they can use to prevent depressive reactions from triggering full-blown depressive episodes. This emphasis on relapse and recurrence prevention is particularly important in depression, given the high risk of relapse and recurrence among depressed youth.[2,22–26] Issues related to termination are also addressed at the end of treatment.

PLANNING INDIVIDUAL COGNITIVE BEHAVIOR THERAPY SESSIONS

Effective CBT clinicians adapt their treatment plans to match the needs of individual youth. Most often, a general CBT session format helps ground treatment in a structure that allows flexibility while encouraging skill building. A typical CBT session begins by setting a session agenda collaboratively with the youth, reviewing homework from the previous week, bridging to the prior session, teaching and practicing the current cognitive-behavioral skill, addressing crises and issues that have arisen in the youth's life over the previous week, helping the youth summarize the skills that have been learned during the session, and developing practice/homework assignments. Treatment dose varies depending on youth and family needs. Although CBT is often provided weekly for 12 to 16 weeks, at times a 12- to 16-week treatment may not be feasible or advisable. For more severely depressed youth, increasing session frequency is encouraged, particularly at the start of treatment if youth present with severe or chronic symptoms. In these instances, an increased CBT dosage can boost effectiveness and promote more optimism regarding the likely benefits of treatment. Extended treatment duration may also be beneficial with more severely depressed youth who show only partial CBT response during the usual acute treatment phase. For youth with milder symptoms or conflicting demands that create a barrier to treatment attendance, a briefer treatment plan may be optimal. Following acute treatment, CBT clinicians often gradually decrease frequency, meeting with the youth biweekly and then monthly over the course of several months to prevent relapse or recurrence. Although data are limited on optimal strategies for continuation and maintenance treatment, continuation treatment is generally recommended for at least 6 to 12 months for youth who respond to acute treatment, and maintenance treatment should be strongly considered among youth at high risk for recurrence.[2]

Different CBT approaches have varied in the amount of parent involvement, and the evidence is unclear regarding the efficacy of different approaches to the family. However, most CBT programs have included some family psychoeducation regarding depression, and many CBT programs have involved family or parent sessions to support generalization of CBT skills beyond the treatment sessions and to assist parents in supporting the youth's recovery.

Here we describe three intervention modules that are commonly included in CBT for youth depression: (1) activities and behavioral activation, (2) cognitive and thought patterns, and (3) communication and problem solving. Our adolescent manual includes four sessions in each module.[27] As we describe these modules, our prototypic depressed youth, Michelle, is used to illustrate the CBT process.

THE ACTIVITY MODULE

This module focuses on examination of the youth's activities and how activities affect moods and lead to downward or upward spirals. Monitoring activities and mood using a "mood and activities diary" can be a powerful therapeutic tool as youth examine what they do each day and whether their activities affect their mood. This process helps youth see that it is often possible to exert some control over negative mood states by altering their own behaviors and activities. Youth learn to become more aware of their mood patterns and to take action to prevent the progression of downward spirals. Primary objectives of this module are to (1) understand the connection between mood and fun activities, (2) set realistic mood and activity goals, (3) develop a plan to reach goals, and (4) refine the plan for sustainability. Additionally, the activity module is used as an opportunity for youth to

---

BOX 8.1
CASE EXAMPLE: ACTIVITY MODULE

Clinician: Today, let's focus on how activities impact our mood. When we're depressed, we often stop doing fun things, making us more depressed. This can become a vicious cycle. One way to break this cycle and begin to feel better is to increase the activities that you enjoy. Let's take a look at how this may work in your life. What day did you feel best in the last week?

Michelle: I guess it was last Saturday when I talked on the phone with my friend, Sarah, and went to a movie with my sister. I gave it a rating of a 6.

C: What was the day you felt worst this past week?

M: Monday. I rated Monday a 2. I felt bad when I woke up so I stayed in bed all day and slept.

C: Do you think there were any links between mood and activities on those days? Let's take a look at your mood diary. Interesting, on Monday you had the lowest mood for the week; whereas on Saturday you had a higher mood rating. Could your mood have been affected by what you did? On Saturday, you said you talked to Sarah, but on Monday you stayed in bed all day?

M: Well, it was nice to talk to Sarah because we were really close when I was at my old school. I guess I was in a better mood after talking with her on the phone. On Monday I missed school by sleeping all day and then I felt even worse.

---

examine the individuals they interact with, individuals who provide social support, and strategies for building social skills and strengthening social support.

Typically, youth discover they are less likely to engage in fun activities when they are feeling depressed, which contributes to downward mood spirals, in which youth engage in even fewer activities, which leads to still lower mood. The first goal in this module is to identify links between mood and activities in the youth's life experience. Throughout therapy, youth are asked to monitor daily mood on a mood diary, in our case using a scale from 1 (lowest mood) to 7 (highest mood). Box 8.1 illustrates how the clinician might guide the youth in discovering links between mood and activities.

After introducing the idea of links between mood and activities, youths are asked to identify activities that are enjoyable or give them a feeling of accomplishment. Generally, these activities fall into two categories: social activities, such as fun times with friends or family (e.g., going to the mall, talking on the phone), and success activities that produce feelings of pride or accomplishment (e.g., helping sister with homework, completing an art project, jogging). Youths are encouraged to identify at least ten activities that are enjoyable, inexpensive, legal/not likely to lead to negative consequences, and feasible/under their control. As a practice/homework assignment, youths are invited to uncover the links between mood and activities by recording activities and mood during the coming week on a mood and activity log.

Figure 8.1 shows Michelle's completed log and a graph showing how her mood and activities relate. Michelle and the clinician would plot this graph during the session. The connection between mood and activities is explored by asking questions such as "Are mood and activities related?" If not, follow-up questions to explore potential explanations for the observed pattern would be offered, such as "What were the activities on the day with the highest mood rating? What were the activities on the day with the lowest mood rating? Which activities (social or success) had the strongest impact on your mood?" In Michelle's case, activities range from 0 to 3, and her mood ranges from 2 to 6, with mood appearing somewhat better on the days she was more active.

The next step is to generate activity goals that are realistic (attainable) and specific. Together, Michelle and the clinician agree to set a goal of two pleasant activities a day to see if that is associated with any improvements in mood. The goal of two activities is selected because it is specific (easy to evaluate) and realistic (because she was able to engage in two activities on 3 days during the prior week). For some youth, the clinician might also set a mood goal. However, because Michelle is severely depressed and mood is more difficult to control than actions, the emphasis is on the activity goal. Michelle is asked to continue tracking mood and activities over the next week with the aim of meeting her activity goal and collecting more data on how activities influence her mood.

Evaluating youth abilities to meet activity goals may highlight areas that need to be addressed to reach the goals (e.g., social support and skills problems). Modifications to the activity list and

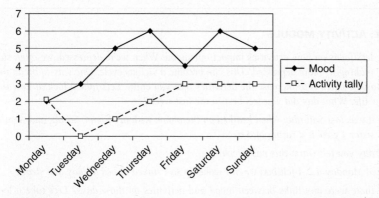

Activity	Mon	Tue	Wed	Thur	Fri	Sat	Sun
Drawing	x						
Walking the dog							x
Watching TV with Mom	x		x	x	x	x	x
Listening to music				x	x	x	
Taking a bubble bath							
Playing board games with sister						x	
Helping Mom prepare dinner					x		x
# Activities	2	0	1	2	3	3	3
Mood	2	3	5	6	4	6	5

■ **Figure 8.1** Example of an activity log that can be assigned as homework (below) with its accompanying chart (above). Adapted from Clarke GN, Lewinsohn PM, Hops H, et al. *Adolescent Coping with Depression Course.* Eugene, Ore: Castalia Press; 1990.

activity goals may be indicated. Important strategies for improving success rates may include making efforts to evaluate progress, scheduling activities in advance, and finding a balance between responsibilities and fun activities. Clinicians can also work with youth to assess situations that make it more difficult to reach goals. For example, although Michelle really enjoys walking her dog, her parents do not like her to do this alone. Consequently, Michelle and her parents can schedule times to walk the dog together. Creating a written contract may also increase success rates because the youth makes a formal commitment to follow through on goals.

THE COGNITIVE MODULE

The cognitive module is rooted in the cognitive model of depression[28] that views depressive symptoms as consequences of negative thought patterns, schemas (patterns of processing information), and cognitive errors that serve to maintain negative beliefs despite the presence of contradictory evidence. This module focuses on helping youth to (1) discriminate between "helpful" thoughts that lead to upward spirals and "unhelpful" thoughts that lead to downward spirals, (2) develop strategies for generating more helpful thoughts that are realistic and relevant to situations or stresses that tend to trigger "unhelpful" thoughts, and (3) practice using these more helpful thought patterns in response to potential stresses/situations.

Depressed youth often interpret situations negatively (e.g., "I got three wrong on my spelling test, which means I'm no good at spelling") and attribute negative intentions to others in ambiguous situations (e.g., "Jane just said she was busy later because she thinks I'm a loser and doesn't want to hang out"). The ways in which depressed youth approach their worlds and themselves with negatively tinted glasses are unique to each youth, but these "thought distortions" can be understood as falling into different categories, such as dichotomous (all or none) thinking, catastrophizing, jumping to conclusions, missing the positive, and taking the blame. The overarching goal of the cognitive component in CBT for youth depression is to teach the youth to identify and dispute negative and irrational cognitions, replacing them with more helpful and realistic counter-thoughts. Box 8.2 provides

BOX 8.2
CASE EXAMPLE: COGNITIVE MODULE

Clinician: So, Michelle, one of the things you added to our agenda for today is "friends." What have you been thinking about friends lately?

Michelle: That it sucks that I don't have any friends.

C: I know that it's been hard for you to move and to make new friends in your current school. I'm wondering, though, if your statement, "I don't have any friends," might relate to what we spoke about earlier today, about unhelpful thoughts.

M: Yeah, the thought is negative, it makes me feel worse, but it's true.

C: I wonder, if someone else were to look at that thought, like we were looking at other thoughts just a little bit ago, might have alternative ways of thinking about the situation?

M: They might think more positively, don't focus on the negative, but this time it's not wrong— I really have no friends.

C: That must be really hard, but you make a good point: We need to carefully look at the situation and see what the evidence is that the thought is true. Let's take a moment and do that now. We'll look for evidence for both sides. Let's start with evidence that "I have no friends" is true.

M: Last weekend I stayed home all weekend.

C: OK, now let's list some evidence against.

M: Well, some girls at my bus stop asked if I wanted to go to the mall on Saturday, but I think they were doing it just for pity.

C: What makes you think that?

M: I don't know, why else would they ask?

C: We can't know for sure why they asked, but it sounds to me like you were right to put that they asked you in the evidence against having no friends, and thinking that they were doing it for pity might be jumping to conclusions.

[At this point, clinician and Michelle would continue to gather pieces of evidence]

C: You see, Michelle, you did a really great job thinking of evidence on both sides, even though at first it seemed (or felt) as if the statement, "I have no friends," was true. I imagine when you're feeling crappy it's a lot easier to think negative.

M: Yeah.

C: Looking at all the evidence for "I have no friends" being true and false, what do you think might be a more helpful way to think about this situation?

M: Maybe, "Even though I don't feel very close to anyone here yet, there are some girls who are very nice and may want to be my friends."

C: How would that thought make you feel?

M: Much better.

C: Is that thought realistic—could it be true?

M: It could be.

C: Now you said earlier that you told them you were busy and then felt even worse at home, going into a downward spiral. What do you think might have happened if you were thinking this more helpful thought?

M: I might have hung out with them and had a good time at the mall.

C: That's a great example of how changing your thoughts could turn a downward spiral into an upward spiral.

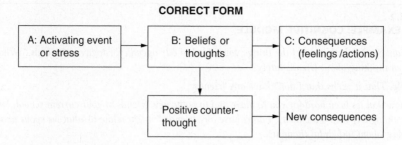

QUESTIONS TO HELP YOU THINK OF A POSITIVE COUNTER-THOUGHT

What are some **OTHER WAYS** to think about this situation?
What is the **EVIDENCE** for and against this belief?

     Evidence **FOR:**
     Evidence **AGAINST:**

If this belief were true,

     what is the **WORST** thing that could happen?
     what is the **BEST** thing that could happen?
     what is the **MOST LIKELY** thing that would happen?

What is a **PLAN OF ATTACK** that you can use to help with this situation?

■ **Figure 8.2** Cognitive Restructuring Form Examining one's cognitive reactions to different situations and generating more positive counter-thoughts can be done by using handouts like this one. Adapted from Clarke GN, Lewinsohn PM, Hops H, et al. *Adolescent Coping with Depression Course.* Eugene, Ore: Castalia Press; 1990.

an example of a discussion in which the clinician guides the youth through this process. Figure 8.2 shows a sample cognitive restructuring form that the youth can complete.

The approach to the cognitive module varies according to clinician and patient characteristics, but we have found the following general tips to be helpful:

1. *Scenarios, examples.* For youth who have difficulty identifying or sharing their own thoughts, examples of situations that could happen to another youth may help them recognize that different reactions are possible in the same situation. For instance, a youth who says "I'm an idiot" when getting a poor grade may handily suggest a more neutral interpretation for another's low test grade (e.g., "maybe he forgot to study").
2. *Games and activities.* Especially for younger children, games and activities may bring energy and understanding to what can be challenging skills for youth to learn and practice. In our work with younger children, sessions were structured around the production of a video to be shown to their parents, providing opportunities to rehearse and practice CBT skills.[16] Games, such as card games, are used. In these, youth turn over cards describing situations and negative thoughts, and they are asked to generate as many helpful thoughts as they can to the situation. Simple principles can be useful, such as "Try to find two helpful thoughts for every unhelpful thought."[19] In another game, the youth gets points by listening to a negative thought and correctly identifying the type of thought distortion, with bonus points for offering a positive counter-thought.
3. *Personalize the approach to the individual youth.* It is critical to tailor the treatment to the individual youth's life situation, behavioral style, cognitive level, and social and problem-solving skills. Youths' individual issues can be related to the concepts of downward and upward spirals; sessions can be structured to support youth in using CBT skills to address real-life problems.
4. *Application training to promote generalization to life situations.* Whatever skill level a youth attains, it is important to apply these new skills to the problems and stressors the youth encounters in daily life. This application helps the youth learn to generalize therapeutic work to nontherapeutic settings, and it increases the likelihood that the youth will use these skills once the therapy concludes.

THE COMMUNICATION AND PROBLEM-SOLVING MODULE

Depressed youth tend to behave in ways that push others away (e.g., irritability). When they argue with family members and friends, they often feel worse. Techniques aimed at enhancing communication and problem-solving skills can help prevent youth from entering these negative cycles. The communication and problem-solving modules aim to equip youth with skills to build and maintain relationships. Youth are taught how to listen actively to others and to communicate feelings in a manner that other people can hear. In addition, youth are taught steps for dealing with interpersonal problems: defining the problem, brainstorming solutions, evaluating possible solutions, picking a solution, and implementing a plan for success.

Clinicians may introduce communication and problem-solving skills with the youth alone and promote generalization through practice/homework assignments, include parents in the session, or work with parents individually. In our work we frequently bring parents in for parts of the session to promote generalization. However, we have also had strong success working with youths individually, often asking them to play the part of their parents in role plays while the clinician plays the part of the youth. This promotes increased understanding of the parents' perspectives on the part of the youth, provides information about the parents to the clinician, and provides a structure for teaching the skills. When parents are informed the youth has homework that involves practicing communication and problem-solving skills learned in therapy, we have found that many times youth and parents effectively practice the skills at home and youth benefit from having opportunities to teach the skills to their parents.

The first step in building communication skills (and consequently building the youth's social network) is to become a better listener. People prefer talking to others who make them feel understood. For instance, in this module Michelle and her mother might be brought together to review strategies for active listening: (1) use nonverbal cues to show you are listening (e.g., nodding head, eye contact), (2) listen carefully before saying what you think, (3) ask clarifying questions to make sure you understand, (4) check out or paraphrase the message to confirm that you understood correctly, and (5) avoid judging the other person or the message.[19,27] Using these simple rules can help promote productive communication and minimize nonproductive behaviors such as accusatory statements, interruptions, and put-downs. Role playing is a particularly helpful format for practice within the session.

In the communication module, Michelle and her mother might be asked to begin practicing active listening on nonthreatening topics such as how they feel about the family dog, what kinds of movies they like, and their favorite flavors of ice cream. The clinician would praise them for using the active listening rules. If Michelle and her mother become judgmental, a common feature in conflictual adolescent–parent interactions, the clinician would remind them that listening does not mean you agree, only that you understand. For instance, the mother might complain the family dog is poorly behaved, in which case the clinician would gently guide Mom toward a less judgmental approach (e.g., the poor dog just doesn't know what to do). To consolidate these skills, assignment/homework would be given for Michelle and her mother to practice active listening three times the next week, recording how it goes.

Learning to identify when, how, and why to share positive and negative feelings with others is another important aspect of successful communication. Sharing positive feelings helps build closer relationships and makes others feel good, whereas sharing negative feelings serves to repair problems in relationships. Although sharing positive feelings is usually beneficial to relationships, youth are encouraged to consider carefully the pros and cons of sharing negative feelings; the assumption is that sharing negative feelings is useful when there is a desire to continue and improve the relationship. If the youth has no interest in maintaining a relationship, avoiding the situation could be the best action. For instance, one of the factors contributing to Michelle's school refusal is that a group of girls tease her. Sharing negative feelings with the girls is unlikely to be productive. Consequently, the clinician and Michelle can explore ways for Michelle to develop sources of support at school and avoid this group of girls.

In contrast to Michelle's feelings about the girls at school, she reports being upset that her parents do not seem to understand how she is suffering at school. Because Michelle's relationship with her parents is very important to her, she wants to address this issue. The clinician could work with Michelle to help her find a way to share these feelings in a way that would help her parents to listen, understand the situation from Michelle's perspective, and find a way to solve her school problems.

The clinician may remind Michelle that sharing negative feelings in a clear, calm, and nonjudgmental manner is likely to help her parents be more willing to change their responses, encouraging Michelle to state both the feeling *and* what specifically happened to elicit the feeling. For example, it is more helpful to say, "I felt hopeless about my situation at school when you told me you expected me to go to school and didn't care how I felt," rather than to simply say, "I felt hopeless." Whereas the later statement only describes the feeling, the first statement is more informative to the listener, clarifies what behaviors cause the emotion, and provides a starting point for helpful change.

Sharing feelings helps youth and parents identify and define problems that need to be addressed. Problems and disagreements are bound to occur in relationships, even with close friends and family members. Because this is normal, it is important for youth and parents to learn how to settle disagreements through problem solving and respond in an open, understanding way when someone states a problem. A general rule of thumb is that dealing with minor problems sooner prevents bigger conflicts later.

In Michelle's case, after identifying her discomfort at school, therapy can move forward to teach strategies for problem solving, beginning with defining the problem, brainstorming solutions, evaluating possible solutions, picking a solution, and implementing a plan for success. General guidelines for defining problems are introduced, including rules for defining problems in a straightforward, positive, and nonjudgmental manner. For instance, the clinician suggests that Michelle (1) begin with something positive to help the other person feel less defensive, (2) describe the behaviors that are creating the problem so there is a clear understanding of the behavioral change requested, (3) be specific about what the problem is, (4) avoid name-calling, (5) express feelings as a reaction to what the other person did, (6) admit her contribution to the problem to show that she accepts some of the responsibility, (7) not accuse or blame the other person, and (8) be brief so she can focus more on developing a solution.[19,27] The clinician and Michelle practice defining a variety of problems, beginning with relatively mild ones, that do not evoke high levels of negative emotions (e.g., deciding what to eat for dinner), and progressing to more challenging conflicts once the youth has practiced more.

After the problem is defined, so that everyone understand what it is, the next step is to brainstorm creatively and list different solutions to the problem. Once several solutions are generated, each solution is evaluated by allowing each person to give a "plus" or "minus" rating, indicating whether the solution is acceptable or not. Next, a solution is chosen that has the most pluses and the fewest minuses or, in other words, the solution that works best for everyone. The importance of compromise is emphasized because compromises that address the needs of each person involved tend to be the most successful solutions. Once a solution is selected, the details are spelled out in terms of how the solution will be implemented. This is often done using a written contract that specifies exactly what each person will do and when, what will happen if a party fails to uphold the agreement, and period of time for which the contract is good. Again, problem-solving skills are taught beginning with mild, nonaffectively charged problems. As the youth's skills develop, the problem-solving skills are applied to address more difficult problems.

BARRIERS TO COGNITIVE BEHAVIOR THERAPY

Barriers common to all psychosocial treatments (i.e., factors impacting attendance to sessions and treatment progress such as stigma, alternative obligations such as parents' work and youths' school schedules, transportation problems, etc.) remain a concern in CBT. Yet some barriers may be particularly important from the perspective of a manualized CBT approach. For instance, limited cognitive abilities are often a barrier to mastering the treatment's cognitive components; we have found that younger children in particular often find behavioral strategies more helpful than cognitive strategies.[16]

A common difficulty in applying manualized CBT is that crises and problems emerge and compete for time with the CBT skills work. The challenge for CBT clinicians is to integrate discussion of these problems within the CBT treatment model—for example, by relating the problem to the concept of downward spirals and encouraging the youth to apply the learned CBT skills to the problem situation. That being said, there will be times when real-world problems will threaten the therapeutic relationship and stability of the therapy situation (e.g., if youth suicidality or other issues trigger out-of-home placement). In these instances, the key goal in treatment will be to stabilize the situation and assess youth and family needs. Although not discussed here, cognitive-behavioral approaches have been developed for strengthening emotion regulation skills and addressing suicidal tendencies to prevent such therapy-threatening crises.[13,29,30]

Another potential barrier to CBT success is not completing the practice/homework assignments. These assignments can be done retrospectively as youth are waiting for the session or during the session. The important point is to emphasize the value of the assignments to promote the use of the CBT skills outside of sessions. If practice/homework lags and youth are not applying CBT skills outside the session, a reevaluation and adjustment of the therapeutic strategy is indicated.

The high level of comorbid disorders and co-occurring problems among depressed youth can also present problems from the perspective of a disorder-specific treatment. Algorithms have been proposed for determining the appropriateness of CBT given comorbidity and complexity among depressed youth[31] and there will clearly be times when it is preferable to treat a comorbid disorder or problem prior to depression. For example, substance dependence might be the initial focus if a youth presents with comorbid substance dependence and depression (see Chapter 18).

DEVELOPMENTAL CONSIDERATIONS

Developmental transitions have important implications for clinicians delivering CBT. One developmental shift is the increase in cognitive capacity to sustain attention, take others' perspectives, discuss abstract concepts, and tackle complex reasoning tasks that occur as youth enter adolescence.[26] Thus adolescents are likely to respond better to cognitive approaches based on adult cognitive therapies than younger children, who may respond better to more concrete tasks and behavioral strategies.

Younger children and adolescents at earlier developmental stages may require a more active play-oriented treatment to enhance rapport building and skill learning, and to optimize therapeutic outcomes (e.g., the already mentioned video production aimed at demonstrating CBT skills).[16] Clinicians working with younger children should consider including interactive activities and present exercises as "games" to facilitate youth motivation and active participation in therapy.[16,32]

A second pivotal change as youth become older is the expansion and diversification of their social world. Although familial relationships may remain central throughout adolescence, peer support and influence account for the most prominent portion of this expanding social network.[33] This may require more emphasis on family work with younger depressed youth. Additionally, given that parents typically seek treatment on behalf of their children, ensure that they attend therapy, and play an important role in whether the youth continues with treatment,[34] establishing an alliance with parents is crucial when working with younger patients.[35] Efforts toward increasing parent commitment may help prevent early dropout, increase motivation for treatment, and ensure more active participation and completion of practice/homework assignments.

Completion of practice/homework assignments is often a challenge, and more concrete reinforcement programs may be useful, particularly for younger children. For instance, a reinforcement program might be developed in which youth earn stickers or prizes (e.g., $10 gift certificate, trip to favorite restaurant with parents) for completing homework. This may help promote a positive attitude toward the practices/homework and improve adherence to this part of treatment. Concrete feedback and reinforcement can also be provided in sessions in the form of tokens or poker chips.[29] Tokens are a form of concrete, positive feedback to the youth, indicating that a comment, idea, or behavior is valued and encouraged.

CONCLUSION

Evidence-based treatments, such as CBT, are currently available for treating depressed youth and offer valuable tools to practicing clinicians. This chapter focuses on strategies for applying CBT and promoting recovery in youth such as Michelle, our prototypic depressed youth. Manuals and training programs are available to assist clinicians in this effort. We encourage clinicians to review available material and obtain training and supervision as they work to adapt cognitive-behavioral approaches to the needs of individual youth and families.

RESOURCES FOR PROFESSIONALS

NIMH's Resources on Depression in Children and Adolescents: http://www.nimh.nih.gov/health/topics/
depression/depression-in-children-and-adolescents.shtml
SAMHSA's National Registry of Evidence-based Programs and Practices: http://www.nrepp.samhsa.gov/

RESOURCES FOR PATIENTS AND FAMILIES

NIMH Pamphlet on Depression: http://www.nimh.nih.gov/health/publications/depression-easy-to-
read.shtml
Association of Behavioral and Cognitive Therapies, Clinician Locator: http://www.abct.org/members/
Directory/Find_A_Therapist.cfm
Academy of Cognitive Therapy: www.academyofct.org
Note: These resources are provided for information. Inclusion in these lists does not imply author
endorsement.

REFERENCES

1. Asarnow JR, Jaycox L, Duan N, et al. Effectiveness of a quality improvement intervention for adolescent depression in primary care clinics: a randomized controlled trial. *JAMA.* 2005;293:311–319.
2. Birmaher B, Brent D, AACAP Work Group on Quality Issues. Practice parameter for the assessment and treatment of children and adolescents with depressive disorders. *J Am Acad Child Adolesc Psychiatry.* 2007;46:1503–1526.
3. U.S. Food and Drug Administration (FDA). Available at: www.fda.gov. Accessed December 1, 2007.
4. Reinecke MA, Ryan NE, DuBois DL. Cognitive-behavioral therapy of depression and depressive symptoms during adolescence: a review and meta-analysis. *J Am Acad Child Adolesc Psychiatry* 1998;37:26–34.
5. Lewinsohn PM, Clarke GN. Psychosocial treatments for adolescent depression. *Clin Psychol Rev.* 1999;19: 329–342.
6. Cohen J. *Statistical Power for the Behavioral Sciences.* Hillsdale, NJ: Erlbaum; 1988.
7. Weisz JR, McCarty CA, Valeri SM. Effects of psychotherapy for depression in children and adolescents: a meta-analysis. *Psychol Bull.* 2006;132:132–149.
8. March J, Silva S, Petrycki S, et al. Fluoxetine, cognitive-behavioral therapy, and their combination for adolescents with depression: Treatment for Adolescents with Depression Study (TADS) randomized controlled trial. *JAMA.* 2004;292:807–820.
9. March JS, Silva S, Petrycki S, et al. The Treatment for Adolescents with Depression Study (TADS): long-term effectiveness and safety outcomes. *Arch Gen Psychiatry.* 2007;64:1132–1143.
10. Curry J, Rohde P, Simons A, et al. Predictors and moderators of acute outcome in the Treatment for Adolescents with Depression Study (TADS). *J Am Acad Child Adolesc Psychiatry.* 2006;45:1427–1439.
11. Goodyer I, Dubicka B, Wilkinson P, et al. Selective serotonin reuptake inhibitors (SSRIs) and routine specialist care with and without cognitive behaviour therapy in adolescents with major depression: randomised controlled trial. *Br Med J.* 2007;335:142–146.
12. Melvin GA, Tonge BJ, King NJ, et al. A comparison of cognitive-behavioral therapy, sertraline, and their combination for adolescent depression. *J Am Acad Child Adolesc Psychiatry,* 2006;45:1151–1161.
13. Brent D, Emslie G, Clarke G, et al. Switching to another SSRI or to venlafaxine with or without cognitive behavioral therapy for adolescents with SSRI-resistant depression. The TORDIA randomized controlled trial. *JAMA.* 2008;299:901–913.
14. Clarke G, Debar L, Lynch F, et al. A randomized effectiveness trial of brief cognitive-behavioral therapy for depressed adolescents receiving antidepressant medication. *J Am Acad Child Adolesc Psychiatry.* 2005;44: 888–898.
15. Byford S, Barrett B, Roberts C, et al. Cost-effectiveness of selective serotonin reuptake inhibitors and routine specialist care with and without cognitive behavioural therapy in adolescents with major depression. *Br J Psychiatry.* 2007;191:521–527.
16. Asarnow JR, Scott CV, Mintz J. Cognitive-behavioral treatments and family interventions for children with depression. A combined cognitive-behavioral family education intervention for depression in children: A treatment development study. *Cogn Ther Res.* 2002;26:221–229.
17. Weisz JR, Thurber CA, Sweeney L, et al. Brief treatment of mild-to-moderate child depression using primary and secondary control enhancement training. *J Consult Clin Psychol.* 1997;65:703–707.
18. Asarnow J, Jaycox LH, Tompson MC. Depression in youth: psychosocial inventions. *J Clin Child Psychol.* 2001;30:33–47.
19. Clarke GN, Lewinsohn PM, Hops H, et al. *Adolescent Coping with Depression Course.* Eugene, Ore: Castalia Press; 1990.

20. Meichenbaum D. *Cognitive Behavioral Modification: an Integrative Approach*. New York: Plenum Press; 1977.
21. Jaycox LH, Reivich KJ, Gillham J, et al. Prevention of depressive symptoms in school children. *Behav Res Ther.* 1994;32:801–816.
22. Birmaher B, Arbelaez C, Brent D. Course and outcome of child and adolescent major depressive disorder. *Child Adolesc Psychiatry Clin N Am.* 2002;11:619–637.
23. Harrington R, Fudge H, Rutter M, et al. Adult outcomes of childhood and adolescent depression. I. Psychiatric status. *Arch Gen Psychiatry.* 1990;47:465–473.
24. Kovacs M, Devlin B, Pollock M, et al. A controlled family history study of childhood-onset depressive disorder. *Arch Gen Psychiatry.* 1997;54:613–623.
25. Kovacs M. Presentation and course of major depressive disorder during childhood and later years of the life span. *J Am Acad Child Adolesc Psychiatry.* 1996;35:705–715.
26. Garber J, Flynn CA. *Vulnerability to Depression in Children and Adolescents*. New York: Guilford; 2001.
27. Asarnow J, Jaycox LH, Clarke G, et al. *Stress and Your Mood: A Manual*. Los Angeles: UCLA School of Medicine; 1999.
28. Beck A, Rush AJ, Shaw BF, et al. *Cognitive Therapy of Depression*. New York: Guilford Press; 1979.
29. Rotheram-Borus MJ, Goldstein AM, Elkavich AS. Treatment of suicidality: a family intervention for adolescent suicide attempters. In: Hofmann SG, Tompson MC, eds. *Treating Chronic and Severe Mental Disorders: A Handbook of Empirically Supported Interventions*. New York: Guilford Press; 2002:191–212.
30. Asarnow J, Berk M, Baraff LJ. *Family Intervention for Suicide Prevention: A Specialized Emergency Department Intervention for Suicidal Youth*. Los Angeles: University of California; 2008.
31. Asarnow JR, Carlson G, Schuster M, et al. *Youth Partners in Care: Clinician Guide to Depression Assessment and Management Among Youth in Primary Care Settings (Adapted from Rubenstein, Unutzer, Miranda, et al. Partners in Care: Clinician Guide to Depression Assessment and Management in Primary Care Settings; 1996.)*. Los Angeles: UCLA School of Medicine; 1999.
32. Stark KD, Herren J, Fisher M. Treatment of childhood depression. In: Mayer MJ, Van Acker R, Lochman J et al, eds. Cognitive Behavioral Interventions for Students with Emotional/Behavioral Disorders. New York: Guilford (in press).
33. Collins WA, Laursen B. Changing relationships, changing youth: interpersonal contexts of adolescent development. *J Early Adolesc.* 2004;24:55–62.
34. Armbruster P, Kazdin AE. Attrition in child psychotherapy. *Adv Clin Child Psychol.* 1994;16:81–108.
35. Hawley KM, Weisz JR. Youth versus parent working alliance in usual clinical care: distinctive associations with retention, satisfaction, and treatment outcome. *J Clin Child Adolesc Psychol.* 2005;34:117–128.

How to Use Interpersonal Psychotherapy for Depressed Adolescents (IPT-A)

LAURA MUFSON, HELENA VERDELI, KATHLEEN F. CLOUGHERTY, AND KAREN A. SHOUM

KEY POINTS

- The goal of IPT-A is to decrease depressive symptoms and help adolescents improve their relationships.
- Monitor depression symptoms and do mood ratings at the beginning of each session.
- Link mood to interpersonal events that have happened during the past week. Always monitor suicidal ideation and behavior weekly.
- Provide psychoeducation about depression and encourage normal activities (especially school responsibilities) as a means to feeling better. Performance will improve as mood improves.
- Stay focused on the interpersonal issues most closely related to the depression: triggers or interpersonal issues that may be maintaining the symptoms.
- Keep the timeframe and time-limited nature of treatment in the foreground as a motivation for working hard in sessions.
- Identify small and manageable "interpersonal experiments" in the middle phase to practice new skills.
- Encourage self-mastery and independence.
- During termination, highlight new interpersonal skills, and promote generalization of specific strategies and identification of warning signs of depression for relapse prevention.

Introduction

Interpersonal psychotherapy (IPT) is an effective, time-limited, manualized psychosocial treatment for depression originally developed for depressed, nonbipolar, nonpsychotic adults.[1] IPT is a product of the interpersonal theorists and their emphasis on the importance of positive interpersonal relationships for mental health, and the belief that people experience distress when disruptions occur in their significant attachments, which result in a loss of social support. IPT identifies the relationship between the onset or maintenance of depressive symptoms and interpersonal events while recognizing that genetic, biologic, and personality factors also contribute to the vulnerability for depression. The IPT therapist intervenes by targeting depressed adolescents' interpersonal skills to improve their relationships and decrease the depression symptoms.

Unlike other psychotherapies, IPT refrains from delving into the adolescent's past and instead focuses on current interpersonal conflicts to improve relationships. IPT and cognitive behavior therapy (CBT) have a number of similar features, such as structure, time limit, focus on the here-and-now, and techniques. However, CBT focuses predominantly on assisting the individual in monitoring and changing behaviors and cognitions to bring about mood change (see Chapter 8). In contrast, IPT focuses on the examination and modification of maladaptive communication patterns and interpersonal interactions in the context of significant relationships and roles that contribute to the onset or maintenance of the depression. Ultimately, IPT alleviates depressive symptoms by reducing current interpersonal stressors.

Based on strong efficacy data for adults, and similarities in symptom presentation between adolescent and adult depression, Mufson and colleagues[2] hypothesized that IPT might also be an effective treatment for adolescent depression. Several characteristics of IPT make it especially relevant for adolescents, including its time-limited nature, which may fit with adolescents' reluctance to seek or stay in treatment. IPT's focus on the interpersonal context, such as major life choices in education, work, and the establishment of intimate relationships (of significant focus at this stage in development), make it especially relevant for treating adolescents. Additionally, in light of the research demonstrating the persistence of interpersonal problems after remission of depression symptoms,[3] a treatment focusing on both the symptoms and the interpersonal domain might be advantageous for facilitating and maintaining improvement in the interpersonal realm after symptom improvement.

Several adaptations have been made to IPT to make it more developmentally appropriate for adolescents. The adolescent version of IPT (IPT-A) is an active treatment with a large psychoeducational component aimed at building the adolescent's competencies and skills. It is structured and organized in such a way that the adolescent can take an increasingly more active role in the treatment as it progresses. IPT-A was adapted specifically to address important developmental tasks of adolescence, such as individuation from parents, development of romantic relationships, peer pressures, and so on, and it may include family members in various phases of the treatment.[4]

SUITABILITY FOR IPT-A

Because depressed adolescents often present with comorbid psychiatric diagnoses and IPT-A is designed to treat adolescents 12 to 18 years of age with nonpsychotic unipolar depression, treatment with IPT-A is suitable for depressed adolescents with comorbid anxiety disorders, attention deficit disorder, and oppositional defiant disorder. However, IPT-A is most effective when depression is the primary diagnosis and comorbid diagnoses are limited. Clinically, IPT-A is used in conjunction with medication for depression for adolescents with severe neurovegetative symptoms to assist them in deriving maximum benefit from the psychotherapy, as well as for adolescents who present with severe symptomatology and impairment. In addition, IPT-A is used with adolescents who are on stable doses of medication for ADHD. However, currently no clinical trials have been conducted on the effects of combined pharmacotherapy and IPT-A. IPT-A is not recommended for adolescents who are mentally retarded, actively suicidal or homicidal, psychotic, bipolar, or actively abusing substances.

Before initiating IPT-A, a complete diagnostic evaluation should be conducted with the adolescent and custodial parent(s) to assess current symptoms and diagnoses, as well as psychiatric, family, developmental, medical, social, and academic history (see Chapter 3). This evaluation is the equivalent to what many clinics refer to as an "intake." The therapist should gather information to assess whether or not the adolescent is suffering from a depressive illness while determining his or her suitability for IPT-A treatment. The therapist also gathers information about possible triggers or factors that maintain the depression symptoms, such as a death in the family, a change in the family or transition for the adolescent, significant disruptions in important relationships, a trauma, or chronic stressors. The therapist revisits and explores these issues further during the initial phase of treatment.

PARENTAL INVOLVEMENT

IPT-A is conceptualized as an individual treatment that recommends (but does not require) parental participation. It is recommended that parents attend at least one session in the initial phase of treatment to become educated about depression and the IPT-A treatment. Parents are also told they may call the therapist if they have any concerns or to report significant events in the adolescent's life that might impact treatment. Parents are treated as "experts" on their children who can contribute information to assist the therapist with the treatment.

ADAPTATIONS FOR ADOLESCENTS

The grief problem area has been adapted to treat adolescents who may be experiencing a severe grief reaction to assist them in mourning the loss and in preventing a delayed or abnormal grief response in the future. Another adaptation is the use of the telephone between sessions to assist in the development of the therapeutic alliance in the initial phase, and to maintain therapeutic momentum in the middle phase, especially if the adolescent is unable to attend a session. In the initial phase, a therapist is encouraged to call the adolescent between sessions to check on his mood, to remind him of the upcoming appointment, and to express interest in seeing him at the next session. Later in treatment, if it is impossible to have a session in a given week, the therapist can conduct the symptom check-in over the phone and facilitate continued work on the identified problem area (Table 9.1).

The concept of the limited sick role (see Session 1 tasks, page 117) is another adaptation in which the adolescent and parent are informed that depression can affect motivation to participate in normal activities as well as influencing performance. The adolescent is encouraged to participate in as many activities as possible with the awareness that performance will improve as the depression remits. The parent is encouraged to help the adolescent engage in his once-typical activities instead of supporting his avoidance and social isolation. The parent is also reminded to refrain from criticizing and blaming the adolescent for poor performance in activities at school (e.g., low grades) and at home (e.g., incomplete chores).

MAIN PHASES OF TREATMENT

The treatment is divided into three phases: initial, middle, and termination. Each phase consists of approximately four sessions. A session-by-session description of the tasks to be covered in each phase is described here.

INITIAL PHASE (SESSIONS 1–4)

Following a comprehensive clinical and psychosocial assessment to determine appropriateness for IPT-A, the initial phase is conducted over four sessions. During these meetings, the therapist aims to (1) educate the adolescent and parent(s) about depression while giving hope, (2) explore how depression affects and, in turn, is affected by the adolescent's significant relationships and roles, and (3) explicitly contract with the adolescent on the interpersonal problem area(s) that will become the focus of the remainder of treatment. Problem areas derive from key aspects of an adolescent's life circumstances or relationships that appear to trigger and/or maintain the current depressive episode.

The four interpersonal problem areas of IPT-A include the following:

- *Grief* (actual death of a significant other, person, or pet)
- *Interpersonal disputes* (parent–child conflicts, arguments with peers, or the breakup of a romantic relationship)
- *Interpersonal role transitions* (difficulty making transitions between stages in life or changes in life circumstances, such as parental divorce, moving to a new town, illness of a sibling, transition to high school)
- *Interpersonal deficits* (social isolation and/or significant communication problems that lead to difficulty in starting or maintaining relationships)

The following is a description of the tasks that typically take place in the initial phase of IPT-A (Sessions 1 through 4).

Session 1

Therapist should administer a *DSM-IV* checklist or other measure of depression (e.g., Hamilton Rating Scale for Depression or Beck Depression Inventory), making sure to cover suicidality (even if denied during past assessment) as well as depression symptoms idiosyncratic to the adolescent (pains/aches, rejection sensitivity, etc.).

Task: Start with a symptom check to be repeated in the beginning of every session. Teach the adolescent how to do a mood rating.

> *"Rate your mood on a scale of 1 to 10, with 1 being the happiest you could feel and 10 being the saddest. How would you rate your mood this past week? Was there a time in the past week when you felt worse than you do now? (Obtain rating). Was there any time you felt better? What happened when you were feeling that way?"*

Task: Educate the adolescent and parent about depression. Explain treatment options (medical model).

> *"Bill, your recent trouble with studying, your cutting back on seeing friends and playing baseball, being easily annoyed with people, trouble with falling asleep (list other symptoms) are symptoms of a depressive episode that started this fall. Depression affects 1 in 10 adolescents; you are not alone. It is a real medical illness. We are all here to help you recover. The good news is that we have a number of treatments that work very well for depression like yours, such as medication and psychotherapy (talk therapy)."*

Task: Assign the "limited sick role" to the adolescent and parent.

> *"Due to your depression, you may have trouble doing a number of things that you want or need to do. If you had broken your leg, you wouldn't expect to run in a week. However, you would need to push yourself to walk around, otherwise your muscles would be weak and your healing would take more time. It's important to do the same here. Try not to miss school but also try hard not to be upset if your grades drop. We have learned that as you begin to feel better, your performance and motivation will improve. The most important thing right now is to get out of this depression. Everything else will follow.*
> *Mrs. Smith, it is important that you recognize that Bill is having trouble doing these things not because he is trying to be difficult and get out of his responsibilities, but rather because he is depressed and that significantly affects his motivation. So it would be really helpful if you can encourage Bill to be active and go to school as much as possible, and be supportive knowing that his performance will improve as he begins to feel better."*

Task: Introduce the basic principles of IPT-A. Obtain a commitment for treatment and explain the goals for session 2. Discuss confidentiality with both parent and adolescent, noting under what circumstances it must be breached. Discuss number, frequency, and duration of IPT-A sessions, and the policy for missed appointments.

> *"Bill, we will try a talk therapy that has had very good results with depression. It's called interpersonal psychotherapy. The idea behind it is that difficulties or changes in important relationships affect an adolescent's mood, and by helping the adolescent manage these better, depression improves."*

Between sessions, liaise with the adolescent's school (see reference 4 for more details).

Session 2

Task: The therapist should start the session with a symptom check/mood rating (see Session 1 task). This should be done at the beginning of every session to monitor closely the clinical course of the depression, which tends to fluctuate in adolescents, and to give the therapist time to deal with any worsening of symptoms or possible emergencies.

Task: Understand the interpersonal context of the depression.

> *"Bill, I'd like to learn more about what happened last fall, when your depression started. Has anyone important to you died recently? Any pets?*
> *Have there been any big changes in your life around that time? Have you had to adapt to anything new yourself, like a new school or new neighborhood? What has been difficult about the change(s)?*
> *Do you have difficulty making friends? In what way?"*

■ **Figure 9.1** Circle of Closeness

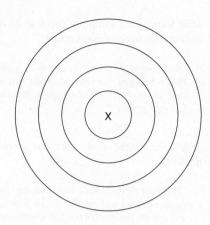

Task: Draw the circle of closeness (Figure 9.1).

> *"This set of circles is a closeness circle. What we are going to do is begin to look at your story of what has been happening to you, and the people who may be related to your depression, a story about your life and your depression. You are in the middle of the circles, and we are going to identify who the main characters in your story are and how they play an important part in your life. We are going to put the people you feel closest/most important to you in the circle closest to you, and those more distant you can put in the outer circles. Close can mean that you have conflict with them but that they are still important to you and your mood, too."*

Task: Conduct the "Interpersonal Inventory." This is a review of the important relationships in the adolescent's life that were identified on the closeness circle. It is intended to fill-in information about people in the adolescent's life who may be triggering or supporting the depression, and it steers the therapist toward a focus on a particular problem area. The therapist wants to get examples of interactions and communications to identify strengths and weaknesses in the adolescent's interpersonal skills. The therapist needs to be a detective to try to understand what interpersonal issues/relationships are most connected to the depression.

Session 3

Task: Start the session with symptom check/mood rating. Continue the inventory.

> *"I'm interested in learning about the important people in your life. Who would you like to start with?*
>
> *What do you like about _____?*
> *What don't you like about _____?*
> *Have you ever told _____ how you feel?*
> *What stops you? What do you think would happen?*
> *Are there any times that you and _____ are together and it is okay? Can you give me an example?*
> *Are there things in your relationship that you would like to change?*
> *How would you feel if those things were different?"*

Session 4

Task: Start the session with symptom check/mood rating. Complete the interpersonal inventory. Connect the depression symptoms to the problem area. Present the interpersonal formulation. Set the treatment contract.

> *"From all the information we gathered these past few weeks, it seems to me that your depression began in the fall when you started your new school. You felt behind the other students academically, felt like you didn't fit in, and missed your old friends and teachers. You became more withdrawn and didn't talk with anyone about how you were feeling. As a result, you began to feel more depressed. Does this sound right to you? Can you explain this to me in your own words and any other thoughts you have about why you became depressed? We'll be talking about this very important change that triggered your depression and we'll try to find ways to help you feel confident to negotiate these changes that have happened—switching*

schools, new friends. I want to remind you that we will be meeting every week for the next eight weeks. It's
important that you come on time and that you reschedule if you need to miss an appointment."

TROUBLESHOOTING

- If the therapist and adolescent do not initially agree on a problem area, the therapist should take more time to explore the adolescent's point of view and find a means to identify the common elements of their viewpoints. The therapist may also consider that the adolescent may be right and adjust his or her focus of treatment appropriately.
- When the parent is unwilling to accept the diagnosis of depression and accuses the adolescent of "laziness," the therapist should take time to provide additional psychoeducation to the parent about the symptoms of depression and how they are manifest in adolescents, exploring resistances to accepting a depression diagnosis.

MIDDLE PHASE (SESSIONS 5–8)

During the *middle phase* of treatment, the therapist teaches the adolescent to link depressive symptoms to difficulties in one or more of these areas, and to link improvement in mood to using effective interpersonal strategies, including constructive and direct communication. Parental participation in the middle phase is flexible, depending on the identified problem area and the treatment targets. Parental participation can be helpful by providing adolescents with opportunities to practice the interpersonal skills they have learned in their individual sessions, with the parents and the therapist present to help facilitate a positive interaction.

If an adolescent is not progressing as expected, the therapist may meet with the parent to obtain more information about possible events occurring outside the sessions that may be preventing the adolescent from progressing as expected. The therapist might ask, *"Do you see any changes at home? How does he seem to be lately? Are there any conflicts or other stressors that may be affecting him?"* This meeting also provides the therapist with the opportunity to assess whether parental problems may be interfering with the progress of treatment. The information gleaned during a parent session is later shared with the adolescent during his session to assist in understanding how best to help him.

At the beginning of each session, regardless of the phase of treatment, the therapist assesses the adolescent's depressive symptoms, noting any changes that occurred over the course of the week and linking changes in symptoms to interpersonal events. Following the review of symptoms, the therapist focuses the session to address the tasks particular to that phase of treatment. In the middle phase, the therapist asks about any particular events in the past week that seem related to the identified interpersonal focus of treatment. Together with the adolescent, the therapist explores the events that occurred and investigates how events could have been managed differently, using the IPT-A techniques to address communication and problem-solving approaches. Table 9.1 lists the four problem areas, along with goals and strategies.

TABLE 9.1 INTERPERSONAL PROBLEM AREAS WITH GOALS AND STRATEGIES

Problem Area	Goals	Strategies
Grief: death of an important person or pet	• Mourn the loss of the important person • Reestablish relationships and interests to substitute for what was lost	• Encourage the adolescent to talk about the loss in great detail • Discuss the sequence of events prior to, during, and after the death, along with associated feelings • Help the adolescent find ways to meet new people and develop new social supports to fill the loss
Interpersonal role disputes: ongoing disagreements with an important person	• Identify the dispute and specific stage[a] • Make some choices about a plan of action • Modify communications • Modify expectations • Find resolution of the dispute	• Explore unrealistic or mismatched expectations and their contributions to the dispute • Assess and modify maladaptive communication strategies • Teach the art of negotiation

(continued)

TABLE 9.1 INTERPERSONAL PROBLEM AREAS WITH GOALS AND STRATEGIES (CONTINUED)

Problem Area	Goals	Strategies
Role transitions: life changes; can be positive or negative	• Mourn the loss of the old role • Find a way to accept and move into the new role with less difficulty • Develop new social skills • Develop new attachments and social support in the new situation/role	• Understand what change means to the adolescent • Identify what is gained and lost in the new role • Master new skills needed to move into the new role
Interpersonal deficits: loneliness and social isolation/difficulty making and sustaining relationships	• Review in detail past and current relationships identifying recurrent patterns, negative and positive • Reduce social isolation by improving social skills • Strengthen current relationships and assist in finding new ones	• Relate depressive symptoms to problem of social isolation • Rehearse new social skills for the formation of new relationships and deepening of existing relationships

[a]Stages of Disputes:
- *Renegotiation:* Adolescent and significant other are still communicating but have faulty skills and have been unsuccessful at resolving dispute. Both want to resolve dispute.
- *Impasse:* Attempts at resolution have failed. Adolescent believes that nothing will get better, and he has stopped trying. A relationship still exists with the significant other, but discussion and even arguments about the dispute have stopped. Therapist attempts to get the two parties talking again.
- *Dissolution:* Adolescent and significant other want to dissolve the relationship. Therapist explores with adolescent whether or not he might make "one last try" at renegotiation. If the adolescent won't agree or if the adolescent tries but no improvement in the dispute is achieved, the therapist helps the adolescent to end the relationship. The dissolution approach is rarely used when the dispute is between the adolescent and his parent(s).

IPT-A techniques are not unique to interpersonal psychotherapy. Although they have been used in other active, time-limited psychotherapies, IPT-A specifically focuses their use on addressing interpersonal issues. Adolescents are taught communication skills to express their feelings regarding conflicts or disappointments in their relationships and life circumstances such as an absent father, an inconsistent father, or conflict about dating rules. The specific interpersonal skills include expression of affect, clarification of expectations for relationships, communication analysis, interpersonal problem solving, and role-playing new methods of interaction.

The techniques listed here are used to help make the link between interpersonal difficulties and mood, analyze the interpersonal problem into its component parts so communication and problem-solving influences can be addressed, and then practice new skills to facilitate improved interactions.

Technique: Link Mood to Event and Event to Mood

> "Bill, you said you felt better after the session on Thursday but sad again last Sunday. What happened between Thursday and Sunday?"

Technique: Communication Analysis

- Teach the adolescent to communicate in a more effective manner by increasing clarity and directness.
- Investigate the specific dialogue or argument that occurred between the adolescent and another person. Focus on a specific situation.

> "Natalia, last week your parents fought a lot in front of you, which made you very sad and angry. Could you think which argument felt worst for you? OK, I'd like to hear from you with as much detail as you can what exactly happened and how you handled the fight. Pretend that we are watching a film of the argument, and describe what happened."

- *How were you feeling before it started?*
- *How did it start?*
- *What did Dad say?*
- *What did Mom say?*

- *Then what happened?*
- *How did you feel?*
- *Could you tell them how you felt?*
- *What stopped you? or Was that the message you wanted to convey?(depending on what happened)*
- *What did you wish you had said? or How do you think it made them feel?*
- *How could you have said it differently?*
- *How do you think she would have felt?*
- *How would you have felt differently?*

Technique: Decision Analysis

Help the adolescent consider various ways to respond to a problem while also assessing the associated consequences:

- Identify the decision that needs to be made.
- Encourage adolescent to generate a list of options.
- Evaluate options by assessing consequences.
- Discuss the "best" option or a combination of options.
- Evaluate the possible outcome as well as the possibility of needing an alternate course of action ("Plan B").

> *"Susan, we have identified that you and Mom disagree about the rules for your curfew. We have discussed that you may need to think about some type of compromise. Let's look at what your options are for changing your curfew with Mom. Let's try to make a list of them together. What would you say they are?*
>
> *1. I have to be able to stay out 'til midnight like everyone else.*
> *2. I could stay out 'til 11 PM on Fridays and midnight on Saturday.*
> *3. I would call you at 11 PM and let you know where I am and then promise to be home by midnight.*
>
> *OK, let's look at these options. How would Mom respond to option 1? What are her concerns? Does this seem likely to work? What about option 2 . . . ?"*

Technique: Role Playing

- Help the adolescent change behavior by rehearsing new ways of behaving with others.
- Select a relevant topic and a small manageable goal.
- Decide who will be playing what role.
- Offer praise and encouragement.
- Ask the adolescent how he thinks it went; ask if he thinks there was anything he could have done differently and how he would have felt in the situation.
- Provide constructive feedback.
- Do not role-play the easiest situation in the office because this is unlikely to occur in the adolescent's life.
- Prepare the adolescent for a range of possible outcomes, and encourage him to come back the following week to discuss what happened regardless of success or failure.

> *"OK, so we have decided option 3 is the best. Let's practice how you can have a conversation with Mom to present and discuss this option with her. How could you start the conversation? What could you say? OK, now we need to practice. We are going to do a role play of the conversation between you and Mom. Who do you want to play first? I will play you first and you can see how I do it and you can play Mom and then we will switch."*

Technique: Work at Home

- Assign work at home in between sessions to help the adolescent practice skills and generalize them to relationships outside of the therapy setting (it is very important to pick something small, specific, and with lower levels of emotionality to ensure likelihood for success as an initial interpersonal experiment). Refer to the skill practice as an interpersonal experiment: There is no success or failure, just more data to help figure out how to improve the relationship.

Here are some examples of possible experiments:

- Initiating a conversation with a peer
- Talking to a parent about going to a movie with a friend

Be sure to check the outcome with the adolescent at the next session.

An outcome of a communication analysis or decision analysis is the identification of an interaction where communication could be improved. The therapist provides psychoeducation about specific communication skills to prepare the adolescent to practice a different interaction in the role play, and eventually for the adolescent to take these newly honed skills into the world. They are the basis of the middle phase's psychoeducation about interpersonal skills and the promotion of positive interactions.

Technique: Using I Statements

Definition: To start a statement using an "I feel" statement.
Example: "*I feel hurt when you don't make an effort to listen to me and when you spend more time with my sister.*"

Technique: Strike While the Iron is Cold

Definition: It is best to have a conversation about a problem when the two people are calm, not when feeling angry.
Example: "*Mom, I really want to talk to you, but we are both so angry at the moment. Can we calm down and talk about it later?*"

Technique: Give to Get

Definition: It is important to let the other person know that you understand their perspective in the situation before stating your own.
Example: "*Mom, I know that you are working lots of hours these days and money is tight, but is there a way for us to find the money so I can go to the prom like my friends?*"

Technique: All in the Timing

Definition: It is very important to figure out the best time to have a conversation—when the other person can focus, and when he is not doing something else simultaneously.
Example: "*Dad, I would like to talk to you about my plans for the summer. Do you think we can talk about this on Sunday after you get home from church?*"

Technique: Do Not Give Up

Definition: It takes more than one try to change your own and others' ways of communicating and interacting, so you have to keep trying strategies over and over again.
Example: "*Your mom didn't respond exactly the way you wanted this time. What do you think might happen if you try to talk to her again?*"

Technique: Be Specific, and Avoid "Always" and "Never"

Definition: When talking with another person, keep the conversation focused on the current time period on which you want to work.
Example: "*I know you worry when I go out with my friends, but I would really like to go on Saturday to the movies with Steve* [versus] *You never let me go out with my friends on the weekend, but I want to go on Saturday.*"

Technique: Be Willing to Compromise and Practice the Art of Negotiation

Definition: When trying to find a compromise between two points of view, it is good to have possible solutions in mind and learn how to meet someone part of the way so that each of you gets part of what you want and avoids a standstill.

Example: *"I know you are worried about my safety when I am out with my friends and that's why you don't want me to go. What if I call you when I get to the theater and call you when I am leaving? Or, what if we arrange to speak twice during the time I am out of the house like at 7 and 9 PM?"*

TERMINATION PHASE (SESSIONS 9–12)

The goal of the *termination phase* is to clarify warning symptoms of future depressive episodes, identify successful strategies used in the middle phase, foster generalization of skills to future situations, emphasize mastery of new interpersonal skills, and discuss the need for further treatment. Session-specific tasks are as follows:

Sessions 9 and 10

Task: Remind the adolescent that three sessions remain after today (this is explicitly discussed in the next three sessions).

"I just want to remind you that we have three sessions after today."

Task: Continue to work on the identified problem area with an eye toward what the adolescent has accomplished and the areas for future and continued work.

Task: Begin this session as you have every other but, rather than exploring the events of the week, talk specifically about mood and symptom change throughout the treatment.

"How would you rate your mood for this past week? Let's talk today about how your symptoms and mood have changed over the last ten sessions. Do you remember what symptoms you had when you first came here? (It is helpful to refer to the original depression rating scale and mood rating). *What do you think has contributed to the change? Which symptoms haven't changed? What have you been doing that has been affecting your symptoms and mood?"*

Task: Assess the status of problem area focus—what has changed, what has not.

"Now I'd like to talk about the interpersonal problem(s) that contributed to your depression. How are things going with (fill in the specific problem)? *or, How are things going between you and your parents? Let's talk about that. What has changed, and what still needs work?"*

Task: Discuss reasons for changes—what the adolescent did and specific skills he used.

"Why do you think things changed? (Refer to the specific interpersonal problem.) *What specifically did you do?* (This should be a discussion about the strategies the adolescent has been trying to use.) *How do you see these changes affecting your mood?"*

Task: The warning signs of relapse of the depression should be discussed. If the symptoms did not completely remit, the therapist needs to address the idea of a partial remission and what the adolescent's options are in order to continue treatment in pursuit of a complete remission.

"As you know, depression may recur. Do you remember what depression symptoms you had when you first came here? (If adolescent does not remember, then the therapist should remind her.) *These are symptoms that you need to watch out for in the future. Of all those symptoms, which are most important to you?"*

Session 11

Task: Invite parents to discuss the adolescent's experience in treatment, effect on family, parents' feelings about termination, and the need for further treatment. This can be done with or without the adolescent present.

> *"As you know, Bill has two more sessions remaining. I'd like to spend part of today talking with you about the work he has done. What changes have you seen in Bill? (Get them to be specific, including symptom and behavioral changes.) How has he accomplished these? What role did you play? What do you think he needs to continue to work on? What are your concerns? How do you feel about his stopping treatment?"* (Address nonresponse and other options if necessary.)

Session 12

Task: Identify future triggers for depression and the specific skills the adolescent will use to counteract these triggers. Discuss feelings about termination (both adolescent and therapist), as well as the need for future treatment should the adolescent encounter difficulties. Options for maintenance treatment sessions should be discussed.

> *"Today is your last session. We'll complete your final mood and symptom check and then talk about what you think may be future triggers for depression, skills you have learned to help you manage those triggers, and your feelings about termination. After that, we'll talk about options you have for psychotherapy in the future. As you look into the future, what situations do you think might be stressful and/or trigger another depression?"*

In addition to what the adolescent discusses, the therapist should be prepared to suggest future situations that she thinks could be stressful enough to trigger a depressive episode. The therapist should use the situation that the adolescent has suggested and ask how he would handle it to foster generalization of skills as a relapse prevention technique.

> *"Now let's talk about your feelings about ending our weekly sessions."*

Process the adolescent's feelings and talk a little about your feelings. Next, talk about continuation or maintenance treatment. If IPT-A has not worked, discuss other possible treatments that the adolescent might try.

MAINTENANCE TREATMENT

Therapists using IPT with adults have found that continuation/maintenance sessions can be helpful in providing opportunities to further consolidate and practice skills learned in the acute phase of treatment. It is generally recommended that treatment continue for at least 6 months following symptom remission to consolidate the treatment response and avoid relapse.[5] However, this is based primarily on adult treatment studies and clinical consensus.

The treatment discussed in this section is for those adolescents who have achieved remission or partial remission. The continuation model usually consists of tapering sessions after the acute phase to two sessions a month for 2 to 3 months, followed by another 3 months of monthly sessions. The maintenance model consists of monthly therapy sessions for 6 to 12 months after the acute treatment has ended. In either model, the therapist continues to emphasize the interpersonal strategies learned and practiced during acute treatment while addressing any current and future interpersonal stressors as a strategy to prevent a recurrence of depressive symptoms.

Currently, there are no clinical trials studying the use of IPT-A as a continuation or maintenance treatment; however, clinical practice suggests it is useful in helping adolescents feel more confident in their skills and abilities, enabling them to generalize the skills to new situations. Testing of this model in clinical trials is needed.

TABLE 9.2 EMPIRICAL EVIDENCE FOR IPT-A

Study	Treatment Modality	Control Condition	Age of Subjects (yr)	N	Diagnosis	Setting	Results
Mufson et al., 1999[6]	Individual IPT-A 12 sessions	Clinical monitoring	12–18	48	DSM-III-R diagnosis of MDD	Clinic	The IPT-A group showed greater reductions in depression and more improvement in social and global functioning than the clinical monitoring control group. No follow-up reported.
Rossello and Bernal, 1999[8]	Individual IPT-A; Individual CBT 12 sessions	Wait list	13–18	71	DSM-III-R diagnosis of MDD	Clinic	The IPT-A and CBT groups improved more than the control group. There was no significant difference in the primary measure between CBT and IPT-A. The IPT-A group showed greatest improvement in social functioning and self-esteem. No significant differences were found between IPT-A and CBT groups at 3-month follow-up.
Mufson et al., 2004[7]	Individual IPT-A 12 sessions	Treatment as usual	12–17	63	DSM-IV diagnosis of MDD, dysthymia, MDD NOS, or adjustment disorder with depressed mood	School-based clinics	Adolescents treated with IPT-A showed significant reductions in depression symptoms by both therapist and self-report measures, as well as significant improvement in overall functioning and in specific domains of social functioning
Young et al., 2006[9]	IPT-AST (Adolescent Skills Training) 8 sessions	Treatment as usual	11–16	41	Subthreshold depression symptoms (no DSM-IV diagnosis)	School (classroom-based school screening)	Adolescents who received IPT-AST had significantly fewer depression symptoms and better overall functioning post-intervention and at 3- and 6-month follow-up. Adolescents in IPT-AST also reported fewer depression diagnoses than adolescents receiving treatment as usual (school counseling).

MDD, major depressive disorder; MDD NOS, major depressive disorder not otherwise specified.

EMPIRICAL EVIDENCE

The efficacy and effectiveness of IPT-A for reducing adolescents' depressive symptoms have been examined in three randomized controlled clinical trials,[6,7,8] and the prevention model has been examined in one randomized controlled clinical trial.[9]

RATING THE EVIDENCE

Table 9.2 summarizes the empirical studies about the effectiveness of IPT-A. A differentiation needs to be made between IPT-A as a theoretical orientation and a specific manualized approach. As a theoretical orientation, IPT-A meets the criteria of a well-established treatment for adolescent depression: (1) its efficacy was demonstrated by two different teams of investigators, (2) it has been described in well-delineated treatment manuals, and (3) it has been compared to a minimal treatment as well as to another active treatment. These studies included moderate sample sizes with detailed sample characteristics. Finally, it is one of the few treatments that has demonstrated transportability and continued effectiveness when delivered by community clinicians in a real-world setting.

However, one of the research teams that replicated its efficacy[6] did not use the same manual as the Mufson team (although they followed the same general IPT strategies and techniques). Thus, technically, the IPT-A manualized protocol (by the Mufson group) meets criteria for a probably efficacious intervention.

RESOURCES FOR PATIENTS AND FAMILIES

Fristad MA, Goldberg-Arnold JS. *Raising a Moody Child: How to Cope with Depression and Bipolar Disorder*. New York: Guilford Press; 2004.

Koplewicz HS. *More Than Moody: Recognizing and Treating Adolescent Depression*. New York: Putnam's Sons; 2002 (also published as a paperback by Penguin).

Mufson L, Dorta KP, Moreau D, et al. *Interpersonal Psychotherapy for Depressed Adolescents*. 2nd ed. New York: Guilford Press; 2004.

Depression and Bipolar Support Alliance (DBSA): www.dbsalliance.org/site/PageServer?pagename=about_depression_lifespan

RESOURCES FOR PROFESSIONALS

References 6, 7, 8, and 9.

For more information about the use of IPT-A for the treatment of adolescent depression, refer to the complete treatment manual (reference 4).

REFERENCES

1. Weissman MM, Markowitz JC, Klerman GL. *A Comprehensive Guide to Interpersonal Psychotherapy*. New York: Basic Books; 2000.
2. Mufson L, Moreau D, Weissman MM, et al. Modification of interpersonal psychotherapy with depressed adolescence (IPT-A): phase I and phase II studies. *J Am Acad Child Adolesc Psychiatry*. 1994;33:695–705.
3. Puig-Antich J, Lukens E, Davies M, et al. Psychosocial functioning in prepubertal depressive disorders II: interpersonal relationships after sustained recovery from affective episode. *Arch Gen Psychiatry*. 1985;42: 511–517.
4. Mufson L, Dorta KP, Moreau D, et al. *Interpersonal Psychotherapy for Depressed Adolescents*. 2nd ed. New York: Guilford Press; 2004.
5. Birmaher B, Brent D, AACAP Work Group on Quality Issues. Practice parameter for the assessment and treatment of children and adolescents with depressive disorders. *J Am Acad Child Adolesc Psychiatry*. 2007;46:1503–1526.
6. Mufson L, Weissman MM, Moreau D, et al. Efficacy of interpersonal psychotherapy for depressed adolescents. *Arch Gen Psychiatry*. 1999;56:573–579.

7. Mufson L, Dorta KP, Wickramaratne P, et al. A randomized effectiveness trial of interpersonal psychotherapy for depressed adolescents. *Arch Gen Psychiatry.* 2004;61:577–584.

8. Rosselló J, Bernal G. The efficacy of cognitive-behavioral and interpersonal treatments for depression in Puerto Rican adolescents. *J Consult Clin Psychol.* 1999;67:734–745.

9. Young JL, Mufson L, Davies M. Efficacy of interpersonal psychotherapy—adolescent skills training: an indicated preventive intervention for depression. *J Child Psychol Psychiatry.* 2006;47:1254–1262.

Using Family Therapy[a]

LEONARD WOODS

KEY POINTS

- Most risk factors for onset, relapse, and recurrence of depression in children and adolescents occur in the family context (e.g., parental depression, poor bonding, divorce, parent–child conflict, abuse, or trauma).
- Instead of prescribing family therapy because "it must be the family causing the depression," family therapy assists the family to cope with the illness and to modify individual, psychological, and interactive factors that may be at play.
- Clinicians should be careful when implying that parental rearing practices, relationships, or psychiatric disorders are the cause of dysfunctional interactions because these problems may be driven, in part, by the child's current psychopathology.
- A family treatment approach seeks to reduce risk factors and enhance protective factors by increasing positive interactions between parents and children, and by increasing understanding of the illness for everyone in the family.
- Providing psychoeducation to the family about the mutual influence between illness, individual and family may facilitate engagement in family treatment.
- Be aware of your beliefs or assumptions about families. They will greatly influence your ability to engage or use the family as a resource to treat a child's or adolescent's depression.
- Obtain the family's perspective and beliefs about the risk factors in their unique situation; a pie chart may be the simplest and quickest way to accomplish this.
- Identify and address risk factors for this unique family.
- Block or interrupt patterns of interaction that are not working.
- Create a space to experience alternative interactions with better outcomes.
- Use in-session enactments to facilitate the direct experience of interacting differently that may result in family members' experiencing successful relationship outcomes.
- Increase supportive mechanisms that serve as protective factors.
- Provide psychoeducation on possible signs of recurrence of the depression and ways to address these if they occur.
- Sensitivity toward issues of race, culture, ethnicity, and gender for specific groups is imperative to treat families from different cultural backgrounds.

[a]Portions of the material come from my collaboration with colleagues and fellow trainers at Western Psychiatric Institute and Clinic of UPMC Presbyterian-Shadyside. Credits to the Family Based Mental Health Training Services: Patricia Johnston QCSW, BCD, Robert Sheen, MA, LMFT, Cynthia Stone, MS, LMFT, and Robert Sukolsky, MS, NCC; as well as colleagues at Western Psychiatric Institute and Clinic, Center for Children and Families who worked with me on preparation of the *Family Therapy Treatment Manual* for our Child and Adolescent Outpatient Clinic: Amy Chisholm, MA, Amy DeMario, LCSW, Bradley Sanders, LCSW.

Introduction   *The two most consistent risk factors for adolescent major depressive disorder (MDD) are being female and a history of MDD in the family.[1,2] A 20-year follow up study by Pilowsky[3] showed that "parental depression is associated with family discord and is a consistent risk factor for offspring major depressive disorder." It further concluded that "family discord factors may be a risk factor for major depressive disorder in offspring of non-depressed parents." Further studies have shown that treating parental depression reduces diagnoses and symptoms in the children.[4] These matters are described in detail in Chapter 2. However, it is worth highlighting that factors predicting or contributing to onset, recurrence, and relapse of MDD in children and adolescents are mostly adverse family environments, such as absence of supportive interactions, poor parental bonding or attachment, harsh discipline, parental divorce, family and parent–child conflict, abuse, rejection, and high expressed emotion.[5–8] Most findings suggest that stresses in young persons' social environment— whether family, peer, or school network—influence the emergence, amelioration, or exacerbation of a depressive episode. Conversely, once adolescents are depressed, they themselves become a significant influence on their own social environment.[9,10]*

EVIDENCE ABOUT EFFECTIVENESS OF FAMILY THERAPY

"It is virtually impossible to successfully treat a child or adolescent patient without the close involvement of parents."[10] Given that most risk factors occur within the family context, it would appear the family would be the natural focus of intervention for most depressed children and adolescents.[11–13]

Diamond and Siqueland conducted a review of randomized clinical trials in which parents were included as primary participants in the treatment of child and adolescent psychiatric disorders. They concluded that "for many disorders, family treatment can be an effective stand-alone intervention or an augmentation to other treatments."[14] Trowell et al.[15] studied the use of family therapy and individual psychodynamic therapy in a group of clinically depressed youth. They reported significant reductions in the rate of disorders with both therapies and a reduction in comorbid conditions. Changes in both treatment groups persisted at the 6-month follow-up. An attachment-based family therapy[16] was more effective in adolescent depression than wait list or no treatment, and improvement was maintained at 6-month follow-up. An influential study of depressed youth, which compared the use of cognitive behavioral therapy (CBT), nondirective supportive therapy (NST), and systemic behavioral family therapy (SBFT), showed that all three interventions were effective.[17] Although CBT performed better for acute treatment, CBT was not superior to SBFT or NST when the effects of maternal depression were taken into account. At 2-year follow-up, SBFT had impacted on family conflict and parent–child relationship problems more than CBT or NST.

Although randomized controlled trials (RCTs) of family therapy are scarce and the empirical evidence weak, what there is indicates that intervening at the level of family risk factors can influence the course and outcome of youth depressive episodes.[12,16,18,19–22]

SYSTEMS THEORY

Before discussing how to use family therapy, it is important to review briefly some of the theoretical underpinnings of this treatment modality. Family therapy has largely evolved from the concepts of systems theory,[23] which conceptualize the family as a system and propose that components of a system are interconnected and interactions regulated by means of "recursive feedback loops," the system attempting always to maintain a balance. That is, individual family members respond to each other to maintain the balance or "homeostasis" within the family system. Any behavior or symptom would thus be understood within the context of the system. Earlier practitioners saw the individual's symptoms as a reflection of dysfunction in the larger system; modifying factors within the family system was the route to eliminating symptoms in the individual. This simplistic view, which used mechanical systems as a model, can easily move from "recursive feedback loops" to "circular causality," and to the covert or overt assumption that because symptoms exist in a family context, interactions within the family *cause* the mental illness, ignoring biologic factors that may also be at play. This type of thinking was quite off-putting to many families.

RECIPROCAL INFLUENCE VERSUS CAUSALITY

Most contemporary family therapy theorists of childhood disorders acknowledge reciprocal influences among genetic, personality, cognitive, behavioral, familial, interpersonal, and sociocultural factors in the emergence and maintenance of the depressive illness.[24,25] Although temperament, personality, and internalized meanings of individual experiences are at play in us all and may become predisposing factors for psychopathology, a person's biologic or genetic makeup also influences and is influenced by systemic interactions. In that context, children can be seen as positively and negatively influencing their families and vice versa—families influencing their children.

Most researchers are also aware of the larger sociocultural influences at play.[26] How we are acculturated to social expectations regarding gender, status as a majority or minority member of our society, our beliefs about mental illness, and so on, influence the range of options we instinctively believe are available to us.

Rather than focusing on causality (i.e., deciding whether the chicken or the egg came first), clinicians can take what already exists and engage families in treatment. Instead of prescribing family therapy because "it must be the family causing the depression," this approach views family treatment as assisting the family to cope with the illness and to modify individual, psychological, and interactive factors that may be at play. This is similar to the situation in families struggling to deal with chronic medical conditions like diabetes.

Research seems to support the view of reciprocal influence versus causality. For example, a study of factors that may influence a group of children and adolescents at risk of developing MDD did not find any that were highly predictive.[27] The authors concluded that "family and peer interactions of the high risk youth were similar to the interactions of the healthy controls" and that dysfunctional family patterns seemed to depend mainly on the child's depressive symptoms. "Clinicians should be careful when implying that parental rearing practices, relationships, and/or psychiatric disorders are the cause of family dysfunctional interactions because these problems may be driven, in part, by the child's current psychopathology" was one of the conclusions.[27]

SKILL LEVELS FOR FAMILY INTERVENTION

Family treatments are broader than just formalized family therapy. Irrespective of the context in which clinicians work (primary care physician, school counselor, inpatient unit, emergency room, etc.), there will be opportunities to engage families. Job context and responsibilities, training and comfort level will all influence the role that one may take with a family, but families can be used in different forms to assist a young person struggling with depression. A continuum of levels of intervention and generic skills necessary to be successful at each level follows.

1. *Giving feedback and information to the family about depression and the treatment of the individual family member (psychoeducation).* One must be willing and open to talk with families and give information about the present diagnosis and treatment of the family member. This includes education about biologic influences, effects of depression on cognitions and of cognitions on depression, influences of depression on relationships (family, marriage, work, school, and social) and of relationships on depression. One needs to remain open and honest to build trust and rapport, as well as to deal with naturally occurring fear and reluctance on the part of family members.

2. *Taking a history to better understand what is happening and make recommendations or referral.* One needs the skills listed in number 1 and the ability to ask questions respectfully about family structure, family's history (biologic, psychological, interactional), strengths, attempted solutions, internal and external resources, and family's beliefs about the illness, the patient, and therapy. One needs the ability to listen empathically, a basic knowledge of family development and transitions, and confidence in identifying and stopping harmful interactions among family members.

2A. *Single session using the family as a consultant to the treatment.* Such a session would require the skills described in numbers 1 and 2, as well as the ability to summarize and give feedback to the family about the content of what they shared with the clinician, and possible hypotheses or additional insights they may have given regarding understanding and treating the patient's depression.

3. *Family meeting to problem-solve interactional issues influencing or being influenced by the depression.* An intervention at this level would require the skills mentioned in the previous headings as well as confidence in clarifying issues and problem solving in a family context. One should also have the ability to recognize when problems are above one's head (e.g., related to "how stuck" a family is in their interactional patterns and in need of referral to someone with more expertise).

4. *Family therapy.* To conduct family therapy, one requires all the skills listed in the previous headings as well as having the training, experience, and supervision in a method of family therapy.

DRAWING A PIE CHART OF THE AREAS OF INFLUENCE

One simple tool for discussing and assessing areas of influence and risk factors that can be used across all levels of intervention is to engage the patient and/or family in drawing a pie chart of the areas of influence (biologic, psychological [thinking], social [interactive]), as seen by them, or to assess their effect in the present situation. This provides a way of educating patients about the complex factors at play simply and efficiently. This task allows clinicians to work with the patient collaboratively by finding about the young person's belief system and to prescribe a treatment consistent with the patient's experience and beliefs rather than reinforcing the clinician's own thinking.

When young persons (or family) recognize that family or interactional patterns are affecting the emergence or maintenance of depression—or that depression is affecting the family—they may be open to family treatment. Similarly, if a patient or family is able to identify a strong biologic component as well as interactional patterns, using medication and family therapy concurrently would not only be consistent with research findings but also match the belief system of the patient and family, thus increasing the probability of adherence.

ENGAGEMENT

Effectiveness research is increasingly showing the strength of the alliance between therapist and client, rather than the model of treatment, is one of the most important factors influencing outcome.[28] Most family therapists pay particular attention to establishing a strong therapeutic alliance with the family as a whole or with particular subsystems like the adolescent or parents. If the therapist is able to maintain a positive view, this will increase the ability to engage a family in a true therapeutic alliance. To engage a family (especially parents) effectively, clinicians must be able to believe in the positive intent of most family interactions (even in the midst of some terrible situations) and view interactions as becoming "stuck" rather than judging individuals for their behaviors.

CORE BELIEFS

One of the most difficult aspects when dealing with families is maintaining a strength-focused or positive perspective. Much of the current health training centers predominantly on disease, dysfunction, illness, and pathology, partly as a result of health insurance reimbursement demands. A biomedical view has become the most commonly held. This creates ambiguous situations (e.g., when a patient does not respond to first-line treatment, usually medication or individual psychotherapy). It is at this point that a referral for family therapy is usually considered, often with the simplistic message (overt or covert) that "if the individual and pharmacological treatments didn't work, it must be the family that is influencing the patient's depression." The next small but unhelpful step is to believe that the family is *causing* the depression or, at the very least, interfering with our efforts to treat it. Conversely, the longer family members struggle unsuccessfully with a child's depression, the more stuck they can become in mutually reinforcing ineffective patterns that can lead the treatment team to see the family in a negative light.

Every clinician carries personal, professional, and sociocultural bias (positive and negative) about families that influence their beliefs and automatic thoughts regarding families and depression. This varies from country to country, but it is important to be aware of and, when needed, to challenge these beliefs if we are to engage families successfully.

Depending on the context in which the family is seen (e.g., child protective services, psychiatric emergency room, juvenile court probation, inpatient unit), one is likely to deal with families at a time of high stress and emotional turmoil, and they can become intimidating and overwhelming to the professionals looking after them. It is easy to understand how—out of self-protection—clinicians may develop ways of thinking about and dealing with these families that are less than positive or strength based. However, the training of psychiatric residents in the United States and elsewhere is increasingly emphasizing the need for skills in family therapy and an appreciation of the potential positive role of the family.

CULTURE AND ETHNICITY

Addressing how racial, ethnic, and cultural backgrounds affect family therapy is beyond the scope of this chapter (see Chapters 23 and 24). However, the cultural assumptions that both family and clinician bring to the therapy process will influence the outcome of treatment. Having a sense of the issues of race, culture, ethnicity, and gender for specific groups is imperative to treat families from different cultural backgrounds. No clinician can be expert in all cultures, so it is critical to educate and sensitize oneself to issues and values across cultures. Excellent resources exist for increasing clinicians' appreciation for this subject.[29] Even if one could become knowledgeable about all cultures, each family should be approached as a unique entity because not all families of Irish, African American, Eastern European, or any other ethnicity or culture are homogeneous. The most important resource for understanding any family's culture is the "expert family" sitting in the room. The golden rule should be this: *When in doubt, trust and ask the family to explain what one needs to know and appreciate in order to work with that unique family.*

An example of how cultural issues impinge on family therapy is the sensitivity of some African Americans to give family information by doing a genogram too early in treatment, before they have established trust with the clinician. Another example is the intergenerational clash in some recently immigrated families over whether to "acculturate" or to keep their culture of origin. This is especially troublesome when the parental generation wants to remain true to their culture of origin and children are fighting to assimilate to the new culture. Not understanding these issues through the lenses of the values of these families can lead to misunderstandings and possibly pathologizing healthy cultural values.

REFRAMING

When one deals with families, one immediately begins to be influenced by them as much as one is influencing them. Families present with interactions or ways of dealing with issues that can be challenging to clinicians and may lead to unhelpful judgments and reactions. Methods of discipline, expressions of anger and hurt, responses to children's mood, to name few, can be perceived by clinicians as having ill intent, leading to attempts to change these persons' methods without understanding the intent. A stance on the part of the clinician that remains "respectfully curious" and looks for a noble intent, rather than becoming critical, is most productive.

A technique known as "reframing" uses a shifting of the perspective or "frame" of a behavior by stating the positive intent behind a behavior to assist the change of focus. An example would be reframing a father's loud and angry tone when his son fails a class as "the way he is attempting to show his concern about his son's future." If the father agrees that this is his *mission* or intention (to influence a positive future for his child), you can engage them in evaluating if this particular method is effective. If both agree that indeed this works and the son improves his performance every time his father yells, it can be assumed the father would continue to employ this method. On the contrary, if they agree it doesn't work or that it has some other negative effects, one could engage them in exploring other more effective methods.

POSITIVE ASSUMPTIONS

Following are some of the beliefs that have been transmitted to me by various mentors, colleagues, and families. I have found these assumptions assist me in working from a positive or strength-based perspective.

- Families do not *cause* mental illness.
- It is a privilege for therapists when a family lets us work with them at such an intimate level as required by family therapy.
- It takes courage and humility for a family to be in treatment.

- People have the potential to change and act or interact differently.
- The family is trying its best to solve and manage this problem.
- Families want what is best for the family but often do ineffective or unhelpful things to achieve it.
- If I can identify the intent or mission and help the family construct an alternative method of accomplishing it (that meets their personal and cultural value system), they will be willing to try.

BALANCING TREATMENT AND SAFETY

Although this may vary according to country and culture, practice in the Unite States requires balancing respect for the independence of the family with the statutory requirements of being a mandated reporter of abuse or neglect, as well as the danger of suicidal or homicidal acts. To balance these two, sometimes competing, demands, I distinguish *control of the family* (what they do, decisions they make) from the *responsibility for providing treatment*. What the family does or does not do is 90% the responsibility of the family and 10% the responsibility of the clinician. The 10% that belongs to clinicians reflects (1) the responsibility as mandated reporters in cases of abuse or neglect, (2) the responsibility of seeking involuntary commitment in cases of clear and present danger owing to mental illness, and (3) the duty to warn in cases of homicidal intent. It is essential to explain this to a family in the first meeting when delineating the parameters of confidentiality.

In regard to the *responsibility for the process of treatment*, I see the therapist as 51% responsible. Clinicians are responsible for providing the expertise and leadership in an informed process in which families may choose to engage to address their struggle with depressive illness. The 49% responsibility of the families reflects (1) their involvement, whether they choose to engage and continue in treatment or not; and (2) bringing the courage and honesty necessary to make the process effective.

ASSESSING TO INDIVIDUALIZE TREATMENT

Once a family is engaged, a template for assessing areas that are influencing or being influenced by the depression is needed. Instead of one particular model of family therapy (each of which focuses on particular aspects of family interaction as the target for intervention), a broader assessment is proposed. The specifics of the intervention can subsequently be chosen based on the family's belief system and expectations as well as therapists' particular skills. This allows for specific targeting of the unique risk factors that may be present.

Some information is obtained from details that people tell you directly, other from observing how the family interacts. Different therapists use different systems to gather data to make an assessment. In the programs in which I am presently involved, several tools are used: genogram,[30] structural maps,[31] family and illness timelines, an eco-map, and observation of family interactions in a structured first interview format (modified from Jay Haley).[32] These tools can be used at the beginning of treatment or later, depending on the family.

GENOGRAM

Genograms are diagrams listing family members and their relationships, ideally to a minimum of three generations. This family history seeks more than just dates and names. It intends to capture a sense of the family's relationships and an appreciation of patterns and values through the generations. Focus may vary (e.g., history of depression and other psychopathologies through the generations, beliefs about causes or treatments for depression, pattern of interactions, parenting practices through the generations, and traumas). Family transitions, attempted solutions to deal with depression or conflicts, and relationships after a divorce are other possible areas of exploration.

TIMELINES

Timelines can be used to track the particular depressive episode as well as influences or events around the time of onset. This may lead to finding connections between happenings within the family and the depression. The onset of a depressive episode may be close to a relocation or some other event. Past losses or traumas may be seen through the timelines as associated with the onset of the depression or that they had not been resolved. It is not uncommon to find many years later that a family is still struggling to resolve an earlier trauma or loss.

STRUCTURAL MAPS

Structural maps are visual representations of the family's interactions, how they relate to each other. The map seeks to capture the hierarchy, subsystems, power, closeness/distance of relationships, as well as the boundaries between and among subsystems and individuals. The structure is then assessed for aspects that assist or hinder the family's goal of helping the depressed child. Resources and strengths are identified as well as ways the family is interacting or organized that may have been effective in the past but now are hindering functioning or causing conflict. A basic tenet of systems theory is the need for families to adjust as situations change (e.g., to accommodate the evolving needs of children growing up). For example, a father and his 11-year-old daughter spend daddy/daughter time by going to the mall on Saturdays. This had become a very enjoyable and predictable pattern that developed between the two. Suddenly, one Saturday at the age of 13, the daughter as usual requests, "Dad, could you drive me to the mall?" The father instinctively prepares himself physically, emotionally and cognitively for an afternoon of quality time with his daughter. When they get to the mall and Father turns the car off, the daughter asks, "Where are you going? I'm going to meet my friends. Didn't Mom tell you? She said I could." Instead of the usual closeness from their typical Saturday together, this could set off misunderstandings and feelings of hurt and anger that may distance the two.

ECO-MAPS

Eco-maps are diagrams of the relationships between and among the other systems involved in the family's life. This includes friends, work, school, place of worship, and so on. For some families, other entities, such as mental health, legal, and child protective services, medical personnel, and welfare agencies, are also relevant. The eco-map graphically represents the family's judgment as to how positive or negative these relationships are. This allows assessing possible collaborations that can be used or negative influences that may be exacerbating the depression or hindering the family's ability to manage the illness better.

Assessing different domains allows an appreciation of each family's unique experience, beliefs, and expectations. A description of each of these areas is beyond the scope of this chapter, but interested readers can find detailed information in the references provided. These are the areas:

1. Family structure or organization[31]
2. Development (individual, couple, family)[33]
3. Biology (medical, genetic, biochemical contributions)[34]
4. Meaning (beliefs, language, myths both implicit and explicit)[35]
5. Patterns of solution/interaction[32,36]
6. Trauma and loss (past and present)[37,38,39]
7. Larger systems (mental health, school, work, etc.)[40]
8. Social constructs (gender, race, economic, stigma, socioeconomic, etc.)[41-46]

OUTLINE OF THERAPY

What follows describes briefly, within the requirements of a book of this kind, what usually transpires during family therapy: goals, stages, issues, and problems. This is neither prescriptive nor representative of all types of family therapy—that vary considerably according to practitioner and theoretical orientation—although the basic skills are similar. Those interested in a deeper understanding can obtain more information from the Resources for Practitioners section.

INVITING KEY PLAYERS

A general rule is to get as many family members as possible present for the first session. Fathers, although a key member of the family, are often unavailable or reluctant. Explaining the rationale for inviting more than just the depressed youth presents the first challenge. Are you asking everyone to attend because you want everyone who might possibly be contributing to the depression? Or because they are the greatest resource to help this youth and the clinician?

PHASE ONE: ORIENTATION AND ASSESSMENT (SESSIONS 1–3)

The first interview usually follows five stages, which are largely self-explanatory: greeting and orientation, social, problem/change, interactional, and summary and treatment planning. The goals for this phase include (1) educating the family about the clinician and treatment modality, (2) establishing therapeutic rapport, (3) initiating family assessment (structural map, genogram, timeline, eco-map, semistructured first interview, assessment of the eight areas of potential influence or risk), and (4) establishing a treatment contract.

One begins the first session by greeting each family member individually (usually from eldest to youngest) and asking how they would like to be referred to, followed by an explanation of who you are and how they may refer to you. Subsequently, clinicians give basic information about themselves, their style, and the rationale for using family therapy, highlighting the limitations to confidentiality.

From the moment of first contact and throughout the rest of treatment, clinicians must struggle to establish and maintain rapport on two levels, hierarchical and lateral. *Hierarchal rapport* is established by showing that the therapist is capable and willing to "deliver the goods." *Lateral rapport* is established when the client feels comfortable because the clinician is perceived as empathetic, respectful, trustworthy, and understanding.

The *social stage* represents a deliberate effort to know each person (competencies, strengths, skills, and positive aspects of each individual as well as the family) and not just problems. Following this, the therapist seeks to gain a clear appreciation of how each member sees the problem and orients toward change by identifying what changes each family member would like to see regarding the problem. This requires asking examples and clarifying what the family has already tried, what worked and what did not.

In the *interaction stage,* clinicians often set up tasks leading toward interaction (diagnostic enactment) among family members to "get the problem in the room"—by saying something like "I'd like to get a feel for how you all get stuck. Would you be willing to talk about x, y, and z?" This is not necessary if enactments have spontaneously occurred already during the interview and have been identified as a focus for treatment.

Establishing a treatment contract requires giving feedback to the family, clarifying the safety plan, negotiating the meeting structure, and the development of the treatment plan in collaboration with the family. Feedback should summarize the therapist's impressions (after gathering the data from the various instruments) about the diagnosis and risk factors present in this unique family. If the family does not agree with the therapists' formulation, a contract can nevertheless be agreed on to deal with the areas that are influencing or being influenced by the depression. Between-session tasks can also be discussed. It is important to administer a depression rating scale (see Chapter 3) to quantify the severity of symptoms at baseline, which can later be used to evaluate progress and outcome. By the end of sessions 2 or 3, it is generally expected for the clinician and family to have developed a treatment plan collaboratively containing measurable goals.

PHASE TWO: INTERVENTION: PUSH FOR CHANGE (SESSIONS 3–8 OR 10)

In this phase the therapist seeks to provide the family with direct, in-session experiences of more satisfying and effective ways of interacting, keeping in mind the following goals: to orient the family toward change and keep treatment focused, to decrease patterns that negatively influence the child's symptoms or family relations, to facilitate in-session positive interactions, and to prescribe between-session tasks (homework).

Each session begins by checking safety issues, setting the agenda, and clarifying whether other topics need to be dealt with. This is followed by discussion of the outcome of experiments or homework. The focus is on "what worked, was successful, positive, or good," always directing the family toward the ultimate goal by reverting to the desired changes that are occurring or not. *Enactment*[31] is the primary tool for facilitating positive in-session experiences. An enactment is an interaction (usually between two family members) that seeks to give participants a different, more satisfying outcome. The therapist also tries to assist the family in blocking negative interactions previously identified, often by deliberately manipulating boundaries between family members or subsystems. This usually requires direct therapist intervention, such as raising a finger (to indicate wait a minute), holding a hand up (stop or stay out), ignoring someone, or deliberately making eye contact with someone.

PHASE THREE: REVIEW AND DISPOSITION (SESSIONS 8–12)

This phase starts with a review of treatment (in about session 8) by readministering depression scales and requesting an assessment by parents and child of progress in meeting the goals of treatment. If the goals have been achieved, the focus changes to the process of termination and strategies for preventing relapse. If goals have not been met but progress was made, the family and clinician may agree to continue with treatment as per phase two. The benefits of continuing with family therapy will need to be reconsidered if progress has not occurred. Appropriate referral options may then be contemplated.

When mental health conditions in parents or sibling come to light during therapy, it may be at this juncture that referral for evaluation and treatment for these family members may be broached. Parents who have been struggling with depression (or other illnesses) and not sought treatment may be open to do so now to help their child. Again, the intent with which such a recommendation is made will greatly increase or decrease the chances of their accepting the recommendation.

If comorbid disorders (such as ADHD, anxiety, etc.) have become known during treatment, it would also be at this point that the family therapy may continue but shift focus to address the comorbid disorder as well. If appropriate, information can be given about referral to another specialist for more specific intervention for conditions such as substance abuse (see Chapter 18), bipolar illness, posttraumatic stress disorder, or obsessive-compulsive disorder.

One of the goals of this stage is *prevention of relapse and recurrence*, particularly important in MDD because of its recurrent nature (see Chapter 1). As part of the review and termination process, it is important to recall what symptoms brought family members into treatment, what changes have been made, and what they did that was effective. This is the beginning of a relapse prevention plan. *Warning signs* that may indicate recurrence are collaboratively identified; highlighting that the quicker they learn to spot these signs, the sooner they can take positive action. Many times the first step is remembering what was effective during treatment and to reapply that if problems recur. Another aspect is to agree on symptoms or interactions that would indicate the need for reapplying solutions, booster sessions, or using emergency services.

It needs to be emphasized that events or situations can occur at any stage of treatment that require a review and consideration of referral. These events include, but are not restricted to, a significant deterioration in the child's depression or mental state, high suicide or homicide risk, poor fit or conflict between therapist and family, and marked family turmoil.

CHALLENGES AND SOLUTIONS, PARTICULARLY WHEN DEALING WITH ADOLESCENTS

- *Stigma.* The stigma of mental health treatment among teens in America—and all over the world—is high. Acknowledging this fact and allowing for a normalization of the teen's concerns may allow him or her to move beyond this and engage in treatment.
- *Therapy as punishment.* Teens may correctly or incorrectly perceive their parents' decision to undertake family therapy as another method of punishing them. If so, it is important to deal directly with this problem so the family can correct misperceptions or to shift the focus to an attempt to make things better for both the teen and the family as a whole.
- *Family influences the therapist to appear aligned with parents or with the adolescent.* It is important in the initial stages of treatment to engage each individual family member explicitly but clearly announce your alliance to the family as a whole. This allows the family to address overtly the issue if indeed the therapist becomes too aligned with one subsystem.
- *After-session repercussions.* For families that have been unable to deal with certain issues or in cases where secrets or previously unacknowledged information (e.g., abuse, trauma) may come forth, it is important to monitor safety (stating the limits of confidentiality and responsibilities as a mandated reporter of abuse during the first session and later if necessary). If one is unsure, asking the family, "Is this safe to do?" is a useful option. At times it is wise to be restrained and let the family

convince the therapist that it is safe by having them describe plans or methods of coping should sensitive material be revealed. It is imperative for the parents to lead this discussion because they are ultimately responsible for providing a safe environment once they leave the session.

- *Loss of time and interference with social or academic commitments.* It is critical to make this an overt concern and acknowledge the sacrifice the adolescent is asked to make. It is also important to ensure that attending sessions does not cause loss of social supports, particularly important in depression. Flexible scheduling to minimize social disruption may be a solution.
- *"What's in it for me?"* Many times the parental goals and the teen's self interest appear totally different. Openly discussing the potential benefits ("What's in it for me?") of treatment with the adolescent can be useful.
- *Individual work with subsystems.* Meeting with the teen alone to increase rapport and identify self-interest goals that may be accomplished in the therapy can occasionally help. This is not individual therapy because the aim of returning to family therapy remains. Similarly, one may in some cases need to do work with the parents alone.
- *Authenticity.* Teens in particular react to authenticity rather than false attempts by clinicians to act in a certain way to establish rapport.
- *Humor.* Using humor—if one is funny and is not contrived—can be of great assistance.
- *Normalization.* A helpful skill is the ability to convey an understanding that the behaviors or feelings expressed could naturally exist given the clients' context (intent or mission), particularly if this is followed by dealing with the effectiveness of the feelings, behavior, or interaction.
- *Learning to agree to disagree.* This can occasionally be the only option on certain issues, even if one thinks the other's position is wrong. This concept is developmentally challenging for adolescents and their parents; making it overt and explicit can help stop ineffective arguments and estrangement of relationship by allowing disagreement but giving a sense of being heard, understood, and connected.
- *"Tell me/don't tell me."* It is common for parents and adolescents to send ambiguous messages, such as "You ask me if I'm having sex because you want to know, but then you lecture me or ground me because I told you the truth. It's better I don't tell you, but then you say I'm lying to you." Ambiguous messages like this can trap parents and children into conflict. Making the ambiguity overt and drawing the dyad into a direct conversation to clarify the issue can sometimes decrease conflict. The clinician does not need to know if the child should tell; it is up to the child and parent to work that out. The clinician facilitates the interaction to allow them to resolve the issue.
- *"Listening without a reaction does not mean I am agreeing or condoning the behavior."* This concept can help parents stop unhelpful and conflict-generating responses, which they feel compelled to carry out for fear that not doing so would convey the message they are condoning the behavior. This may pave the way for a more productive and mutually satisfying communication.
- *Independence and privacy.* Another universal developmental issue that affects families is teens' desire for independence and privacy. Different cultures vary in the degree of personal independence and privacy versus family identification that is considered appropriate. If the struggle for more independence appears to be a factor influencing parent–teen interactions and possibly affecting the depression, it would be the clinician's responsibility to present this struggle to the family and to assist family members to find the appropriate balance for that unique family and culture.
- *Goodness of fit of interventions.* Four principles should be kept in mind when deciding to use an intervention so that it meets the needs of this particular family: Is it developmentally appropriate? Does it recognize the mutual influence of the depression, family, and individuals on each other? Does it address the level of risk present? Does it leave parents in charge and connected to their child?

RESOURCES FOR PATIENTS AND FAMILIES

Gottman J. *Raising an Emotionally Intelligent Child: The Heart of Parenting.* New York: Simon & Schuster; 1997.

National Alliance on Mental Illness: http://www.nami.org.

Nelson J, Lott L. *Positive Discipline for Teenagers: Resolving Conflict with your Teenage Son or Daughter.* Rocklin, Calif: Prima Publishing; 1990. Also available at: http://www.Positivediscipline.com.

Walsh F. *Strengthening Family Resilience.* 2nd ed. New York: Guilford Press; 2006.

RESOURCES FOR PROFESSIONALS

To find a family therapist: American Association for Marriage and Family Therapy (Available at: http://www.AAMFT.org); http://www.TherapistLocator.net.

Carter B, McGoldrick M, eds. *The Expanded Family Life Cycle.* 3rd ed. Boston: Allyn & Bacon; 1999.

Haley J. *Problem-Solving Therapy.* San Francisco: Jossey-Bass; 1976.

McGoldrick M, Gerson R, Shellenberger S. *Genograms: Assessment and Intervention.* 2nd ed. New York: Norton; 1999.

McGoldrick M, Giordano J, Garcia-Presto N, eds. *Ethnicity and Family Therapy.* 3rd ed. New York: Guilford Press; 2005.

Minuchin S. *Families and Family Therapy.* Cambridge, Mass.: Harvard University Press; 1974.

Rolland J. *Helping Families with Chronic and Life-Threatening Disorders.* New York: Basic Books; 1994.

REFERENCES

1. Weissman MM, Warner V, Wickramaratne PJ, et al. Offspring of depressed parents. 10 years later. *Arch Gen Psychiatry.* 1997;54:932–940.
2. Weissman MM, Warner V, Wickramaratne PJ, et al. Offspring at high risk for anxiety and depression: preliminary findings from a three generation study. In: Gorman J, ed. *Fear and Anxiety: Benefits of Translational Research.* Washington, DC: American Psychiatric Association Press; 2004:65–85.
3. Pilowsky DJ, Wickramaratne P, Nomura Y, et al. Family discord, parental depression, and psychopathology in offspring: 20-year follow-up. *J Am Acad Child Psychiatry.* 2006;45:452–460
4. Weissman MM, Pilowsky PA, Wickramaratne P, et al. Remissions in maternal depression and child psychopathology: a STAR*D-child report. *JAMA.* 2006;22:1389–1398.
5. Birmaher B, Arbelaez C, Brent D. Course and outcome of child and adolescent major depressive disorder. *Child Adolesc Psychiatr Clin N Am.* 2002;11:619–637.
6. Cole DA, McPherson AE. Relation of family subsystems to adolescent depression: implementing a new family assessment strategy. *J Fam Psychol.* 1993;7:119–133.
7. Whitbeck LB, Hoyt DR, Simons RL, et al. Intergenerational continuity of parental rejection and depressed affect. *J Person Soc Psychol.* 1992;63:1036–1045.
8. Miklowitz DJ, George EL, Axelson DA, et al. Family-focused treatment for adolescent with bipolar disorder. *J Affect Disord.* 2004;82(suppl):S113–S128.
9. National Institute of Clinical Excellence (NICE), National Collaborating Center for Mental Health. Depression: Management of Depression in Primary and Secondary Care. 2004 Clinical Guideline 23. Available at: http://www.nice.org.uk.
10. American Academy of Child and Adolescent Psychiatry. Practice parameter for the assessment and treatment of children and adolescents with depressive disorders. *J Am Acad Child Psychiatr.* 2007;46:1503–1526.
11. McQuillan CT. Psychotherapy of the child and adolescent with depression. *Bol Asoc Med P R.* 2003;95:21–28, 33–41.
12. Sanford M, Boyle M, McCleary L. A pilot study of adjunctive family psychoeducation in adolescent major depression: feasibility and treatment effect. *J Am Acad Child Adolesc Psychiatry.* 2006;45:386–495.
13. Goodman D, Happell B. The efficacy of family intervention in adolescent mental health. *Int J Psychiatr Nurs Res.* 2006;12:1364–1377.
14. Diamond G, Siqueland L. Current status of family intervention science. *Child Adolesc Psychiatr Clin N Am.* 2001;10:641–661.
15. Trowell J, Joffe I, Campbell J, et al. Childhood depression: a place for psychotherapy: an outcome study comparing individual psychodynamic psychotherapy and family therapy. *Eur Child Adolesc Psychiatry.* 2007;16:157–167.
16. Diamond GS, Reis BF, Diamond GM, et al. Attachment-based family therapy for depressed adolescents: a treatment development study. *J Am Acad Child Adolesc Psychiatry.* 2002;41:1190–1196.
17. Brent DA, Kolko D, Birmaher B, et al. Predictors of treatment efficacy in a clinical trial of three psychosocial treatments for adolescent depression. *J Am Acad Child Psychiatry.* 1998;37:906–914.
18. Asarnow JR, Goldstein MJ, Tompson M, et al. One-year outcomes of depressive disorders in child psychiatric in-patients: evaluation of the prognostic power of a brief measure of expressed emotion. *J Child Psychol Psychiatry.* 1993;34:129–137.
19. Birmaher B, Brent DA, Kolko D, et al. Clinical outcome after short-term psychotherapy for adolescents with major depressive disorder. *Arch Gen Psychiatry.* 2000;57:29–36.
20. Garber J, Keiley MK, Martin NC. Developmental trajectories of adolescents' depressive symptoms: predictors of change. *J Consult Clin Psychol.* 2002;70:79–95.
21. Hammen C, Brennan PA, Shih JH. Family discord and stress predictors of depression and other disorders in adolescent children of depressed and nondepressed women. *J Am Acad Child Psychiatry.* 2004;43:994–1002.

22. Nomura Y, Wickramaratne PJ, Warner V, et al. Family discord, parental depression, and psychopathology in offspring: ten-year follow-up. *J Am Acad Child Psychiatry.* 2002;41:402–409.

23. Von Bertalanffy L. *General Systems Theory: Foundations, Development and Applications.* New York: George Braziller; 1968.

24. Wamboldt MZ, Wamboldt FS. Role of the family in the onset and outcome of childhood disorders: selected research findings. *J Am Acad Child Psychiatry.* 2000;39:1212–1219.

25. Keitner GI, Archambault R, Ryan CE, et al. Family therapy and chronic depression. *J Clin Psychol.* 2003; 59:873–884.

26. White M. *Re-authoring Lives: Interviews and Essays.* Adelaide, Australia: Dulwich Centre Publications; 1995.

27. Birmaher B, Bridge J, Williamson D, et al. Psychosocial functioning in youths at high risk to develop major depressive disorder. *J Am Acad Child Psychiatry.* 2004;43:839–846.

28. Hubble MA, Duncan BL, Miller SD. Directing attention to what works. In: Hubble MA, Duncan BL, Miller SD, eds. *The Heart and Soul of Change: What Works in Therapy.* Washington, DC: American Psychological Association Press; 1999:407–448.

29. McGoldrick M, Giordano J, Garcia-Presto N, eds. *Ethnicity and Family Therapy.* 3rd ed. New York: Guilford Press; 2005.

30. McGoldrick M, Gerson R, Shellenberger S. *Genograms: Assessment and Intervention.* 2nd ed. New York: Norton; 1999.

31. Minuchin S. *Families and Family Therapy.* Cambridge, Mass: Harvard University Press; 1974.

32. Haley J. *Problem-Solving Therapy.* San Francisco: Jossey-Bass; 1976.

33. Carter B, McGoldrick M, eds. *The Expanded Family Life Cycle.* 3rd ed. Boston: Allyn & Bacon; 1999.

34. Rolland J. *Helping Families with Chronic and Life-Threatening Disorders.* New York: Basic Books; 1994.

35. Hoffman L. A constructivist position for family therapy. *Irish J Psychol.* 1988;9:110–129.

36. de Shazer S. *Clues: Investigating Solutions in Brief Therapy.* New York: Norton; 1988.

37. Figley C. *Trauma and Its Wake: The Study and Treatment of Post-Traumatic Stress Disorder.* New York: Brunner/Mazel; 1985.

38. Andrews B. Bodily shame as a mediator between abusive experiences and depression. *J Abnorm Psychol.* 1995;104:277–285.

39. Trad PV. Save our children. *Am J Psychother.* 1994;48:175–178.

40. Imber-Black E. *Families and Larger Systems: A Family Therapist's Guide Through the Labyrinth.* New York: Guilford Press; 1988.

41. Gergen K. The social constructionist movement in modern psychology. *Am Psychol.* 1985;40:266–275.

42. Gergen K. The saturated family. *Fam Ther Network.* 1991;15:26–35.

43. Hare-Musten RT. A feminist approach to family therapy. *Fam Process.* 1978;17:181–194.

44. Burnam MA, Stein JA, Golding JM, et al. Sexual assault and mental disorders in a community population. *J Consult Clini Psychol.* 1988;56:843–850.

45. Harris TL, Molock SD. Cultural orientation, family cohesion, and family support in suicidal ideation and depression among African American college students. *Suicide Life Threat Behav.* 2000;30,341–353.

46. Bassuk EL, Buckner JC, Perloff JN, et al. Prevalence of mental health and substance use disorders among homeless and low-income housed mothers. *Am J Psychiatry.* 1998;155:1561–1564.

Dynamic Psychotherapy for the Treatment of Depression in Youth

RACHEL Z. RITVO

KEY POINTS

- To undertake dynamic therapy with a depressed child or adolescent, clinicians need to know the basic principles of dynamic psychology, the dynamics of depression, be able to construct a dynamic formulation, and be competent in structuring therapy and using dynamic therapy techniques.
- The dynamic formulation focuses on understanding the patient in terms of psychodynamic psychology, the dynamics of depression, and the current developmental challenges. A dynamic formulation is akin to the patient's personal story told from a psychologically minded perspective.
- For children and adolescents, the dynamic formulation should always include the developmental challenges facing the patient.
- The dynamics of depression arise from threats to relationships and/or to self-esteem. Anger and rage in response to these threats may be masked by the depressive sadness and slowing of behavior.
- Traditionally, dynamic therapy has been an individual therapy, but increasingly there are models for dyadic treatments of the child and parent together.
- Dynamic therapy has customarily been long term and open ended, but increasingly there are models for brief focused dynamic therapy for depression in children and adolescents.
- Dynamic therapy is expressive, that is, aimed at allowing patients to express as much of their feelings as they are comfortable and able to express. Thus patients need to feel secure in the treatment setting. Clinicians need to maintain an empathic, nonjudgmental attitude and to hold the young person's feelings of anger, pain, loss, and so on.
- Dynamic therapy for children can be done through play.
- Psychodynamic psychotherapy is hypothesized to work through the caring, understanding relationship that is established between therapist and patient, through the insight gained by the patient into the psychological roots of the depression, and through the development of more mature, adaptive defenses and internal representations.
- Dynamic therapy can be used in conjunction with medication and additional psychosocial interventions.

Introduction

Shannon, 3 years old, is referred for evaluation because she is biting her peers and caregivers at her child-care center. Observing Shannon at the center, the evaluator notices Shannon spends long periods of time alone in a corner, wrapped in her "blankey," sucking her thumb, and watching the other children at play, the very image of a sad, depressed preschooler. Shannon's parents reported that Shannon's life had been disrupted recently by an unusual number of stressors: Her mother went back to work for the first time in her life and Shannon went to child care, a baby brother was born 9 weeks earlier, a new nanny had been hired for the brother, the family had moved to a new house, and the parents were experiencing threats of downsizing at their jobs.[1]

What distinguishes Shannon's sadness from normal sadness? The normally sad child might be subdued at child care but would not be sitting off in the corner day after day. Shannon might be diagnosed as having an adjustment disorder with depressed mood, rather than major depression, if she had only been symptomatic for a few weeks and an active, albeit ineffective, coping process was evident. Shannon's symptoms are severe. She has been at child care for nearly 3 months and is increasingly withdrawn. She takes no pleasure in peers, her irritability and sadness spill over at home, and developmental progression in toileting and sleep routines has halted or even regressed. Major depression is the appropriate diagnosis.[2]

The consultant offered several interventions: The couple works to reduce marital stress, stabilizing bedtime and other routines, special time with each parent, and a behavior program to decrease the biting at child care. In addition, he met with Shannon weekly for one-on-one dynamic play therapy. That dynamic therapy gave Shannon a chance to express her feelings of anger and sadness over all the changes in her life and to master those feelings in the play setting. Additionally, the therapist provided a reliable, caring person who attended to Shannon's feelings, helped her understand them, and, by getting to know Shannon's feelings better, could help her parents understand them too.

EMPIRICAL EVIDENCE FOR PSYCHODYNAMIC TREATMENT OF DEPRESSION IN YOUTH

Psychodynamic approaches to the treatment of emotional and behavioral disturbances of childhood and adolescence have developed over the past 100 years, beginning with Freud's report on "Little Hans" in 1909.[3] A systematic retrospective chart review of 763 cases treated at the Anna Freud Centre in London identified 352 youths with emotional disorders.[4] Nearly three quarters of these patients showed improvement in adaptation at the end of treatment. Children younger than 11 years were more likely than older children to be fully in remission at discharge. Youths with more severe pathology did better in psychoanalysis (four or more sessions per week) than with less frequent (one or two) sessions per week.

Research studies testing manualized psychodynamic psychotherapy for depressed and anxious youth have only recently been undertaken. Muratori et al.[5] used an active treatment versus community services model to examine the short- and long-term effects of time-limited psychodynamic psychotherapy for children meeting *DSM-IV* criteria for depressive and anxiety disorders. The psychodynamic treatment condition achieved an effect size of 0.73 on the Children's Global Assessment Scale (C-GAS). From end of treatment to 2-year follow-up, youth who received psychodynamic therapy showed continued improvement on the Child Behavior Checklist (CBCL). This continued improvement after completion has been found in adults treated with psychodynamic psychotherapy[6] and is referred to by Muratori et al.[5] as a "sleeper effect."

Time-limited (30 sessions) psychodynamic psychotherapy for youths 9 to 15 years of age with major depression, dysthymia, or both was compared with family therapy in a randomized multisite trial that enrolled 72 patients.[7] At the end of treatment, 74.3% of cases in individual treatment were no longer clinically depressed. At follow-up 6 months after treatment, 100% of youths in the psychodynamic treatment group were not clinically depressed. Drawing on the extensive clinical material recorded in the course of the studies, Trowell et al.[8] published a qualitative analysis of two patients that provides a rich elaboration of the dynamics of depression in childhood and the stresses experienced by therapists providing time-limited treatment to severely distressed youths.

Although there are too few efficacy studies of psychodynamic therapy for children and adolescents to do a meta-analysis, there are sufficient studies in adults. Leichsenring et al.,[6] in a meta-analysis of 17 studies of short-term psychodynamic psychotherapy (STPP) for treatment of specific psychiatric disorders, found STPP to be effective. The Anna Freud Centre chart review[4] suggested that long-term intensive psychodynamic psychotherapy is more effective than shorter treatments. This finding has not been tested further in youths, but a 3-year randomized effectiveness trial has compared long- and short-term psychodynamic psychotherapy with solution-focused therapy in a sample of 326 adult outpatients seeking treatment for mood disorder (84.7%) or anxiety disorder (43.6%).[9] Although no significant difference in outcome was noted between the short-and long-term therapies in the first

2 years, by the third year patients in the long-term treatment group showed statistically significant (14% to 37%) lowering of symptom scores on the Hamilton Depression Rating Scale, Beck Depression Inventory, Symptom Check List Anxiety Scale, and the Hamilton Anxiety Rating Scale.

HOW TO USE DYNAMIC PSYCHOTHERAPY

A therapist needs three basic skill sets to undertake a dynamic therapy with a depressed child or adolescent:

- Knowledge of the basic principles of dynamic psychology and the dynamics of depression
- Ability to construct a dynamic formulation
- Competence structuring therapy and using dynamic therapy techniques

BASIC PRINCIPLES OF DYNAMIC PSYCHOLOGY

1. "There is more than meets the eye." Conscious thoughts, feelings, and behaviors are determined by complex mental processes (e.g., memories, beliefs, wishes, defenses) that are outside of conscious awareness.
2. Symptoms, thoughts, and behaviors are "overdetermined;" that is, they arise from more than one unconscious source. Thus every communication or behavior has multiple meanings.
3. Templates (usually called internal representations) of relationships and of the "real world" are built from the child's experience with parents, siblings, other significant persons, and the "real world." These internal representations, largely unconscious, shape the child's basic assumptions and expectations.
4. Transference is the repetition or reenactment, in a relationship with a new person, of the internalized relational patterns of past experience with parents or other significant persons. Transference in the patient–therapist relationship provides an opportunity to observe, understand, and revise these internalized relational patterns in the here-and-now of the sessions.
5. Internal, usually unconscious, conflicts occur in a person's mind between competing urges, impulses, and desires and between these drives and internalized parental and societal prohibitions.
6. Defenses are unconscious patterns of thought or behavior that maintain psychological balance (homeostasis) and reduce anxiety and awareness of internal conflict[10,11] (Table 11.1).

TABLE 11.1 DEFENSES COMMONLY EXHIBITED BY CHILDREN IN PSYCHODYNAMIC THERAPY

Denial	The disavowal of intolerable external reality factors or of urges, thoughts, feelings, and wishes.
Displacement	The transfer of emotions, ideas, or wishes from the original object to a more acceptable substitute.
Externalization	The attribution of internal conflicts to the external environment and a search for environmental solutions. In therapy, the therapist is used to represent the patient's problem.
Reaction formation	The adoption of affects, ideas, or behaviors that are the opposites of impulses harbored either consciously or unconsciously.
Repression	The exclusion of unacceptable ideas, fantasies, affects, or impulses from consciousness. Repressed material emerges in disguised form in thought, speech, and actions.
Suppression	The *conscious* effort to control and conceal unacceptable impulses. Suppression is the exception to the rule that defenses are unconscious processes.
Somatization	The transfer of tension from drives or affects into disturbances of bodily functions or rhythms.
Turning passive to active	The management of affects and impulses stirred by a passive experience with a more powerful "other" by playing out in action or story the active "other's" role. This includes identification with the aggressor.

Information from Edgerton J, Campbell RJ, eds. *American Psychiatric Glossary.* Washington, DC: American Psychiatric Press; 1994, Freud A. *The Ego and the Mechanisms of Defense.* New York: International Universities Press; 1936, and Freud A. *Normality and Pathology in Childhood: Assessments of Development.* New York: International Universities Press; 1965.

TABLE 11.2 DYNAMICS OF DEPRESSION

Interpersonal/Anaclitic Symptoms	Self-Critical/Introjective Symptoms
• Fears of abandonment	• Worthlessness
• Helplessness	• Guilt
• Weakness	• Sense of failure
• Depletion	• Rage
• Clinging	• Sadness
• Demanding attention	
• Rage	
• Sadness	

7. Emotions are signals. Dynamic psychology is particularly interested in signals of internal distress, conflict, and loss of internal balance. Anxiety and depression are typical affect signals of internal distress.

These principles are common to all psychodynamic and psychoanalytic treatments. In the United States, the term *psychoanalysis* is used only for treatments that occur three or more times per week and are performed by a clinician trained in psychoanalysis. Psychoanalysis, where available, might be offered to a child or adolescent who is engaged in psychotherapy but has not improved with a less intensive treatment. In other parts of the world "psychoanalysis" may refer to any therapy based on these principles.

THE DYNAMICS OF DEPRESSION

The dynamic precipitants of depression can be conceptualized as disruptions and frustrations occurring in one *or both* of two parallel lines of personality development: the line of development of stable, mutually-satisfying interpersonal relations (the anaclitic line) and the line of development of a realistic and positive self-identity (the introjective line)[12–14] (Table 11.2). Depressed youths are struggling to contain anger, disappointment, frustration, and shame or guilt.

When meeting a depressed adolescent or child, the dynamic clinician ascertains whether there is stress or disruption in the youth's relationships to psychologically important persons. Are there threats to the youth's feeling of security in her most important relationships? Are his needs for dependency and intimacy being met? Sometimes the threat comes from within the youth. For example, it may be triggered by a maturational surge. Dynamic theory suggests that the frequency of depression at the onset of adolescence is related to the youth's need to become more autonomous in relation to parents and the feelings of loss this may cause.

The clinician wants to determine if there have been threats to the youth's positive sense of self. Again it must be considered that these threats may be internal and possibly unconscious, buried in fantasies. (Once conscience develops, children or adolescents can feel guilt over fantasized transgressions.) Threats to self-esteem may be caused by disappointment in one's own body (e.g., frailty, learning disabilities).

When treating a youth whose depression seems out of proportion to current stressors, the clinician should consider whether the depression is being fed by memories and feelings from an earlier, troubled time.[15,16] Disruptions on either the relational or the self-esteem lines of personality development that may not have reached clinical significance at the time they occurred, or may not have been recognized, can contribute to depression later in life.[17] Most difficult to recognize are feelings reactivated from difficulties that occurred before the age at which the child developed narrative memory. If Shannon had been punished for her biting and her depression ignored, her depression might recur later in life when developmental demands or life events reawakened her pain over loss of closeness with her mother.

DYNAMIC FORMULATION

Case formulation is the process whereby a clinician organizes the clinical data on a given patient, including the differential diagnosis, and generates hypotheses to understand and explain the individual patient's condition in order to propose a treatment plan and make a prognosis. Of the several current models for case formulation in psychiatry,[18,19] dynamic formulation fits most comfortably in the biopsychosocial model[20] in which it is the "psychological" component. The dynamic formulation focuses on understanding the patient and explaining the patient's condition in terms of the principles of psychodynamic psychology and the dynamics of depression. With children and adolescents, the dynamic formulation should always include the developmental challenges facing the patient.

It may be easiest for practitioners to think of the dynamic formulation as the patient's personal story told from a psychologically minded perspective. Let's think about Shannon. We can hypothesize that this 3-year-old feels suddenly abandoned at the child-care center by her mother who has always been with her. She is both angry with her mother and longing to be reunited with her. Shannon is also likely to be angry about sharing her parents with her baby brother while also being fascinated by the baby and enjoying his interest in his big sister. She uses displacement as a defense. She does not attack her brother or her mother but instead directs her angry and competitive feelings at the children she bites at the child-care center. Shannon is struggling with the developmental challenge of entry into a school-like setting. Most 3-year-olds can do this with a bit of initial struggle, but Shannon's development is hindered by the stress of the changes in her life. She defensively withdraws when she misses her mother rather than being able to use the teachers or the other children for stabilization.

This formulation prepares the clinician for what might come out in Shannon's dynamic play therapy. Themes of abandonment and loss, competition, anger, and loneliness can be looked for in her play. The clinician will also be looking to revise this understanding of Shannon if other themes emerge in the therapy. For instance, Shannon might, in her play, have a theme about a bad child who is punished for being disruptive, hurtful, and competitive. The therapist would expand his or her formulation to include a description of Shannon's emerging development of conscience and the loss of self-esteem that is contributing to her depression.

STRUCTURING THERAPY

Actions speak louder than words. Although dynamic therapy is often called talk therapy, dynamic therapists are very aware of the impact on the therapeutic process of all the nonverbal interactions between the clinician and the patient (and family).

Dynamic therapy is an expressive therapy aimed at allowing the patient to express as much of his feelings as he is comfortable and able to express. The patient needs to feel secure in the treatment setting. The clinician maintains an empathic and nonjudgmental attitude. The clinician must be able to hold the child's or adolescent's feelings of anger, pain, loss, and so on, neither brushing them aside nor fanning the flames, but rather understanding their roots in the child's struggle to adapt. The clinician explains to the child or adolescent that the patient's behavior and communications in the session will be kept confidential and only relayed to parents as generalized assessments of the patient's status or themes to help the parents understand the patient. Particularly with depressed patients, the clinician should clarify that the patient's safety is paramount. If the patient is in immediate danger from suicidal impulses or risk-taking behavior, the clinician and the patient would discuss how to inform the parents in order to secure the patient's safety. Whether the suicidality or risk taking require parental notification or not, the therapist will work with the youth to understand the meaning of the behaviors and the internal conflicts that motivate them. The therapist will work on the alliance with the patient's desire to mature and to be self-regulating.

The room should be comfortable and able to withstand age-appropriate behaviors and some loss of behavioral control. A modest collection of age-appropriate toys, games, and simple art materials serve as vehicles for expression and for putting the patient at ease. The clinician strives to be dependable, keeping regular appointments. Sessions should be frequent enough for the child or adolescent to feel connected to the clinician and not abandoned between sessions. Commonly this means weekly sessions, but for younger children early in the treatment and for older children and adolescents when symptoms are severe, twice-weekly sessions are indicated.

Although dynamic therapy has traditionally been an individual therapy, research supports models for therapy of the child and parent together.[5] The clinician always keeps in mind the child's point of view and feelings of vulnerability stemming from the natural dependency of childhood. Dyadic therapy in which the mother and child are seen together is the preferred model in treating children younger than 3 years.[21-23] The clinician must also assess whether the parent is in need of mental health treatment of his or her own.

Psychodynamic group therapy is increasingly hard to find in the United States where psychoeducational and social skills groups are now the most available group therapies. Many depressed youths are reluctant to join a group. Group therapy can be very beneficial for youth who are isolated and have difficulty forming peer relationships. For adolescents whose developmental need to feel autonomous from adults is strong, a group experience can allow them to hear from their peers what they might not hear from a therapist.

Clinicians find it helpful to think about dynamic therapy as having three phases: opening, middle, and closing (termination).[24] In the opening phase, the therapist develops a working alliance with the patient and the family and expands the dynamic formulation of the depression. In the middle phase, the patient and therapist work together to elaborate and address the many strands of the patient's inner conflicts and developmental struggles that have fueled the depressive affect and kept the depressive state going. Ideally, the closing phase begins when the therapist, the patient, and the family all agree that the depression is in remission and the causative, destabilizing issues in the patient's life or inner-self have been resolved. Even if such agreement is not reached, the closing phase begins whenever planning for ending treatment starts. Because termination may stimulate feelings of loss or abandonment by the therapist, it can reignite the depressive symptoms. Some time should be planned for working with these feelings. Scheduling follow-up contact is appropriate.

Length of treatment can vary greatly. Evidence indicates that treatments as short as 24 or 30 weekly sessions have positive outcomes.[5,7] In the Anna Freud Centre retrospective chart review of 352 children and adolescents treated for anxiety or depressive disorders, 72% of those treated for at least 6 months showed clinically significant improvement.[4] Traditionally, treatments have lasted 18 to 24 months or longer depending on the degree of psychopathology in the child and the family.

Combining dynamic psychotherapy with the use of medication is a common practice. Guidelines for the use of antidepressants in children and adolescents should be followed (see Chapter 6). Hospitalized patients are likely to begin medication before therapy. In less severe cases, dynamic therapists usually prefer to complete the opening phase of treatment (evaluation, formulation, and initiation of the alliance) before starting medication. The child or adolescent may respond to the therapy and not require medication. If medication is required, or recommended, the therapist is in a better position to work with the child and the family on understanding both the youth's depression and the decision to add medication. The use of medication should be presented in an age-appropriate fashion. For young children, it may be presented as a choice made by the parents and therapist/physician that the child has feelings and opinions about. Older children and adolescents should be active participants in the medication decision. At all ages the medication may be presented as a tool that is used to aid recovery. The therapist tries to clarify and understand what the pill means to the patient as treatment goes forward.

TECHNIQUES

Psychological understanding develops in children from the experience of "doing" more than through abstract thought. Through play, children deal with experience by creating model situations and master reality through experimentation. Only in adolescence does the capacity for abstract and verbal understanding catch up with the power of play and action. The individual child may have a preference for particular play activities: imaginary play, games with rules, art projects, or physical activities. The therapist develops skill at playing with the child while attending to both the content and, most importantly, the process of the play. For example, when playing a board game, the therapist is interested in *how* the child plays and what this manner of play reveals about the child's depressive conflicts and relational patterns.[25,26] In the play process it is useful to observe when the play becomes repetitious, disrupted, or reaches satisfaction or completion. Repetitions show where the child is stuck, and the therapist can begin to think how to put the stuck feelings into words in order to think together about other ways the action could go. Disruptions indicate that the feelings were becoming too much for the patient. The therapist can look for ways to go at the problem more gradually or to provide more support. Satisfying conclusions generally indicate that the patient has mastered the difficulty and is getting ready to move on developmentally and in the therapy.

Two defensive patterns are so common in the play of children in dynamic therapy that they can be considered core techniques for the novice therapist. The imaginary play, game, or art project can be considered as a symbolic, metaphoric representation of the child's subjective experience. Rather than bringing the content back directly to refer to the child, the therapist can stay with the child and work in the metaphor. The metaphor is essentially a form of defensive displacement. Thus if Shannon played with a puppy figure being left by a mommy dog, the therapist would talk about the feelings of the puppy and the mommy dog, even though the allusion to Shannon's own situation is fairly transparent.

Commonly when playing with the therapist, a child creates a role reversal that uses the defense of turning passive to active.[10] Shannon might become the mother leaving the therapist, her child, at the child-care center. The therapist could then give voice to how the child might feel. As the therapy progresses, the therapist might, from within the child/passive role, begin to model solutions like asking to sit in the staff member's lap, playing with another child, or making a picture for mommy.

Preteens and early adolescents may shy away from play as too childish and yet be uncomfortable talking about their problems. A game of cards or checkers may serve as an icebreaker. Just as the younger children use displacement, and turning passive to active, to get some defensive distance that makes it possible to examine topics that might otherwise be overwhelming, the older child or adolescent may need to start with safer topics (e.g., about friends or areas of special interest), only gradually moving closer to sensitive relational issues or deeper worries about self that are at the root of his or her depression. The therapist needs to listen to both process and content to pick out the patterns and themes that are reflective of the dynamic formulation of the youth's depression. As these patterns emerge the therapist can begin to point them out gently and gauge the patient's ability to see them.

The verbal techniques used in dynamic therapy of depression lie on a continuum from those that are most supportive of the patient's strengths and current adaptations to those that lead to expression of deeper feelings and bring the patient's inner conflicts and issues into the discussion (Table 11.3). The bulk of the work is done with clarifications, encouragement to elaborate, and empathic validation. The therapist may restate what the patient has told him or her to give coherence to statements that have been vague or disconnected. The clarification is a way both of checking whether the therapist understood correctly and of giving patients an opportunity to "hear" what they have been saying. A play therapy clarification frequently used when the child gives the therapist a role to play is the "stage whisper." The therapist playing the puppy left behind by Shannon's mommy dog might "stage whisper" "Should the puppy cry for mommy to come back? Or should he say 'I am a tough puppy' and go meet the other puppies?" With an older patient who is telling about events outside the therapy session, clarifications include questions about the history given. "Tell me more about that . . ." is a straightforward type of encouragement to elaborate. When patients are unable to elaborate, the clinician must judge whether this is defensive turning away from a hot spot. If so, the therapist will go more carefully, supporting the defense while looking for a gentler approach to the issue. Empathic validation says, "I can see why you feel that way." Empathic validations often facilitate further elaboration, particularly with older children and adolescents who are talking and not playing.

Developmental assistance is given when a child is struggling to achieve a new developmental achievement. With a very young child, the therapist might be helping the child separate from the mother or caretaker by first having the mother in the room. Next the therapist introduces the idea

TABLE 11.3 EXPRESSIVE-SUPPORTIVE CONTINUUM OF VERBAL INTERVENTIONS

Most expressive

Interpretation
Confrontation
Clarification
Encouragement to elaborate
Empathic validation
Developmental assistance
Psychoeducational interventions
Advice and praise

Most supportive

of mother leaving and works with the child on figuring out what is needed to make that possible. With an adolescent, developmental assistance might be encouraging the adolescent who cannot envision life beyond high school to begin talking about specific plans for after graduation. At a deeper level the therapist is always thinking about the developmental challenge facing the particular child or adolescent and how it feeds the depression. The therapist considers what steps the patient needs to make to meet the challenge and tries to foster growth in that direction.

Confrontation and interpretation are intended to give patients a greater explicit understanding of their difficulties. Confrontations draw the patient's attention to something they know but are avoiding recognizing or speaking about. Because a confrontation may be experienced as critical or aggressive, the clinician wants to be tactful and, if the patient responds angrily, be prepared to work calmly but empathically with their distress. For example, a teenager who drives himself to therapy may consistently come late. The clinician would want to inquire about this and understand with the patient the factors making the patient late. Adolescents frequently need adults to present the constraints of reality on their imaginative constructions of plans of action in their journey to becoming independent.[27] In the healthy adolescent, this may take the form of reality checks such as a parent or therapist questioning where the adolescent intends to get the money for a planned ski-trip. For the depressed adolescent, a therapist may have to confront him with the idea that if he commits suicide to revenge himself on his parents for their flaws and perceived mistreatment, he won't be around to see them suffer. Of course such a confrontation must be done carefully, with empathy for his angry disappointment and concern for his well-being and survival.

Interpretations take clarifications and observations about the patient's behavior, comments, expressed feelings, or gestures and connect them to a possible explanation. An interpretation for Shannon in the puppy play might be "I wonder if that puppy was so angry when his mommy left that when the other puppy bumped him in play, all the anger blew up inside him and he just had to bite the other puppy." Interpretations should typically be proposed as hypotheses, "Do you think it could be that?" Often if the interpretation is close but off the mark, the patient will correct the therapist and bring it to the mark. "She bit that puppy because he was a boy and she doesn't like boys," Shannon might say, telling her therapist that she is struggling to accept her brother's role in the family. At other times, if the interpretation is premature or incorrect, the patient may simply dismiss it.

A special group of interpretations are called reconstructions. A therapist may want to help the patient see how earlier experiences have laid the ground for the current depression. If Shannon, at age 17, became angry and depressed as she approached departure for college, her therapist at that time might say, "I wonder if you feel so sad and angry now because being away from your mother brings back all the feelings from when you were 3 and went to child care." If this made sense to a teenage Shannon, then the therapist would also point out how now Shannon is the active party and has many more abilities with which to cope with being away from her mother.

Psychodynamic psychotherapy works both through the caring, understanding relationship that is established between therapist and patient and through the insight gained by the patient into the psychological roots of the depression. Research with adults suggests that in patients with relational/anaclitic depressions, the relationship with the therapist carries most of the therapeutic effect, whereas for patients with self-critical/introjective depressions, interpretation may carry more of the effect.[13] In children, attention to their developmental challenge in the context of a caring relationship and the therapist's interventions as a model for understanding and speaking about feelings and inner conflicts contribute to the therapeutic effect and to the development of more mature and adaptive defenses and internal representations.[4,8]

DYNAMIC THERAPY IN THE REAL WORLD

In the real world, few children present with a pure case of depression and no complicating factors. Dynamic therapists treat the whole child or adolescent and not just the specific diagnosis. Comorbid disorders such as learning disabilities, attention deficit hyperactivity disorder (ADHD), or eating disorders would be evaluated and integrated into the dynamic formulation and addressed with the depressive dynamics in the therapy. If required, consultation would be recommended for management of the comorbid disorder such as tutoring for learning disorders, medication for ADHD, or nutritional counseling and pediatric supervision for an eating disorder. Substance-abusing adolescents who cannot maintain abstinence often need to be referred to a program that will monitor for drug use.

Dynamic therapists speak with whomever the therapist, patient, or parents feel it would be beneficial to contact. The therapist may contact the teacher or pediatrician for history. Often teachers or school officials are eager to have the therapist's assistance in understanding the youth's condition and tailoring the school's response to meet the youth's needs and manage behavior more effectively. Such contacts should be made with the patient's awareness and input. A psychoanalyst seeing a child or adolescent in a classical multiple-sessions-per-week psychoanalysis may choose not to speak directly to teachers, coaches, or others in the youth's life.

RESISTANT DEPRESSION

When a youth fails to improve, or shows only limited improvement, reassessment is indicated. Frequently the problem is that sessions are being held too infrequently.[28] For patients who are not improving with twice-per-week therapy, referral for evaluation for intensive psychoanalysis could depend on the availability of resources for such a treatment.

In addition to considering increasing the frequency of sessions, the clinician reexamines the biopsychosocial data to determine what elements are driving the depressive dynamics. For instance, an inappropriate school placement may need correcting. Remember Shannon? If she remained depressed despite therapy, she might have been taken out of an all-day child-care program and placed in a morning nursery school with aftercare at home with her brother and the nanny.

Projective testing can help uncover dynamics the clinician has not fully perceived. A reassessment may include a consultation with a more experienced psychodynamic clinician for a second opinion. As stated earlier in this chapter, antidepressant medication is frequently considered for cases in which the depressive symptoms persist and are disrupting the youth's functioning. Similarly, additional therapies including family therapy or inpatient treatment maybe indicated (see Chapter 16).

MAKING THE REFERRAL TO A DYNAMIC THERAPIST

Dynamic therapy may be the therapy of choice for depressed children younger than 7 years, an age group for whom medication and cognitive-behavioral approaches are less suitable. Dynamic therapy appeals to youths and parents who are psychologically minded. For youths with complex chronic difficulties and comorbidities complicating their depression, dynamic therapy is a good choice because of its foundation in a comprehensive psychological theory, emphasis on assisting developmental progress, and tradition of long-term treatments.

Dynamic therapists can be found in all the mental health disciplines. Local professional societies can provide referrals. Other sources for locating a dynamic therapist are training programs. These may be university-based graduate programs in psychology or social work or free-standing educational institutions providing postgraduate training. See the Resources for Professionals section for more information.

RESOURCES FOR PATIENTS AND FAMILIES

Axline VM. *Play Therapy*. New York: Ballantine; 1969.
Fassler DG, Dumas LS. *"Help Me, I'm Sad:" Recognizing, Treating, and Preventing Childhood and Adolescent Depression*. New York: Viking; 1997.
Fraiberg S. *The Magic Years*. New York: Fireside; 1996.

RESOURCES FOR PROFESSIONALS

The International Psychoanalytic Association (www.ipa.org) provides contact lists for national psychoanalytic institutes and societies.
Most psychoanalytic institutes train psychotherapists as well as psychoanalysts. The Association for Child Psychoanalysis (www.childanalysis.org) lists members both in the United States and internationally.
The American Psychoanalytic Association (www.apsa.org) provides contact information for psychoanalytic organizations in the United States.

The American Academy of Psychoanalysis and Dynamic Psychiatry (www.aapdp.org) provides referrals to its members who are dynamic psychiatrists.

Axline VM. *Play Therapy*. New York: Ballantine; 1969.

Lewis JM, Blotcky MJ. *Child Therapy: Concepts, Strategies, and Decision Making*. Washington, DC: Brunner/Mazel; 1997.

Novick KK, Novick J. *Working with Parents Makes Therapy Work*. Lanham, Md: Jason Aronson; 2005.

Sandler J, Kennedy H, Tyson RL. *The Technique of Child Psychoanalysis: Discussions with Anna Freud*. Cambridge, Mass: Harvard University Press; 1980.

REFERENCES

1. Fassler DG, Dumas LS. *"Help Me, I'm Sad:" Recognizing, Treating, and Preventing Childhood and Adolescent Depression*. New York: Viking; 1997.
2. Zero to Three. *Diagnostic Classification of Mental Health and Development Disorders of Infancy and Early Childhood: DC:0–3R*. Washington, DC: National Center for Clinical Infant Programs; 2005.
3. Freud S. Analysis of a phobia in a five-year-old boy. In: Strachey JE, ed. *The Standard Edition of the Complete Psychological Works of Sigmund Freud*. Vol. 10. London: Hogarth Press; 1955:3–149.
4. Target M, Fonagy P. Efficacy of psychoanalysis for children with emotional disorders. *J Am Acad Child Adolesc Psychiatry*. 1994;33:361–371.
5. Muratori F, Picchi L, Bruni G, et al. A two-year follow-up of psychodynamic psychotherapy for internalizing disorders in children. *J Am Acad Child Adolesc Psychiatry*. 2003;42:331–339.
6. Leichsenring F, Rabung S, Leibing E. The efficacy of short-term psychodynamic psychotherapy in specific psychiatric disorders. *Arch Gen Psychiatry*. 2004;61:1208–1216.
7. Trowell J, Joffe I, Campbell J, et al. Childhood depression: a place for psychotherapy. *Eur Child Adolesc Psychiatry*. 2007;16:157–167.
8. Trowell J, Rhode M, Miles G, et al. Childhood depression: work in progress. *J Child Psychother*. 2003;29:147–169.
9. Knekt P, Lindfors O, Härkänena T, et al. Randomized trial on the effectiveness of long- and short-term psychodynamic psychotherapy and solution-focused therapy on psychiatric symptoms during a 3-year follow-up. *Psychol Med*. 2008;38:689–703.
10. Blackman JS. *101 Defenses: How the Mind Shields Itself*. New York: Brunner-Routledge; 2004.
11. Cramer P. *Protecting the Self: Defense Mechanisms in Action*. New York: Guilford Press; 2006.
12. Blatt SJ. Levels of object representation in anaclitic and introjective depression. *Psychoanal Study Child*. 1974;29:107–157.
13. Blatt SJ. The differential effect of psychotherapy and psychoanalysis with anaclitic and introjective patients: the Menninger psychotherapy research project revisited. *J Am Psychoanal Assoc*. 1992;40:691–724.
14. Blatt SJ. Contributions of psychoanalysis to the understanding and treatment of depression. *J Am Psychoanal Assoc*. 1998;46:723–752.
15. Ritvo S. Double dipping: child analysands return as young adults. In: Cohen J, Cohler BJ, eds. *The Psychoanalytic Study of Lives over Time*. New York: Academic Press; 2000:333–345.
16. Weiss S. Child analysis: its impact on later development. In: Cohen J, Cohler BJ, eds. *The Psychoanalytic Study of Lives over Time*. New York: Academic Press; 2000:209–225.
17. Blatt SJ, Homann E. Parent-child interaction in the etiology of dependent and self-critical depression. *Clin Psychol Rev*. 1992;12:47–91.
18. Henderson SW, Martin A. Formulation and integration. In: Martin A, Volkmar FR, eds. *Lewis' Child and Adolescent Psychiatry: A Comprehensive Textbook*. Philadelphia: Wolter Kluwer/Lippincott Williams & Wilkins; 2007:377–382.
19. Winters NC, Hanson G, Stoyanova V. The case formulation in child and adolescent psychiatry. *Child Adolesc Psychiatr Clin N Am*. 2007;16:111–132.
20. Gabbard GO. *Long-Term Psychodynamic Psychotherapy: A Basic Text*. Washington, DC: American Psychiatric Publishing; 2004.
21. Toth S, Maughan A, Manly JT, et al. The relative efficacy of two interventions in altering maltreated preschool children's representational models: implications for attachment theory. *Dev Psychopathol*. 2002;14:877–908.
22. Lieberman AF, Van Horn P, Ippen CG. Toward evidence-based treatment: child-parent psychotherapy with preschoolers exposed to marital violence. *J Am Acad Child Adolesc Psychiatry*. 2005;44:1241–1248.
23. Lieberman AF, Ippen CG, Van Horn P. Child-parent psychotherapy: 6-month follow-up of a randomized controlled trial. *J Am Acad Child Adolesc Psychiatry*. 2006;45:913–918.
24. Ritvo RZ, Ritvo S. Psychodynamic principles in practice. In: Martin A, Volkmar FR, eds. *Lewis' Child and Adolescent Psychiatry: A Comprehensive Textbook*. Philadelphia: Wolter Kluwer/Lippincott Williams & Wilkins; 2007:826–842.

25. Bellinson J. Shut up and move: the uses of board games in child psychotherapy. *J Infant Child Adolesc Psychother.* 2000;1:23–41.
26. Bellinson J. *Children's Use of Board Games in Psychotherapy.* Northvale, NJ: Jason Aronson; 2002.
27. Winnicott D. Adolescent process and the need for personal confrontation. *Pediatrics,* 1969;44:752–756.
28. Target M. The problem of outcome in child psychoanalysis: contributions from the Anna Freud Centre. In: Leuzinger-Bohleber M, Target M, eds. *Outcomes of Psychoanalytic Treatment: Perspectives for Therapists and Researchers.* New York: Brunner-Routledge; 2002:240–251.

How to Use Complementary and Alternative Medicine Treatments

JOSEPH M. REY

KEY POINTS

- Use of complementary and alternative medicine (CAM) is widespread. For example, St. John's wort is the most commonly prescribed antidepressant for children in Germany.
- A host of CAM interventions have been recommended or used for the treatment of depression. Hardly any are supported by credible evidence of effectiveness, particularly in children and adolescents.
- CAM remedies have to satisfy less rigorous efficacy and safety criteria than prescription drugs, lack standardized preparation, and are more prone to contamination, adulteration, and inaccurate dosage, among other problems.
- Excessive concern about liability is unwarranted. An open, informed stance by clinicians often leads to disclosure of use by patients, acknowledgment of patients' dislikes and beliefs, and better patient education and outcomes.
- Clinicians recognize patients' and families' interest in CAM therapies, but they often do not feel comfortable asking about, discussing, or recommending them.
- Clinical evaluation should include routine questioning about CAM use.
- Despite heterogeneous findings, extrapolation of adult data showing that omega-3 fatty acids are effective and safe appears to justify their use for the treatment of depression and bipolar disorder in children and adolescents.
- Inconsistencies notwithstanding, it appears that St. John's wort is helpful for mild depression. It may be useful when parents or adolescents refuse taking or have not benefited from conventional antidepressant treatment and after discussion of risks.
- Treatment with St. John's wort requires monitoring because of side effects and, more importantly, a multitude of potential interactions with other treatments, such as the contraceptive pill, selective serotonin reuptake inhibitors (SSRIs), and anticoagulants.
- Although S-adenosyl methionine (SAMe) appears to be effective and well tolerated in adults, little data are available for children and adolescents. SAMe could be used by extrapolating adult findings, but it should be done with close supervision.
- Although lacking empirical evidence in childhood depression, physical exercise is such a well known health-enhancing practice that appropriate physical activity should be part of any management plan for depressed children and adolescents.

Introduction

Alternative medicine refers to a collection of treatments—often very disparate—that exists largely outside the institutions where mainstream health care is provided.[1] Alternative medicine is increasingly seen as complementing standard medical practice and often referred to as "complementary and alternative medicine" (CAM). The boundary between CAM and conventional medicine is becoming blurred because of some clinicians using CAM treatments, inclusion in health insurance packages, incorporation in medical curricula, and a growing use of the scientific method (e.g., randomized, placebo-controlled trials) to test the effectiveness of these treatments. So-called integrative medicine[2] combines treatments from mainstream medicine and from CAM. In Asia, CAM (e.g., Chinese, Ayurvedic) is often a component of primary health care: Scientific medicine is used to suppress symptoms and traditional medicine to restore the body to its "natural balance." Many studies show high rates of CAM use in Western countries, including the United States, particularly to deal with chronic conditions.[3] For example, St. John's wort is by far the most commonly prescribed antidepressant for children in Germany.[4]

Herbal remedies have contributed greatly to the advancement of medicine (e.g., aspirin, quinine) and psychopharmacology. For example, *Rauwolfia serpentina* was used in Indian medicine for centuries. The active alkaloid, reserpine, was introduced into Western medicine as an antipsychotic in 1954. Although effective, side effects lessened its popularity. The ability of reserpine to induce depression and deplete brain amines became one of the foundations of the biogenic amine theory of mood disorders.[5]

Clinicians treating children and adolescents ought to have a good working knowledge of CAM for the following reasons:

- CAM remedies are consumed extensively in the community, and use is growing.[3] For example, a survey of over 2,000 persons in the United States reported a 45% increase in use from 1990 to 1997.[6]
- Many patients (or their parents) are interested in CAM.
- Knowingly or not, clinicians often treat children and adolescents who are taking CAM substances. That is, concurrent use of CAM and prescription medicines is common.[3]
- Some CAM interventions might be effective and useful.
- CAM treatments may induce side effects and interact with prescription drugs.

In spite of this and although recognizing patients' interest in CAM, many physicians do not feel comfortable asking about, discussing, or recommending CAM treatments and wish to know more about them.[7] Negative physicians' attitudes and prejudice can occasionally be a problem and may result in not inquiring about CAM use, resulting in avoidable harmful interactions with prescription drugs, and alienation of patients.

The U.S. government established the National Center for Complementary and Alternative Medicine (NCCAM) in 1998 to explore CAM practices in the context of rigorous science, train CAM researchers, and disseminate authoritative information to the public and professionals.[8] State-supported organizations with similar aims exist in many other countries. NCCAM[8] groups CAM practices into these categories:

- *Whole medical systems*, which are built on a body of theory and practice, such as homeopathic medicine (which seeks to stimulate the body's ability to heal itself by giving very small doses of highly diluted, often toxic substances) and naturopathic medicine (that aims to support the body's ability to heal itself through the use of dietary and lifestyle changes together with therapies such as herbs, massage, and joint manipulation). Non-Western systems include traditional Chinese medicine (based on the concept that disease results from imbalance in the forces of yin and yang, among others) and the Indian-origin Ayurveda (which aims to integrate body, mind, and spirit to prevent and treat disease).
- *Mind-body medicine* uses a variety of techniques designed to enhance the mind's capacity to affect bodily function and symptoms, such as meditation and the use of art, music, or dance.
- *Biologically based practices* use substances found in nature, such as herbs, foods, and vitamins. Examples include dietary supplements and herbal remedies.
- *Manipulative and body-based practices* include chiropractic or osteopathic manipulation and massage.
- *Energy medicine* involves the use of energy fields. Biofield therapies seek to influence energy fields that supposedly surround and penetrate the human body. Bioelectromagnetic-based therapies involve the use of electromagnetic fields.

This chapter focuses on biologically based treatments, particularly herbal products and supplements, which are of more relevance to child and adolescent mental health practitioners.

SAFETY

Many people believe that natural remedies—because they are natural—are safe this is often not the case. One of the main concerns refers to the fidelity of botanical and nutritional products. Apart from having to satisfy less rigorous efficacy and safety criteria than prescription drugs, herbal remedies and dietary supplements lack standardized preparation and are more prone to contamination, substitution, adulteration, incorrect packaging and storage, wrong dosage, and inappropriate labeling and advertising.[9] That is, consumers often cannot be sure they are ingesting the amount they are supposed to take or an uncontaminated substance; this has been a particular problem in products sourced from India and China. Examples include contamination of anti-inflammatory Chinese herbal remedies with the plant *Aristolochia* (aristolochic acid is a potent nephrotoxic, carcinogenic, and mutagenic agent, which has caused the so-called Chinese herb nephropathy and several deaths) and lead and other heavy metal contamination in Ayurvedic herbal medicines. Of all the dietary supplements, preparations containing ephedra have caused the most adverse events,[10] so much so that the Food and Drug Administration banned them in 2004. Ephedra, an alkaloid obtained from the plant *Ephedra sinica*, is of limited direct relevance for mental health. However, many adolescents use ephedra preparations to enhance performance in sports or, more often, to lose weight.[3]

LIABILITY

Although malpractice liability exists in theory, it has been extremely rare in practice.[11] It may include prescribing supplements known to be ineffective or unsafe or clinicians directing patients to a negligent CAM practitioner. In these cases, clinicians may also be disciplined by their professional body. One of the most important considerations is whether the use of alternative medicine treatments deprives the child of an effective mainstream therapy, occasionally resulting in the child's death; questions of child abuse or neglect have arisen in these circumstances.[11]

To avoid problems, Cohen and Kemper[11] suggest asking the following questions:

- Do parents elect to abandon effective care when the child's condition is serious or life threatening?
- Will use of the CAM therapy deprive the child from imminently necessary conventional treatment?
- Are the CAM therapies selected known to be unsafe and/or ineffective?
- Have the proper parties consented to the use of the CAM therapy?
- Is the risk/benefit ratio of the proposed CAM therapy acceptable to a reasonable clinician?
- Does the therapy have at least minority acceptance or support in the medical literature?

COMPLEMENTARY AND ALTERNATIVE MEDICINE REMEDIES USED FOR DEPRESSION

A huge number of CAM interventions are recommended or used for the treatment of depression; some of the more popular are listed in Appendix 12.1. Apart from case reports, none of them are supported by credible evidence of effectiveness. Table 12.1 summarizes CAM interventions for which there is some evidence of effectiveness for the treatment of depression, generally in adult patients. It is emphasized that, at this time, systematic evidence is largely lacking for children and adolescents. The ratings and recommendation in Table 12.1 are extrapolated from adult data to a greater or lesser extent.

OMEGA-3 FATTY ACIDS

There is growing interest in the possible benefits of long-chain polyunsaturated fatty acid supplementation in childhood mental disorders as well as in many other health problems. Neuronal membranes are rich in these compounds, called "essential" because the body does not manufacture them and must therefore be acquired through the diet. It is well known that changes in the Western diet

TABLE 12.1 COMPLEMENTARY AND ALTERNATIVE MEDICINE TREATMENTS[a]

Treatment	Quality of Evidence	Strength of Recommendation	Comments
Omega-3 fatty acids (EFAs)	**	✓✓✓	Several RCTs in adults of heterogeneous quality but few in children.[12] Meta-analyses suggest that EFAs are effective.[13,14]
St. John's wort (*Hypericum*)	**	✓✓	Many RCTs in adult patients, mostly with mild depression. Results inconsistent; larger, better designed studies with more severely depressed patients show negative results more often than smaller ones.[15] Very limited data for children.[16] *Hypericum* might be as beneficial as antidepressants in mild depression.
S-Adenosyl methionine (SAMe)	**	✓✓	Adult data, of inconsistent quality, showing that SAMe might be as effective as tricyclic antidepressants.[17,18] No evidence for children.

[a]Treatments listed here are those with some evidence of effectiveness, generally in adult patients, for the treatment of depression.
EFA, essential fatty acid; RCT, randomized controlled trial.
***Multiple high-quality scientific studies with homogeneous results.
**At least one relevant high-quality study or multiple adequate studies.
*Expert opinion, case studies, or standard of care.
✓✓✓Useful and effective.
✓✓Weight of evidence/opinion is in favor.
✓Usefulness not established.

have resulted in a reduced intake of essential fatty acids (EFAs), which are hypothesized as a factor contributing to an increase in the rates of depression. Also, epidemiologic studies suggest that a diet rich in EFAs is associated with lower rates of depression.[12]

EFFICACY

The mechanisms of action are not known, but consumption of a combination of eicosapentaenoic acid (EPA) and docosahexaenoic acid (DHA) is associated with best results. It is of note that α-linolenic acid, an omega-3 EFA found in plant products such as flaxseed oil, is not efficacious.[13]

At this point there is only one randomized controlled trial (RCT) in youth (6 to 12 years of age) with major depression, reporting a significant reduction of depressive symptoms with EFAs compared with placebo.[12] Studies in adults with major depression show an overall benefit. For example, a meta-analysis of 10 RCTs of variable quality including 329 patients found treatment with EFAs to be superior to placebo in adults with major depression (effect size, 0.61).[14] Effectiveness did not differ according to dosage, but results varied substantially among studies, some positive and some negative.[13,14] This, together with their safety, makes use of omega-3 supplements justified for the treatment of depression and bipolar disorder in children and adolescents, but more RCTs are needed.

SAFETY AND SIDE EFFECTS

Excessive amounts of EFAs (e.g., more than three servings of fish per day) can cause bleeding. EFAs can also interact with anticoagulant drugs (e.g., warfarin, clopidogrel) and may cause nuisance symptoms such as a fishy smell, flatulence, bloating, and diarrhea.[13] Little is known about long-term unwanted effects in children; a potential hazard is contamination with heavy metals or pesticides.

DOSAGE AND ADMINISTRATION

The best approach is to obtain EFAs from the diet. It has been suggested that adults eat fish at least twice a week.[13] However, young children (and pregnant women) should avoid eating large amounts of fish because of its potential contamination with mercury. The main dietary sources of EFAs are fatty fish (e.g., salmon, halibut, sardines), plant oils (e.g., flaxseed, canola), and nut oils. As noted, EFAs from plant oils (e.g., α-linolenic acid, flaxseed oil) do not seem to be efficacious.

EFAs can also be taken as fish oil capsules (a wide variety of doses and compositions are available). The dose is based on the amount—which varies according to manufacturer—of eicosapentaenoic acid (EPA) and docosahexaenoic acid (DHA), not on the quantity of oil. Adult patients with mood disorders should consume at least 1 g of EPA + DHA per day.[13] Daily doses of 400 mg of EPA and 200 mg of DHA resulted in significant benefit and no side effects in depressed children 6 to 12 years of age.[12] Fish oils should be kept refrigerated, and it is important to purchase supplements made by reputable companies that certify they are free of contaminants.

Little is known about how long treatment should last. Human and animal models suggest that the time required to restore EFAs in cerebral membranes after chronic deficiency is usually longer than the standard duration of treatment trials.[13] It would appear that once improvement is achieved, consumption of EFAs should continue indefinitely (e.g., eating fish at least twice a week or a slightly reduced amount of fish oil supplements).

ST. JOHN'S WORT

St. John's wort (*Hypericun perforatum*), also known as *Hypericum,* is one of the oldest, better studied, and most widely used CAM treatments for depression, although data for children and adolescents are limited.[16] St. John's wort is a top-selling herbal product in the United States, Germany, and other countries. Many constituents with potential biologic activity have been extracted from the flowers and leaves, the parts of the plant used for medicinal purposes. The mechanism of action is not known but is probably serotonergic.[9]

EFFICACY

There are many positive RCTs in adults with mild depression—mostly European and of variable quality[15]—and three large RCTs conducted in the United States, two negative and one that showed St. John's wort to be superior to fluoxetine but not to placebo for moderate to severe depression. One of these trials, funded by the National Institute of Mental Health,[19] found that St. John's wort was not superior to placebo, but neither was sertraline, used in one of the treatment arms. An open-label study in youths 6 to 16 years of age with major depression showed good response and tolerability.[20]

Because of the inconsistent and heterogeneous quality of the evidence, experts disagree about whether St. John's wort should be used. The National Institute of Clinical Excellence in the United Kingdom[21] concluded that St. John's wort should not be prescribed owing to lack of data in young people, the potential for drug interactions, and because it is not a licensed medicine. Although more studies are required to clarify the situation, a pragmatic view is that the effectiveness of St. John's wort is sufficiently supported by adult data to be recommended for mild depression:

- When parents or adolescents refuse taking or have not benefited from conventional antidepressant treatment
- After discussion of risks and side effects
- After the acknowledgment that treatment requires monitoring owing to side effects and, more importantly, interactions with other drugs

SAFETY AND SIDE EFFECTS

It is important for clinicians to know if patients, whether depressed or not, are taking St. John's wort because of its potential to influence the metabolism of other medications. Table 12.2 presents the more important interactions. Although limited information is available about the mechanisms involved, the common view is that St. John's wort extracts activate the cytochrome P450 system, mostly CYP3A4.[22] In particular, St. John's wort should *not* be used concurrently with antidepressants because of the risk of triggering a serotonergic syndrome. *Hypericum* also has been found to interact with drugs metabolized via other pathways. Other side effects, such as increased sensitivity to sunlight (requiring the wearing of sunglasses), gastrointestinal symptoms, fatigue, and headaches, are uncommon at therapeutic doses.

TABLE 12.2 SOME CLINICALLY SIGNIFICANT INTERACTIONS OF ST. JOHN'S WORT WITH PRESCRIPTION DRUGS

Interacting Agent	Clinical Effect/Presentation
SSRIs and similar drugs (e.g., citalopram, fluoxetine, fluvoxamine, paroxetine, sertraline)	Increased serotonergic effects and increased likelihood of adverse reactions (e.g., serotonergic syndrome).
Oral contraceptives	Reduced blood levels with risk of breakthrough bleeding. Possible failure to prevent conception.
Anticonvulsants (e.g., carbamazepine, phenytoin)	Reduced blood levels. Lowered anticonvulsant action.
Cyclosporin, tacrolimus	Reduced blood levels. Risk of rejection of transplant.
Warfarin	Reduced blood levels. Reduced anticoagulant effect.
Theophylline	Reduced blood levels and bronchodilator action.
Digoxin	Reduced blood levels and effectiveness. Toxicity upon cessation of St. John's wort.
HIV protease inhibitors (e.g., indinavir, nelfinavir, ritonavir)	Reduced blood levels with possible loss of HIV suppression. Resistance.
HIV nonnucleoside reverse transcriptase inhibitors (e.g., efavirenz, nevirapine)	Reduced blood levels with possible loss of HIV suppression. Resistance.
Triptans (e.g., sumatriptan, naratriptan, zolmitriptan)	Increased serotonergic effects and increased likelihood of adverse reactions.
Irinotecan (and possibly other drugs used to treat cancer)	Reduced blood levels and reduced myelosuppression.

Reproduced from Rey JM, Walter G, Soh N. Complementary and alternative medicine (CAM) treatments and pediatric psychopharmacology. *J Am Acad Child Adolesc Psychiatry.* 2008;47:364–368.

DOSAGE AND ADMINISTRATION

St. John's wort is available as tablets, capsules, drops, and teas. Multiple brands exist, and *Hypericum* is widely available in health food stores or via the Internet. Many St. John's wort preparations marketed also have other ingredients and should be avoided.

The adult dose of St. John's wort traditionally recommended for treating depression is 300 mg of plant extract orally three times daily (plant extracts are usually standardized to 0.3% hypericin), which can be increased to 1200 mg/day. There are no data about the optimal dose in young people. Clinicians often start with half the adult dose and increase the amount up to 300 mg three times daily after 3 or 4 weeks, if the herb is well tolerated and there is no improvement.[20] Clinical experience shows this regime results in few unwanted effects in the young.[20]

As with prescription antidepressants, there is a 2- or 3-week lag in onset of action. If side effects are marked, or if at 6 to 8 weeks *Hypericum* is deemed to be ineffective, the patient can be weaned off and another treatment considered. Unfortunately, there are no data about washout periods following discontinuation of St. John's wort. A conservative approach would be to wait 1 or 2 weeks after ceasing St. John's wort before beginning another agent.

S-ADENOSYL METHIONINE

SAMe has been used throughout Europe since the 1970s for the treatment of a variety of ailments such as depression, osteoarthritic pain, and liver problems, and it is a prescription medication in Italy, Spain, and Germany. Use as an over-the-counter dietary supplement in the United States has grown in recent years.

SAMe is a metabolite synthesized from l-methionine and present in most tissues. SAMe plays a key role in the synthesis of a variety of important molecules, such as norepinephrine, dopamine, and serotonin, through transmethylation and other processes. Although the mechanisms of action are not yet known, low SAMe levels are reported in the cerebrospinal fluid of depressed individuals and higher plasma levels are associated with a reduction in depressive symptoms.[23]

EFFICACY

RCTs—mostly European—are available for adult patients with major depression of various levels of severity; meta-analyses have concluded that SAMe is superior to placebo (causing a significant reduction in depressive symptoms of about 6 points in the Hamilton Rating Scale for Depression) but similar to other antidepressants (mostly tricyclics).[17,18] More recently, SAMe has been used as an augmenting treatment for adult patients who did not respond or responded partially to SSRIs.[24] There are hardly any data published in English for children and adolescents, apart from a few case reports.[25]

In summary, although trials involving children and adolescents are lacking, extrapolation of adult data suggests that SAMe may be effective in young people and that it may be recommended with similar provisos to those mentioned for St. John's wort. SAMe might be contraindicated in bipolar depression for there are several reports of manic switching.[26]

SAFETY AND SIDE EFFECTS

Reporting of unwanted events in SAMe treatment studies has been poor. Based on these data, the most that can be said is that side effects are not life threatening.[17] However, SAMe can occasionally cause manic switching[26]—likely to be a bigger problem in children than in adults—and serotonergic syndrome, making the combination with SSRIs potentially risky. There are no reports of significant interactions between SAMe and other medications.[23] Other side effects reported include insomnia, loss of appetite, constipation, nausea, dry mouth, sweating, dizziness, and nervousness. As is the case with herbal remedies and supplements, it is important to purchase products from reputable manufacturers.

DOSAGE AND ADMINISTRATION

SAMe can be administered parenterally, but recent studies use oral preparations. It is relatively expensive ($0.75 to $1.25 US for a 400-mg tablet). Daily doses in adults range from 400 mg to 1,600 mg. In the absence of specific research to guide prescription in the young, doses should probably be lower in children and adolescents (e.g., starting with 200 mg/day and building up the amount gradually, depending on response and tolerance).[25]

PHYSICAL EXERCISE

There has been growing interest on the potential antidepressant effect of physical exercise. Several RCTs in adult and elderly patients, although of variable quality, show enduring benefits in mood, particularly in older patients.[27,28] For example, Blumenthal et al.[28] showed in a group of 202 adults (mean age, 52 years) that physical exercise resulted in a reduction of depressive symptoms similar to treatment with sertraline and greater than to placebo. There are also suggestions that regular exercise may be protective. For example, a German prospective study of a large community sample of adolescents and young adults showed that regular exercise significantly reduced the risk of dysthymia and reduced the rate of major depression after 4 years, although the latter was not statistically significant.[29] Although there are no studies yet involving children and adolescents, this does not mean that clinicians should wait for that evidence. Physical exercise is such a well-known health- and well-being-enhancing practice that appropriate physical activity should be part of any management plan for depressed young people.

OTHER COMPLEMENTARY AND ALTERNATIVE MEDICINE TREATMENTS

Studies are lacking showing that massage, relaxation, art therapy, yoga, or meditation result in a lasting improvement in mood.[16] However, these interventions may improve young people's emotional state in the short term. There is a meta-analysis of bibliotherapy (providing patients with appropriate reading materials for therapeutic purposes, e.g., self-help) for clinically significant depression in adults, which concluded that bibliotherapy is more effective than waiting list or no treatment.[30]

RESOURCES FOR PATIENTS AND FAMILIES

Complementary and Alternative Medicine; a New Zealand website that aims to provide clear, precise, and up-to-date evidence-based information to the public about complementary and alternative medicine; available at: http://www.cam.org.nz/

The Research Council for Complementary Medicine; a United Kingdom group; available at: http://www.rccm.org.uk/default.aspx?m=0

The National Centre for Complementary and Alternative Medicine (NCCAM) website has detailed up-to-date information for practitioners and consumers; available at: http://www.nccam.nih.gov/

University of Maryland, Complementary and Alternative Medicine Index (CAM); available at: http://www.umm.edu/altmed/

Quackwatch; a website maintained by a nonprofit corporation whose purpose is to combat health-related fraud, myths, fads, fallacies, and misconduct is useful; available at: http://www.quackwatch.com/

RESOURCES FOR PROFESSIONALS

The National Centre for Complementary and Alternative Medicine (NCCAM) website has detailed up-to-date information for practitioners and consumers; available at: http://nccam.nih.gov/

The Complementary and Alternative Medicine Evidence Online (CAMEOL) database of the Research Council for Complementary Medicine has a section on depression; available at: http://www.rccm.org.uk/cameol/include/login.aspx?ReturnUrl=%2fcameol%2fDefault.aspx

House of Lords of the United Kingdom, Select Committee on Science and Technology Sixth Report: Complementary and Alternative Medicine; available at: http://www.publications.parliament.uk/pa/ld199900/ ldselect/ldsctech/123/12301.htm

Bandolier, an independent journal about evidence-based health care, has much information about CAM; available at: http://www.jr2.ox.ac.uk/bandolier/booth/booths/altmed.html

References 9, 11, 13, 15, 16, and 23

REFERENCES

1. Zollman C, Vickers A. What is complementary medicine? *Br Med J.* 1999;319:693–696.
2. University of Maryland, Center for Integrative Medicine: http://www.umm.edu/cim/.
3. Wilson KM, Klein JD, Sesselberg TS, et al. Use of complementary medicine and dietary supplements among U.S. adolescents. *J Adolesc Health.* 2006;38:385–394.
4. Fegert JM, Kolch M, Zito JM, et al. Antidepressant use in children and adolescents in Germany. *J Child Adolesc Psychopharmacol.* 2006;16:197–206.
5. Lopez-Munoz F, Bhatara VS, Alamo C, et al. Historical approach to reserpine discovery and its introduction in psychiatry. *Actas Esp Psiquiatr.* 2004:32:387–395.
6. Eisenberg DM, Davis RB, Ettner SL. Trends in alternative medicine use in the United States, 1990–1997: results of a follow-up national survey. *JAMA.* 1998;280:1569–1575.
7. Kemper KJ, O'Connor KG. Pediatricians' recommendations for complementary and alternative medical (CAM) therapies. *Ambul Pediatr.* 2004;4:482–487.
8. The National Centre for Complementary and Alternative Medicine: http://nccam.nih.gov/.
9. Rey JM, Walter G, Horrigan JP. Complementary and alternative medicine in pediatric psychopharmacology. In: Martin A, Scahill L, Charney D, et al., eds. *Pediatric Psychopharmacology. Principles and Practice.* New York: Oxford University Press; 2003:365–376.
10. Dennehy CE, Tsourounis C, Horn AJ. Dietary supplement-related adverse events reported to the California Poison Control System. *Am J Health-Sys Pharm.* 2005;62:1476–1482.
11. Cohen MH, Kemper KJ. Complementary therapies in pediatrics: a legal perspective. *Pediatrics.* 2005;115:774–781.
12. Nemets H, Nemets B, Apter A, et al. Omega-3 treatment of childhood depression: a controlled, double-blind pilot study. *Am J Psychiatry.* 2006;163:1098–1100.
13. Freeman MP, Hibbeln JR, Mischoulon D, et al. Omega-3 fatty acids: evidence for treatment and future research in psychiatry. *J Clin Psychiatry.* 2006;67:1954–1967.
14. Lin PY, Su KP. A meta-analytic review of double-blind, placebo-controlled trials of antidepressant efficacy of omega-3 fatty acids. *J Clin Psychiatry.* 2007;68:1056–1061.
15. Linde K, Berner M, Egger M, et al. St John's wort for depression. Meta-analysis of randomized controlled trials. *Br J Psychiatry.* 2005;186:99–107.

16. Jorm AF, Allen NB, O'Donnell CP, et al. Effectiveness of complementary and self-help treatments for depression in children and adolescents. *Med J Aust.* 2006;185:368–372.

17. Hardy M, Coulter I, Morton SC, et al. *S-Adenosyl-L-Methionine for Treatment of Depression, Osteoarthritis, and Liver Disease.* Evidence Report/Technology Assessment Number 64 (prepared by Southern California Evidence-Based Practice Center under Contract No. 290–97–0001). AHRQ Publication No. 02-E034. Rockville, Md: Agency for Healthcare Research and Quality; October 2002. Available at: http://www.ncbi.nlm.nih.gov/books/bv.fcgi?rid=hstat1a.chapter.2159.

18. Papakostas GI, Alpert JE, Fava M. S-adenosyl-methionine in depression: a comprehensive review of the literature. *Curr Psychiatry Rep.* 2003;5:460–466.

19. Hypericum Depression Trial Study Group. Effect of *Hypericum perforatum* (St. John's wort) in major depressive disorder: a randomized, controlled trial. *JAMA.* 2002;287:1807–1814. Full-text available at: http://jama.amaassn.org/cgi/content/full/287/14/1807?maxtoshow=&HITS=10&hits=10&RESULTFORMAT=&fulltext=hypericum&searchid=1&FIRSTINDEX=0&resourcetype=HWCIT.

20. Findling RL, McNamara NK, O'Riordan MA, et al. An open-label pilot study of St. John's wort in juvenile depression. *J Am Acad Child Adolesc Psychiatry.* 2003;42:908–914.

21. National Institute for Health and Clinical Excellence. *Depression in Children and Young People: Identification and Management in Primary, Community and Secondary Care.* National Clinical Practice Guideline No. 28. Leicester, UK: The British Psychological Society; 2005:11–12. Available at: http://www.nice.org.uk/nicemedia/pdf/cg028fullguideline.pdf.

22. Ernst E. Second thoughts about safety of St John's wort. *Lancet.* 1999;354:2014–2016.

23. Mischoulon D. Update and critique of natural remedies as antidepressant treatments. *Psychiatr Clin N Am.* 2007;30:51–68.

24. Alpert JE, Papakostas G, Mischoulon D, et al. S-adenosyl-L-methionine (SAMe) as an adjunct for resistant major depressive disorder: an open trial following partial or nonresponse to selective serotonin reuptake inhibitors or venlafaxine. *J Clin Psychopharmacol.* 2004;24:661–664.

25. Schaller JL, Thomas J, Bazzan AJ. SAMe use in children and adolescents. *Eur Child Adolesc Psychiatry.* 2004;13:332–334.

26. Carney MWP, Chary TNK, Bottiglieri T. Switch mechanism in affective illness and oral S-adenosylmethionine (SAM). *Br J Psychiatry.* 1987;150:724–725.

27. Jorm AF, Christensen H, Griffiths CM, et al. Effectiveness of complementary and self-help treatments for depression. *Med J Aust.* 2002;176:S84–S96.

28. Blumenthal JA, Babyak MA, Doraiswamy PM, et al. Exercise and pharmacotherapy in the treatment of major depressive disorder. *Psychosom Med.* 2007;69:587–596.

29. Ströhle A, Höfler M, Pfister H, et al. Physical activity and prevalence and incidence of mental disorders in adolescents and young adults. *Psychol Med.* 2007;37:1657–1666

30. den Boer PC, Wiersma D, Van den Bosch RJ. Why is self-help neglected in the treatment of emotional disorders? A meta-analysis. *Psychol Med.* 2004;34:959–971.

Complementary and Alternative Medicine Treatments Often Recommended for Depression with No Evidence of Effectiveness for Child and Adolescent Depression

Medicines and Homeopathic Remedies
- 5-Hydroxy-L-trytophan
- American ginseng (*Panax quinquefolius*)
- Ashwagandha (*Withania somnifera*)
- Astragalus (*Astragalus membranaceous*)
- Bach flower remedies (including Rescue Remedy)
- Basil (*Ocimum* spp.)
- Biotin
- Black cohosh (*Actaea racemosa* and *Cimicifuga racemosa*)
- Borage (*Borago officinalis*)
- Brahmi (*Bacopa monniera*)
- California poppy (*Eschscholtzia californica*)
- Catnip (*Nepeta cataria*)
- Cat's claw (*Uncaria tomentosa*)
- Chamomile (*Anthemis nobilis*)
- Chaste tree berry (*Vitex agnus castus*)
- Chinese medicinal mushrooms (reishi or Lingzhi) (*Ganoderma lucidum*)
- Choline
- Chromium
- Clove (*Eugenia caryophyllata*)
- Coenzyme Q10
- Cowslip (*Primula veris*)
- Damiana (*Turnera diffusa*)
- Dandelion (*Taraxacum officinale*)
- Flax seeds (linseed) (*Linum usitatissimum*)
- Foti-tieng (Chinese herbal tonic)
- Folate
- γ-Aminobutyric acid (GABA)
- Ginger (*Zingiber officinale*)
- Ginkgo biloba
- Ginseng (*Panax ginseng*)
- Gotu kola (*Centella asiatica*)
- Hawthorn (*Crataegus laevigata*)
- Homeopathy
- Hops (*Humulus lupulus*)
- Hyssop (*Hyssopus officinalis*)
- Inositol
- Kkampo (Japanese herbal therapy)
- Kava (*Piper methysticum*)
- Lecithin
- Lemon balm (*Melissa officinalis*)
- Lemongrass leaves (*Cymbopogon citrates*)
- Licorice (*Glycyrrhiza glabra*)
- Melatonin
- Milk thistle (*Silybum marianum*)
- Mistletoe (*Viscum album*)
- Motherwort (*Leonurus cardiaca*)
- Nettles (*Urtica dioica*)
- Nicotinamide
- Oats (*Avena sativa*)
- Para-aminobenzoic acid (PABA)
- Passionflower (*Passiflora incarnata*)
- Peppermint (*Mentha piperita*)
- Phenylalanine
- Purslane (*Portulaca oleracea*)
- Rehmannia (*Rehmannia glutinosa*)
- Rosemary (*Rosmarinus officinalis*)
- Sage (*Salvia officinalis*)
- Schizandra (*Schizandra chinensis*)
- Selenium
- Siberian ginseng (*Eleutherococcus senticosus*)
- Skullcap (*Scutellaria lateriflora*)
- Spirulina (*Arthrospira platensis*)
- St. Ignatius bean (*Ignatia amara*)
- Suanzaorentang
- Taurine
- Thyme (*Thymus vulgaris*)
- Tissue salts
- Tyrosine
- Valerian (*Valeriana officinalis*)
- Vervain (*Verbena officinalis*)
- Vitamins B, D, and E
- Wild yam (*Dioscorea villosa*)
- Wood betony (*Stachys officinalis*, *Betonica officinalis*)

- Yeast
- Zinc
- Zizyphus (*Zizyphus spinosa*)

Physical Treatments
- Acupuncture
- Air ionization
- Aromatherapy
- Hydrotherapy
- Reflexology

- Alexander technique
- Autogenic training
- Color therapy
- Humor
- LeShan distance healing
- Meditation
- Music therapy
- Pets
- Tai chi
- Yoga

Slightly modified from Jorm AF, Allen NB, O'Donnell CP, et al. Effectiveness of complementary and self-help treatments for depression in children and adolescents. *Med J Aust.* 2006;185:368–372. ©Copyright 2006. *The Medical Journal of Australia.* Reproduced with permission.

Managing Acute Depressive Episodes: Putting It Together in Practice

RAPHAEL G. KELVIN, PAUL O. WILKINSON, AND IAN M. GOODYER

KEY POINTS

- "Specialized treatment as usual" (STAU) for depression should be the default management approach for all cases of moderate and severe depressive illness.
- STAU requires a broad-based, expert, multimodal approach that addresses the relevant causal factors, as ascertained by the assessment.
- Specific therapies, such as cognitive behavior therapy (CBT), interpersonal psychotherapy (IPT), family therapy, and medication, when necessary, should be used selectively in addition to STAU.
- Medication treatment should not be dissociated from the other aspects of STAU.
- When applying multimodal treatment, good liaison between the professionals involved is essential to maintain coherence in case management.
- Attention should be paid to both the internal *and* the external worlds of the patients, as well as the wider system: school, peers, neighborhood, social care system, and, most of all, parents.
- Psychoeducation of the young persons, their parents, and other responsible adults is a key element in treatment and relapse prevention.
- The basic clinical skills of listening and empathy are essential, especially when risk becomes an issue.
- Performing repeated risk assessments alone identify the risk but do not change it. Therapists should focus instead on understanding the dangers and on actions to modify risk.
- The depression should be placed within the "lived experience" of the patients and their families, with the particular developmental stage of patients and their families woven into this understanding.
- Up to 20% of cases respond in the first 4 weeks of STAU.
- Overall, approximately 65% of moderate to severe depressive episodes show good response, but about 35% respond partially or are resistant to treatment.

Introduction

This chapter addresses the management of acute unipolar major depressive episodes in patients between 7 and 18 years of age. Although the focus is on cases of moderate to severe illness, reference is also made to milder episodes. Clinic-referred depression is usually heterogeneous and often presents with comorbid conditions; one isolated treatment such as cognitive behavior therapy (CBT) or interpersonal psychotherapy (IPT) may be insufficient to effect remission. Indeed, most services worldwide do not have the resources to provide such specific therapies. This chapter looks at the whole range of help child and adolescent mental health services should offer to patients presenting with acute depression. In many cases, specialized treatment as usual for depression (for brevity, referred to as STAU) is sufficient to resolve the episode, so that scarce specific therapy resources can be targeted to adolescents with more severe or treatment-resistant illnesses.[1,2] The main body of the chapter describes STAU, whose principles can be easily transferred to primary care settings because depression at all levels of severity shares common risk and

> protective factors (see Chapter 2) and elements of effective treatment. Chapter 19 specifically examines treatment in primary care settings. The term parent or parents is used to mean parents, guardians, and caregivers.

"STAU" SPECIALIST TREATMENT AS USUAL

STAU includes the full package of assessment, formulation, case management, engaging the young persons and their parents, and treatment planning and delivery. Most of these issues were discussed in earlier chapters in detail and are mentioned here briefly to present a coherent picture of the treatment of an acute episode.

ACTIVATION

Key themes in the psychology of depression include learned helplessness, impaired problem solving, distorted conflict resolution, and a tendency to ruminate negatively.[3,4] *Activation* is used here to describe the process of reversing such mindsets or cognitive styles. Clinicians must be aware that dysfunctional mindsets may evolve in the individual with depression and *also* in those in contact with the patient, potentially reinforcing the patient's negative cognitions. Activating the patient, their parents, teachers, and friends, if required, involves reflection on what led to the depression and what is required to find solutions. *Activation* here describes a shifting of mental orientation in the patient and others, from a sense of helplessness and inertia to one of action and solution. It is important to differentiate the use of the term *activation* in this context from the potential adverse effects of specific selective serotonin reuptake inhibitors (SSRIs).

CASE MANAGEMENT

A key aspect of STAU is case management. To develop and implement a management plan, the clinician needs to understand the components of case management and formulation, which include the following:

- Engaging with the young persons and their parents
- Accurately diagnosing depression and comorbid conditions
- Understanding the impairments and consequences of symptoms—the "lived experience"—including effects in other settings such as school or peer relationships
- Conducting a careful and accurate risk assessment
- Identifying risk and protective factors
- A psychoeducative process that aims at all points to *activate* patients, their parents, and the social system around patients
- A management plan arising from the assessment

Although it can be helpful to think of assessment and treatment as separate, in reality elements of treatment are part of assessment, and assessment often continues during treatment.

FORMULATION

A formulation includes (1) a summary of the presentation; (2) statements regarding diagnosis, severity, and differential diagnosis; (3) statements regarding risk; (4) statements of possible etiological, resilience, and protective factors; and (5) a decision about where and when to intervene based on a dialogue between the clinician and the patient and their parents. An understanding of what has helped as well as what makes things worse is crucial.

SEVERITY AND COMPLEXITY

The treatment plan largely depends on the severity and complexity of the case (described in Chapters 1 and 3), which have treatment and prognostic significance.[5–8] Severity may be indexed by the seriousness of functional impairment, the number of depressive symptoms, and the coexisting disorders or problems complicating the presentation, along with the length of time the disorder was present before treatment.[8–10] The presence of psychosis may indicate increased risk of bipolar disorder.[6] Although severity is important, so is *complexity*. Certain co-occurring problems or disorders—such as hopelessness, major family conflict, current abuse or undisclosed previous abuse, obsessive compulsive disorder, anxiety, attention deficit hyperactivity disorder (ADHD), conduct disorder, persistent suicidal plans and behaviors[6,9–11]—can complicate assessment and treatment. Similarly, parental mental disorder, the level of family support, and the existence of a close confiding relationship[12] have an impact on how treatment is delivered and probably on the chances of success.

RATING SCALES

Chapter 3 describes rating scales for the measurement of depressive symptoms[13] and impairment in detail. A host of other potentially useful measures and questionnaires are available to assess family relationships, parental mental health, family stress, peer relationships, life events, adversities, and so forth, but their use may often not be feasible in routine clinical practice.

It needs to be emphasized that measures such as the Mood and Feelings Questionnaire (MFQ)[14] are to be used as adjuncts to the face-to-face clinical assessment, not instead of it. Using a measure of impairment—for example, the Children's Global Assessment Scale (CGAS)—alongside a depression rating scale such as the MFQ is particularly useful. For example, a severe episode typically has a CGAS rating of <41.[15–18]

Where the self-rating scores or individual items differ significantly from current face-to-face clinical assessment, the clinician should discuss the reasons with the patient. The review may lead either to a reevaluation of the clinical assessment or of the self-ratings. Self-report scales like the MFQ may reveal unsuspected levels of self-harm ideation or plans. To manage such disclosures, clinicians are advised where possible to administer the rating scale during the clinical interview and review the results with patients and their parents. Where questionnaires are sent out in advance and the completed scales received by mail, clinicians must have in place a care pathway to ensure they can act urgently if the questionnaire or rating scale indicates a high risk of self-harm.

ASSESSING AND MANAGING RISK TO SELF AND OTHERS

Because depression is a major risk factor for completed suicide and nonsuicidal deliberate self-harm, often severity related, assessing and managing this risk is essential (described in detail in Chapters 3 and 15). In the authors' experience, there are cases where the level of suicidality or self-harm is greater than and inconsistent with the severity of the depression (e.g., where unhappy, distressing family circumstances are driving the self-harming thoughts and behavior). Continued self-harm may be perceived as evidence of failure of treatment of the depression. This assumption, when incorrect, can lead to a vicious cycle of unhelpful inpatient admissions or use of complex medication regimes in the presence of mild or even minimal depressive symptoms. In such cases treatment should address the family relationships, for example through work with the family (see Chapter 10). As highlighted in Chapters 3 and 15, in rare circumstances, a depressed young person may pose a risk to others. Clinicians should be aware of their duty to disclose this risk.

RISK AND PROTECTIVE FACTORS

Table 13.1 lists some risk factors and methods to address them. In addition, by helping all involved to understand the consequences of these risk factors, we provide *psychoeducation* and start relapse prevention work.

DEVELOPMENTAL CONSIDERATIONS

Case management ought to be adjusted to the emotional, cognitive, social, and physical development of the patient and the life cycle of the family. For example, adolescents have an increasing need for independence and a sense of themselves as evolving young adults; younger children need to feel safe and secure. In both cases, the experience of depression can have a regressive effect, which needs to be counteracted by clinicians.

TABLE 13.1 EXAMPLES OF COMMON RISK FACTORS, THEIR CONSEQUENCES, AND AREAS OF INTERVENTION

	Consequences	Treatment	Modality of Delivery
Parental conflict	• Low self-esteem • Splitting between parents: "all good" or "all bad" • Divided loyalties—leading to rumination • Lack of support from parents to child	• Psychoeducation of patient, parents, and other involved adults • Parental conflict resolution by mediation or couples work • Activate all by alerting to consequences for child • Opportunities for validation to child from each parent	• Family work • Separate treatment of parents' depression, substance abuse, and so on
Bullying	• Fear and low self-worth • Rumination on fear if not dealt with • Can sometimes resonate with other maltreatment (e.g., in the family)	• Activate all concerned to action • Ask parents to be involved in liaison with school to address bullying • Address issues in the family if bullying at school is mirrored by bullying at home	• School liaison • Family consultation • Individual work regarding coping and trauma processing
Disappointment and loss event (e.g., friendship breakdown)	• Grief and bereavement response • Loss of intimacy • Helplessness • Identification with the loss and withdrawal from current life opportunities • Loss of self-worth, guilt	• Psychoeducation about grief to all concerned • Enable expression of loss and linked feelings • Encourage actions to restart working through the loss • Emphasize importance to self-worth and current function of living in the present	• Same as above
Family history of depressive disorder	• Increased chances of developing depression • Possibly familial cultural style of relating and thinking linked to effects on development of parent being depressed	• Psychoeducation about this tendency • Place epidemiology and increased risk in context • Advise about managing this liability, relapse prevention, emotional hygiene, and early help seeking if symptoms develop	• In any of the individual modalities (STAU, CBT, IPT, BPP) • Treatment of depression in family members • Family consultations or family therapy
High neuroticism or emotionality	• Same as above	• Same as above • Enhance self-awareness and strategies to manage emotional hygiene	• In any of the individual modalities (STAU, CBT, IPT, BPP) • Family consultations, family therapy
Substance misuse: drugs and alcohol	• Direct chemical effects on mood • In vulnerable individuals may act as precipitant factor • Loss of usual relationships • Induction to crime and dishonesty • Increased risk-taking behaviors with associated hazards of adversity and loss that compound risk for depression	• Psychoeducation about drugs and alcohol and depression • Consider involvement of substance misuse service • Beware of risk of substance and medication interactions and advise accordingly	• Same as above

(continued)

TABLE 13.1 EXAMPLES OF COMMON RISK FACTORS, THEIR CONSEQUENCES, AND AREAS OF INTERVENTION (CONTINUED)

	Consequences	Treatment	Modality of Delivery
Maltreatment or very traumatic event (e.g., sexual assault)	• Guilt, confusion, loss of trust, anger and aggression often against the self • Repeated self-harm • Repeated risk-taking behaviors	• Ensure safety as necessary (e.g., by involving social services or protective agencies) • Assist in processing of trauma and helping change self-perception • Help patient develop appropriate trust in others • Help patient become active in making current relationships right and not remaining a victim by repeating the trauma	• Bringing posttrauma and safety work together with managing the depression • May require specific therapy and multisystem liaison
Ruminating cognitive style (this may operate as a predisposing or perpetuating factor)	• Tendency to stick with the negative • Failure to resolve problems • Conflict avoidance • Loss of self-worth	• Psychoeducation of patient, parents, and other involved adults • Assist problem solving and conflict resolution • Activate patient and their close others	• STAU • Specific evidence for CBT[27] • Family consultations or family therapy • Medication can help with breaking ruminatory cycles

BPP, brief psychodynamic therapy; CBT, cognitive behavior therapy; IPT, interpersonal psychotherapy; STAU, specialized treatment as usual for depression.

ENGAGING YOUTH AND PARENTS

Although this topic is described in detail in Chapter 5, it is essential to repeat that effective engagement is especially important as we seek to understand, assess, and provide helpful interventions. Barriers to this include clinicians focusing too much on their own agenda (e.g., asking questions) and too little on the patients' needs or not using listening and reflective skills. Understanding is enhanced by knowledge of *how it is for the patient*. Clinicians should never underestimate the importance of feeling understood, especially for depressed youth.

CONFIDENTIALITY AND TRUST

Trust is hard to earn yet easily broken, for example by injudicious breaches of confidentiality. With adolescents in particular, it is advisable to be clear from the outset about what can be kept confidential and what cannot. The clinician should explicitly state that appropriate adults must be informed if patients reveal something that concerns the clinician about their safety or the safety of others (see Chapter 3 for more details).

INTERVIEWING THE FAMILY OR THE INDIVIDUAL IN THE EARLY PHASES

There are reasons in favor of individual as well as family interviewing, and the ideal situation is to make both an option in case management. Joint interviews can help patients remember, especially the younger ones. They can be useful for opening up previously blocked communication between parents and children, can lead to parents describing their concern and bewilderment at what has happened, and help young persons start feeling more positive toward their parents again. Young persons describing their mental state and their experiences in front of the parents can lead parents to understand better what their child is going through. Tears are not unusual at this point and can be the beginning of an effective treatment.

TABLE 13.2 POTENTIAL MISPERCEPTIONS ARISING AS A CONSEQUENCE OF DEPRESSION

	Self	Parents	Siblings	Peers	Teachers
Depressed mood	Lower self-esteem	Guilt, anger, confusion	Loser, guilt, anger	Boring, lose interest	Not interested
Anhedonia	Fewer achievements, no pleasure	As above	As above	As above	As above
Irritability	Angry feelings	Anger	Anger	Anger	Difficult
Loss of concentration	Fewer achievements	Not listening	Not listening	What's wrong with him?	Not paying attention; falling behind
Appetite loss	No pleasure	What's wrong with my food?	Being difficult to mother	Less interaction at mealtimes	Skipping lunches
Suicidality, self-harm	Desperation	Attention seeking?	Attention seeking?	Attention seeking?	Attention seeking?

Many adolescents prefer to be seen alone because they want to say things to the therapist that they are afraid to say in front of the parents and want to feel independent. Sometimes there are so many conflicts with the parents that at the beginning it is better to see parents and child separately. They will argue during the initial interview and the child or parents may refuse to come back as a consequence.

THE "LIVED EXPERIENCE OF DEPRESSION"

It is not sufficient in specialist care just to know the symptoms of depression. To really understand depressed patients, clinicians must link the impairments associated with the particular symptoms for that individual. For example, one patient finds his schoolwork deteriorating owing to loss of concentration; another finds her sports performance diminished by loss of motivation and energy. In each case the effect is amplified through a negative feedback loop. Clinicians need to understand this, use these losses as targets for rehabilitation, and convey to the patient that they understand and together the clinician and patient can do something about it. From the patient's perspective, he may have been criticized by his teacher for not completing his schoolwork or she may be disparaged by her sports coach. For each symptom there can be associated impairments. Table 13.2 lists some further examples.

CHAIN ANALYSIS

Chain analysis can be useful in managing self-harm in young people and is equally applicable to other aspects of the depressive presentation. Chain analysis consists of naming elements in a chain of events and seeing them link together. This is a powerful method of capturing some of the three-dimensional aspects of the patient's lived experience. For example, patients are asked to relay an episode of self-harm. Often the answer is they just "felt bad" and found cutting themselves, overdosing, or risk taking with no obvious reason. Working through the events of the preceding period—minutes, hours, or days—the therapist can identify salient happenings. The salience can be highlighted by either the patient or the therapist. Once salient points are identified, they are noted on a piece of paper. Eventually, a sort of map of the chains of events (with associated emotions) emerges. A copy of the map is offered to the patient for own reference and reflection; if agreed, it can be shared with important others. This process is a form of psychoeducation and helps develop the emotional literacy of patients. Solutions may be identified by examining triggers and factors that reinforce the process.

TREATMENT PLANNING AND DELIVERY

Treatment options are discussed with the youth and family. Except in extreme circumstances, the approach is to respect their choices but also explain their likely consequences. These issues may need to be reexamined as treatment progresses and circumstances change. In the most severe cases, for example in psychotic depression or when there is severe suicide risk, involuntary treatment may be required.

OPTIMAL TREATMENT SETTING

Most cases of child or adolescent depression can be treated safely and effectively on an outpatient basis. This is contingent on having access to the range of skills and knowledge necessary and to frequent review for high-risk cases or in periods of crisis. Although admission to an inpatient unit can be seem as a safe alternative, it also poses risks. Admission may lead to a reduced sense of self-responsibility and inpatients may learn or amplify maladaptive coping strategies—such as self-harm—from each other. However, inpatient admission is the appropriate option when (1) the depression is severe and not responding to outpatient treatment; (2) it is not possible to manage the suicidal or, more rarely, homicidal risks safely despite best efforts; (3) there are doubts about diagnosis and a more close observation is needed; or (4) aspects of the home environment seem to play a major role but cannot be clarified in the outpatient setting.

Day patient or partial hospitalization offers a halfway option that can be useful where it seems important for young people to be at home or in their community in the evenings and weekends, if admission is not acceptable to the patient or family, and when a brief day-patient admission can be used for more intensive assessment or as a prelude to inpatient care.

PSYCHOEDUCATION

Psychoeducating the young person and their parents can and should be integral to the treatment. Each interaction is an opportunity to help patients and parents learn about themselves, the disorder, and how they can become experts in helping themselves recover and remain well. This includes describing the symptoms and how they affect the individual patient, discussing with the family what seems to make them better, what makes them worse, how commonly depression occurs in the community, typical time course of treatment, and what may happen if untreated. An indication should be given of what the clinician expects will occur. False optimism is not helpful, but clinicians need to look for opportunities to instill hope. Sometimes it is helpful to remember the importance of *harm minimization* and not to seek a full "cure" at any cost (e.g., where circumstances indicate it is unrealistic). Toward the end of a successful treatment, there should be discussion regarding risks in the medium and longer term (e.g., risk of recurrence), what to do to prevent recurrences, and the importance of acting early. When medication is used, appropriate information and psychoeducation regarding the medication should be part of the care.

SCHOOLS

Letting teaching staff know—after obtaining patients' and parents' consent—what the young person is going through can relieve patients' anxieties. The message conveyed depends on the severity of the depression. In milder cases, the advice may be to become aware the youth is more vulnerable, may have lapses in concentration or be more irritable, but should be able to manage school with support. In moderate to severe cases, school and family need to be helped to strike a balance between supporting attendance and schoolwork with lower achievement or, in more severe cases, partial or no attendance with reduced teachers' and parents' expectations. This needs reviewing as treatment proceeds and impairment changes. Bullying may either be a precursor or arise following the onset of depression. If so, activation of the parental and school systems to invoke effective antibullying measures is necessary.

ORGANIZATION OF STAU SESSIONS

Assessment sessions typically take 1 to 2 hours and often require more than one session. Elements of active intervention and psychoeducation should be weaved into every step. In some cases it is necessary to start medication early; in others this can be considered after four to six sessions. Frequency of sessions depends on the severity of the illness and patients' or families' ability and willingness to attend. Ideally, this should be weekly at first, decreasing in frequency as depression improves. Infrequent maintenance sessions should continue for 6 to 12 months after recovery. In some cases care can be transferred to the nonspecialist or primary care setting after recovery.[6,19] Length of sessions usually ranges from 30 to 60 minutes. Clinicians need to set aside time to write in the medical record and communicate with other professionals involved. Even when it is not felt that family sessions are necessary, feedback, discussion, education, and problem solving with the parents should be maintained from time to time.

When it is necessary to add one or more of the specific psychotherapies—CBT (see Chapter 8), ITP (see Chapter 9), and, even if there is little hard evidence, brief psychodynamic therapy (BPP) (see Chapter 11) and family therapy (see Chapter 10)—to STAU, the organization of the sessions is modified to accommodate the requirements of the specific therapy (e.g., CBT, ITP), although the other components of STAU (e.g., psychoeducation, discussion with parents, and liaison with other professionals) remain. This may be undertaken within the specific therapy sessions or as separate sessions by another team member. Thus a typical CBT intervention requires 12 weekly sessions of 45 to 60 minutes, followed by less frequent maintenance sessions (see Chapter 8). In our view, family therapy is best used alongside individual STAU or one of the specific individual psychotherapies.

SPECIFIC PSYCHOTHERAPY INPUT INTO STAU

After considering the available evidence—including the Treatment for Adolescents with Depression Study (TADS)[20] and the Adolescent Depression Antidepressant and Psychotherapy Trial (ADAPT)[1,2] studies along with the American Academy of Child and Adolescent Psychiatry[6] and National Institute for Health and Clinical Excellence (NICE) guidelines[19]—our conclusion is that specific psychotherapies such as CBT and IPT should be used for moderate to severe depression as follows: The initial approach to patients and families should be based on STAU. Subsequent to assessment, the default care package should be STAU with or without medication. Clinicians may opt for the addition of a specific therapy if the assessment indicates this may be advisable over and above STAU. The next phase in which the clinician should consider opting for the addition of a specific treatment is if STAU plus medication is not producing the desired improvement after 8 to 12 weeks. One British study suggests there is no clinical or economic benefit in adding CBT to STAU combined with medication for adolescents with severe major depressive disorder (MDD) over the short to medium term (7 to 8 months).[1,2]

There is little empirical evidence to guide us as to when specific therapies are likely to be useful. Advice is therefore based largely on clinical experience. The availability of practitioners who can deliver these therapies competently limits what can be offered in each clinic setting; patients' or families' preference should also be taken into account.

Indications for specific psychotherapies overlap; CBT may be indicated where there are high levels of anxiety or a comorbid anxiety disorder, comorbid obsessive-compulsive disorder (OCD), or a highly negative thinking style with significant cognitive distortions.[11] IPT may be indicated in cases of significant interpersonal relationship problems, losses, or changes in relationships.[21] BPP may be indicated in patients with a history of significant loss and trauma with associated distortions to the sense of self, or when CBT or IPT cannot be used.[22] We believe that formal family therapy is a useful adjunct in the treatment of moderate to severe depression[6,11,19] alongside individual treatment. There is a continuum, from involving the family in consultations, which should always take place in STAU, to formal family therapy (see Chapter 10). Indications for family work include high levels of family conflict not resolving early in the assessment process, severe misunderstandings about the youth's presentation, and family adversities (e.g., bereavements or chronic illness). Concerns regarding abuse or neglect need addressing also through the appropriate social care agencies and statutory processes. Parents who suffer from depression or other conditions should also be referred for treatment in their own right.

MEDICATION

Chapters 6 and 16 address the use of medication in detail, so that information is not repeated here. Note that medication is not advised as an initial treatment for mild depressive disorder when episodes present alone (as often occurs in community and primary care settings) or in cases where a mild depressive episode is comorbid with another primary-presenting condition such as conduct disorder. The situation with dysthymia is less clear.

Antidepressant medication should be considered—always in conjunction with STAU— in moderate or severe depressive episodes if there is no or minimal improvement with STAU after 4 to 6 weeks, if there is deterioration, or if improvement plateaus with substantial symptoms or impairment persisting after an initial improvement. Medication should be considered from the outset for patients who present with a very severe disorder (e.g., psychotic depression) and serious risk of self-harm. Clinicians should be wary of rushing to prescribe in a crisis, such as in the first hours after an episode of self-harm. Where possible, the patient should be seen soon for a second time before starting medication. This is because the therapeutic content of the initial assessment or the family's response to the crisis often leads to an improvement in symptoms. Fluoxetine should be the first choice (because it has more studies and of better quality). If after an adequate trial of fluoxetine there is no response, alternative medications should be considered. In the United Kingdom the suggested second-line treatments are sertraline and citalopram.[19]

Youth's wishes regarding their treatment are a crucial consideration. Some have clear ideas about the treatment they want or do not want. For example, a teenager may want medication and not talking treatment or vice versa. Clinicians need to ascertain these views during assessment and treatment planning and discuss their pros and cons. In helping patients and their families to decide on the best treatment, it is necessary to inform them of the risks (e.g., the rare but significant risk that antidepressants may worsen suicidality and self-harm).[23] Current risk/benefit analysis suggests that for young people with MDD, the potential benefits outweigh the risk for fluoxetine[6,19] and possibly for sertraline, citalopram, and escitalopram[24] (see also Chapters 6 and 14).

In the United Kingdom, NICE recommends that only specialist practitioners (child and adolescent psychiatrists) should initiate antidepressant treatment in children and adolescents. Nonspecialists may prescribe after a specialist's recommendation and in consultation with the specialist. This is a challenging policy that has profound implications on service delivery, and some would disagree about it being the best use of resources. The policy is aimed at accomplishing these goals:

- Curbing inappropriate prescription of SSRIs
- Encouraging adequate monitoring, which may detect and manage emerging problems earlier
- Ensuring that medication is not used as the default treatment for child and adolescent depression but encouraging a "stepped care" approach; the first step being appropriate psychosocial treatment
- Making sure that when medication is used, it is *only* used as part of an integrated care package and *not* in isolation
- Highlighting the risks in managing youth with MDD
- Encouraging appropriate service development

EXERCISE, SLEEP, AND DIET

Some evidence indicates that exercise is an antidepressant for milder episodes in adults, and the same may be true in adolescents and children[19] and should be encouraged until further research is available (see Chapter 12). Common sense is necessary; for example, in the early treatment of a melancholic adolescent with retardation, expecting physical exercise may simply be asking too much.

Sleep problems can be integral to the picture of depression. Poor sleep exacerbates irritability, loss of energy, and concentration problems. Advice on basic sleep hygiene, often linked with advice on exercise and diet, is useful.

Although evidence on the effects of diet is rather limited, there are indications that unhealthy diets can have negative effects on mood, sleep patterns, and concentration.[19,25] Some foods and drinks such as alcohol, caffeine, and chocolate are considered to influence mood. A healthy diet should be part of the management plan, particularly if there is evidence of very poor diet or poor knowledge in this regard (with the added benefit that it may prevent obesity). Preliminary evidence indicates that fish oil supplementation may be effective in treating childhood depression[26] (see Chapter 12).

REFERRING TO SPECIALIST SERVICES

A stepped care approach, summarized in Table 13.3, is advocated by the current NICE guidelines in the United Kingdom.[19] Organization of services in other parts of the world is different; the UK model is presented as an example.

TABLE 13.3 THE NICE[a] STEPPED CARE MODEL

Focus	Action	Responsibility
Detection	• Risk profiling	• Primary care (Tier 1[b])
Recognition	• Identification of disorder	• All tiers primary to tertiary care (Tiers 1–4[b])
Mild depression	• Watchful waiting • Nondirective supportive therapy • Problem solving and understanding • Group CBT • Guided self-help	• Primary care up to outreach and community-based specialist care (Tier 1–2[b])
Moderate to severe depression **Select cases of mild depression with high complexity or risk**	• STAU • Specific individual therapy and family consultation • Consider family therapy as adjunct • Fluoxetine if appropriate	• Specialist care (Tiers 2–3[b])
Depression unresponsive to treatment **Recurrent depression** **Psychotic depression**	• Intensive longer term therapy • Fluoxetine, sertraline, or citalopram • For psychosis, consider augmenting with antipsychotic	• Specialist outpatient (Tier 3[b]) • Inpatient care (Tier 4[b])

[a]NICE, National Institute for Health and Clinical Excellence.[19]
[b]Tier 1: Services that have primary or direct contact with youth for reasons other than mental health (e.g., general practice, general pediatrics, social services, health visitors, schools). Tier 2: Specialist child and adolescent mental health (CAMHS) professionals working in community-based settings alongside Tier-1 workers. Tier 3: Multidisciplinary teams of CAMHS professionals working in specialist CAMHS facilities. Tier 4: Highly specialized multidisciplinary services (often inpatient) for very severe depression or for those who need very intensive treatment or supervision.
CBT, cognitive behavior therapy. STAU, specialist treatment as usual for depression.

OUTCOMES

Among patients with MDD referred to specialist clinics, 20% are likely to respond to the first 2 to 4 weeks of assessment and early intervention (early STAU for depression).[1] A further 50% to 60% of the reminder is likely to respond over the next 12 to 28 weeks to a combination of STAU and medication. Data regarding longer term outcome are sparse. Most longer term studies have found a group of treatment-resistant patients comprising about 20% of cases by 12 months.[7,8] These treatment-resistant patients are the focus of Chapter 16.

The evidence to date indicates that our treatments are bringing forward the onset of recovery when compared with naturalistic outcomes without active care. Studies of untreated samples suggest the median length of an episode is around 7 to 8 months.[8] However, there is a subgroup of youth who will have disorders that may last years if untreated, perhaps around 20%.[7,8]

RESOURCES FOR PRACTITIONERS

References 10 and 19.
Goodyer IM, ed. *The Depressed Child & Adolescent*. 2nd ed. Cambridge, UK: Cambridge University Press; 2000.
Hawton K, James T. Suicide & deliberate self harm in young people: ABC of Adolescence series. *BrMed J* 2005;330:891–894.

RESOURCES FOR PATIENTS AND FAMILIES

Graham P, Hughes C. *So Young So Sad So Listen*. London: Gaskell Press; 2005.
National Institute for Health and Clinical Excellence. Depression in children and young people: Information for the public. Available at: http://www.nice.org.uk/guidance/index.jsp?action=download&o=29860.

Young Minds: a British charity with a lot of information about depression. Available at: http://www.youngminds.org.uk/publications/all-publications/publications-by-subject/depression/?searchterm=depression.

REFERENCES

1. Goodyer I, Dubicka B, Wilkinson P, et al. Selective serotonin reuptake inhibitors (SSRIs) and routine specialist care with and without cognitive behaviour therapy in adolescents with major depression: randomized controlled trial. *Br Med J.* 2007;335:142–146.
2. Byford S, Barrett B, Roberts C, et al. Cost-effectiveness of selective serotonin reuptake inhibitors and routine specialist care with and without cognitive-behavioural therapy in adolescents with major depression. *Br J Psychiatry.* 2007;191:521–527.
3. Seligman ME. Learned helplessness as a model of depression. Comment and integration. *J Abnorm Psychol.* 1978;87:165–179.
4. Nolen-Hoeksema S. Ruminative coping with depression. In: Heckhausen J, Dweck CS, eds. *Motivation and Self-Regulation Across the Lifespan.* Cambridge: Cambridge University Press; 1998:237–256.
5. Goodyer IM, Herbert J, Secher SM, et al. Short-term outcome of major depression: I. Comorbidity and severity at presentation as predictors of persistent disorder. *J Am Acad Child Adolesc Psychiatry.* 1997;36:179–187.
6. Birmaher B, Brent D, AACAP Work Group on Quality Issues. Practice parameter for the assessment and treatment of children and adolescents with depressive disorders. *J Am Acad Child Adolesc Psychiatry.* 2007;46:1503–1526.
7. Dunn V, Goodyer IM. Longitudinal investigation into childhood- and adolescence-onset depression: psychiatric outcome in early adulthood. *Br J Psychiatry.* 2006;188:216–222.
8. Harrington RC, Dubicka B. Natural history of mood disorders in children and adolescents. In: Goodyer I, ed. *The Depressed Child and Adolescent.* 2nd ed. Cambridge: Cambridge University Press; 2001:311–343.
9. Goodyer IM, Herbert J, Secher SM, et al. Short-term outcome of major depression: I. Comorbidity and severity at presentation as predictors of persistent disorder. *J Am Acad Child Adolesc Psychiatry.* 1997;36:179–187.
10. Curry J, Rohde P, Simons A, et al. Predictors and moderators of acute outcome in the Treatment for Adolescents with Depression Study (TADS). *J Am Acad Child Adolesc Psychiatry.* 2006;45:1427–1439.
11. Brent DA, Kolko DJ, Birmaher B, et al. Predictors of treatment efficacy in a clinical trial of three psychosocial treatments for adolescent depression. *J Am Acad Child Adolesc Psychiatry.* 1998;37:906–914.
12. Goodyer IM. Life events: their nature and effects. In: Goodyer IM, ed. *The Depressed Child and Adolescent.* 2nd ed. Cambridge: Cambridge University Press; 2001:204–232.
13. Poznanski EO, Grossman JA, Buchsbaum Y, et al. Preliminary studies of the reliability and validity of the children's depression rating scale. *J Am Acad Child Adolesc Psychiatry.* 1984;23:191–197.
14. Burlesson Davis W, Birmaher B, Melham NA, et al. Criterion validity of the Mood and Feelings Questionnaire for depressive episodes in clinic and non-clinic subjects. *J Child Psychol Psychiatry.* 2006;47:927–934.
15. Shaffer D, Gould MS, Brasic J, et al. A children's global assessment scale (C-GAS). *Arch Gen Psychiatry.* 1983;40:1228–1231.
16. Schorre BE, Vandvik IH. Global assessment of psychosocial functioning in child and adolescent psychiatry. A review of three uni-dimensional scales (CGAS, GAF, GAPD). *Eur Child Adolesc Psychiatry.* 2004;13:273–286.
17. Dyrborg J, Larsen FW, Nielsen S, et al. The Children's Global Assessment Scale (CGAS) and Global Assessment of Psychosocial Disability (GAPD) in clinical practice—substance and reliability as judged by intraclass correlations. *Eur Child Adolesc Psychiatry.* 2000;9:195–201.
18. Cooper P J, Goodyer IM. A community study of depression in adolescent girls: I. Estimates of symptom and syndrome prevalence. *Br J Psychiatry.* 1993;163:367–374.
19. National Institute for Health and Clinical Excellence. *Depression in Children and Young People: Identification and Management in Primary, Community, and Secondary Care.* National Clinical Practice Guideline No. 28. Leicester, UK: The British Psychological Society; 2005.
20. March J, Silva S, Petrycki S, et al. Fluoxetine, cognitive behaviour therapy and their combination for adolescents with depression. Treatment for Adolescents with Depression Study (TADS) randomised controlled trial. *JAMA.* 2004;292:807–820.
21. Mufson L, Dorta KP, Wickmaratne P, et al. A randomised effectiveness trial of interpersonal psychotherapy for depressed adolescents. *Arch Gen Psychiatry.* 2004;61:577–584.
22. Trowell J, Joffe I, Campbell J, et al. Childhood depression, a place for psychotherapy: an outcome study comparing individual psychodynamic psychotherapy and family therapy. *Eur Child Adolesc Psychiatry.* 2007;16:157–167.
23. Dubicka B, Hadley S, Roberts C. Suicidal behaviour in youths with depression treated with new-generation antidepressants: meta-analysis. *Br J Psychiatry.* 2006;189:393–398.

24. Bridge JA, Iyengar S, Salary CB, et al. Clinical response and risk for reported suicidal ideation and suicide attempts in pediatric antidepressant treatment: a meta-analysis of randomized controlled trials. *JAMA.* 2007; 297:1683–1696.
25. Gesch CB, Hammond SM, Hampson SE, et al. Influence of supplementary vitamins, minerals and essential fatty acids on the antisocial behaviour of young adult prisoners. Randomised, placebo-controlled trial. *Br J Psychiatry.* 2002;181:22–28.
26. Nemets H, Nemets B, Apter A, et al. Omega-3 treatment of childhood depression: a controlled, double-blind pilot study. *Am J Psychiatry.* 2006;163:1098–1100.
27. Wilkinson PO, Goodyer IM. The effects of cognitive-behavioural therapy on mood-related ruminative response style in depressed adolescents. *Child Adolesc Psychiatry Ment Health.* 2008;2:3.

Preventing, Detecting, and Managing Side Effects of Medications

STANLEY KUTCHER, AINSLIE MCDOUGALL, AND ANDREA MURPHY

KEY POINTS

- Treatment emergent adverse events (side effects) are a complicating factor in psychopharmacologic treatment and need to be properly managed and, if possible, avoided.
- Side effects can be physiological, emotional, or behavioral.
- Educating the patient and appropriate caregivers about common side effects and rare but serious side effects and what to do if they occur is an integral component of psychopharmacologic treatment.
- The use of a side effects checklist applied at baseline and at subsequent visits can provide the clinician and patient with a good framework for identification and management of treatment-emergent adverse events.
- A number of successful strategies to manage side effects can be employed, thus increasing the likelihood of treatment adherence and improved therapeutic outcomes.
- Side effects of antidepressants include, among others, suicidality, activation, manic switch, and serotonin syndrome.

Introduction

Medications play a necessary but often insufficient role in the treatment of most child and adolescent mental disorders. Unlike psychological, social, or other types of interventions, medications are regulated by agencies responsible for the safety, efficacy, and quality of these products. These include the Food and Drug Administration (FDA) (USA), Health Canada (Canada), Medicines and Healthcare Products Regulatory Agency (MHRA) (UK), European Medicines Evaluation Agency (EMEA) (European Union), and the Therapeutic Goods Administration (Australia). Although the process for medication approval may vary from one agency to another, requiring clinical trials that demonstrate the safety and efficacy of the medications is compulsory. Many medications used in treating children and adolescents, including those with mental disorders, have initially received approval for use in adult populations prior to manufacturers seeking regulatory approval for indications relevant to pediatric patients. In many instances where approval in children or adolescents has not been sought, medications are used in an "off-label" fashion (see also Chapter 4). Off-label use of a drug has been described as prescribing a medication for uses that are not included in the product information.[1] Some clinicians also consider the use of doses that are higher than recommended as off-label. As few as a quarter of marketed medications can be deemed to have met regulatory criteria for safety and efficacy in pediatric populations.[2] This is not an uncommon phenomenon in populations in which research is sparse, for a variety of reasons including legal and ethical concerns. More recently, the number of medication studies conducted in child and adolescent mental disorders has increased and so too has the number of medications that have received regulatory approval.[3,4]

Of particular importance in the regulatory process is the determination of treatment-emergent adverse events (referred to in this chapter as "adverse events" or "side effects") that have been systematically collected for those compounds registered. Adverse events can be defined as symptoms that onset during treatment and arise from that treatment.[5] Although this has served to better inform clinicians about side effects of various medications, the research is limited in children and adolescents.[6] The "off-label" use of many medications poses significant challenges for clinicians because information regarding their therapeutic value and side effects may be less readily available.[2] Also, information related to side effects collected by regulatory agencies and in the public domain may be based on data from adults. As such, information about child and adolescent-specific adverse effects may be lacking and not listed in medication information provided to or by regulatory authorities.[2]

Many studies of medication use in various child and adolescent mental disorders are relatively short term with limited follow-up periods. Thus, although there may be reasonably good information about adverse events in the acute intervention phase, there may be fewer data about side effects that occur later in the course of treatment. The information captured during these trials can also be limited to a priori specific questionnaires or scales that do not incorporate all possible side effects. Some information on longer term adverse events may be available through postmarketing surveillance, but it is not clear how this is captured for medications used "off-label." In Canada, for example, reporting of adverse reactions regardless of how the medications are used (i.e., "off label" or for approved indications) remains a voluntary process. The situation in most other countries is similar. Although viewed as a professional responsibility, the decision to report is at the discretion of the clinician, and for a variety of reasons (e.g., lack of time, unrecognized adverse reaction) reporting may be suboptimal. Other sources of information are observational studies—including case reports, case series, or case-control and cohort studies—published in journals, bulletins, web pages, or newsletters distributed by regulatory agencies. It is unlikely these can adequately capture the variety and frequency of adverse events. Nor is it likely that all practitioners will be informed about these adverse events using these methods of information distribution.

These issues notwithstanding,[7,8] substantial data pertaining to adverse events in young people are available. Although it is beyond the scope of this chapter to list all those that have been identified, resources are available to the practicing clinician in which this information can be found. These include both textbook and online sources and are listed in the resources section at end of this chapter. The purpose here is to provide a framework by which to understand and address treatment-emergent adverse events pertaining to the treatment of depression in young people.

The evidence for pharmacologic treatment of depression in children and adolescents is growing but still limited (see Chapter 6). At this time it is reasonable to consider the use of selective serotonin reuptake inhibitors (SSRIs)—especially fluoxetine—as first-line pharmacotherapy.[9-11] Every treatment decision is based on a benefit/risk evaluation, where the benefit should outweigh the risk.[5] Many medications used for the treatment of depression in adults have either not undergone sufficient

TABLE 14.1 USE AND AVOIDANCE OF ANTIDEPRESSANTS FOR CHILDREN AND ADOLESCENTS[a]

USE[b]	AVOIDANCE		
Evidence Available to Support Use	Not Extensively Studied or Negative Evidence	Ineffective	Substantial Risk of Side Effects
Fluoxetine	Mirtazapine	Imipramine	All tricyclic antidepressants
Citalopram[c]	Fluvoxamine	Desipramine	All monoamine oxidase
Sertraline[c,d]	Escitalopram	Amitriptyline	inhibitors (MAOIs)
	Reversible inhibitor of monoamine oxidase-type A (RIMAs)	Venlafaxine	Venlafaxine
	Bupropion		
	Paroxetine		

[a]Table contents based on meta-analyses and systematic reviews of efficacy and safety included in this chapter.
[b]Only fluoxetine has received regulatory approval in the United States and some other countries for the treatment of pediatric depression (see also Chapter 6).
[c]Considered second line to fluoxetine.
[d]Data favor adolescents.

evaluation in children and adolescents, have not shown to be significantly more effective than placebo, or have a side-effect profile that makes their risk generally unacceptable in young people. Table 14.1 summarizes this information. Accordingly, this chapter primarily focuses on side effects associated with antidepressants that have the best available evidence for efficacy in this population.

WHAT ARE TREATMENT-EMERGENT ADVERSE EVENTS?

Adverse events can be defined as any effect (physical, emotional, or behavioral) that is unwanted, caused by the medication, and has a negative or deleterious effect on the well-being or functioning of the individual. It is essential that the identified adverse effect is caused by the medicine. All therapeutic interventions may elicit adverse effects—even placebo! Therefore, it may be difficult to determine in the individual patient if the adverse event is caused by the medication or not.[5] This complexity is demonstrated in Table 14.2. As a result, tables that list side-effect prevalence rates (i.e., 12% reporting headaches) are not very useful for clinicians. What would be more useful is an indication of how much more frequently specific side effects occur compared with placebo. Unfortunately, such data are not easily available.

Side effects can be classified in many ways, for example (1) organ system involved (cardiovascular, digestive, locomotor, etc.); (2) impact on the individual (from nuisance [minor discomfort, such as morning drowsiness] to severe [necessitating discontinuation of treatment, or causing the onset of a debilitating illness, or a fatal result, such as an anaphylactic reaction]); (3) biochemical effects (such as anticholinergic or antihistaminic); and (4) domain in which symptoms manifest themselves (physical, emotional, or behavioral). Frequently, more than one classification is used concurrently (i.e., a minor behavioral event). Regardless of the schemata used, side effects should be described according to their frequency, severity, and duration, with adequate detail of onset and outcome. Side effects can also arise as a result of the cessation or withdrawal of treatment and are described similarly.

Adverse events arise from pharmacokinetic (what the body does to the drug, including absorption, distribution, metabolism, and elimination) or from pharmacodynamic (what the drug does to the body) interactions.

TABLE 14.2 COMBINED TREATMENT-EMERGENT ADVERSE EVENTS INCIDENCE[a] FOR PATIENTS TREATED WITH PROZAC VERSUS PLACEBO FOR DEPRESSION, OBSESSIVE-COMPULSIVE DISORDER, AND BULIMIA COMBINED

Adverse Event	Prozac (N = 2,444)	Placebo (N = 1,331)
BODY AS A WHOLE		
Headache	21	20
Asthenia[b]	12	6
Flu syndrome	5	4
Fever	2	1
CARDIOVASCULAR SYSTEM		
Vasodilation	3	1
Palpitation	2	1
DIGESTIVE SYSTEM		
Nausea[b]	23	10
Diarrhea	12	8
Anorexia[b]	11	3
Dry mouth	10	7
Dyspepsia	8	5

[a]Percentage of patients reporting event.
[b]Difference of ≥5%.
Adapted from reference 12.

PHARMACOKINETIC INTERACTIONS

For kinetic interactions, it is important to establish whether manipulations such as adding, stopping, or dosage adjustments of concomitant medications—including prescription, nonprescription, natural health products, and illicit substances—can cause new side effects or potentiate preexisting effects. These interactions often result from changes in absorption, metabolism, or elimination and less so for distribution interactions (e.g., protein binding) with concurrent use of several medications. For absorption interactions, medications may affect physiologic parameters, such as the gastric pH (e.g., antacids) or motility and transit time (e.g., laxatives).

There is a lack of documentation regarding clinically relevant interactions with the SSRIs that result from altering gastric pH. Some medications used to treat dyspepsia symptoms, including histamine-2 receptor antagonists (e.g., cimetidine) and proton pump inhibitors (e.g., omeprazole), may interact with some antidepressants, but this typically occurs by inhibiting the hepatic metabolism of the psychotropic. In excretion interactions, where the kidneys are primarily responsible for the elimination of a medication, it is often necessary to consider how other medications affect renal blood flow (e.g., nonsteroid anti-inflammatories and lithium), fluid and electrolyte homeostasis (e.g., diuretics and lithium), and whether the medication itself has been associated with causing nephrotoxicity (e.g., lithium). With concomitant lithium therapy it is essential to examine how the combination of medications may affect lithium's clearance.

When medications are combined, unanticipated changes in the serum level of drugs (e.g., decreases or increases) and adverse events can result from interactions involving the hepatic cytochrome P450 (CYP450) system in which medications are substrates (i.e., metabolized by) and competing for the same enzyme, or in cases where one medication influences (i.e., induces or inhibits) the metabolism of another. Some medications (e.g., carbamazepine, St. John's wort, modafinil) activate the CYP450 system (also called induction), resulting in an increased metabolism of other drugs metabolized by the same enzyme, typically resulting in reduced serum concentrations and a potential loss of effectiveness. A well-known example of this is carbamazepine, which has the ability to induce its own as well as the metabolism of other drugs (e.g., bupropion).[13] Another example of the same process that is common in young people is cigarette smoking.[14] St. John's wort, a natural health product, is an inducer of the CYP450 system, particularly CYP3A4[15] (see Table 12.2).

Definitive guidelines for dosage adjustments of medications are not readily available for many CYP450 interactions. It can also be difficult to judge the clinical relevance of some interactions; although many are theoretically possible, data are often nonexistent, and frequently such interactions occur without significant clinical impact.

The commonsense approach when little or no data regarding interactions are available is to recognize the potential for interaction and increase vigilance in terms of frequency of monitoring at the initiation of use, with dosage change, and when other medications are added. Involving parents and other health care providers in monitoring can also facilitate collecting information on whether or not the effects of an interaction are clinically significant. Similarly, individual differences in the efficiency of drug metabolism may create different levels of drug metabolites that may have different effects on specific body organs (e.g., carbamazepine and its major metabolite). Some studies have noted individual differences in metabolic rates between Asian versus white patients;[16,17] others are inconclusive.[18]

PHARMACODYNAMIC INTERACTIONS

Pharmacodynamic interactions usually result from the use of two or more medications that act as either agonists or antagonists at the same receptor group. The consequence can be potentiation of a side effect or emergence of new adverse effects. Examples include the following:

- Taking together two drowsiness-inducing medicines may cause excessive sedation (e.g., fluoxetine plus an antihistamine, lorazepam and mirtazapine).
- Taking medications with anticholinergic side effects concurrently can cause severe anticholinergic reactions, such as urinary retention, constipation, blurred vision, tachycardia, or confusion (e.g., imipramine and benztropine, chlorpromazine and benztropine).

"START LOW, GO SLOW, BUT GO"

Many side effects are dose related, and every medication has a toxic dose. It is important to recognize that because of individual differences, side effects can arise at different doses for different people. Receptor sensitivities can also vary from one person to another. Thus it is difficult to determine a priori what possible side effects (if any) an individual may experience as a result of taking a specific medication at any specific dose. A common approach when starting medications and titrating to the therapeutic dose is to "start low, go slow, but go;" this allows clinicians and patients to determine the individual tolerability of the medication.

As mentioned previously, side effects can also occur with placebo treatment. In many cases, double-blind, placebo-controlled trials (randomized controlled trials [RCTs]) demonstrate no statistically significant differences among reported rates of side effects between drug and placebo. It is not clear if this is owing to different methods of reporting (spontaneous or structured) or to physiologic, emotional, or behavioral changes induced by the placebo. Thus, for any individual, it may be difficult to determine if complaints following the onset of medication are the consequence of the medication itself. This is particularly true of mild to moderate symptoms. It does not seem to be as common with severe or life-threatening adverse events (personal experience of authors).

TYPES OF SIDE EFFECTS

PHYSICAL

Physical side effects include any manifestation pertaining to physical health, such as headaches, palpitations, orthostatic hypotension, dizziness, tremors, restlessness, drowsiness, dystonia, abdominal pain, diarrhea, skin rashes, anorgasmia, erectile dysfunction, and so on. Changes in laboratory parameters owing to medication but without physical symptoms are a subcategory of the physical side effects. Examples of this are increased thyroid-stimulating hormone (TSH) with lithium, elevated prolactin (PRL) levels with antipsychotic medications, increased heart rate, or prolongation of the QT interval with tricyclic antidepressants (TCAs). In some cases, changes in laboratory values may predict the onset of physical symptoms such as hypothyroidism with increased TSH, and galactorrhea with increased PRL. In many cases, these laboratory-identified changes are asymptomatic and of no clinical significance; in others, they can have substantial consequences in the long run (e.g., metabolic syndrome if olanzapine is added to an SSRI in the treatment of psychotic depression). In young people, it is not well known what long-term consequences (if any) of subclinical changes in these measures may herald. A final issue, especially in children, is that some medications (such as psychostimulants) may affect growth negatively (i.e., height and weight). This occurs over time and may not be noticed unless growth and weight are plotted over the course of treatment.

The SSRI antidepressants are, as a group, unlikely to cause clinically significant endocrine, metabolic, or cardiovascular side effects or significant changes in laboratory parameters. As a result, laboratory monitoring of SSRI treatment is not necessary; the exception is routine pregnancy testing in sexually active young women.

EMOTIONAL/BEHAVIORAL

Any medication that affects the central nervous system has the potential to induce emotional or behavioral adverse effects (e.g., mood changes such as depression or manic symptoms, anxiety or agitation, lethargy, hyperactivity). Some medications may cause unwanted effects on cognition, such as problems with attention or concentration, and difficulties with memory. All of these symptoms may be induced by antidepressant medicines, although they are relatively uncommon and usually mild.

PREVENTION OF SIDE EFFECTS

The first step in prevention is a good working knowledge of several issues pertaining to the pharmacokinetics and pharmacodynamics of specific medications, which include the following:

1. What adverse events are most likely to arise with a particular medication? For example, medications that exhibit substantial antihistaminic effects such as mirtazapine and quetiapine often induce drowsiness.
2. What side effects are most likely to arise because of drug–drug interactions associated with another medication the patient is taking? It should be remembered that over-the-counter and herbal remedies can interact with prescription medicines. For example, the combination of St. John's wort and an SSRI can lead to serotonin syndrome.[19]
3. What is the expected time course of the onset of side effects in relation to dosing? For example, when does drowsiness usually occur after taking mirtazapine, or when do symptoms of activation occur after taking bupropion?
4. What severe or potentially harmful adverse events do clinicians need to counsel patients about? Do they know what to do if these events occur? For example, does the patient know what to do if a dystonic reaction as a result of antipsychotic treatment occurs? Can the patient and caregivers recognize suicidal ideation, behaviors, and warning signs of suicide during antidepressant treatment? Allergic reactions are an adverse event that always needs to be considered, regardless of the medication.
5. What medications are being used together? Are they necessary? Whenever possible, monotherapy is preferred to polypharmacy. Antidepressant monotherapy optimally applied is typically used to treat depression in young people. However, some situations may require polypharmacy, such as psychotic depression (SSRI plus an antipsychotic), augmentation of therapeutic response (SSRI plus lithium or T4), when there are comorbid conditions (such as attention deficit hyperactivity disorder [ADHD] where a stimulant might be added to an SSRI), or short-term therapeutic layering (where an anxiolytic, such as clonazepam, may be added to an SSRI in a depressed patient suffering from panic attacks).

Another potential measure for preventing side effects is testing for CYP450 polymorphism. Variability in enzyme metabolic activity may result from polymorphisms in CYP450 genes and lead to a variability of response to SSRIs. Although testing is currently available in some jurisdictions, screening for genotype polymorphisms to guide treatment is not yet supported by evidence.[20] As new data emerge, this technology may become routine practice.

Once these issues have been considered, the clinician can deal with side-effect prevention in the following manner:

1. For compounds with specific properties that may be distressing to the patient, a therapeutic alternative (if available) may be prescribed. For example, an 18-year-old man receiving bupropion for depression and smoking cessation is unable to tolerate "jitteriness" and "insomnia"; bupropion is discontinued and fluoxetine is prescribed as an alternative.
2. Medications known to interact with another drug the patient is taking should be avoided or dose adjustments made in anticipation. The clinician should always inquire about over-the-counter medications, natural health products, and illicit or recreational drug use when prescribing.
3. The timing of doses must be considered. For example, a medication that causes drowsiness (e.g., amitriptyline) can be given at night, a medication that decreases appetite (e.g., bupropion) can be given after meals.
4. Dosing that is appropriate for the age and size of the child or adolescent may also help minimize adverse events, although not all adverse reactions are dose related. Few medications in children and adolescents have dosing guidelines well supported by pharmacokinetic and clinical trial data. Dosing of medications for children, and in some instances adolescents, is often done according to weight (e.g., mg/kg) or body surface area. For many psychotropics, mg/kg-dosing data for children and adolescence are not available. In these cases, a combination of the "start low, go slow, but go" approach, clinical experience, and consulting literature that outlines suggested starting doses and titration schedules is advisable.[21]

Knowledge of who to contact or when to access emergency services for certain side effects is important and necessary to discuss with patients. Some clinicians find it useful to outline the urgency related to some adverse reactions in terms of "can wait until the next appointment" versus "see a doctor immediately." Then it is necessary to discuss with patient and caregiver what side effect should be considered under each category (i.e., an allergic reaction to an SSRI or a seizure with bupropion would need immediate attention). Providing patients and families with a phone number for immediate contact is helpful. A World Health Organization website can be consulted to locate poison control centers around the world and emergency information.[22]

Another strategy is to anticipate side effects and initiate counteracting interventions before they occur. For example, prophylactic anticholinergic medicines (such as benztropine) may be given concurrently with typical antipsychotics when these are initiated. No such strategy is necessary for SSRIs.

As a rule of thumb, the lower the initiation dose, the less likely it is to cause side effects. Similarly, smaller dose escalations are less likely to lead to adverse events. Thus the often repeated "start low and go slow" is a useful directive that may help prevent side effects. This is particularly important in nonurgent situations such as the pharmacotherapy of depression. In the "start low and go slow" strategy, both dose initiations and increments can be lower than the manufacturer's recommendations, and the time between dose changes can be prolonged somewhat. For example, an antidepressant medication might be initiated at half-the-recommended starting dose, and the time to reach the anticipated therapeutic dose may be 2 weeks instead of 1 week.

DEALING WITH ANXIOUS PATIENTS AND CAREGIVERS

Another piece of clinical lore (albeit with some data to support it) alerts the clinician to the possible effects of anticipation or anxiety about the expression of adverse events. High levels of anxiety are associated with high rates of side-effect reporting. Similarly, patient (or sometimes parent) anticipation of side effects may be associated with high rates of side-effect reporting.

Highly anxious patients or caregivers may benefit from "microdose" initiation. For example, instead of starting fluoxetine at 10 mg, the initial dose could be 5 mg (obtained by cutting the 10 mg tablet in half). There are occasional patients in whom anxiety about medication is so high that even microdose initiation strategies do not seem to decrease the rates of self-reported side effects. In these cases, a placebo run-in or a placebo-controlled "N of one" approach may prove useful. If this is chosen as a strategy, it is essential that the patient (and caregiver) be informed participants in the process.

A PLACEBO RUN-IN STRATEGY

The patient (and caregiver) agree to start a treatment that may be either the medication or a placebo. Informed consent of patient and caregiver must be obtained. The purpose is to help them and the clinician differentiate effects that arise from the medicine from effects that are mainly driven by anxiety. A placebo is initiated, and spontaneously reported side effects are recorded. This is a "single-blind" approach in that the clinician knows the patient is taking a placebo but the patient does not. The clinician must be careful not to influence the self-reporting of symptoms. Once the placebo-induced side effects are identified and recognized by both the patient/caregiver and the clinician, the medication can be introduced using the microdose initiation method. Lack of availability of placebo or legal considerations may mitigate against the use of this strategy in some jurisdictions.

EDUCATION

Anticipation of side effects is an important issue that should be addressed in the education of patient/caregiver about the medication and its use. Open and guided discussion about anticipated therapeutic effect, time to therapeutic effect, and possible side effects (ranging from nuisance to severe) are an essential component of preventing or ameliorating the experience of negative effects. This should be supported by best available evidence that can be provided as patient handouts or as answers to frequently asked question lists. Many seasoned clinicians find it useful to begin medication treatment after the patient/caregiver has self-researched details (often using the Internet) about the medication suggested. This is important because many patients/caregivers have heard "horror stories" or read exaggerated or misinformed media reports about antidepressant medications. The clinician should encourage the sharing of this information in a nonjudgmental and respectful manner and deal with misperceptions or factual inaccuracies. Only following this discussion should medication treatment be initiated.

A useful clinical tool, called MedED, was designed to facilitate this type of discussion by two of the authors of this chapter along with other colleagues. MedED is a youth-friendly book that uses a "frequently asked questions" approach to address issues of efficacy, tolerability, safety, and therapeutic use. The resource also includes easy-to-follow monitoring sheets for functional improvements and side effects. A smaller companion, Med Ed Passport, uses similar features and allows youth to have the components of MedED in a portable format. These resources are meant to be used by patients, caregivers, and clinicians alike and provide the framework for informed and consumer-empowered discussions about medications and their use. The passport is meant to be used in every clinical situation in which medications are initiated or monitored and provides a useful, practical, and interactive framework for ongoing discussion and evaluation of efficacy, tolerability, and safety of treatment.[23] Further information about MedED can be obtained at www.teenmentalhealth.org.

Gardner and colleagues[24] have devised graphic illustrations of the expected time course for side effects and therapeutic effect of psychotropic medications (Figure 14.1). The authors have found this tool helpful in educating patients about what to expect, and patient/caregiver feedback has been positive. The take-home message is that side effects usually occur relatively early in treatment and that many if not all will spontaneously resolve as the body "gets used to the medicine." However, the expected therapeutic effect may occur later in treatment (exceptions to this rule are psychostimulants and benzodiazepines in which therapeutic effects occur more quickly). This enhances patient/caregiver understanding of the pharmacotherapy, helps clinicians and patients/caregivers to address collaboratively the issue of side effects, and improves adherence.

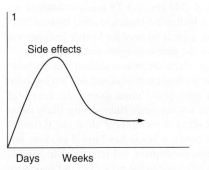

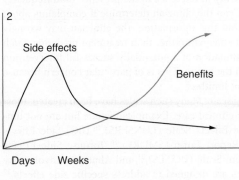

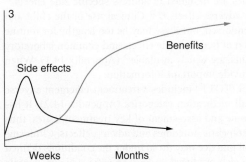

■ **Figure 14.1 The Health Professional's Antidepressant Communication Tool.** Created by D. M. Gardner, Dalhousie University, and adapted from Newman S, Gardner DM, Brown L, et al. Improving the use of antidepressants in the community: the design of a cohort and intervention study evaluating antidepressant epidemiology and adherence (ACHIEVA). *Can Pharm J.* 2007;140:175–179. Reproduced with permission.

DETECTING TREATMENT-EMERGENT ADVERSE EVENTS

A proactive approach to detecting side effects must be assumed and begins with the systematic base-line assessment of symptoms and laboratory values covering a large area of somatic dimensions prior to the initiation of any medication.[5] In the absence of this, it is simply not possible to determine if the symptom that the patient describes is new, different, or the same as was present before the med-ication was taken. Thus the traditional method of open-ended questions about side effects com-monly used by clinicians is unlikely to provide information about true adverse events. Simply put, spontaneous reporting of symptoms is not as useful as systematic questioning. Similarly, it is not possible to determine if a laboratory value is substantially different, slightly different, or unchanged if a baseline value is not established.

The baseline assessment of side effects consists of laboratory measures of physiologic parameters that are known to be affected by the medication to be prescribed. If the medication is not known to affect a particular measure, there is no reason to obtain it. For example, lithium carbonate is known to affect thyroid functioning, and thus TSH and free T4 serum levels must be taken at baseline and at appropriate time points thereafter. However, lithium carbonate treatment does not affect prolactin serum levels; thus prolactin measurement is unnecessary. Neither the SSRI medications nor bupro-pion are known to affect any laboratory measures substantially.

The clinician should not confuse laboratory testing conducted to establish or confirm a diagnosis with that undertaken for monitoring physiologic measures known to be affected by treatment. Thus, if on the basis of medical history and physical examination, a clinician suspects that a depressed patient may be suffering from hypothyroidism, the determination of TSH and free T4 levels at baseline are appropriate, even if the patient is being treated with a SSRI, which is not known to affect thyroid func-tioning. In such a case, once the diagnosis has been clarified, there is no need for further investigation of this physiologic parameter unless the clinical condition of the patient suggests this is necessary.

Establishing causality can be difficult; therefore adverse effects are best evaluated when a base-line measure of symptoms known to occur with a particular medication is obtained and not by spon-taneous reporting.[25–27] This measure is then repeated at appropriate times during the course of treatment. Changes can then be used to interpret whether or not the medication was the likely cause of the change. For example, headache may occur as a side effect of medication. However, if the cli-nician does not know whether or not the patient is experiencing headaches (and if so, how fre-quently and how intensely) prior to medication treatment, subsequent self-reports of headaches cannot be evaluated in relation to the medication. Only in reference to the presence (and frequency and intensity) of headaches before medication use can the clinician determine if complaints about headaches are new, different, or unchanged. Without this information, the clinician may wrongly conclude that the patient's symptoms are treatment emergent rather than treatment predating. Such an erroneous conclusion could lead to the discontinuation of a potentially successful intervention and prevent the patient's access to that treatment in the future. This is of particular concern because in some mental disorders, treatment options are not limitless.

The most parsimonious method is to use a rating scale. Many such scales have been created, most for use in research, but some have been applied to clinical care. Examples include but are not lim-ited to the Liverpool University Neuroleptic Side Effects Scale (LUNSERS),[28] UKU Side Effects Rating Scale,[29] Safety and Monitoring Uniform Report Form (SMURF),[26] Toronto Side Effects Scale (TSES),[30] Dosage Records Treatment Emergent Scale (DOTES),[31] and Abnormal Involuntary Movement Scale (AIMS).[32,33] Although some scales are designed to address specific side effects,[32] others are more general and address whole-body adverse effects.[26,31] Clinical use of the child and adolescent whole-body side effects scales can be endorsed, but these may be too lengthy for routine clinical use. Other scales, addressing a combination of frequent side effects and common laboratory tests while allowing patient self-report of complaints, are widely available[21] (Appendix 14.1). When applied in routine clinical care, these tools can provide important information.

The Mental Health Therapeutic Outcomes Tool (TOT)[34] includes a treatment-emergent adverse events detection scale[35] that can be used across all medication categories (Appendix 14.2). It has the added advantage of including treatment outcome and assessment of key treatment issues, thus providing a single instrument to evaluate both therapeutic outcomes and adverse effects. Clinicians who wish to use this scale in their everyday clinical practice may do so under the conditions defined by the scale's authors (Appendix 14.2). Kutcher[21] also produced an SSRI-specific side-effects scale that is available for reproduction and use. One clinical pearl regarding the use of these scales is that the clinician and patient/caregiver need to come to an agreement about what the various ratings mean. For example, when the clinician describes a side effect as "mild," it must correspond to what the patient considers to be "mild." Spending extra time at the baseline visit clarifying how symptoms are measured is necessary for optimal use of the scale. In the TOT, the anchor points for each score are defined on the scale and combine frequency, intensity, and impact of symptom for severity rating.

MANAGING SIDE EFFECTS

Even with the best initiation methods and education, adverse events may occur. Once side effects have been properly identified and characterized, it is possible to address them clinically. Serious adverse events (physical, emotional, or behavioral) need to be dealt with immediately. If they occur, the medication should be immediately discontinued and proper medical attention sought. One exception is psychotic depression, where an antipsychotic-induced acute dystonia can be treated with benztropine, the dose of the antipsychotic decreased, or an alternative agent prescribed. In settings where atypical antipsychotics are unavailable and typical antipsychotics are generally used, coadministration of benztropine at the time of medication initiation is advised. If the patient is concurrently taking an antidepressant with substantial anticholinergic effects, additional anticholinergic medication may not be needed.

Mild side effects can often be ameliorated by simple interventions while the clinician and patient/caregiver wait for their impact to decrease spontaneously. These interventions include but are not limited to the following:

- Taking medications with meals if they cause gastric upset
- Asking the patient to chew sugarless gum if medications cause dry mouth
- Taking the medication at night if it causes drowsiness
- Taking the medication in the morning if it is alerting
- Taking the medication at bedtime if it causes headaches or nausea

If the mild side effect is believed to be dose related and treatment is not urgent, a temporary dose reduction or slowing the rate of titration may be beneficial. Usually these commonsense approaches lead to their resolution and treatment discontinuation is not necessary.

Moderate side effects cause a clinical dilemma. The clinician and patient/caregiver must balance the immediate and ideally short-term negative impact of the medication against the expected long-term benefit. Before medication discontinuation is chosen, several strategies can be employed:

- The same interventions used to treat mild side effects should be instituted.
- Dose reduction to a level where the side effects are tolerable. Clinical experience indicates that some patients respond to doses lower than those suggested by the manufacturers. Therefore, if side effects limit dosing, it may be prudent and realistic to continue the patient on a dose below that which produces difficult-to-tolerate side effects. This dose could then be continued for the expected duration of initial treatment with occasional attempts to increase the dose slightly at reasonable intervals. If this strategy still elicits difficult-to-tolerate side effects, then the best tolerated dose can be maintained.
- Changing the medication to a long-acting compound or to a preparation with a different delivery system, if available (e.g., side effects related to the short half-life of stimulants and the potential to switch to slow-release preparations).
- Discontinuing the medication and using an alternative. This is more difficult when efficacy is more compelling for one medication over the alternatives (such as fluoxetine compared with other SSRIs).
- Although not advocated for long-term use and for every adverse effect, concomitant medications can sometimes be used to manage adverse effects. As an example, headache could be treated with analgesics.

These options can be discussed with the patient/caregiver and a decision as to which one to pursue made jointly.

DEALING WITH SPECIFIC ADVERSE EFFECTS OF ANTIDEPRESSANTS

SUICIDALITY CONTROVERSY WITH SSRIS

Since 2003, a great deal of debate has surrounded the treatment of child and adolescent depression.[36-43] Overall, the data demonstrate that SSRI treatment is associated with a decrease in suicidality as demonstrated in clinical trials and population studies.[41] Based on current best available evidence, the number needed to treat depression with an SSRI are estimated to be 10; the number needed to harm is 143.[41] Clinicians need to monitor their depressed patients for suicide ideation and attempts throughout treatment[43-45] and should inform their patients (and their caregivers) of the complex relationship of suicidality, depression, and its pharmacotherapy. Prudent monitoring includes frequent follow-up (e.g., weekly) after treatment initiation and with any dosage adjustments (see Chapter 15).

ACTIVATION SYNDROME VERSUS MANIC SWITCHING

It is important for clinicians to be aware of phenomena such as behavioral activation and manic switching or conversion when treating patients with medications for depression, regardless of the class. Behavioral activation can present as a constellation of symptoms, including akathisia, hostility, irritability, and agitation.[46] Differentiating these symptoms from mania-like symptoms in the child or adolescent can be difficult.

SEROTONIN SYNDROME

Serotonin syndrome has rarely been reported in the absence of a drug interaction or one serotonergic agent. Serotonin syndrome is characterized by a constellation of symptoms. including neuromuscular excitation (e.g., hyperreflexia, myoclonus, clonus, rigidity), autonomic stimulation (e.g., hyperthermia, tachycardia, diaphoresis, tremor, flushing), and altered mental status (e.g., agitation, confusion).[47,48] Depending on the severity of symptoms, it can be a life-threatening medical emergency, and appropriate medical care should be sought immediately. It is important to be aware of what medications a patient is taking to avoid interactions that may result in serotonin syndrome. Patients should be educated regarding seeking professional advice before taking any medications (including natural health products, over-the-counter medications, etc.) and counseled to seek medical advice immediately if the symptoms just listed occur.

CARDIAC-ADVERSE EVENTS

Cardiovascular-adverse events commonly considered in clinical practice with antidepressants primarily relate to TCAs and their ability to create dysrhythmias. TCAs can cause prolongation of the QT interval, which can lead to fatal arrhythmias such as torsades de pointes.[49] Detailed medical and family history (e.g., syncopal episodes, palpitations, renal disease or other causes for electrolyte abnormalities, family history of long QT syndrome, etc.), concurrent medications (to consider dynamic or kinetic interactions that can increase the risk), and physical examination (e.g., murmurs, etc.) are required when considering prescribing these agents. A physical examination as well as inquiring about any new medications or suspicious symptoms (e.g., fainting, palpitations) should be conducted at each visit. For a variety of reasons, patients with depression may also receive concurrent treatment with other psychotropics, including antipsychotics, alpha agonists, or psychostimulants, which have all been associated with various cardiovascular related effects including prolonged QT. The approach of preventative measures and comprehensive follow-ups remains the same. The importance of detailed medical histories and physical assessments should not be underestimated.

METABOLIC SYNDROME

As previously indicated, the SSRIs as a group, are unlikely to cause clinically significant endocrine, metabolic, or cardiovascular side effects, or significant changes in laboratory parameters. However, for some patients with psychotic depression, antipsychotics may be required as a concomitant treatment.

Metabolic and related side effects (e.g., hyperglycemia, hypercholesterolemia, weight gain, etc.) associated with some of the atypical antipsychotics (e.g., olanzapine) require careful consideration of risks and benefits. Adequate baseline investigations and monitoring during follow-up are required to determine the severity of these side effects if they occur.

BLEEDING

The debate about SSRIs and their potential to increase the risk of bleeding endures. Several investigators have examined the risks of bleeding with SSRIs alone and in combination with nonsteroidal anti-inflammatories (NSAIDs).[50–55] An increased risk has been demonstrated in several studies, but data are not currently available for children and adolescents. Very little guidance exists in terms of preexisting medications or diseases that may increase the risk of this potential side effect. Clinicians should obtain histories as to bleeding disorders in the patient and family members and consider illnesses that may increase the risk of bleeding (e.g., hepatitis C). Although not based on evidence from children and adolescents, the use of medications such as NSAIDs should occur with the supervision of a physician. Because these agents can be purchased without a prescription in many countries, it is advisable to counsel patients that the use of pain relievers, cough and cold remedies, or other products that may contain analgesics should not be contemplated without seeking the advice of a health provider. This approach should also be recommended for natural health products because several agents (e.g., ginkgo biloba) have been reported to have antiplatelet activity.

SEXUAL SIDE EFFECTS

Although sexual side effects of SSRIs are fairly common among adults (e.g., decreased libido, delayed orgasm, erectile dysfunction, anorgasmia), they are considerably less common for children and adolescents. Research into this area in young people is scarce,[56] but clinically these side effects may interfere with treatment adherence and not be openly discussed by sexually active youth. It is essential that clinicians enquire about sexual activity and possible sexual side effects if young people are treated with SSRIs.

PREGNANCY AND LACTATION

Another important group of adverse effects to consider related to some psychotropics, including antidepressants, is in relation to the reproductive system, pregnancy, and lactation. Clinicians who treat women of childbearing age need to be aware of these issues, regardless of the patient's age. It is important to consider the risks versus benefits of treatment for both the mother and the developing infant. Recent data suggest that some SSRIs (e.g., paroxetine) may increase the risk of malformations, particularly cardiovascular effects within the first trimester. Further long-term data are also required to assess the long-term neurologic and developmental effects in children exposed in utero to antidepressant medications. For breastfeeding mothers, it is necessary to consider the extent that medications pass into breast milk and the potential implications this has for the infant. Information on benefits and harms in pregnancy and lactation is rarely examined prospectively in controlled trials. Therefore clinicians should have up-to-date, credible resources that examine these issues; databases addressing this issue are available.[57] Other specialists (e.g., obstetricians) and health care providers (e.g., pharmacists, drug information specialists) may help determine the best therapeutic alternative and management plan during pregnancy or lactation when medication is a necessary component of care or when an in utero exposure to medication has occurred. Some manufacturers also keep registries with data regarding medication use and pregnancy outcomes.[58]

DOCUMENTING ADVERSE REACTIONS

Clinicians should document side effects accurately in the medical record. This includes what the adverse effect "looked" like, when did it happen (in relation to starting the medication, dosage changes, or stopping the medication), what interventions were necessary (what made it better or worse, were emergency services required), and what was the final outcome. Answering these key questions provides a good starting point for other clinicians involved in a patient's care who may consider prescribing certain medications.

CONCLUSION

Medication management is a combination of the science and art of medicine. The use of systematically applied measurement tools such as side-effect scales in the context of a solid knowledge of the pharmacokinetics and pharmacodynamics of the medicine used plus a supportive, collaborative decision-making approach to pharmacotherapy can be expected to enhance patient care and optimize treatment outcomes.

RESOURCES FOR PATIENTS AND FAMILIES

Psychiatric Medication for Children and Adolescent under *Facts for Families* (Nos. 21, 29, 51). Available at the American Academy of Child and Adolescent Psychiatry: http://www.aacap.org.

Koren G, Motherisk Program. *The Complete Guide to Everyday Risks in Pregnancy & Breastfeeding: Answers to your Questions About Morning Sickness, Medications, Herbs, Diseases, Chemical Exposures & More.* Toronto: R. Rose; 2004.

RESOURCES FOR PRACTITIONERS

World Health Organization. The International Programme on Chemical Safety (IPCS), World Directory of Poison Centres: www.who.int/ipcs/poisons/centre/directory/en/.

Bezchlibnyk-Butler KZ, Virani AS. *Clinical Handbook of Psychotropic Drugs for Children and Adolescents.* 2nd ed. Toronto: Hogrefe & Huber; 2007.

Medscape from MedMD: http://www.medscape.com/druginfo/druginterchecker.

National Institute of Mental Health (NIMH): http://www.nimh.nih.gov/.

Briggs GG, Freeman RK, Yaffe SJ. *Drugs in Pregnancy and Lactation: A Reference Guide to Fetal and Neonatal Risk.* 6th ed. Philadelphia, Pa; London: Lippincott Williams & Wilkins; 2002.

Eberhard-Gran M, Eskild A, Opjordsmoen S. Use of psychotropic medications in treating mood disorders during lactation: practical recommendations. *CNS Drugs.* 2006;20:187–198.

Koren G. *Medication Safety in Pregnancy & Breastfeeding : The Evidence-Based, A–to–Z Pocket Guide.* New York: McGraw-Hill; 2007.

Motherisk, treating the mother, protecting the unborn. The Hospital for Sick Children: http://www.motherisk.org/women/index.jsp. Accessed January 14, 2008.

REFERENCES

1. Gazarian M, Kelly M, McPhee JR, et al. Off-label use of medicines: consensus recommendations for evaluating appropriateness. *Med J Aust.* 2006;2:379–380.
2. Carleton BC, Smith MA, Gelin MN, et al. Pediatric adverse drugs reaction reporting: understanding and future directions. *Can J Clin Pharmacol.* 2007;14:e45–e57.
3. Laughren T. Regulatory issues in pediatric psychopharmacology. *J Am Acad Child Adolesc Psychiatry.* 1996; 34:1276–1282.
4. Benjamin DR, Smith PB, Murphy MD, et al. Peer-reviewed publication of clinical trials completed for pediatric exclusivity. *JAMA.* 2006;296:1266–1273.
5. Kutcher S, Chehil S. Physical treatments. In: Rutter M, Bishop D, Pine D, et al., eds. *Rutter's Child and Adolescent Psychiatry.* 5th ed. Oxford, UK: Blackwell; 2008.
6. Vitiello B. Research in child and adolescent psychopharmacology: recent accomplishments and new challenges. *Psychopharmacology.* 2007;191:5–13.
7. Vitiello B, Jensen PS. Developmental perspectives in pediatric psychopharmacology. *Psychopharmacol Bull.* 1995;31:75–81.
8. Vitiello B, Riddle. MA. How can we improve the assessment of safety in child and adolescent psychopharmacology? *Rutter's Child and Adolescent Psychiatry.* 2003;42:634–641.
9. Cheung AH, Emslie GJ, Mayes TL. The use of antidepressants to treat depression in children and adolescents. *Can Med Assoc J.* 2006;174:193–200.
10. Cheung AH, Emslie GJ, Mayes TL. Review of the efficacy and safety of antidepressants in youth depression. *J Child Psychol Psychiatry.* 2005;46:735–754.

11. Cheung AH, Zuckerbrot RA, Jensen PS, et al. Guidelines for Adolescent Depression in Primary Care (GLAD-PC): II. Treatment and ongoing management. *Pediatrics.* 2007;120:e1313–e1326.

12. Canadian Pharmacists Association. *Compendium of Pharmaceuticals and Specialties, The Canadian Drug Reference for Health Professionals.* Ottawa: Canadian Pharmacists Association; 2007.

13. Ketter TA, Jenkins JB, Schroeder DH, et al. Carbamazepine but not valproate induces bupropion metabolism. *J Clin Psychopharmacol.* 1995;15:327–333.

14. Desai HD, Seabolt J, Jann MW. Smoking in patients receiving psychotropic medications: a pharmacokinetic perspective. *CNS Drugs.* 2001;15:469–494.

15. Madabushi R, Frank B, Drewelow B, et al. Hyperforin in St. John's wort drug interactions. *Eur J Clin Pharmacol.* 2006;62:225–233.

16. Caraco Y, Wilkinson GR, Wood AJJ. Differences between white subjects and Chinese subjects in the in vivo inhibition of cytochrome P450s 2C19, 2D6, and 3A by omeprazole. *Clin Pharmacol Ther.* 1996;60:396–404.

17. Smits KM, Smits LJM, Schouten JSAG, et al. Influence of SERTPR and STin2 in the serotonin transporter gene on the effect of selective serotonin reuptake inhibitors in depression: a systematic review. *Mol Psychiatry.* 2004;9:433–441.

18. Hong Ng, Easteal, S, Tan, S, et al. Serotonin transporter polymorphisms and clinical response to sertraline across ethnicities. *Prog Neuro-Psychopharmacol Biol Psychiatry.* 2006;30:953–957.

19. Hu Z, Yang X, Ho PC, et al. Herb-drug interactions: a literature review. *Drugs.* 2005;65:1239–1282.

20. Evaluation of Genomic Applications in Practice and Prevention (EGAPP) Working Group. Recommendations from the EGAPP working group: Testing for cytochrome P450 polymorphisms in adults with nonpsychotic depression treated with selective serotonin reuptake inhibitors. *Genet Med.* 2007;9: 819–825.

21. Kutcher S. *Child and Adolescent Psychopharmacology.* Toronto: Saunders; 1997.

22. World Health Organization. World directory of poison centres. 2008. Available at: http://www.who.int/ipcs/poisons/centre/directory/en/.

23. Kutcher S, Murphy A, Gardner D, et al. The development of a psychopharmacotherapeutic tool for mentally ill youth and their caregivers. Poster presented at the 58th Annual Canadian Psychiatric Association Conference, Montreal, Quebec, November 2007.

24. Newman SC, Gardner D, Brown L et al. Improving the use of antidepressants in the community: the design of a cohort and intervention study evaluating antidepressant epidemiology and adherence (ACHIEVA). *Can Pharm J.* 2007;140:175–179.

25. Brent D. Antidepressants and suicidal behavior: cause or cure? *Am J Psychiatry.* 2007;164:989–991.

26. Greenhill LL, Vitiello B, Fisher P, et al. Comparison of increasingly detailed elicitation methods for the assessment of adverse events in pediatric psychopharmacology. *J Am Acad Child Adolesc Psychiatry.* 2004; 43:1488–1496.

27. Jordan S, Knight J, Pointon D. Monitoring adverse drug reactions: scales, profiles and checklists. *Int Nurs Rev.* 1995;166:650–653.

28. Day JC, Wood G, Dewey M, et al. A self-rating scale for measuring neuroleptic side-effects. Validation in a group of schizophrenic patients. *Br J Psychiatry.* 1995;166:650–653.

29. Lingjaerde O, Ahlfors UG, Bech P, et al. The UKU side effect rating scale. A new comprehensive rating scale for psychotropic drugs and a cross-sectional study of side effects in neuroleptic-treated patients. *Acta Psychiatr Scand Suppl.* 1987;334:1–100.

30. Vanderkooy JD, Kennedy SH, Bagby RM. Antidepressant side effects in depression patients treated in a naturalistic setting: a study of bupropion, moclobemide, paroxetine, sertraline, and venlafaxine. *Can J Psychiatry.* 2002;47:174–180.

31. Fleischhaker C, Heiser P, Hennighausen K. Clinical drug monitoring in child and adolescent psychiatry: side effects of atypical neuroleptics. *J Child Adolesc Psychopharmacol.* 2006;16:308–316.

32. Guy WA. Abnormal Involuntary Movement Scale (AIMS). *ECDEU Assessment Manual for Psychopharmacology.* Washington, DC: U.S. Department of Health Education and Welfare; 1976:534–537.

33. Munetz MR, Benjamin S. How to examine patients using the Abnormal Involuntary Movement Scale. *Hosp Comm Psychiatry.* 1988;39:1172–1177.

34. Chehill S, Kutcher S. Mental Health Therapeutic Outcomes Tool (MHTOT), 2007 (see Appendix 14.2).

35. Kutcher S. Practitioner review: the pharmacology of adolescent depression. *J Child Psychol Psychiatry.* 1997;38:755–767.

36. Hammad TA, Laughren T, Racoosin J. Suicidality in pediatric patients treated with antidepressant drugs. *Arch Gen Psychiatry.* 2006;63:332–339.

37. Hetrick S, Merry S, McKenzie J, et al. Selective serotonin reuptake inhibitors (SSRIs) for depressive disorders in children and adolescents. *Cochrane Database Syst Rev (Online).* 2007;3.

38. Kaizar EE, Greenhouse JB, Seltman H, et al. Do antidepressants cause suicidality in children? A bayesian meta-analysis. *Clin Trials.* 2006;3:73–98.

39. Dubicka B, Hadley S, Roberts C. Suicidal behavior in youths with depression treated with new-generation antidepressants: meta-analysis. *Br J Psychiatry.* 2006;189:393–398.

40. Mann JJ, Emslie G, Baldessarini RJ, et al. ACNP task force report on SSRIs and suicidal behavior in youth. *Neuropsychopharmacology.* 2006;31:473–492.
41. Bridge JA, Iyengar S, Salary CB, et al. Clinical response and risk for reported suicidal ideation and suicide attempts in pediatric antidepressant treatment: a meta-analysis of randomized controlled trials. *JAMA.* 2007;297:1683–1696.
42. Sharp SC, Hellings JA. Efficacy and safety of selective serotonin reuptake inhibitors in the treatment of depression in children and adolescents: practitioner review. *Clin Drug Invest.* 2006;26:247–255.
43. Kutcher S, Gardner D. Use of selective serotonin reuptake inhibitors and youth suicide: making sense of a confusing story. *Curr Opin Psychiatry.* 2008;21:65–69.
44. TADS Team. The treatment for adolescents with depression study (TADS): long term effectiveness and safety outcomes. *Arch Gen Psychiatry.* 2007;64:1132–1143.
45. March J, Silva S, Petrycki S, et al. Fluoxetine, cognitive-behavioral therapy, and their combination for adolescents with depression: treatment for adolescents with depression study (TADS) randomized controlled trial. *JAMA.* 2004;292:807–820.
46. Rey JM, Martin A. Selective serotonin reuptake inhibitors and suicidality in juveniles: review of the evidence and implications for clinical practice. *Child Adolesc Psychiatric Clin N Am.* 2006;15:221–237.
47. Isbister GK, Buckley NA, Whyte IM. Serotonin toxicity: a practical approach to diagnosis and treatment. *Med J Aust.* 2007;187:361–365.
48. Dunkley EJ, Isbister GK, Sibbritt D, et al. The Hunter serotonin toxicity criteria: simple and accurate diagnostic decision rules for serotonin toxicity. *Q J Med.* 2003;96:635–642.
49. Blair J, Taggart B, Martin A. Electrocardiographic safety profile and monitoring guidelines in pediatric psychopharmacology. *J Neural Trans.* 2004;111:791–815.
50. Dalton SO, Johansen C, Mellemkjaer L, et al. Use of selective serotonin reuptake inhibitors and risk of upper gastrointestinal tract bleeding: a population-based cohort study. *Arch Intern Med.* 2003;163:59–64.
51. de Abajo FJ, Jick H, Derby L, et al. Intracranial haemorrhage and use of selective serotonin reuptake inhibitors. *Br J Clin Pharmacol.* 2000;50:43–47.
52. de Abajo FJ, Rodriguez LA, Montero D. Association between selective serotonin reuptake inhibitors and upper gastrointestinal bleeding: population based case-control study. *Br Med J.* 1999;319:1106–1109.
53. Kharofa J, Sekar P, Haverbusch M, et al. Selective serotonin reuptake inhibitors and risk of hemorrhagic stroke. *Stroke.* 2007;38:3049–3051.
54. Tata LJ, Fortun PJ, Hubbard RB, et al. Does concurrent prescription of selective serotonin reuptake inhibitors and non-steroidal anti-inflammatory drugs substantially increase the risk of upper gastrointestinal bleeding? *Aliment Pharmacol Ther.* 2005;22:175–181.
55. Loke YK, Trivedi AN, Singh S. Meta-analysis: gastrointestinal bleeding due to interaction between selective serotonin uptake inhibitors and non-steroidal anti-inflammatory drugs. *Aliment Pharmacol Ther.* 2008;27:31–40.
56. Scharko AM. Selective serotonin reuptake inhibitor-induced sexual dysfunction in adolescents: a review. *J Am Acad Child Adolesc Psychiatry.* 2004;43:1071–1079.
57. Motherisk, treating the mother, protecting the unborn. The Hospital for Sick Children. Available at: http://www.motherisk.org/women/index.jsp. Accessed January 14, 2008.
58. GlaxoSmithKline Pregnancy Registries: Bupropion Pregnancy Registry. Available at: http://pregnancyregistry.gsk.com/bupropion.html. Accessed January 4, 2008.

Side Effects of Antidepressants

Name: _____   Date: _____

Medication: _____   Dose: _____

Circle the number that best describes how the patient has experienced *each* of the following possible side effects over the past week:

Subjective side effects	Never		Somewhat		Constantly
Trouble sleeping	0	1	2	3	4
Heart racing	0	1	2	3	4
Heart pounding	0	1	2	3	4
Feeling dizzy	0	1	2	3	4
Feeling tense inside	0	1	2	3	4
Restlessness	0	1	2	3	4
Numbness of hands or feet	0	1	2	3	4
Tingling in hands and feet	0	1	2	3	4
Trouble keeping balance	0	1	2	3	4
Dry mouth	0	1	2	3	4
Blurred vision	0	1	2	3	4
Seeing double	0	1	2	3	4
Constipation	0	1	2	3	4
Diarrhea	0	1	2	3	4
Delays when urinating	0	1	2	3	4
Itchiness	0	1	2	3	4
Light hurting eyes	0	1	2	3	4
Nausea	0	1	2	3	4
Vomiting	0	1	2	3	4
Increased/poor appetite	0	1	2	3	4
Stomach pains	0	1	2	3	4
Drowsy	0	1	2	3	4
Leg spasms at night	0	1	2	3	4
Sweating	0	1	2	3	4
Tremor	0	1	2	3	4
Headache	0	1	2	3	4
Sexual: _____	0	1	2	3	4
Other: _____	0	1	2	3	4

Objective side effects (to be determined from the appropriate clinical examination)

BP sitting: _____   Pulse: _____   Weight: _____

BP standing: _____

EKG report summary: _____

Signature: _____

Mental Health Therapeutic Outcomes Tool

NAME: _____ Tele: _____

File# _____

Informant (name & relation): _____

Tele: _____

ΨDx:		Med Dx:	
ΨMedications:		Medications:	

ΨMEDICATION TARGET SYMPTOMS (rate over past week)	*Rating 0–3		ΨMEDICATION TARGET SYMPTOMS (rate over past week)	*Rating 0–3	
	Patient	Informant		Patient	Informant

FOR PATIENTS ON ANY PSYCHIATRIC MEDICATION – RATE SIDE EFFECTS (SE) OVER THE PAST WEEK:															
*SIDE EFFECT	0	1	2	3	*SIDE EFFECT	0	1	2	3	*SIDE EFFECT	0	1	2	3
Headache					Change in Weight					Sleep Problems				
Daytime Drowsiness					Stomachaches					Nightmares				
Foggy Head/Spaced Out					Dry Mouth					Nervousness/ Anxiety				
Confusion					Diarrhea					↑ Irritability/ Crankiness				
Blurry Vision					Constipation					↑ Mood Swings				

(continued)

Feeling Unsteady/Dizzy				Sweating					↑ Suicidal Ideation			
Nausea				Skin Rash					Trouble Urinating			
Vomiting				Fatigue/Lethargy					↓ Interest in Sex			
Change in Appetite				Acne					↓ Sexual Function			

OTHER:

FOR PATIENTS ON ANTIPSYCHOTIC MEDICATION – RATE SIDE EFFECTS (SE) OVER THE PAST WEEK:

*SIDE EFFECT	0	1	2	3	*SIDE EFFECT	0	1	2	3	*SIDE EFFECT	0	1	2	3
Tremor					Restlessness/Agitation					Slurred Speech				
Stiffness					Dystonia					Menstrual Problems				
Drooling					Balance Problems					Breast Enlargement				
Slowed Down					Odd Movements					Nipple Discharge				

OTHER:

*SAFETY	YES	NO	*SAFETY	YES	NO	*SAFETY	YES	NO
Poor Compliance			Suicide Ideation			Self-Harm Behavior		
Poor Insight			Suicide Intent			Aggression		
Substance Use			Suicide Plan			Risk Behavior		

OTHER:

(continued)

*Symptom Rating: 0 = Absent   1 = Present/not problematic   2 = Problematic/Ø impairment   3 = Problematic/ + impairment

PHYSICAL EXAM: Weight: _____   HR: _____   BP: _____

Temp:_____   ECG: Yes _____ No _____

PHYSICAL EXAM FOR PATIENTS ON ANTIPSYCHOTIC MEDICATIONS

EPS EXAM	0	1	2	3	EPS EXAM	0	1	2	3	EPS EXAM	0	1	2	3
Bradykinesia					Tongue Movements					Stiffness				
Akathisia					Tremor					Accentuation	Y	N		
Abnormal Movements					Balance					Abnormal Gait				

NOTES:

CLINICAL CHANGE RATING	Rate change since last assessment based on patient, informant, and clinician impression (–2 to +2)
	–2: much worse –1: little worse 0: no change +1: little better +2: much better

DOMAIN	PATIENT RATING					INFORMANT RATING					CLINICIAN RATING				
Symptoms	–2	–1	0	+1	+2	–2	–1	0	+1	+2	–2	–1	0	+1	+2
Side effects	–2	–1	0	+1	+2	–2	–1	0	+1	+2	–2	–1	0	+1	+2
School/work function	–2	–1	0	+1	+2	–2	–1	0	+1	+2	–2	–1	0	+1	+2
Family function	–2	–1	0	+1	+2	–2	–1	0	+1	+2	–2	–1	0	+1	+2
Peer function	–2	–1	0	+1	+2	–2	–1	0	+1	+2	–2	–1	0	+1	+2
Recreation function	–2	–1	0	+1	+2	–2	–1	0	+1	+2	–2	–1	0	+1	+2
Self care	–2	–1	0	+1	+2	–2	–1	0	+1	+2	–2	–1	0	+1	+2
Safety	–2	–1	0	+1	+2	–2	–1	0	+1	+2	–2	–1	0	+1	+2
Summary (since last assessment)	–2	–1	0	+1	+2	–2	–1	0	+1	+2	–2	–1	0	+1	+2

(continued)

OVERALL IMPROVEMENT Since Initiation of Intervention or Mental Health Contact	Patient Overall Rating					Informant Overall Rating					Clinician Overall Rating				
	−2	−1	0	+1	+2	−2	−1	0	+1	+2	−2	−1	0	+1	+2

NOTES:

_____

_____

_____

_____

_____

_____

_____

_____

_____

_____

_____

_____

IMPRESSION/PLAN: _____

_____

_____

_____

FOLLOW-UP DATE/TIME: _____

ASSESSMENT COMPLETED BY:

SIGN _____DATE _____

The Mental Health Therapeutic Outcomes Tool (TOT) may be used by experienced clinicians in their care of patients. Any other use requires express written consent of its authors. They can be reached at skutcher@dal.ca or sonia.chehil@dal.ca. The TOT is also available online at: http//:www.teenmentalhealth.org under the practitioner section.

Managing Crises and Emergencies in the Course of Treatment

AVA T. ALBRECHT

KEY POINTS

- Life-threatening emergencies in the field of child and adolescent psychiatry are uncommon. When they occur, almost half are for suicidal threats or behavior, and nearly a quarter for violent or destructive behaviors, symptoms that often occur in depression.
- Additional crises include nonadherence, treatment refusal, sudden deterioration, school refusal, family instability, and peer and school problems.
- Have a means of being contacted urgently for crisis situations.
- Assess the nature of the crisis or emergency over the telephone first.
- Counseling and reassurance may be all that is needed to stabilize a crisis.
- Refer to the emergency room if there is concern for suicidality or dangerousness and the child cannot be seen in a timely manner, using emergency medical services or police if necessary.
- Distinguish between nonsuicidal self-injury and suicide attempt (consider intent, lethality, and chronicity of behavior).
- Assess medication compliance at every visit.
- Coordinate with other providers caring for the child (e.g., therapists, school counselors, case managers, pediatricians).
- Address family crises (e.g., divorce, violence, financial instability, abuse), which can precipitate a deterioration.
- Family psychopathology may require referral of parent or parents for treatment.
- Assess academic functioning and facilitate appropriate school-based services.
- Monitor substance use.

Introduction

Life-threatening emergencies in the field of child and adolescent psychiatry are uncommon. When they occur, almost half are for suicidal threats or behavior, and nearly a quarter for violent or destructive behaviors.[1] Emergencies and crises that present during the course of treatment often are related to the perceptions of the persons involved in the supervision of the child (usually parents, but school personnel and other providers as well), and thus they may be secondary to circumstances apart from the child, such as stressors within the family. Although crises can occur with any psychiatric illness, they are common in depressive disorders, particularly suicidal behaviors. The prevention of crises and emergencies is facilitated by a comprehensive evaluation of patients and their environment, looking for risks, close management, and follow-up during the treatment phase, and timely response to new problems or new stressors. Table 15.1 outlines various crisis situations that can occur in the treatment of depressed children and notes potential adverse outcomes if they are not addressed judiciously.

TABLE 15.1 CRISES, POTENTIAL ADVERSE OUTCOMES, AND INTERVENTIONS

Crisis	Potential Adverse Outcome	Initial Intervention
Suicidal behavior	Suicide attempt or completion	Evaluation for safety and treatment plan adjustments • Emergency department (ED) versus office visit • Consider medication adjustment • Consider increase in freqency of therapy
Homicidal behavior or violence	Serious injury to others/legal problems	Evaluation for safety and treatment plan adjustments • ED versus office visit • Consider medication adjustment • Consider other disorders
Sudden deterioration	Hospitalization	Reevaluate treatment plan • Assess adherence • Consider medication adjustment • Assess for new stressors
Nonadherence with treatment	Treatment refusal/untreated depression complications	Regular monitoring of adherence • Psychoeducation • Simplify dosing schedules • Behavioral interventions for refusal
School conflicts	Academic delay/dropout	Assess academic needs • Communicate with school personnel • Facilitate requests for accommodations if needed
Family instability	Increased stress within support group	Family sessions • Closely monitor in presence of family discord • Refer parents for individual treatment as needed

Unquestionably, suicidal behaviors, homicidal ideation, aggression, and violence are the most urgent crises to manage. Other crises that are often encountered include running away from home, manic switching, sudden deterioration, the emergence of psychotic symptoms, school crises (e.g., dropping out), family conflict (e.g., abuse), and substance use. Timely intervention is important because these situations can spiral out of control for both patient and family leaving them feeling hopeless and overwhelmed, and potentially resulting in worse outcomes. Crises may be directly related to the child's depressive illness or owing to other factors. Additionally, because the treatment for depression typically extends into a year or more, new crises can present that were absent at the start of treatment.

Phone contact with the concerned party (e.g., parent, patient, school professional) is the simplest and quickest method to avoid and manage crises. The clinician must be available to respond to urgent calls, so that early telephone intervention can be initiated, and the clinician's call policy should be known to the patient at the start of treatment. The nature of the crisis and the level of risk can often be assessed through the phone call. To evaluate if an emergency exists, it is important to clarify the exact circumstances and antecedents. Some crises can thus be managed over the telephone with support and counseling and a plan for follow-up. Other crises may require bringing the child or adolescent to the emergency department. In some countries or areas with well-developed community mental health services, specialist teams can conduct home visits, evaluate the crisis, and provide appropriate treatment and support without the need to use emergency department services. Almost always a follow-up appointment is needed as soon as possible. The more common crises are discussed in the paragraphs that follow. The word *child* is used to refer to children and adolescents unless specified otherwise; *parent* is used to mean parents, guardians, or caregivers.

SUICIDAL BEHAVIOR

Depressive disorders carry an increased risk for suicidal behavior, which ranges from ideation, through threats and attempts, to completion. Both the initial and ongoing assessment of depression should always include an evaluation of suicide risk (see Chapter 3). Suicide attempts and completion are among the most significant consequences of major depressive disorder (MDD) in youth, with approximately 60% reporting having thought about suicide and 30% actually attempting suicide.[2] Prepubertal children are at lower risk for suicide attempts than adolescents, with completed suicides becoming gradually more frequent with increasing age, even within adolescence.[3] In the United States, suicide is the third leading cause of death for both the 10 to 14 years and the 15 to 19 years age groups, representing 7.2% and 11.8% of all deaths, respectively.[4] A recent review by Kloos et al.[5] examines the nature of prepubertal suicidality, the relative dearth of information regarding the screening of this age group, and risk factors for suicide attempts, noting that even in the younger age groups, screening should take place for suicidal behaviors, especially in the presence of depression. Family psychopathology appears to be a contributing risk for childhood suicide that continues into adolescence.[3,5,6]

Assessment of suicide risk, particularly suicidal intent, is complex and unreliable. The Columbia Classification Algorithm for Suicide Assessment (C-CASA), a standardized suicidal rating system developed for the evaluation of suicidality in antidepressant trials, is reliable (intraclass correlation coefficient, 0.89) and transportable, and the Food and Drug Administration (FDA) has mandated its use in psychotropic and other drug trials.[7] Although this is a research instrument, it may also be useful in clinical practice, at least by standardizing the terminology. Appendix 15.1 lists C-CASA definitions and examples.

A suicidality assessment should be done for all patients with depression, encompassing both a risk assessment and an evaluation of the safety systems present or needed to minimize risk. Although ongoing assessment of suicidality is obviously required when present at the start of treatment, it is not always evident that it requires continued reassessment even if absent at the outset. A review of symptoms during follow-up visits should include questions regarding the presence or absence of suicidal thoughts. This is particularly important with the initiation of pharmacotherapy, discussed in detail in Chapter 6. Should suicidal behavior arise during the course of treatment, knowledge of the initial presentation will guide an assessment of any additional interventions. The presence of suicidal behavior may come to the treatment provider's attention via a telephone call or during a follow-up visit. If through a phone call, an initial assessment over the phone is necessary to determine if the child needs to be brought to the emergency department for immediate evaluation or to the office or clinic for further assessment (which also depends on how soon the child can be seen, the judged level of acute risk, and the level of supervision; when in doubt, an emergency department referral is the safest option). Based on knowledge of the patient and the parent's ability to provide close monitoring of the child, a decision to evaluate in the office may be made. If a suicide attempt is reported, the most prudent action would be an immediate evaluation in the emergency department to determine if hospitalization is warranted. If the parent is not able to transport the child to an emergency department safely, emergency medical services and/or police can be contacted for assistance. Supervision of the child should be continuous until help arrives. Nonsuicidal self-injurious behavior may not require an emergency assessment (see further discussion later).

Various factors need to be considered when assessing suicide risk. The risk increases if these situations are present:

- A history of suicide attempts
- Comorbid psychiatric disorders (e.g., disruptive disorders, substance abuse)
- Impulsivity and aggression
- Availability of lethal agents (e.g., firearms)
- Exposure to negative events (e.g., physical or sexual abuse, violence)
- Substance abuse
- Family pathology and family history of suicidal behavior
- Hopelessness
- Psychosis
- Reduced level of support

The availability of lethal means of suicide should be assessed because firearms, suffocation, and poisoning were the top three methods used in the United States for suicide in both the 10-to-14 and the 15-to-19 age brackets,[4] with suffocation the top choice for the younger age group and firearms for the older group (the relative frequency of the means used for suicide vary from country to country; see Chapter 24).

Keep in mind that adolescents may not initially reveal thoughts of suicide, which will probably need to be drawn out using indirect questions (e.g. "Do you ever have thoughts that you'd rather not live or wish you'd never been born?"). Acknowledgment of more "passive" means of dying or suicide are more readily elicited and can further enable accurate reporting to questions about intent or plans. Here are some questions for assessing suicidal ideation:

- Did you ever wish you weren't born?
- Did you ever wish you could disappear?
- Did you ever wonder about death?
- Did you ever consider hurting yourself?
- Did you ever have thoughts about killing yourself?
- Did you ever think of a plan to kill yourself?
- What sort of plans have you considered?
- Do you want to die?
- What keeps you from killing yourself?

Further suicide assessment should include questions about whether or not the child has considered a plan in the past or more recently, as well as an assessment of suicidal intent, which examines the desire to die versus to live. As noted earlier, access to guns or medications should be ascertained from the child and the parent and eliminated. Ultimately, if a child presents with a specific plan, and with the intention to carry the plan out, hospitalization is probably warranted. With lesser degrees of intent, the need for hospitalization depends on the balance of risk and protective factors, as well as the ability of parents to provide round-the-clock supervision while the treatment plan is adjusted.

In addition to hopelessness, hostility, negative self-concept and isolation are also proposed as psychosocial factors to consider when assessing risk.[8] Higher risk periods for suicide occur following discharge from hospital, after a medication change, or during an absence of the therapist. With an adequate support system in place, a child may be safely monitored as an outpatient with daily phone calls and weekly, or more frequent, visits. Once a child has been in treatment for some time, knowledge of the child will make it easier to manage these eventualities.

When onset occurs during the course of treatment, the effectiveness of the treatment ought to be reviewed. Emergent suicidality may be owing to a new disorder, a side effect, or lack of efficacy of the medication. If the suicidal ideation is new and treatment was recently started, continuation of the treatment plan (with adequate monitoring and safeguards, such as close supervision at home and school, regular telephone contact, and more frequent office visits) may simply be required. The suicidal behavior can also be contrasted with the symptoms present during the evaluation phase to determine if the treatment is working. If symptoms have been in remission, the occurrence of suicidal behavior may be a signal that a relapse is occurring and medication or therapeutic modality require adjustment, such as increased medication dosage, change of medicine, increased frequency of therapy sessions, or changes to the modality of therapy (e.g., family conflicts as a precipitant for suicidal behavior may be a signal for the use of family therapy). Figure 15.1 presents a basic overview of the management of a suicidal patient.

NONSUICIDAL SELF-INJURY

Suicidal behavior needs to be differentiated from other types of self-harm—often identified as nonsuicidal self-injury (NSSI), deliberate self-harm, or self-injurious behavior without suicidal intent—whose goal is hypothesized to be relieving negative emotions (assessing the intention in specific cases is often very difficult). This behavior most commonly involves repetitive self-cutting to relieve anger, distress, or loneliness rather than seeking to end one's life.[9] Nonsuicidal self-injurious acts can occur in suicidal individuals as well. Superficial cutting or burning of the skin often occurs without suicidal intent, although such actions can result in emergency department referrals. Intentional self-injury typically serves to reduce tension in the short-term, with many individuals who practice such

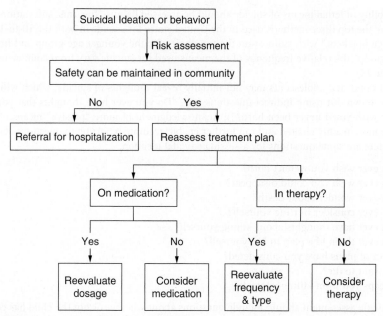

■ **Figure 15.1** Flowchart summarizing the approach to the suicidal patient in an outpatient setting. The text provides more details regarding each step in the algorithm, in particular the factors to consider in determining whether safety can be maintained in the community.

behaviors describing a feeling of *relief of emotional pain* as a consequence. More common in adolescents than in children, nonsuicidal self-injury is often associated with mood disorders, in particular depression. Most studies on NSSI have been done in the adult population. Efforts to better understand NSSI and its relationship to suicide attempts in adolescents are ongoing. Brunner et al.[10] examined differences between occasional (one to three times per year) and repetitive forms (four or more times per year) of self-injurious behaviors in a group of German adolescents. They found that social factors, like school-related and family-related variables, demonstrated a strong association with occasional self-injurious behavior and that psychological factors seemed to be more strongly associated with repetitive self-injurious behavior. Suicidal behavior (suicidal ideation and suicide attempts) was associated with both the occasional and repetitive forms of self-injurious behavior (although more strongly in the repetitive type). Lloyd-Richardson et al.[11] investigated a community sample of U.S. adolescents for self-injurious behavior and found that some form of it was endorsed by 46% of adolescents within the previous year. The 28% who endorsed more moderate or severe forms of self-injurious behavior was the group more likely to have a history of psychiatric treatment and past or current suicidal ideation. The most common reasons cited for self-injury were "to try to get a reaction from someone," "to get control of a situation," and "to stop bad feelings." In a study of adolescent inpatients, Nock et al.[12] found that those who engaged in NSSI reported more frequently doing so to regulate their own emotions rather than to influence the behavior of others. A review[13] found a prevalence of NSSI between 13% and 23% among studies that included only adolescents. Adolescents from various samples and levels of psychopathology reported engaging in NSSI to regulate—typically to decrease but sometimes to increase—emotions; MDD occurred in 42% to 58% of patients with NSSI; if all depressive disorders were included, up to 89% of the participants engaged in NSSI.

When learning of new cutting behavior, it is important to assess the lethality of the action to determine if an emergency consultation is needed. The adolescent needs assessment of the behavior as soon as possible and, if new or recurrent, it may suggest a depressive relapse and need for a review of treatment. To differentiate between NSSI and a suicide attempt, it can be useful to consider the intent, lethality of the method, and chronicity of the behavior. These factors have been cited by Muehlenkamp[14] as a few of the means of discriminating between NSSI and suicide attempt based on adult studies; clinical experience suggests these can be helpful in assessing NSSI in adolescents as well. If recurrent and well known to the treatment provider, cutting should still be assessed for unique features of the action not previously present. Clinicians working with depressed adolescents should routinely assess for NSSI in addition to suicidal thoughts and behaviors, being aware that a child may be engaging in NSSI in the absence of suicidal ideation. It should also be kept in mind that with the initiation of antidepressant medication, there is a similar small increased risk for self-injury as there is for suicidal ideation.

Self-injurious behavior, although a symptom of borderline personality disorder, can occur in many depressed adolescents in the absence of other personality disorder traits (personality disorders are not usually diagnosed until adulthood). Dialectical behavior therapy (DBT) is a form of psychotherapy that reduces suicidality and self-injurious behavior in adults with borderline personality disorder. Although there are no randomized controlled trials in adolescents, noncontrolled studies have shown some promise for the adaptation of DBT in the suicidal adolescent,[15] and thus possibly could be beneficial for adolescents with NSSI as well.

VIOLENT BEHAVIORS

Violent behaviors can range from aggression (e.g., fighting, destroying property) to homicidal ideation, to homicidal plans, to homicide attempt. Aggression can co-occur with depression and other mood disorders. In fact, both suicidal and homicidal ideation can occur in the same person, and thus a similar evaluation should be conducted for homicidality as for suicidality.[2]

Because depression in children can be characterized by irritability and impulse control is not fully developed, children are more susceptible to acting on their angry impulses in the context of depression. Frequently, aggression and fighting are viewed as owing to externalizing disorders, but the possibility of depression must be considered as well. Once depression is diagnosed, its treatment should address underlying symptoms that drive the aggressive behavior unless there are comorbid conditions, such as substance abuse or disruptive behavior disorders. Depressive symptoms are predictive of violent behavior, although the nature of that relationship is unclear[16] and may reflect exposure to risk factors for violence that can also cause depression. In a group of hospitalized patients, depression was not an independent predictor of violence, but some characteristics of and conditions associated with depression did appear to be predictive, such as hopelessness, impulsivity, drug abuse, and suicide risk. Violence risk and suicide risk were independent predictors of each other.[17] In practice, because of similar risk factors, the assessment for risk of violence is also important during the evaluation of depression.

Similarly to suicidal ideation, the presence of homicidal ideation may warrant hospitalization if there appears to be acute danger. In assessing aggressive or homicidal ideation, it is important to distinguish wish or fantasy from intent. The ability to reflect on and provide insight into the consequences of aggressive actions (such as legal sanctions, feelings of remorse) can provide information as to strength of intent and therefore risk. Clinical experience suggests that the consideration of adverse consequences and punishment can serve as deterrents, and treatment can continue on an outpatient basis. If, however, real homicidal risk is suspected, in most jurisdictions clinicians are obligated to notify the intended victim and/or the police of the threat.

Apart from depression-related irritability, aggressiveness in a depressed youth can be a sign of a comorbid condition such as a disruptive behavior disorder, substance abuse, psychosis, or personality disorder. In addition, the possibility of bipolar disorder should be considered. A full review of symptoms to ascertain the likely condition that is causing the violent ideation or actions is indicated, and treatment may require adjustment. If another condition is suspected, reevaluation of the medication and the therapy is indicated. Keep in mind, however, that aggression and violence as problems in society are more complex in their origins than merely being symptoms of mental illness. For example, although depression is often comorbid with conduct disorder, a number of mechanisms may account for the associations between the two conditions, including early deprivation or other childhood experiences that predispose to both depression and antisocial behavior.[18]

Given recent highly publicized violent events perpetrated by young people, it is more common that threats of any level in certain environments (such as in schools) are taken seriously and frequently result in referral to the emergency department. A psychiatric evaluation is often required in these circumstances in order to return to school.

NONADHERENCE TO TREATMENT

During the course of treatment, a relapse or recurrence of symptoms may be observed after a period of apparent response (see Chapter 16 on treatment-resistant depression for more information). When considering reasons for lack of response or recurrence, poor compliance should be taken into account because medication nonadherence is a significant problem in medical practice.[19] Potential reasons for nonadherence with both medication and therapy include the following:

- Ambivalence
- Active or passive resistance (oppositionality)
- Forgetfulness
- Peer pressure
- Complicated dosing schedule
- Adverse medication effects
- Therapy conflicts with other activities
- Comorbid conditions such as substance use
- Lack of parental oversight
- Treatment not considered helpful, family beliefs, cultural/religious issues

For most children and many adolescents, going on medication or being in therapy is a decision made by the parents. The child may not think treatment is indicated, may recognize a problem but feel uneasy about what treatment means (e.g., "taking medicine means I'm crazy"), as well as have worries about stigmatization (see Chapter 4). Ambivalence and resistance can be lessened by spending time educating and involving children from the beginning in all the treatment decisions affecting them. In a group of adults on antidepressant medication, adherence to treatment was associated with a lower perceived stigma of depression.[20] Providing education regarding the origins of depression can facilitate reducing the feelings of shame some people experience when getting treatment.

Forgetfulness has been cited as the most common reason for missing antidepressant doses in adults,[19] and this probably applies to youth also. Clinical experience shows that forgetfulness is common in adolescents and often ties in with unconscious ambivalence, passive resistance, or lack of parental oversight. Premature discontinuation of antidepressant medication is common in adults[21] and can result in relapse or recurrence of the illness. Although not specifically studied in children, similar concerns may apply. The older the child, the more likely some parents will place responsibility for taking medication in the hands of the child. Some parents leave the medicine out and expect their adolescent to take it on the way out the door in the morning or after dinner. Although taking responsibility for the medication is a reasonable expectation in many youth, it is important to find out if it works in practice.

Adolescents sometimes stop medication without telling anyone, and unless they are asked specifically they do not volunteer this information. In addition, patients often do not report missed dosages—because they do not think that a couple of missed tablets per week might be significant—or may run out of medication and be without it for some time before requesting a refill. For these reasons, it is important to ask both the child and the parents specifically how the medicine is being taken and if any dosages are missed. This should be done during all visits. These problems can by lessened by:

- Educating child and parents about the medication.
- Asking both the child and the parent specifically how the medicine is taken and if any dosages are missed.
- Asking parents to oversee the ingestion of medication where appropriate.
- Suggesting methods to help remembering and compliance (e.g., daily pill boxes, alarm watches, coordination with another routine).
- Simplifying dosing schedules.
- Switching to an antidepressant with a longer half-life, such as fluoxetine.

Reports of missed doses also warrant inquiring about adverse effects the patient is not reporting; experiencing side effects may be one of the reasons for nonadherence. Adolescents, for example, often do not report a decrease in sexual functioning and need to be asked about this directly.

Sometimes real-life issues can result in missed appointments. Children and adolescents often have busy after-school schedules, and they are not typically desirous of missing contacts with friends to attend therapy sessions. These issues should be discussed openly in therapy and a compromise reached regarding the timing of sessions.

Comorbidity can contribute to poor adherence. For example, in substance abuse, dosages may be missed because of intoxication or deliberately, to avoid the adverse effects of combining medication with substances of abuse. Other factors can be situations at home or in relationships that make it difficult to comply with treatment (e.g., moving between divorced parents' homes, acting out anger toward a parent, peer pressure).

If nonadherence is suspected but the patient does not acknowledge it, some medications are readily monitored by blood levels. Other medications can be checked for metabolites in the blood (see Chapter 16).

REFUSAL OF TREATMENT

One outcome of nonadherence can be outright treatment refusal. This can mean either refusing medication, therapy, or both. Treatment refusal is more likely with older adolescents because they are more apt to rebel against their parents' wishes, although children can "refuse" via temper tantrums or other behavior problems when the time to go to the clinician approaches. In the case of children, a behavioral plan with rewards and consequences can be useful. For adolescents, it is important to establish a working alliance with the teenager at the start of treatment in order to avoid refusal of treatment at a later date. In this way, even if refusing to comply with parents wishes, the adolescent may be prepared to consider the clinician's advice. Knowing the adolescent's worries may allow finding solutions to keep the teenager in treatment. This may entail negotiating changes to the treatment plan, which may give teens some sense of control and thus gain their participation. With the use of rewards, parents can facilitate their child's initial cooperation with the treatment.

The fit between the clinician and the child should also be considered. Perhaps the adolescent would be willing to see a different professional for another opinion. Ultimately, if children continue to refuse treatment, forcing them to remain in therapy or on medication will be futile. In rare cases, when risk is high, and depending on the level of need, other resources may warrant consideration, such as hospitalization or residential care.

SUDDEN DETERIORATION

Reasons for deterioration need to be explored when a previously stable patient presents with a recurrence of severe depressive symptoms. Sudden deterioration can occur under the following circumstances:

- New psychosocial stressor
- Stopping medication or poor adherence
- Medication no longer efficacious
- Substance abuse
- Comorbidity
- Manic switch
- Psychosis
- Medical/neurologic illness

Whenever a parent or patient reports deterioration, the existence of new stressors related to family, school, or peer group should be explored because deterioration can be owing to an adjustment reaction rather than a depressive recurrence. Parental divorce, physical or sexual abuse, a new sibling, change of school, and bullying or peer rejection are examples of situations that could result in deterioration. In that context, it needs to be determined whether to increase or change medication. Increasing the frequency of visits can often be helpful in the early stages.

Suddenly stopping the medication can result in a discontinuation syndrome that can look like a sudden worsening; lack of compliance over time can cause a recurrence of the depression. Premature discontinuation of medication often occurs after symptoms improve because of the belief that treatment is no longer necessary. The reasons for nonresponse and strategies to deal with them are discussed in detail in Chapter 16.

Sudden deterioration may also occur as a result of a switch from depression to mania—in youth presenting with depression who actually have a bipolar disorder—or as a side effect of antidepressant medication (see Chapter 14). The emergence of psychotic symptoms is also a sign of deterioration and may occur as part of a bipolar disorder, in connection with worsening depression, as a result of substance use, or as a manifestation of a primary psychotic disorder. In cases where either mania or psychosis emerges, it is more likely that hospitalization will be necessary. Diagnosis will need to be reviewed and alternative or additional medications considered, such as mood stabilizers or antipsychotics.

SCHOOL CRISES

Issues can arise during treatment that may require intervention at the school level, such as plummeting grades and conflict with teachers or peers; these may be because of the depression or something else. Notification of school difficulties may come from parents or from school personnel directly. If the school initiates contact, it is important to have consent from the parents as well as the adolescent—if possible before communicating with teachers, guidance counselors, or principals. Consent may have been obtained at the start of treatment, but if new issues arise, it is reasonable to clarify the situation with the parents first to determine who the clinician might speak with at the school and what information he or she may provide. School personnel may also need psychoeducation to help them understand and provide for the needs of a depressed child (see Chapter 5). The clinician, along with the family, may advocate for some accommodations (e.g., changes in schedule, workload) to the patient's current difficulties until recovery is achieved. If academic difficulties persist after recovery, then subsyndromal depression or other comorbid conditions should be considered.[2] When accommodations are requested, the treating clinician needs to document the disorder and the impairments for which the accommodations are being sought. Laws in the United States mandate that accommodations be made at school for children with disabilities, which would include depression. Letters may be needed for the school to excuse missing work or frequent absences.

Nowadays, schools also refer children and adolescents to a physician for "psychiatric clearance" to return to school if suicidal or homicidal threats have been made, regardless of the circumstances. The child may not be able to return to school until such a clearance is obtained, which typically means a letter from a mental health practitioner stating it is safe for the child or adolescent to return to school.

If a school placement does not meet the child's needs, parents may need assistance in requesting alternative placement or services for their child. Referral to an educational specialist can be helpful if parents are unsure about how to work with educational authorities in their community. A mental health evaluation with recommendations may be required by the school district to determine appropriate services. For behavioral disturbances that are occurring over the course of treatment, the clinician needs to determine if the depression is the cause, and thus in need of optimized treatment, and may need to communicate this information to school personnel so there is a better understanding of the student's difficulties.

SCHOOL REFUSAL

School refusal is the avoidance of school because of emotional distress. This is different from truancy, which is not necessarily owing to emotional distress but to conduct or social problems, such as preference to spend time with truant friends or selling or using drugs. When secondary to emotional distress, either physical or emotional symptoms are often reported when children have to attend school. If symptoms are not present on weekends or during holidays, an emotional problem is likely. If physical complaints are used to avoid school, liaising with a pediatrician to rule out medical conditions may be necessary. School refusal can be considered a crisis because the longer the child stays out of school the more difficult it will be to resume attendance.[22] Although typically associated with anxiety disorders, school refusal can also occur in depression and disruptive behavior disorders. Untreated depression may present with school refusal. If avoidance of activities occurs on weekends as well as on school days, then the school refusal is more likely to be a result of depression and may resolve when depression improves. However, because school refusal is complex in its origins, continued school avoidance may occur as a result of persistent or new worries (such as fear of being behind in the schoolwork, facing the peer group after an extended absence, bullying), or learning disorders that preceded the depressive episode.

Once depressive symptoms are in remission, it is important to facilitate return to school as soon as possible and not to enable school refusal with unnecessary letters of excuse. Persistent school refusal will probably need family and behavioral therapy. Parents should be informed of the legal consequences for failure to attend school, such as charges of educational neglect. In the United States, the board of education is required to find a suitable educational environment and can often obtain alternative school placements, such as partial hospitalizations, day programs, or home instruction.

FAMILY INSTABILITY

The most common factor precipitating a crisis for the child is a crisis in the family, such as abuse, divorce, abandonment, illness, or death.[1] Family psychopathology, such as parental depression, also has a significant impact on children.[23] Family instability may be present at the start of treatment or become apparent at a later date. It is not uncharacteristic for adolescents and their parents to have difficulty in communication and arguments. Sometimes parents have difficulty separating normal adolescent behavior from signs of worsening depression (e.g., may believe there is a crisis when their adolescent child exhibits any sign of defiance). A phone consultation regarding the circumstances can help determine if an urgent appointment is needed or if reassurance is adequate. However, if familial conflict is thought to be exacerbating the patient's depressive disorder, rather than being a consequence of it, family therapy may be needed. Wedig and Nock[24] recently examined parental expressed emotion as a possible mediator for adolescent self-injury. Although the sample size was small, there was a connection between high parental criticism and parental overinvolvement with both suicidal behaviors and NSSI. Early identification of dysfunctional family patterns and their impact on the child can facilitate setting up a plan to avoid its adverse consequences. Frequent family meetings, family therapy, or referral of one or both parents for treatment (of depression, substance abuse, etc.) can be helpful in preventing or addressing family instability and the consequences of untreated parental psychopathology.

A crisis may precipitate or result from the child running away, a behavior that is more common in late adolescence. More than a million youth run away each year in the United States. The National Runaway Switchboard mentions that family dynamics is the most common problem given by crisis callers,[25] and a poor parent–child relationship is the most consistent finding in the home of runaways.[26] Runaway adolescents can be difficult to treat, but establishing a safe living arrangement is the initial priority. If able to return home, family therapy may be necessary and can be helpful if the family is relatively stable and in acute crisis. If running away is more chronic or the home situation is deemed unsafe (e.g., owing to neglect or abuse), organizing alternative living arrangements through social service agencies may be needed (e.g., group homes, residential centers, or shelters). Identification and treatment of specific psychiatric disorders, particularly depression, which occurs at a high rate in runaway youth,[27] are especially important.

Sexual or physical abuse is a crisis for the child and family that can result in development of a depressive episode or deterioration in a patient already in treatment for depression. The safety of the child needs to be assessed and the appropriate authorities notified. Most states and countries have laws mandating professionals who have regular contact with children to report suspected cases of neglect or abuse.

SUBSTANCE USE

If there is significant substance use or abuse, the treatment plan should address these issues together with the depression. Oftentimes, however, substance use becomes apparent during the course of treatment, either because of new-onset use or because that information was concealed at the start of treatment. New-onset substance use can complicate the treatment by increasing missed dosages of medication (caused by forgetting or fear of interactions) and by making nonadherence or lack of response to treatment more likely. A detailed discussion about substance use in depressed children and adolescents can be found in Chapter 18.

RESOURCES FOR PATIENTS AND PARENTS

The hotlines listed can be contacted by both individuals in crisis or concerned persons:

National Youth Crisis Hotline: 24-hour service providing counseling and referral to local treatment centers for callers in crisis. Phone: 1-800-442-HOPE; www.hopeline.com.

National Hopeline Network: 24-hour service for anyone thinking about suicide; calls are connected to a certified crisis center in the caller's area. Phone: 1–800-SUICIDE; www.hopeline.com.

National Suicide Prevention Lifeline: 24-hour service available to anyone who is in suicidal crisis, providing access to a crisis worker and referrals for services in the caller's area. Phone: 1-800-273-TALK; www.suicidepreventionlifeline.org.

National Runaway Switchboard: This center can be contacted for assistance by someone who is contemplating running away or who is currently on the run. Referrals to local services and agencies can be obtained. Phone: 1-800-621-4000; www.1800runaway.org.

In cases of overdose, the local poison control center can be contacted. There is now a national number (1-800-222-1222) that automatically redirects callers to their local poison control center. For more information, see the website for the American Association of Poison Control Centers at www.aapcc.org.

RESOURCES FOR PROFESSIONALS

Berman AL, Jobes DA, Silverman MM. *Adolescent Suicide: Assessment and Intervention.* 2nd ed. Washington, DC: American Psychological Association; 2005.

Dimeff LA, Koerner K, eds. *Dialectical Behavior Therapy in Clinical Practice: Applications Across Disorders and Settings.* New York: Guilford Press; 2007.

Jacobson CM, Gould M. The epidemiology and phenomenology of non-suicidal self-injurious behavior among adolescents: a critical review of the literature. *Arch Suicide Res.* 2007;11: 129–147.

Miller AL, Rathus JH, Linehan MM. *Dialectical Behavior Therapy with Suicidal Adolescents.* New York: Guilford Press; 2006.

Pilowsky DJ, Wickramaratne P, Nomura Y, et al. Family discord, parental depression, and psychopathology in offspring: 20-year follow-up. *J Am Acad Child Adolesc Psychiatry.* 2006;45:452–460.

REFERENCES

1. Tomb DA. Child psychiatric emergencies. In: Lewis M, ed. *Child and Adolescent Psychiatry: A Comprehensive Textbook.* 2nd ed. Baltimore: Williams & Wilkins; 1996:929–934.
2. Birmaher B, Brent D, AACAP Work Group on Quality Issues. Practice parameter for the assessment and treatment of children and adolescents with depressive disorders. *J Am Acad Child Adolesc Psychiatry.* 2007;46:1503–1526.
3. Brent DA, Baugher M, Bridge J, et al. Age- and sex-related risk factors for adolescent suicide. *J Am Acad Child Adolesc Psychiatry.* 1999;38:1497–1505.
4. Centers for Disease Control and Prevention. Leading causes of death reports. *WISQARS,* 2005. Available at www.cdc.gov/ncipc/wisqars/ http://www.cdc.gov/ncipc/wisqars/.
5. Kloos AL, Collins R, Weller RA, et al. Suicide in preadolescents: who is at risk? *Curr Psychiatry Rep.* 9:2007;89–93.
6. Beautrais AL. Risk factors for suicide and attempted suicide among young people. *Aust N Z J Psychiatry.* 2000;34:420–436.
7. Posner K, Oquendo MA, Gould M, et al. Columbia Classification Algorithm of Suicide Assessment (C-CASA): classification of suicidal events in the FDA's pediatric suicidal risk analysis of antidepressants. *Am J Psychiatry.* 2007;164:1035–1043.
8. Rutter PA, Behrendt AE. Adolescent suicide risk: four psychosocial factors. *Adolescence.* 2004;39:295–302.
9. American Academy of Child and Adolescent Psychiatry. Practice parameter for the assessment and treatment of children and adolescents with suicidal behavior. *J Am Acad Child Adolesc Psychiatry.* 2001;40(suppl): 24S–51S.
10. Brunner R, Parzer P, Haffner J, et al. Prevalence and psychological correlates of occasional and repetitive deliberate self-harm in adolescents. *Arch Pediatr Adolesc Med.* 2007;161:641–649.

11. Lloyd-Richardson EE, Perrine E, Dierker L, et al. Characteristics and functions of non-suicidal self-injury in a community sample of adolescents. *Psychol Med.* 2007;37:1183–1192.
12. Nock MK, Prinstein MJ. A functional approach to the assessment of self-mutilative behavior. *J Consult Clin Psychol.* 2004;72:885–890.
13. Jacobson CM, Gould M. The epidemiology and phenomenology of non-suicidal self-injurious behavior among adolescents: a critical review of the literature. *Arch Suicide Res.* 2007;11:129–147.
14. Muehlenkamp JJ. Self-injurious behavior as a separate clinical syndrome. *Am J Orthopsychiatry.* 2005; 75:324–333.
15. Lynch TR, Trost WT, Salsman N, et al. Dialectical behavior therapy for borderline personality disorder. *Ann Rev Clin Psychol.* 2007;3:181–205.
16. Blitstein JL, Murray DM, Lytle LA, et al. Predictors of violent behavior in an early adolescent cohort: similarities and differences across genders. *Health Ed Behav.* 2005;32:175–194.
17. Becker DF, Grilo CM. Prediction of suicidality and violence in hospitalized adolescents: comparisons by sex. *Can J Psychiatry.* 2007;52:572–580.
18. Wolff JC, Ollendick TH. The comorbidity of conduct problems and depression in childhood and adolescence. *Clin Child Fam Psychol Rev.* 2006;9:201–220.
19. Bulloch AG, Adair CE, Patten SB. Forgetfulness: a role in noncompliance with antidepressant treatment. *Can J Psychiatry.* 2006;51:719–722.
20. Sirey JA, Bruce ML, Alexopoulos GS, et al. Perceived stigma and patient-rated severity of illness as predictors of antidepressant drug adherence. *Psychiatr Serv.* 2001;52:1615–1620.
21. Akincigil A, Bowblis JR, Levin C, et al. Adherence to antidepressant treatment among privately insured patients diagnosed with depression. *Med Care.* 2007;45:363–369.
22. Fremont W. School refusal in children and adolescents. *Am Fam Physician.* 2003;68:1555–1560.
23. Pilowsky DJ, Wickramaratne P, Nomura Y, et al. Family discord, parental depression, and psychopathology in offspring: 20-year follow-up. *J Am Acad Child Adolesc Psychiatry.* 2006;45:452–460.
24. Wedig MM, Nock MK. Parental expressed emotion and adolescent self-injury. *J Am Acad Child Adolesc Psychiatry.* 2007;46:1171–1178.
25. National Runaway Switchboard. National runaway switchboard call content data report January-December 2007. *National Statistics,* 2007. Available at www.1800runaway.org/news_events/call_stats.html http://www.1800runaway.org/news_events/call_stats.html.
26. Tomb DA. The runaway adolescent. In: Lewis M, ed. *Child and Adolescent Psychiatry: A Comprehensive Textbook.* 2nd ed. Baltimore: Williams & Wilkins; 1996:1080–1085.
27. Whitbeck LB, Hoyt DR, Bao W. Depressive symptoms and co-occurring depressive symptoms, substance abuse, and conduct problems among runaway and homeless adolescents. *Child Dev.* 2000;71:721–732.

List of C-CASA Definitions and Examples

Classification/Category	Definition	Training Examples
SUICIDAL EVENTS		
Completed suicide	A self-injurious behavior that resulted in fatality and was associated with at least some intent to die as a result of the act.	(1) After a long argument with his girlfriend, which resulted in the end of their relationship, the patient collected a rope and rode his bike to an isolated area where he fatally hanged himself. A suicide note was later found. (2) After four documented attempts at suicide, the patient stole his uncle's gun and shot himself and was fatally injured.
Suicide attempt	A potentially self-injurious behavior, associated with at least some intent to die as a result of the act. Evidence that the individual intended to kill himself or herself, at least to some degree, can be explicit or inferred from the behavior or circumstance. A suicide attempt may or may not result in actual injury.	(1) After a fight with her friends at school, in which they stopped speaking to her, the patient ingested approximately 16 aspirin and 8 other pills of different types on the school grounds. She said that she deserved to die, which was why she swallowed the pills. (2) The patient used a razor blade to lacerate his wrists, his antecubital fossae, and his back bilaterally. He told his therapist that the "main objective was to stop feeling like that," and he knew that he could die but didn't care. According to the patient, he also ingested a bottle of rubbing alcohol because in his health class he heard "that the medulla will get more suppressed that way," thereby increasing the chances that he would be "successful" and die.
Preparatory acts toward imminent suicidal behavior	The individual takes steps to injure himself or herself but is stopped by self or others from starting the self-injurious act before the potential for harm has begun.	(1) The patient had run away from home overnight because his father had gone to school and retrieved a recent "bad" report card. He was fearful of his father's reaction. Upon his return home, a 5- to 6-hour argument with his parents ensued, and he took a vegetable (broad, sharp) knife and went to his room. He reported putting the knife to his wrist but never puncturing the skin. (2) The patient stated that he "couldn't stand being depressed anymore" and "wanted to die." He decided to hang himself. He tied a telephone cord to the door knob and placed the cord loosely around his neck. Then he stopped himself and did not follow through with the attempt.

(continued)

Classification/Category	Definition	Training Examples
Suicidal ideation	Passive thoughts about wanting to be dead or active thoughts about killing oneself, not accompanied by preparatory behavior.[a]	(1) Active: The patient reported to the doctor that he was thinking about hanging himself in the closet. He was taken to the hospital and admitted. (2) Passive: The patient reported ideas about wanting to be dead but denied acting on these feelings.
NONSUICIDAL EVENTS		
Self-injurious behavior, no suicidal intent	Self-injurious behavior associated with no intent to die. The behavior is intended purely for other reasons, either to relieve distress (often referred to as "self-mutilation"; e.g., superficial cuts or scratches, hitting/banging, or burns) or to effect change in others or the environment.	(1) The patient was feeling ignored. She went into the family kitchen where her mother and sister were talking. She took a knife out of the drawer and made a cut on her arm. She denied that she wanted to die at all ("not even a little"), but she just wanted them to pay attention to her. (2) The patient reported feeling agitated and anxious after a fight with her parents. She went into her room, locked the door, and made several superficial cuts on the inside of her arms. She stated that she felt relieved after cutting herself and that she did not want to die. She reported that she had done this before at times of distress and it usually helped her feel better. (3) The patient was in class, where a test was about to begin, and stabbed himself with a pencil in order to be taken to the nurse's office. (4) A 14-year-old girl wrote her name on her arm with a penknife and said that she often does so to reduce her anxiety. (5) The patient was noted to have multiple superficial burns on his arms. Upon questioning, he denied trying to kill himself.
Other; no deliberate self-harm	No evidence of any suicidality or deliberate self-injurious behavior associated with the event. The event is characterized as an accidental injury, psychiatric or behavioral symptoms only, or medical symptoms or procedure only.	(1) The patient had a cut on the neck from shaving. (2) The patient was hospitalized for worsening of obsessive-compulsive disorder or depressive symptoms with no suicidal thoughts or actions or aggressive behavior. Hospitalization was because of an infection, rhinoplasty, or pregnancy.
INDETERMINATE OR POTENTIALLY SUICIDAL EVENTS		
Self-injurious behavior; suicidal intent unknown	Self-injurious behavior where associated intent to die is unknown and cannot be inferred. The injury or potential for injury is clear, but why the individual engaged in that behavior is unclear.	(1) The patient cut her wrists after an argument with her boyfriend. (2) The patient was angry at her husband. She took 10 to 15 diazepam tablets and flushed the rest down the toilet. Her husband called the police for help, and she was taken to the hospital. She was groggy and stayed overnight in the hospital. (3) A 9-year-old patient had spoken about suicide frequently. After learning that his baseball coach was retiring, he began scratching his arm with a pencil.

(continued)

Classification/Category	Definition	Training Examples
Not enough information	Insufficient information to determine whether the event involved deliberate suicidal behavior or ideation. There is reason to suspect the possibility of suicidality but not enough to be confident that the event was not something other, such as an accident or psychiatric symptom. An injury sustained on a place on the body consistent with deliberate self-harm or suicidal behavior (e.g., wrists), without any information as to how the injury was received, would warrant placement in this category.	(1) A child "stabbed himself in [the] neck with a pencil." The event may have been deliberate as opposed to accidental, as suggested by "stabbed," but not enough information was provided to determine whether the event was deliberate. (2) A cut on the neck.

[a]If ideation is deemed inherently related to a behavioral act, a separate rating is not given. However, if there is no clear relationship to a behavioral event, a separate classification or ideation is warranted.

From Posner K, Oquendo MA, Gould M, et al. Columbia Classification Algorithm of Suicide Assessment (C-CASA): classification of suicidal events in the FDA's pediatric suicidal risk analysis of antidepressants. *Am J Psychiatry.* 2007;164:1035–1043. Reprinted with permission from the American Journal of Psychiatry (Copyright 2007). American Psychiatric Association.

Treatment-Resistant Depression

BORIS BIRMAHER AND DAVID A. BRENT

KEY POINTS

- The main aim of treatment is to achieve remission and not only response.
- No or partial response to treatment is commonly encountered in children and adolescents with major depressive disorder.
- Before considering a patient a partial responder, nonresponder, or treatment resistant, it is imperative to evaluate all potential factors (individual, patient, family, other environmental) and clinicians' specific factors that may contribute to the patient's poor response.
- Promote and assure adherence to psychotherapy and/or pharmacotherapy during the acute and maintenance phases of the treatment.
- The management of a depressed child or adolescent who partially responds or does not respond to treatment should included education, psychotherapeutic, psychopharmacologic, and sometimes other biologic interventions.
- Psychoeducation that promotes parental and child hopefulness in the context of realistic expectation about treatment is warranted.
- Each new treatment needs to be done methodically and carried out step by step.
- The first step is to optimize the current treatment by increasing the dose and/or increasing the length of treatment. If the patient does not respond or tolerate the treatment, consider switching or augmentation strategies depending on the case and preferences of child and family.
- In general, for partial responders, augment treatment with a different class of antidepressant, other type of medications (e.g., lithium or triiodothyronine [T_3]), or psychotherapy.
- The only RCT for adolescents who did not respond to a single treatment with a SSRI showed that the combination of a different SSRI plus CBT was the best next strategy.
- Monitor side effects, give hope, and include parents as co-therapists. This may reduce dropouts, which are common among treatment-resistant cases.
- Manage comorbid disorders and give patients and their families the tools to manage and cope with ongoing family, school, friends, and other environmental stressors.
- To improve the child's outcome, encourage parents to seek treatment for their own psychopathology.
- Treating difficult cases is hard on clinicians who can become disheartened and may benefit from seeking advice or support from colleagues.

Introduction

Pediatric major depressive disorder (MDD) is a recurrent familial psychiatric illness that causes significant disruption to the child's normal psychosocial development and continues into adulthood. MDD is usually accompanied by interpersonal, academic, behavior, and occupational problems, as well as a high risk for substance abuse, legal problems, suicidal behavior, and completed suicide.[1–3] Therefore, the proper treatment of pediatric depression can have a profound impact on the depressed youth's developmental trajectory.

As described in Chapters 6, 8 and 9, current randomized controlled trials (RCTs) have shown that the selective serotonin reuptake inhibitors (SSRIs) and psychotherapy (mainly cognitive behavior psychotherapy and interpersonal psychotherapy) alone or in combination are efficacious for the acute treatment of children and adolescents with MDD.[4,5] However, at least 40% of depressed youth do not respond or do not show an adequate clinical response to these interventions. Moreover, only up to 30% show complete symptomatic remission to acute treatment. Consequently, a substantial proportion of depressed youth remain symptomatic despite exposure to adequate first-line treatment, with considerable impairment in their psychosocial functioning and with increased risk for suicide, substance abuse, behavior problems, and subsequent episodes of major depression.

This chapter discusses the definition, associated factors, and management of youth with "treatment-resistant depression." Because there are very few pediatric treatment-resistant depression studies, the adult literature is cited, but treatments found efficacious for the management of treatment resistant depression in adults may not apply to youth. In this chapter, the term *youth*, unless specified otherwise, applies to both children and adolescents.

Table 4.1 (and reference 3) describe current definitions of response, partial response, remission, relapse, and recurrence. However, several studies have used their own definitions of outcome. For example, it is routine in pharmacologic studies to define remission by certain cutoff scores in a clinician-based rating scale, without taking into account the length of time the subject has been with minimal or no symptoms.

DEFINITION OF TREATMENT-RESISTANT DEPRESSION IN PEDIATRIC MAJOR DEPRESSIVE DISORDER

Given the consequences of diagnosing a child with treatment-resistant depression, it is important to have a clear definition of this condition. However, as noted earlier, existing acute RCTs have shown that up to 50% of depressed youth fail to show significant clinical response to treatment and only a third show complete remission. Can we call these children treatment resistant after only one treatment, or do they need at least two trials with two antidepressants at standard doses for an appropriate period of time? Do the two antidepressants need to be from different classes or the same class? Finally, how should treatment resistance be defined in youth treated with psychotherapy?

These questions require further investigation. Furthermore, to diagnose a patient as nonresponsive or treatment resistant, the field needs to be in agreement about the definition of an adequate pharmacotherapy or psychotherapy treatment. For example, based in some, child and adult RCTs, an adequate treatment of depression with antidepressants has been defined as at least 8 weeks of treatment, at least 4 of which are at the equivalent of 20 mg of fluoxetine per day, and the second 4 weeks at an increased dose, failing an earlier response.[6–12] However, recent adult studies have recommended 6 weeks of treatment before increasing the dose and at least 12 weeks of treatment.[13] "Adequate" psychotherapy appears to require the implementation of one of two interventions for which there is some empirical evidence for efficacy, namely cognitive behavioral therapy (CBT) or interpersonal therapy (IPT), at a "dosage" of 8 to 16 sessions, for a complete course of treatment.[5,14–16]

The only existing RCT for depressed adolescents who did not respond to a trial with a SSRI, the Treatment of SSRI-Resistant Depression in Adolescents study (TORDIA),[8] defined treatment-resistant depression or no response as a clinically significant depression: Child Depression Rating Scale-Revised (CDRS-R)[17] total score ≥40 and a Clinical Global Impression-Severity (CGI-S)[18] subscale ≥4 (at least moderate severity)—despite one appropriate pharmacologic treatment. TORDIA did not evaluate treatment resistance to psychotherapy. However, the "dosage" of psychotherapy in clinical trials of either CBT or IPT in depressed children or adolescents ranged from a low of 5 to 8 sessions of CBT to 12 to 16 individual or group sessions in other studies of CBT and IPT.[14–16,19] Therefore, a reasonable minimum adequate "dose" of evidence-based psychotherapy is approximately 8 to 12 sessions. Longer-term follow-up of psychotherapy studies indicates that even among those who initially respond, many require additional booster sessions or additional types of mental health services, or they experience relapses, which again supports the view that even given "adequate" exposure, many depressed youth will require additional intervention.[20–22]

In summary, there is not clear agreement regarding the definition of treatment resistance. Some experts have defined "treatment-resistant depression" as failure to respond to an adequate course of treatment with an antidepressant or psychotherapy. However, given that in child and adolescent MDD acute RCTs, the response rate to either antidepressants or psychotherapy is around 60%, this would be defining a very high proportion of patients as "resistant." Some might argue that treatment-resistant depression should be defined after failure to respond to 12 weeks of combination therapy (e.g., CBT plus a SSRI)—which would include 30%, still a large proportion. Thus, until these issues are resolved, the following working definition of treatment-resistance in routine clinical practice is proposed:

A youth whose symptoms of MDD and functional impairment persist after:

- 8–12 weeks of optimal pharmacological treatment consisting of:
  - At least 6 weeks of 20 mg of fluoxetine per day (or an equivalent dose of an alternative SSRI)
  - Dose subsequently increased, depending on tolerance, for another 4 to 6 weeks.
- And a further 8 to 12 weeks of an alternative antidepressant or augmentation therapy with other medications or evidence-based psychotherapy.

OR

- 8 to 16 sessions of CBT or IPT
- And a further 12 weeks of pharmacologic treatment consisting of:
  - At least 6 weeks of 20 mg of fluoxetine a day (or an equivalent dose of an alternative SSRI)
  - Dose subsequently increased, depending on tolerance, for another 4 to 6 weeks.

Treatment could be more aggressive in severe cases treated in specialist settings, particularly if the life of the patient were at risk. In all cases, these treatments are complemented with patient and family education, support, and case management.

FACTORS ASSOCIATED WITH POOR OR NONRESPONSE TO TREATMENT

Given the high rate of partial or nonresponse to the existing treatments in youth, it is helpful for clinicians to have a framework to help them determine the particular factors contributing to treatment failure or resistance in each patient and guidelines on how to intervene and increase the likelihood of remission.[1,2,10] Even though these factors overlap, for simplicity's sake they are divided into clinician, individual, family, and other environmental factors. Although nonexhaustive, Figure 16.1 shows some of the common variables associated with no or partial response.

INDIVIDUAL

Individual factors associated with no or partial response include, among others, early age of onset, hopelessness, low psychosocial functioning, poor motivation toward treatment, or poor adherence (for factors associated with poor adherence, see Chapter 15). In the case of medication, this means incomplete adherence to the prescribed regime. When patients are treated with medications with shorter half-lives, such as sertraline, skipping dosages can result in withdrawal symptoms, which in turn can be associated with clinical deterioration and further nonadherence. With regard to psychotherapy, patients are required to practice and apply skills learned within the session. Other predictors of poor response include indicators of severity (high symptom ratings of depression, suicidal ideation, low functioning), chronicity (long duration), and complexity (e.g., presence of psychosis or comorbid conditions such as disruptive behavior disorders, anxiety, eating, and substance abuse disorders), personal identity issues (such as concern about same-sex attraction), and socioeconomic factors (e.g., poverty and poorer response to CBT[23]). Also, use of other medications (e.g., steroids, contraceptives, interferon, and/or retinoic acid) and medical illness such as hypothyroidism, anemia, mononucleosis, folate or B_{12} deficiency and other chronic conditions can produce symptoms that overlap with the depressive symptoms or contribute to treatment nonresponse. Although relatively few studies have examined ethnicity and treatment response, there is some suggestion that IPT may have greater benefit in some domains than CBT for depressed Hispanic adolescents;[24] conversely, response rates to CBT are better in Whites than in minority depressed youth.[25] Hopelessness is

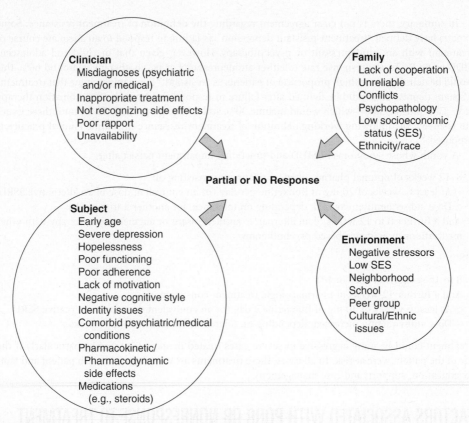

Clinician
- Misdiagnoses (psychiatric and/or medical)
- Inappropriate treatment
- Not recognizing side effects
- Poor rapport
- Unavailability

Family
- Lack of cooperation
- Unreliable
- Conflicts
- Psychopathology
- Low socioeconomic status (SES)
- Ethnicity/race

Partial or No Response

Subject
- Early age
- Severe depression
- Hopelessness
- Poor functioning
- Poor adherence
- Lack of motivation
- Negative cognitive style
- Identity issues
- Comorbid psychiatric/medical conditions
- Pharmacokinetic/ Pharmacodynamic side effects
- Medications (e.g., steroids)

Environment
- Negative stressors
- Low SES
- Neighborhood
- School
- Peer group
- Cultural/Ethnic issues

■ **Figure 16.1** Factors associated with partial or no response.

associated with both a poorer treatment response and dropout, at least in some psychotherapy trials.[26,27] In addition, pharmacokinetic (e.g., absorption, rapid or slow metabolism, intolerance at adequate dosage) and pharmacogenetic (presence of certain polymorphisms, such as the less functional variant of the serotonin transporter) as well as medication side effects may contribute to poor response or poor adherence to antidepressant treatment.[28]

CLINICIAN

Among the first issues a clinician should consider when a patient is not responding to treatment is the possibility of misdiagnosis (e.g., bipolar-II versus unipolar depression) or that the patient has an unrecognized or untreated comorbid psychiatric or medical condition (e.g., anxiety, dysthymia, ADHD, eating, substance use, personality disorder, early-onset schizophrenia) or is using medications that are contributing to depressive symptomatology. Because most youth with a bipolar diathesis present in their first episode as major depression, one of the most problematic differential diagnosis is between unipolar and bipolar depression.[1-3,29] However, the presence of psychosis, a family history of bipolar disorder, or pharmacologically induced hypomania may help the clinician suspect the presence of bipolar instead of unipolar depression.[1-3] Also, the presence of recurrent periods of elation, euphoria, and agitation above and beyond what it is expected for the child's age and cultural background may indicate the presence of bipolar disorder.

Clinicians should also consider that the pharmacotherapy or psychotherapy offered is not appropriate or that the length or dosage is inadequate for the specific child who is not responding to treatment. The presence of unrecognized medication side effects or ongoing exposure to chronic or severe life events (such as sexual abuse or ongoing family conflict) should be taken in consideration. Finally, the clinician may be an inadequate fit with the child, has poor motivation to help, or poor skills as a pharmacotherapist or psychotherapist.

FAMILY

Family psychopathology, ongoing family conflict, or violence are associated with the onset and persistence of depressive symptoms in youth.[21,27,30,31] Specifically, ongoing family conflict is associated with a slower and less complete response to either antidepressants or CBT; maternal depressive symptoms are associated with a less vigorous response.[27,30,31] A history of sexual abuse was associated with poorer response to medication and better response to psychotherapy in one study of adults.[32,33] In adolescents, a history of sexual abuse was associated with a poorer response to CBT and also a greater likelihood for recurrent episodes.[34] In addition, lack of parental cooperation, lack of knowledge regarding the child's psychopathology or available treatments, and unreliability keeping appointments and following treatment recommendations may render a child resistant to any type of treatment. Conversely, a strong parent–child attachment and adequate parental supervision may be protective.[35] The close family relationships in some ethnic, racial, or cultural groups as well as beliefs about mental illness and its treatment may also influence children's acceptance of treatment, adherence, and ultimately their response.

OTHER ENVIRONMENTAL FACTORS

Other factors that may influence the child's response to treatment include, among others, living in poverty or poor neighborhoods, attending unsatisfactory schools, the quality and availability of friends, lack of supportive networks, exposure to ongoing negative stressors (e.g., violence, abuse), and cultural/ethnic issues. For example, greater exposure to neighborhood violence is associated with greater background symptomatology, including higher depression and anxiety.[36] Living in neighborhoods with higher poverty and social disarray has been associated with greater serotonergic dysfunction in adults.[37] Having an antisocial peer group is also a risk factor for the onset, maintenance, and recurrence of depression because membership in such a group is likely to result in more stressful life events, such as arrest, which may precipitate or interfere with recovery from depression.

   The following case vignettes describe instances of what could be qualified as "treatment-resistant" depressed youth and their response to interventions, targeting factors that could explain poor response.

- BF is a 10-year-old girl with a 9-month episode of major depression. Despite good adherence to treatment with an SSRI and psychotherapy for 3 months, she continues to fulfill criteria for MDD and has very poor functioning. Her mother is also depressed, and there are continuous conflicts at home. Mother was referred for treatment. Several months after her mother's depression remitted, BF also began to feel better, and her school and social functioning slowly recovered.
- TM is a 15-year-old girl with two prior major depressive episodes that lasted several months and disappeared without any specific treatment. Currently, she is experiencing a 10-month episode of major depression that has not responded to an adequate trial with two SSRIs plus psychotherapy. Further evaluation revealed that TM has hypothyroidism. Treatment of this condition resulted in improvement of her mood.
- JP is a 14-year-old boy with an unremitting single episode of depression. Despite two adequate trials with antidepressants, he continues to complain about poor concentration, lack of motivation for school activities, and continuous interpersonal problems. Although currently JP does not fulfill criteria for ADHD, when he was younger he used to be more active, very fidgety, and impulsive. On further inquiry, parents remembered that they could not take him to church or a restaurant because he could not sit still. A trial with a long-acting stimulant was implemented with excellent response.
- CB is a 17-year-old boy with recurrent episodes of major depression occurring every 2 to 4 weeks and accompanied by agitation, insomnia, poor concentration, and sometimes suicidal ideation. Two trials with a SSRI helped somewhat but induced severe sexual dysfunction. Because he showed mild recurrent "hypomanic" episodes, valproate was tried without success. For the last 6 years, he has been euthymic on lamotrigine (200 mg/day).
- LM is a 15-year-old girl with a 12-month history of unremitting depression despite interpersonal psychotherapy and two trials with antidepressants. LM revealed ongoing conflicts at home and a history of sexual abuse. Appropriate management of these problems resulted in improvement of her mood.

- CF is a 14-year-old boy with recurrent depressions that are accompanied by suicidal ideation and very poor performance at school. His family background and cultural beliefs are interfering with appropriate treatment. After requesting help from the community pastor, the family began to cooperate, and CF showed improvement in his depressive symptoms.

TREATMENT

GENERAL ISSUES

Despite the high frequency of partial response and nonresponse and the serious consequences of persistent depression in this age group, very few empirical studies are available to guide clinicians regarding the management of depression in children and adolescents who failed to respond to an adequate trial of antidepressants or psychotherapy.[3,10]

Before initiating changes in the treatment, it is necessary to reevaluate the case carefully, taking into account all the factors associated with treatment nonresponse just discussed. This reevaluation should be done in conjunction with the child and the family and using all the information available, such as details provided by prior clinicians or people involved in the treatment and other sources of information such as relatives and teachers. Changes should be implemented *one at a time*.

Patients who have been chronically depressed often have difficulty judging improvement unless assessment is anchored to concrete markers or symptoms. This may be aided by the use of standardized assessments to patients, their families, and sometimes their teachers. These assessments may be clinician based, such as the Children's Depression Rating Scale-Revised (CDRS-R),[17] or self-report scales, like the Beck Depression Inventory (BDI),[38] the Mood and Feelings Questionnaire (MFQ) (parent and child versions),[39] or the Reynolds Adolescent Depression Scale (RADS)[40] (see Chapter 3 for more information regarding evaluation and rating scales for depression in youth).

Importantly, before concluding that a patient is a "nonresponder," the clinician must evaluate whether the patient has adhered to the pharmacologic or psychotherapeutic treatment. To evaluate this for medication, the clinician can use medication diaries, pill counts or, if appropriate, medication blood levels. Even if we do not know yet the significance of the blood level of certain medications, very low levels may imply poor adherence to treatment. Also, a low level of a parent medication with a high level of its metabolite may suggest rapid metabolism, whereas a high level of the parent medication and very little of its metabolite may suggest "white coat compliance" (i.e., the patient may have taken a larger amount of medication prior to testing the drug levels to simulate adherence). Finally, some laboratories have been offering inexpensive and fast genotyping tests to evaluate the person's cytochrome P-450 capacity to metabolize medications. These tests may be useful because a child may not respond to treatment because of very rapid metabolism or stop the treatment owing to side effects because of the slow metabolism of the medication administered.

The treatment of a child with treatment-resistant depression may be divided into education, psychotherapy, pharmacotherapy, and other biologic treatments.[3,10] In addition, once response and, even better, remission has been obtained, maintenance treatment is necessary to prevent relapse or recurrences (see Chapter 6). Finally, the parents' psychopathology needs to be addressed; otherwise the child will either remain at risk of new psychiatric disorders or will not improve.[27,30]

EDUCATION

Education and support to children and family is crucial to avoid misunderstandings, self-blaming, and to reduce the potential for children and their families to become hopeless. Patient and family should be seen as partners in the management of the child's ongoing depressive symptoms.

Because different patients respond to different type and amount of intervention, the sequence of treatment needs to be laid out and clarified with patient and family. Reasons for nonresponse should be discussed in a supportive and nonblaming fashion. Also it is important that family and child understand that the management of a person who is not responding to treatment requires a continuous process of reappraisal and rediagnosis as well as trials with different medications and psychotherapy to find the best treatment. Both prognosis and patient and family nonadherence issues may need to be discussed and addressed.

PSYCHOTHERAPY

Establishing a treatment alliance with patient and parents as partners and collaborators is critical for success. The clinician should (1) provide sustained and hopeful support for patients and their families. This may require the involvement of school and sometimes friends, religious and community organizations; (2) address the patient's hopelessness, frustration, anger, and negative attributions; (3) take a problem-solving approach and recommend activities; and (4) set short-term goals to increase a sense of mastery and accomplishment. Interventions such as CBT and IPT—described in Chapters 8 and 9— have been developed for depressed youth in individual and group formats.[3] CBT combined with pharmacotherapy has been found efficacious for adolescents who failed to respond to one SSRI trial.[8]

Although the efficacy of family therapy for the treatment of youth with MDD has not been well studied, family therapy may be indicated to help the family resolve, cope, and problem-solve ongoing conflicts and to manage the child's depressive symptomatology (see Chapter 10). Clinicians must try to understand children's and families' frustration and anger with the situation. This is particularly important when there are family or child factors that may explain the child's poor response to treatment but the patient and family are unaware of them or using maladaptive defense mechanisms, such as denial or projection, to explain the situation (e.g., it is the clinician's or teachers fault that the child is not getting better). Clinicians also need to be aware of their own reactions and countertransference and may need to consult with colleagues or consider joining a peer supervision or support group to deal with them.

PHARMACOTHERAPY

Even if the clinician opts for pharmacologic management, supportive treatment is necessary. Moreover, the use of psychotherapeutic techniques—aimed at helping patients with their negative attributions, denial, short-term goals, daily activities, adherence to treatment, and problem solving regarding psychosocial, educational, and family issues—is recommended.

Pharmacologic strategies to manage children with treatment-resistant depression include optimization, switching, augmentation, and other biologic treatments.[3,10] Definition of these terms can be found in Table 4.1 and description of the various medications in Chapter 6. Each of these strategies needs to be carried out systematically and one step at a time. Optimization and augmentation strategies are often used when patients have shown a partial response to the current regimen; switching is used when patients have not responded or cannot tolerate the medications, but no studies have validated these practices in children.

Optimization is increasing the medication (or psychotherapy) to a maximum dose or lengthening the duration of treatment. This is the first strategy to consider unless the patient has side effects or is reluctant to continue the treatment. Increasing the dose is effective in adults as well as in the scanty child literature.[3,10,11] Increasing the daily dose of fluoxetine from 10 to 20 mg to 40 to 60 mg after 9 weeks of treatment was associated with higher response in children and adolescents with MDD.[9] Also, some evidence indicates that adequate exposure to SSRIs, resulting in at least 70% serotonin reuptake inhibition, makes response much more likely in depressed adolescents.[41] Similarly, at least for depressed youth treated with bupropion, response is related to having an adequate drug plus active metabolite concentration.[42] In depressed adults, if a modest improvement was present (e.g., $\geq 20\%$ reduction in symptoms), an increase in dosage at 6 weeks and longer duration of treatment enhanced response rate and remission by 12 weeks of treatment.[13] Naturalistic studies in depressed adults and youth have also demonstrated that the proportion of patients who achieve remission increases with greater length of antidepressant treatment.[43] However, it is not clear whether this increase is because of the treatment itself or due to the natural course of the depression.

In summary, the studies just noted emphasize the importance of maximizing the dose and duration of treatment to achieve the ultimate goal: remission.

AUGMENTATION VERSUS SWITCHING

If optimization strategies do not work or are not tolerated, there is the possibility of either augmenting or switching treatments. Augmenting the current treatment can be done with another type of medication (e.g., lithium, another class of antidepressant, T_3).[3,9,11] Also, if the patient is

TABLE 16.1 POTENTIAL ADVANTAGES AND DISADVANTAGES OF SWITCHING AND AUGMENTATION STRATEGIES

SWITCHING VS. AUGMENTATION		AUGMENTATION VS. SWITCHING	
Potential Advantages	*Potential Disadvantages*	*Potential Advantages*	*Potential Disadvantages*
• Different mechanism of action • Fewer drug–drug interactions • Fewer side effects • Better adherence • Less cost	• Need to discontinue initial medication • Lag in response • Loss of partial response to initial medication • Loss of drug–drug synergy	• Maintaining any partial response • Avoiding lag in response • Obtaining drug–drug synergy • Targeting comorbid disorders	• Drug–drug interactions • Additional side effects • Greater cost • Reduced adherence

not receiving an evidence-based psychotherapy, augmentation can be done with CBT or IPT. The switching is carried out by stopping or cross-tapering (reducing gradually one drug while the other is progressively introduced). The switch can be to (1) a different compound of the same class (e.g., an SSRI for another SSRI), (2) a different class of antidepressant (e.g., a SSRI to a serotonin-norepinephrine reuptake inhibitor [SNRI] or to bupropion), or (3) psychotherapy (without medication).

Clinicians need to be familiar with the advantages and disadvantages of switching versus augmentation and to educate patients and families so they can be informed collaborators in the decision-making process (Table 16.1 presents the advantages and disadvantages of each). In any case, as shown by the Sequenced Treatment Alternatives to Relieve Depression (STAR*D) study,[13] the patient (and in the case of children, their families) will have a lot to say about whether to switch or augment based on their own preferences, prior experiences, and presence of side effects.

Little research is available on adolescents with treatment-resistant depression to inform clinicians as to whether to choose augmentation or switching and, if switching, whether to choose the same class or a different class of drug for a particular patient.[3,10,11] Usually, the general rule is to augment with another medication if the current medication is partially helping the patient and not causing significant side effects. Although not well studied in youth, augmentation with lithium, T_3, and atypical antipsychotics has been moderately successful with medium size effects in adults.[3,10,11] Other strategies include augmentation with a second antidepressant or other mood stabilizers (e.g., lamotrigine, valproate, or carbamazepine).

Small open studies using lithium and monoamine oxidase inhibitor (MAOI) augmentation for adolescents with treatment resistant depression have shown contradictory results.[3,10] Also, it is not easy to administer MAOIs to youth. There is only one RCT that studied 334 adolescents with MDD who had been depressed for approximately 2 years and unresponsive to one adequate SSRI trial.[13] Subjects were randomized to one of four treatments: (1) switch to an alternative SSRI, (2) switch to venlafaxine, (3) switch to another SSRI plus addition of CBT, or (4) switch to venlafaxine and addition of CBT. Although longer-term results of the study are not yet available, at 12 weeks, the addition of CBT to either medication strategy resulted in a better rate of clinical response (55% versus 41%), with no difference between the response rates of the two medication strategies (48% for venlafaxine versus 47% for SSRI). However, venlafaxine was associated with more side effects, particularly increased blood pressure and pulse, although these effects were rarely of clinical import. These findings support the use of combination treatment for depressed adolescents who have not responded to an adequate trial with an SSRI; however, because patients in this study received both a medication switch and psychotherapy, the effectiveness of simply adding CBT to existing medication treatment was not evaluated.

Although the results of adult studies cannot always be extrapolated to children and adolescents and there are methodological differences with TORDIA, a landmark study of treatment-resistant depressed adults (STAR*D) reported findings that are consistent with those of TORDIA.[13] In this study, a large sample of adults were treated with citalopram for 12 to 14 weeks; if they experienced intolerable side effects or did not achieve remission, they were offered a switch to sertraline, bupropion-SR, or venlafaxine-XR, or augmentation with bupropion-SR or buspirone. Participants could also switch to, or augment with CBT, although only a third of the participants agreed to randomization. If patients did not respond or experienced intolerable side effects to these treatments, they were offered to switch to mirtazapine or to a different class of antidepressant, nortriptyline. Also, they had the option of augmenting with lithium or T_3). Finally, patients who did not achieve remission to these last treatments were taken off all medications and randomly switched to a MAOI (tranylcypromine) or to the combination of venlafaxine XR with mirtazapine. It is important to note that, although there was randomization with a class of treatment strategy (e.g., switch or augmentation), the findings of the switching and augmentation approaches cannot be directly compared because in STAR*D most patients did not agree to be randomly assigned to one or the other treatment strategies.

In summary, about 50% of participants in STAR*D remitted after two treatment strategies, and over the course of all four treatments; almost 70% of those who did not withdraw from the study became symptom free. However, the rate at which participants withdrew from the trial was substantial. The results from STAR*D suggest that if a first treatment with one SSRI fails, about one in four people who choose to switch to another medication will get better, regardless of whether the second medication is another SSRI or an antidepressant of a different class. If patients choose to add a new medication to the existing SSRI, about one in three people will get better. It appears that it does not make much difference whether the second antidepressant is from a different class or a medication to augment the effect of the SSRI. After two treatment failures, about one in seven people will get better after switching to a different antidepressant, and about one in five will get better when adding a new medication to the existing one. Finally, for patients with the most treatment-resistant depression, a final trial with a different class of antidepressants or a combination of two different classes may benefit another 10% of patients. Therefore, patients with difficult-to-treat depression should be encouraged to try several treatment strategies and not lose hope. However, the odds of remitting diminish with every additional treatment strategy needed, particularly for patients who only showed symptom improvement and not remission, and for those with comorbid psychiatric and/or medical conditions.

Other adult studies have also reported that a combination of medication plus CBT is superior to medication management alone for the treatment of partial responders and for the prevention for relapse.[32,44] Finally, a switch from one modality of treatment to another (medication to psychotherapy or vice versa) has been found helpful for some chronically depressed adults who have failed one monotherapy.[45]

OTHER BIOLOGIC TREATMENTS

Other biologic treatments that need to be considered for youth with treatment-resistant depression include electroconvulsive Therapy (ECT), light therapy, and, to a lesser extent, more experimental interventions, such as transcranial magnetic stimulation (TMS) and vagal nerve stimulation (see Chapter 7). In addition, intravenous clomipramine was found superior to placebo in a small study of adolescents with treatment-resistant depression.[46]

Except for one RCT using light therapy,[47] there is no study demonstrating effectiveness in adolescents of any of these treatments. If seasonal affective disorder is suspected, the light box can be tried. It appears that light therapy is best if it is used in the early morning. However, this might create another source of conflict at home with the parent trying to wake up the adolescent early in the morning. Anecdotally, some adolescents have benefited from using the light box later in the day. There are also case reports for efficacy of ECT in adolescents, but it is not clear what dose, duration, or unilateral versus bilateral should be tried, and there are concerns about the possibility of long-term adverse effects of ECT on the new circuits being formed in the brain of adolescents (see reference 48 and Chapter 7). Studies from case series suggest that adolescents most likely to respond to ECT are those with bipolar depression and less likely are those with comorbid personality disorder traits.[49] If ECT proves effective, then there are questions about what to do afterward to prevent a relapse and whether to use antidepressant medications or maintenance ECT, but there are no studies to guide clinicians' choices.

RESOURCES FOR PROFESSIONALS, PATIENTS AND FAMILIES

Please see these sections in Chapters 6 to 10.

REFERENCES

1. Birmaher B, Ryan ND, Williamson DE, et al. Childhood and adolescent depression: a review of the past ten years. Part I. *J Am Acad Child Adolesc Psychiatry.* 1996;35:1427–1439.
2. Birmaher B, Ryan ND, Brent DA, et al. Childhood and adolescent depression: A review of the past ten years. Part II. *J Am Acad Child Adolesc Psychiatry.* 1996;35:1575–1583.
3. Birmaher B, Brent DA, AACAP Work Group on Quality Issues. Practice parameter for the assessment and treatment of children and adolescents with depressive disorders. *J Am Acad Child Adolesc Psychiatry.* 2007;46:1503–1526.
4. Bridge JA, Iyengar S, Salary CB, et al. Clinical response and risk for reported suicidal ideation and suicide attempts in pediatric antidepressant treatment. A meta-analysis of randomized controlled trials. *JAMA.* 2007;297:1683–1696.
5. Weisz JR, McCarty CA, Valeri SM. Effects of psychotherapy for depression in children and adolescents: a meta-analysis. *Psychol Bull.* 2006;132:132–149.
6. Emslie GJ, Rush AJ, Weinberg WA, et al. Fluoxetine in child and adolescent depression: acute and mainte- nance treatment. *Depress Anxiety.* 1998;7:32–39.
7. Emslie GJ, Heiligenstein JH, Hoog SL, et al. Fluoxetine treatment for prevention of relapse of depression in children and adolescents: a double-blind, placebo-controlled study. *J Am Acad Child Adolesc Psychiatry.* 2004;43:1397–1405.
8. Brent DA, Emslie GJ, Clarke GN, et al. Switching to venlafaxine or another SSRI with or without cognitive behavioural therapy for adolescents with SSRI-resistant depression: the TORDIA randomized control trial. *JAMA.* 2008;299:901–913.
9. Heiligenstein JH, Hoog SL, Wagner KD, et al. Fluoxetine 40–60 mg versus fluoxetine 20 mg in the treatment of children and adolescents with a less-than-complete response to nine-week treatment with fluoxetine 10–20 mg: a pilot study. *J Child Adolesc Psychopharmacol.* 2006;16:207–217.
10. Hughes CW, Emslie GJ, Crismon ML, et al. Texas Consensus Conference Panel on Medication Treatment of Childhood Major Depressive Disorder: Texas Children's Medication Algorithm Project: update from Texas Consensus Conference Panel on Medication Treatment of Childhood Major Depressive Disorder. *J Am Acad Child Adolesc Psychiatry.* 2007;46:667–686.
11. American Psychiatric Association. Practice guidelines for the treatment of patients with major depressive disorder (revision). *Am J Psychiatry.* 2000;157(suppl):1–45.
12. Nierenberg AA, McLean NE, Alpert JE, et al. Early nonresponse to fluoxetine as a predictor of poor 8-week outcome. *Am J Psychiatry.* 1995;152:1500–1503.
13. Rush AJ. STAR*D: what have we learned? *Am J Psychiatry.* 2007;164:201–204.
14. Brent DA, Holder D, Kolko D, et al. A clinical psychotherapy trial for adolescent depression comparing cog- nitive, family, and supportive treatments. *Arch Gen Psychiatry.* 1997;54:877–885.
15. Mufson L, Dorta KP, Wickramaratne P, et al. A randomized effectiveness trial of interpersonal psychotherapy for depressed adolescents. *Arch Gen Psychiatry.* 2004;61:577–584.
16. Mufson L, Weissman MM, Moreau D, et al. Efficacy of interpersonal psychotherapy for depressed adoles- cents. *Arch Gen Psychiatry.* 1999;56:573–579.
17. Poznanski EO, Mokros HB. *Children's Depression Rating Scale, Revised (CDRS-R) Manual.* Los Angeles, Calif: Western Psychological Services; 1995.
18. Guy W. *ECDEU Assessment Manual for Psychopharmacology* (DHEW Publication ADM 76–338). Rockville, Md: U.S. Dept of Health, Education, and Welfare; 1976.
19. Clarke G, Debar L, Lynch F, et al. A randomized effectiveness trial of brief cognitive-behavioral therapy for depressed adolescents receiving antidepressant medication. *J Am Acad Child Adolesc Psychiatry.* 2005;44:888–898.
20. Clarke GN, Lewinsohn PM, Rohde P, et al. Cognitive-behavioral group treatment of adolescent depression: efficacy of acute group treatment and booster sessions. *J Am Acad Child Adolesc Psychiatry.* 1999; 38:272–279.
21. Birmaher B, Brent DA, Kolko D, et al. Clinical outcome after short-term psychotherapy for adolescents with major depressive disorder. *Arch Gen Psychiatry.* 2000;57:29–36.
22. Kroll L, Harrington R, Jayson D, et al. Pilot study of continuation cognitive-behavioral therapy for major depression in adolescent psychiatric patients. *J Am Acad Child Adolesc Psychiatry.* 1996;35:1156–1161.
23. Curry J, Rohde P, Simons A, et al. Predictors and moderators of acute outcome in the Treatment for Adolescents with Depression Study (TADS). *J Am Acad Child Adolesc Psychiatry.* 2006;45:1427–1439.
24. Rossello J, Bernal G. The efficacy of cognitive-behavioral and interpersonal treatments for depression in Puerto Rican adolescents. *J Consulting Clin Psychol.* 1999;67:734–745.

25. Rohde P, Clarke GN, Mace DE, et al. An efficacy/effectiveness study of cognitive-behavioral treatment for adolescents with comorbid major depression and conduct disorder. *J Am Acad Child Adolesc Psychiatry.* 2004;43:660–668.

26. Clarke G, Hops H, Lewinsohn PM, et al. Cognitive-behavioral group treatment of adolescent depression: Prediction of outcome. *Behav Ther.* 1992;23:341–354.

27. Brent DA, Kolko D, Birmaher B, et al. Predictors of treatment efficacy in a clinical trial of three psychosocial treatments for adolescent depression. *J Am Acad Child Adolesc Psychiatry.* 1998;37:906–914.

28. Kronenberg S, Apter A, Brent D, et al. Serotonin transporter (5HTTLPR) polymorphism and citalopram effectiveness and side effects in children with depression and/or anxiety disorders. *J Child Adolesc Psychopharmacol.* 2007;17:741–750.

29. Kowatch RA, Fristad MA, Birmaher B, et al. Child Psychiatric Workgroup on Bipolar Disorder. Treatment guidelines for children and adolescents with bipolar disorder. *J Am Acad Child Adolesc Psychiatry.* 2005;44:213–235.

30. Weissman MM, Pilowsky PA, Wickramaratne P, et al. Remissions in maternal depression and child psychopathology: a STAR*D-child report. *JAMA.* 2006;22:1389–1398.

31. Lewinsohn PM, Rohde P, Seeley JR. Major depressive disorder in older adolescents: prevalence, risk factors, and clinical implications. *Clin Psychol Rev.* 1998;18:765–794.

32. Keller MB, McCullough JP, Klein DN, et al. A comparison of nefazodone, the cognitive behavioral-analysis system of psychotherapy, and their combination for the treatment of chronic depression. *N Engl J Med.* 2000;342:1462–1470.

33. Nemeroff CB, Heim CM, Thase ME, et al. Differential responses to psychotherapy versus pharmacotherapy in patients with chronic forms of major depression and childhood trauma. *Proc Natl Acad Sci USA.* 2003;100:14293–14296.

34. Barbe RP, Bridge J, Birmaher B, et al. Lifetime history of sexual abuse, clinical presentation, and outcome in a clinical trial for adolescent depression. *J Clin Psychiatry.* 2004;65:77–83.

35. Resnick MD, Bearman PS, Blum RW, et al. Protecting adolescents from harm: findings from the National Longitudinal Study on Adolescent Health. *JAMA.* 1997;278:823–832.

36. Singer MI, Anglin TM, Song LY, et al. Adolescents' exposure to violence and associated symptoms of psychological trauma. *JAMA.* 1995;273:477–482.

37. Manuck SB, Bleil ME, Petersen KL, et al. The socio-economic status of communities predicts variation in brain serotonergic responsivity. *Psychol Med.* 2005;35:519–528.

38. Steer RA, Kumar G, Ranieri WF, et al. Use of the Beck Depression Inventory-II with adolescent psychiatric outpatients. *J Psychopathol Behav Assess.* 1998;20:127–137.

39. Daviss WB, Birmaher B, Melhem NA, et al. Criterion validity of the mood and feelings questionnaire for depressive episodes in clinic and non-clinic subjects. *J Child Psychol Psychiatry.* 2006;47:927–934.

40. Reynolds WM. The Reynolds Adolescent Depression Scale-Second Edition (RADS-2). In: Hilsenroth MJ, Segal DS, eds. *Comprehensive Handbook of Psychological Assessment.* Hoboken, NJ: John Wiley; 2004:224–236.

41. Axelson DA, Perel JM, Birmaher B, et al. Platelet serotonin reuptake inhibition and response to SSRIs in depressed adolescents. *Am J Psychiatry.* 2005;162:802–804.

42. Daviss WB, Perel JM, Brent DA, et al. Acute antidepressant response and plasma levels of bupropion and metabolites in a pediatric-aged sample: an exploratory study. *Ther Drug Monit.* 2006;28:190–198.

43. Birmaher B, Arbelaez C, Brent D. Course and outcome of child and adolescent major depressive disorder. *Child Adolesc Psychiatr Clin N Am.* 2002;11:619–637.

44. Fava GA, Ruini C, Rafanelli C, et al. Six-year outcome of cognitive behavior therapy for prevention of recurrent depression. *Am J Psychiatry.* 2004;161:1872–1876.

45. Schatzberg AF, Rush AJ, Arnow BA, et al. Chronic depression: medication (nefazodone) or psychotherapy (CBASP) is effective when the other is not. *Arch Gen Psychiatry.* 2005;62:513–520.

46. Sallee FR, Vrindavanam NS, Deas-Nesmith D, et al. Pulse intravenous clomipramine for depressed adolescents: a double-blind, controlled trial. *Am J Psychiatry.* 1997;154:668–673.

47. Swedo SE, Allen AJ, Glod CA, et al. A controlled trial of light therapy for the treatment of pediatric seasonal affective disorder. *J Am Acad Child Adolesc Psychiatry.* 1997;36:816–821.

48. American Academy of Child and Adolescent Psychiatry. Practice parameter for the use of ECT with adolescents. *J Am Acad Child Adolesc Psychiatry.* 2004;43:1521–1539.

49. Walter G, Rey JM. An epidemiological study of the use of ECT in adolescents. *J Am Acad Child Adolesc Psychiatry.* 1997;36:809–815.

Managing Young People With Depression and Comorbid Conditions

MARYANN O. HETRICK, KIRTI SAXENA, AND CARROLL W. HUGHES[a]

KEY POINTS

- Depression is often comorbid with other disorders, particularly anxiety disorders, attention deficit hyperactivity disorder (ADHD), and disruptive behavior disorders.
- Detecting comorbid conditions early in the assessment process is an important aspect of a comprehensive assessment and needs to be taken into account when planning treatment.

Principles for Treating Childhood Depression and Comorbid Disorders

- Alleviate symptoms of the most severe disorder first.
- Improvement in the specific symptoms of depression and the respective comorbid disorder(s) should be systematically monitored by objective measures to assess response to treatment, rather than monitoring global functioning in isolation. Measures should include multiple sources, such as clinician-, parent-, and child- or adolescent-rated forms.
- The potential for suicidality should be assessed at every treatment visit, particularly when individuals present with comorbid disorders that might exacerbate the symptoms of depression or there are previous suicide attempts, impulsivity, substance abuse, and so on. Safety plans should be developed and implemented, as needed.
- Patients and their parents should be advised to contact the practitioner if symptoms become more severe, suicidal ideation or suicidal gestures begin, or if medication side effects become problematic.
- With the consent of legal guardians, communication should be open and frequent among different treating clinicians (e.g., psychiatrist, psychologist, school personnel, etc.) to ensure treatment integrity.

Pharmacotherapy

- Begin with a single medication when possible. Then make one medication change or addition at a time and allow adequate time for response and possible dose adjustments.
- If the patient shows minimal to no improvement in symptoms, and dose has been increased, a change in medication may be warranted after 4 to 8 weeks of treatment. However, if the patient appears to be responding in some fashion to the medication, remission may still be achieved by 12 weeks.
- Those with residual symptoms after 12 weeks might benefit from augmentation or changing to a different treatment in order to achieve complete remission.
- Patients should have more frequent visits early in the treatment. This allows the practitioner to provide psychoeducation to the family, enhance rapport, monitor changes in symptoms, identify risk for suicidality, monitor adverse effects, and adjust the dose of medications.

[a]Carroll Hughes receives research support and is a consultant to BioBehavioral Diagnostics, Inc. Neither Maryann Hetrick nor Kirti Saxena has any competing interests to report.

- If side effects pose concerns, the dosage should be lowered or a different medication prescribed. Treating side effects of one medication with another medication should be avoided because it can increase the risk of drug interactions, resulting in more side effects or decreased benefit (see Chapter 14).
- If the use of multiple medications is clinically warranted (e.g., to treat the comorbidities), clinicians should be knowledgeable and vigilant about potential negative interaction effects.

Psychotherapy

- Goals should be collaboratively established and agreed upon with the patient and his or her parents.
- Goals should be clear and measurable to allow for effective monitoring of improvement.
- Therapeutic interventions should have specific symptom targets/issues.
- In case of failure to respond to initial treatment, reassessment is essential.

Introduction

Although major depressive disorder (MDD) may occur in isolation, oftentimes that is not the case. It is estimated that 40% to 90% of children and adolescents diagnosed with MDD also have one comorbid psychiatric disorder, and 20% to 40% have two or more, which compromise further their ability to function.[1,2] According to the American Academy of Child and Adolescent Psychiatry,[1] anxiety disorders are the most common disorders that present with depression, whereas other disorders, such as ADHD[3-5] or other disruptive behavior disorders, occur less frequently. More specifically, approximately 30% to 80% of depressed youth are also diagnosed with an anxiety disorder, whereas 10% to 80% have a comorbid disruptive behavior disorder. Although the developmental trajectory of comorbid conditions depend on several individual factors, it appears that certain types of psychiatric disorders, such as anxiety disorders or ADHD, are more likely to develop before symptoms of MDD.[2] Additionally, base rates of specific comorbid conditions vary according to developmental phases of life (e.g., childhood versus adolescence).[6] Other disorders comorbid with depression include eating disorders, pervasive developmental disorders (including Asperger syndrome) (see Chapter 22), and substance abuse (see Chapter 18), but they occur less frequently.

Establishing the timeline of onset of the respective disorders is an important part of the assessment and differential diagnostic process. For example, anxiety symptoms occurring only within a depressive episode are not considered to meet *DSM-IV* diagnostic criteria, as opposed to onset before the MDD. In terms of developmental age, the rate of comorbid MDD and separation anxiety disorder is high in childhood, whereas the rates of comorbid MDD and conduct disorder, social phobia, and generalized anxiety disorder are higher in adolescence. Given the differential rates of comorbidity by age, practitioners are advised to consider base rates of co-occurring disorders when treating depressed youth and assessing potential comorbid conditions. Additionally, practitioners should be familiar with the overlap of symptoms among these disorders because this knowledge can aid in differential diagnosis and accurate identification of comorbid diagnoses. Table 17.1 presents a summary of the symptom clusters for various psychiatric disorders, which shows how easy it can be to mistake one disorder for another in a quick, cursory review of presenting complaints if symptoms for individual disorders are not reviewed carefully.[7] It would still be worse to stop the clinical interview after confirming a single diagnosis and to begin treatment without considering the possibility of other comorbid disorders that may warrant a different management. Finally, one would be remiss not to consider possible substance abuse or medical conditions that are contributing to or causing the symptom profile that needs to be addressed first.

Accurate diagnosis is critical, so a method for reviewing all of the major childhood disorders systematically is essential and always part of good practice. Recognizing that it is not economically feasible for the majority of practitioners to use one of the structured diagnostic interviews, a diagnostic checklist that reviews the symptom profile for each disorder should be used as a minimum. There are some computerized diagnostic assessments (e.g., Diagnostic Interview for Children and Adolescents [DICA]) and behavioral problem summaries (e.g., Behavioral Assessment System for Children [BASC]) commercially available that can be completed by the parent and/or older child prior to the assessment visit. This also applies to disorder-specific self-reports.[8] They not only help clarify the differential diagnosis but place current symptoms in focus, which is important for an ongoing objective assessment of treatment outcome.

TABLE 17.1 A LIST OF POSSIBLE OVERLAPPING SYMPTOMS IN DIFFERENT CHILDHOOD PSYCHIATRIC DISORDERS

Symptom	Major Depression	Anxiety Disorders	ADHD[a]	Bipolar Illness	ODD/Disruptive Behavior Disorders	Substance Abuse	Medical Conditions
Dysphoria	X	X		X	X	X	X
Irritability	X	X	X	X	X	X	X
↓ Concentration/ ↑ Distractibility	X	X	X	X		X	X
Fatigue	X	X				X	X
Restlessness	X	X	X	X	X	X	X
Sleep disturbance	X	X	X	X		X	X
Poor self-concept	X	X	X			X	X
Suicidal ideation	X			X		X	X
Appetite	X	X	X			X	X
Social withdrawal	X	X	X			X	X

[a]ADHD medications can also present with sleep and appetite changes.
ADHD, attention deficit hyperactivity disorder; ODD, oppositional defiant disorder.

When a child or adolescent presents with MDD and a comorbid condition, clinicians are advised to consider both disorders when devising a treatment plan and to focus initially on the more severe. Additionally, it is best to consider biopsychosocial factors, which warrant clinical attention and may guide treatment planning. Concern has been raised that common life events (e.g., a setback in school for some reason, breaking up with boyfriend or girlfriend, injury preventing continuing participation in a sport or other physical activity, etc.) associated with short-term depressive symptoms are sometimes too hastily described as MDD and would be better characterized as time-limited dysphoria not meriting antidepressant medication. Instead of initiating medication, "watchful waiting" can be a useful strategy.[9] Further, specific treatment approaches differ depending on the type of comorbid diagnosis, which diagnosis is the primary or most severe, and the age of the patient (e.g., child versus adolescent). The specific therapies chosen and the order in which they are implemented depend on the combination of disorders, given that different therapies are more effective for certain disorders. It has increasingly become good practice to combine pharmacotherapy and psychotherapy for optimal treatment.[10] A discussion of assessment methods and treatment modalities for different comorbid disorders (i.e., anxiety disorders, ADHD, and disruptive behavior disorders) follows.

With regard to pharmacotherapy, treatment of comorbid disorders with MDD has become more complicated because of concerns that risk for suicidal ideation may increase for a minority of those treated with selective serotonin reuptake inhibitors (SSRIs)[11] when compared with placebo (see Chapters 7 and 14 for more details).

DEPRESSION AND COMORBID ANXIETY

As noted earlier, the probability of treating a depressed child or adolescent with a comorbid anxiety disorder is higher than that of any other childhood comorbid psychiatric disorder. As such, the presence of anxiety disorders should be screened carefully in depressed children and adolescents to ensure the most appropriate treatment is implemented. Each of the 14 different types of anxiety disorder included in *DSM-IV* has a unique set of symptoms, and interventions can differ substantially, emphasizing the importance of careful assessment of the full spectrum of possible types of anxiety. Fortunately, pharmacotherapy for anxiety is frequently similar to that for depression, as discussed later. Comorbid anxiety may be detected using rating scales in conjunction with a thorough clinical interview (see Chapter 3). However, not all rating scales are equally valid and reliable. Pavuluri and Birmaher[12] evaluated child and adolescent rating scales for depression and anxiety to guide their use; Table 17.2 provides a brief summary. Pavuluri and Birmaher underscore the importance of using clinician as well as parent reports and child self-reports to ensure a thorough assessment of symptoms.

TABLE 17.2 SUMMARY OF SOME AVAILABLE ANXIETY RATING SCALES

Scale	Rater	Disorder or Symptom Assessed	Total Number of Items (Time to Complete and Score)	Strengths	Weaknesses
Multidimensional Anxiety Scale for Children	Parent Child Adolescent	Generalized anxiety disorder Social phobia Separation anxiety disorder	39 Items (20 min) or 10-Item Version (5–10 min)	• Excellent discrimination between depression and anxiety	• Poor agreement between child and parent ratings
Screen for Child Anxiety-Related Emotional Disorders	Parent Child Adolescent	Panic disorder Generalized anxiety disorder Separation anxiety disorder Social phobia	41 Items (15 min)	• Excellent discrimination between anxiety and disruptive disorders • Moderate discrimination between depression and anxiety • Sensitive to treatment effects	• Normative data in United States are pending
Social Anxiety Scale for Children—Revised	Child Adolescent	Social anxiety	18 Items (20 min)	• Ability to measure a child's perception of social anxiety	
Fear Survey Schedule for Children—Revised	Child Adolescent	Wide array of fears	80 Items (30 min)	• Can be used with intellectually impaired children and adolescents • Tested with culturally diverse populations	• High correlation among the subscales
Pediatric Anxiety Rating Scale	Clinician	Social phobia Generalized anxiety disorder Separation anxiety disorder	50 Items (45 min)	• Developed to track response to pharmacotherapy	• Interview and scoring process is lengthy
Children's Yale-Brown Obsessive-Compulsive Scale	Clinician		22 Items (120 min)	• Optional self-rating scale to augment the clinical interview • Assesses symptoms and severity • Sensitive to effects of pharmacotherapy and cognitive behavioral therapy	• Items measuring resistance are developmentally inappropriate • Interview and scoring process is lengthy

Adapted from Pavuluri M, Birmaher B. A practical guide to using ratings of depression and anxiety in child psychiatric practice. *Curr Psychiatry Rep.* 2004;6:108–116.

They specifically recommend the Pediatric Anxiety Rating Scale (PARS), the Multidimensional Anxiety Scale for Children (MASC), or the Screen for Child Anxiety-Related Emotional Disorders (SCARED).

As with many disorders, a multimodal treatment is recommended, which may consist of medication, cognitive behavioral therapy (CBT), and involvement of the parents and family. However, the specific treatment components and the timing/order in which each component is implemented depend on many factors, such as the nature and severity of the symptoms. For instance, if a child or adolescent has marked dysfunction as a part of severe depression, he or she may experience difficulty engaging in the CBT process[2] because of lack of energy, difficulty concentrating, and pervasive negative cognitions. In such cases, it is recommended that treatment of depression via medication be implemented first, with the aim of alleviating the severity of depressive symptoms.[2] Once depressive symptoms improve, the child or adolescent will be more likely to engage in the CBT, increasing the likelihood of success.

Medication algorithms have been developed to guide physicians treating individuals with various disorders, such as comorbid MDD and ADHD or ADHD and anxiety.[13,14] Figure 17.1 illustrates the algorithmic approach for childhood anxiety and ADHD as comorbid disorders. Although a medication algorithm has been developed for the treatment of obsessive-compulsive disorder[15] and for ADHD with comorbid anxiety, one for the treatment of comorbid depression and anxiety disorders is yet to be developed. It is conceivable that such an algorithm would combine the features of Figures 17.1 and Figure 6.1 (see Chapter 6) using the hierarchical approach of addressing the most severe disorder first.

The results of double-blind, placebo-controlled studies provide empirical evidence for guidelines for the treatment of MDD with anxiety disorders. These studies have shown that SSRIs are an effective treatment for anxiety and depression, making them the ideal medication to use when the two disorders present simultaneously.[2] When anxiety symptoms are moderate or severe, impairment makes participation in psychotherapy difficult, or psychotherapy results in partial response, treatment with medication is recommended.[16,17] In particular, recent randomized controlled trials (RCTs) have compared the short-term effectiveness of SSRIs with placebo, finding that SSRIs are an effective treatment for generalized anxiety disorder, social phobia, seasonal affective disorder,[18–21] social anxiety,[22] selective mutism with social phobia,[23] and obsessive compulsive disorder.[24–26] Table 17.3 lists

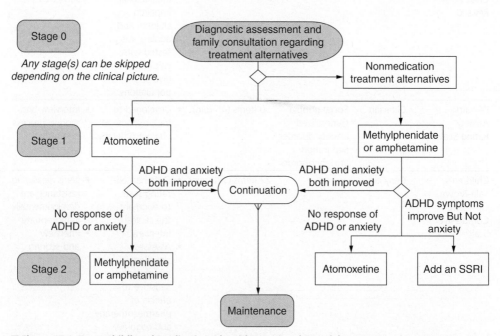

■ **Figure 17.1 Texas Childhood Medication Algorithm Project (CMAP) for ADHD and anxiety.** (Reprinted from Pliszka SR, Crismon ML, Hughes CW, et al. Texas Children's Medication Algorithm Project: a revision of the algorithm for the pharmacotherapy of childhood attention-deficit/hyperactivity disorder. *J Am Acad Child Adolesc Psychiatry.* 2006;45:642–647, with permission from the Texas Department of State Health Services.) *ADHD = Attention Deficit Hyperactivity Disorder, SSRI = Selective Serotonin Reuptake Inhibitor*

TABLE 17.3 MOST FREQUENTLY RECOMMENDED MEDICATIONS FOR DEPRESSION WITH COMORBID DISORDERS

COMORBID ANXIETY: SSRIs[1,2]

Generic Class/Brand Name	Dose Form	Typical Starting Dose	FDA Max/Day	Off-Label Max/Day	Comments	Special Precautions
Fluoxetine (GAD, OCD, PTSD, panic)	10-, 20-, 40-mg cap 10-mg tab 20 mg/5 mL sol	10 mg	20–40 mg	60 mg	Potential side effects: mild, transient gastrointestinal, headaches, increased motor activity, insomnia, possible disinhibition, agitation, anxiety, decreased libido, delayed ejaculation, diarrhea, dizziness, dry mouth, fatigue, decreased appetite, nausea, rash, tremor, vision problems, vomiting	Black box warnings for increased suicidality; should not be taken with MAO inhibitors
Fluvoxamine (OCD) Note: Not FDA approved for MDD	25-, 50-, 100-mg tab	25 mg for children 50 mg for adolescents	200–250 mg	300 mg		
Sertraline (panic, OCD, PTSD)	25-, 50-, 100-mg tab 20 mg/mL sol	12.5–25 mg	50–100 mg	200 mg		
Paroxetine (OCD, panic, GAD, social phobia, PTSD)	10-, 20-, 30-, 40-mg tab 12.5-, 25-, 37.5-mg tab CR 10 mg/5 mL sol	10 mg	20–40 mg	50 mg		

Note: Tricyclic antidepressants avoided because of toxic side effects; benzodiazepines avoided because of abuse potential.

COMORBID ADHD[3]

AMPHETAMINE PREPARATIONS: SHORT ACTING

Adderall[5]	5-, 7.5-, 10-, 12.5-, 15-, 20-, 30-mg tab	3–5 yr: 2.5 mg QD ≥6 yr: 5 mg QD–BID	40 mg	>50 kg: 60 mg	Short-acting stimulants often used as initial treatment in small children (<16 kg) but have disadvantage of BID–TID dosing to control symptoms throughout day	
Dexedrine[5]	5-mg tab 10-mg tab 5 mg/mL elixir	3–5 yr: 2.5 mg QD ≥6 yr: 5 mg QD–BID				
DexroStat[5]	5-, 10-mg tab					

AMPHETAMINE PREPARATIONS: LONG ACTING

Dexedrine Spansule	5-, 10-, 15-mg cap	≥6 yr: 5–10 mg QD–BID	40 mg	>50 kg: 60 mg	Longer acting stimulants offer greater convenience, confidentiality, and compliance with single daily dosing but may have greater problematic effects on evening appetite and sleep; Adderall XR may be opened and sprinkled on soft foods	
Adderall XR	5-, 10-, 15-, 20-, 25-, 30-mg cap	≥6 yr: 10 mg QD	30 mg	>50 kg: 60 mg		
Lisdexamfetamine	30-, 50-, 70-mg cap	30 mg QD	70 mg	Not known		

(continued)

TABLE 17.3 MOST FREQUENTLY RECOMMENDED MEDICATIONS FOR DEPRESSION WITH COMORBID DISORDERS (CONTINUED)

Generic Class/Brand Name	Dose Form	Typical Starting Dose	FDA Max/Day	Off-Label Max/Day	Comments	Special Precautions
METHYLPHENIDATE PREPARATIONS: SHORT ACTING						
Focalin	2.5-, 5-, 10-mg cap	2.5 mg BID	20 mg	50 mg	Short-acting stimulants often used as initial treatment in small children (<16 kg) but have disadvantage of BID–TID dosing to control symptoms throughout day	
Methylin[5]	5-, 10-, 20-mg tab	5 mg BID	60 mg	>50 kg: 100 mg		
Ritalin[5]	5, 10, 20 mg	5 mg BID	60 mg	>50 kg: 100 mg		
METHYLPHENIDATE PREPARATIONS: INTERMEDIATE ACTING						
Metadate ER	10-, 20-mg cap	10 mg q AM	60 mg	>50 kg: 100 mg	Longer acting stimulants offer greater convenience, confidentiality, and compliance with single daily dosing but may have greater problematic effects on evening appetite and sleep; Metadate CD and Ritalin LA caps may be opened and sprinkled on soft food	
Methylin ER	10-, 20-mg cap	10 mg q AM	60 mg	>50 kg: 100 mg		
Ritalin SR[5]	20 mg	10 mg q AM	60 mg	>50 kg: 100 mg		
Metadate CD	10, 20, 30, 40, 50, 60 mg	20 mg q AM	60 mg	>50 kg: 100 mg		
Ritalin LA	10, 20, 30, 40 mg	20 mg q AM	60 mg	>50 kg: 100 mg		
METHYLPHENIDATE PREPARATIONS: LONG ACTING						
Concerta	18-, 27-, 36-, 54-mg cap	18 mg q AM	72 mg	108 mg	Swallow whole with liquids; nonabsorbable tablet shell may be seen in stool	
Daytrana patch	10-, 15-, 20-, 30-mg patches	Begin with 10-mg patch QD, then titrate up by patch strength	30 mg	Not known		
Focalin XR	5-, 10-, 15-, 20-mg cap	5 mg q AM	30 mg	50 mg		
SELECTIVE NOREPINEPHRINE REUPTAKE INHIBITOR						
Atomoxetine-Strattera	10-, 18-, 25-, 40-, 60-, 80-, 100-mg cap	Children and adolescents <70 kg: 0.5 mg/kg/day for 4 days; then 1 mg/kg/day for 4 days; then 1.2 mg/kg/day	Lesser of 1.4 mg/kg or 100 mg	Lesser of 1.8 mg/kg or 100 mg	Not a schedule II medication; consider if active substance abuse or severe side effects of stimulants (mood lability, tics); give q AM, or divided doses BID (effect on late evening behavior; do not open capsule	Monitor closely for suicidal thinking and behavior; monitor for hepatoxicity

(continued)

TABLE 17.3 MOST FREQUENTLY RECOMMENDED MEDICATIONS FOR DEPRESSION WITH COMORBID DISORDERS (CONTINUED)

Generic Class/Brand Name	Dose Form	Typical Starting Dose	FDA Max/Day	Off-Label Max/Day	Comments	Special Precautions
COMORBID AGGRESSION/DISRUPTIVE BEHAVIOR DISORDERS[4]						
Risperidone–Risperdal[6]	0.25-, 0.5-, 1-, 2-, 3-, 4-mg tab 25-, 32.5-, 50-mg ampoule	0.25 mg QID for children 0.5 mg QID for adolescents	1.5–2 mg for children 2–4 mg for adolescents		Weight gain, insulin resistance, sedation, akathisia, orthostatic hypotension, dizziness, increased triglycerides, extrapyramidal side effects; constipation; dizziness; dizziness or fainting when getting up suddenly from a lying or sitting position; drowsiness; dryness of mouth; headache; runny nose; vision problems; weakness; weight gain	Dyskinetic disorders
Olanzapine–Zyprexa	2.5-, 5-, 7.5-, 10-, 15, 20-mg tab 5-, 10-, 15-, 20-mg wafers	2.5 mg for children 2.5–5 mg for adolescents	10–20 mg	60 mg		

Others to consider: clozapine, quetiapine, ziprasidone (Pappadopulos E, Macintyre JC, Crismon ML, Crismon ML, et al. Treatment recommendations for the use of antipsychotics for aggressive youth [TRAAY] II. *J Am Acad Child Adolesc Psychiatry.* 2003;42:145–161).

ADHD, attention deficit hyperactivity disorder; CR, controlled release; FDA, Food and Drug Administration; GAD, generalized anxiety disorder; MAO, monoamine oxidase; MDD, major depressive disorder; OCD, obsessive-compulsive disorder; PTSD, posttraumatic stress disorder; SSRI, selective serotonin reuptake inhibitor.

[1]See Emslie GJ, Hughes CW, Crismon ML, et al. A feasibility study of the childhood depression medication algorithm: the Texas Children's Medication Algorithm Project (CMAP). *J Am Acad Child Adolesc Psychiatry.* 2004;43:1–9, Chapter 6, Tables 6.1 and 6.2, for SSRIs.

[2]Adapted from AACAP. Practice parameters for the assessment and treatment of children and adolescents with anxiety disorders. *J Am Acad Child Adolesc Psychiatry.* 2007;46:267–283.

[3]Adapted from Pliszka SR, Crismon ML, Hughes CW, et al. The Texas Children's Medication Algorithm Project: revision of the algorithm for pharmacotherapy of attention-deficit/hyperactivity disorder. *J Am Acad Child Adolesc Psychiatry.* 2006;45:642–657, and AACAP. Practice parameter for the assessment and treatment of children and adolescents with attention-deficit/hyperactivity disorder. *J Am Acad Child Adolesc Psychiatry.* 2007;46:894–921.

[4]Adapted from TRAY II (Pappadopulos E, Macintyre JC, Crismon ML, et al. Treatment recommendations for the use of antipsychotics for aggressive youth (TRAAY) II. *J Am Acad Child Adolesc Psychiatry.* 2003;42:145–161); and AACAP practice parameter for the prevention and management of aggressive behavior in child and adolescent psychiatric institutions, with special reference to seclusion and restraint. *J Am Acad Child Adolesc Psychiatry.* 2002, 41(2 Supplement):4S–25S.

[5]Generic formulation available.

[6]There is little information to guide dosing strategies for aggression. However, for aggressive children treated with risperidone, doses are about half that of the usual antipsychotic dose (Schur SB, Sikich L, Findling RL, et al. Treatment recommendations for the use of antipsychotics for aggressive youth (TRAAY). Part I. A review. *J Am Acad Child Adolesc Psychiatry.* 2003;42:132–144; and Pappadopulos E, Macintyre JC, Crismon ML, et al. Treatment recommendations for the use of antipsychotics for aggressive youth (TRAAY) II. *J Am Acad Child Adolesc Psychiatry.* 2003;42:145–161).

227

a summary of the best studied medication interventions with recommended doses. SSRIs are well tolerated by children and adolescents with only mild and transient side effects, such as gastrointestinal symptoms, increased motor activity, headaches, and insomnia. Disinhibition is much less frequent (see Chapter 14). It is important to obtain family history of bipolar illness along with bipolar (I or II) as a possible disorder in the child as a part of assessment before initiation of SSRIs.

The volume of research is considerably smaller for pharmacologic interventions with posttraumatic stress disorder (PTSD). However, studies appear to support the use of SSRIs to manage PTSD in adults. Similarly, no controlled trials are available for the treatment of childhood panic disorder. One open trial of SSRIs in adolescents[27] and a chart review in adolescents[28] indicated improvement with SSRIs. It is noted that use of SSRIs for anxiety is advantageous because these drugs—unlike traditional anxiolytics (e.g., benzodiazepines)—do not pose risk for abuse and are not cardiotoxic—unlike tricyclic antidepressants (TCAs).[29] The guidelines[2] indicate no strong empirical evidence for choosing one SSRI over another. Clinically, the choice is based on side-effect profile, duration of action, or response to a particular SSRI in a first-degree relative with anxiety.[30] Fluoxetine is the only SSRI with Food and Drug Administration (FDA) approval for treating childhood depression and was one of the initial medications recommended at the MDD algorithm consensus conference.[13]

Nonpharmacologic treatments have been empirically tested and are well established for the treatment of anxiety and depression.[31] A review of RCTs of CBT for anxiety and depression supported CBT as the treatment of choice.[32] As such, CBT should be considered when the two disorders present comorbidly.[30,32] The specific CBT techniques used vary depending on the disorder or symptoms being addressed (e.g., depression versus anxiety, social phobia versus generalized anxiety disorder, etc.). An overview of CBT for the treatment of depression is provided in Chapter 8. Although a comprehensive coverage of CBT for the various anxiety disorders is beyond the scope of this chapter, certain guidelines can be provided. Table 17.4 summarizes five general components of CBT for the treatment of anxiety disorders. The specific content of these components vary by disorder, need to be individualized for developmental age, and each may be differentially emphasized depending on the disorder. To date, cognitive restructuring models have been predominantly studied and used for adolescents, where there is a greater prevalence of anxiety and intellectual development is further advanced.

When treating a child with a specific phobia, systematic desensitization is emphasized as a means of extinguishing the response to the phobic stimuli. In systematic desensitization, individuals are exposed in a hierarchical and gradual manner, either in vivo or in imagination, to the anxiety-provoking stimuli while simultaneously being exposed to stimuli that elicit incompatible responses

TABLE 17.4 TREATMENT COMPONENTS OF COGNITIVE BEHAVIORAL THERAPY FOR ANXIETY DISORDERS

Psychoeducation (with the child and family)
- Provide information about the nature of the symptoms associated with the disorder
- Recommend books/literature to parents

Somatic management skills training
- Relaxation exercises
- Diaphragmatic breathing
- Self-monitoring of own somatic symptoms

Cognitive restructuring
- Challenge negative thoughts/expectations and replace with more adaptive/positive ones
- Engage in positive self-talk
- Teach thought-stopping techniques

Exposure (imaginal and/or in vivo)
- Systematic desensitization

Relapse prevention
- Booster sessions

Adapted from AACAP Practice Parameters for Anxiety Disorders, Reference 2.

(i.e., relaxation). Clinicians generally begin with teaching progressive muscle relaxation, then ordering the anxiety-provoking stimuli in a hierarchy, from least to most feared, and finally exposing the patient gradually to the stimuli, starting with the least feared, while in a relaxed state.[32] Compton and colleagues[32] warn that young children may experience difficulty with this process and that using aids, such as workbooks, may help them grasp the concepts and engage in systematic desensitization. It appears that the most effective component of systematic desensitization is the exposure to the various stimuli, as opposed to progressive muscle relaxation. Consequently, some clinicians choose to use a pure exposure-based treatment. However, the cooperation of the child is always important.[32]

In addition to exposure and relaxation, cognitive interventions focusing on coping skills, changing negative self-talk, unrealistic fears, modeling (the therapist or parent model successful/nonfearful interactions with the anxiety-provoking stimulus), and problem-solving skills are effective components of CBT; actively involving a child's family in treatment can help maintain therapeutic gains over time and across domains (e.g., home, school, etc.).[2,32]

DEPRESSION AND COMORBID ATTENTION DEFICIT HYPERACTIVITY DISORDER

Given the limited number of RCTs examining the treatment of comorbid MDD and ADHD, experts participated in a consensus conference to update the treatment of child and adolescent ADHD and, in a separate conference, for MDD. Both addressed the issue of treating depression comorbid with ADHD.[13,14] One of the recommendations was to emphasize the importance of using instruments to aid in the assessment of symptom severity. Commonly used rating scales of ADHD are the various forms of the Child Behavior Checklist (CBCL) and the Conners Parent and Teacher Rating Scales.[33] The use of such tools helps screening for the presence of ADHD before conducting the clinical interview, as well as allowing the monitoring of response to treatment. Free rating instruments are available at http://www.adhd.net/.

The consensus conference recommended that pharmacotherapy should focus on the most severe disorder first (e.g., the disorder causing the most impairment), given that symptoms associated with the secondary disorder often improve with treatment of the primary condition (or in this case, the most severe disorder [Figure 17.2]). For example, if a child or adolescent has a diagnosis of MDD and comorbid ADHD but shows depressed mood almost every day for several hours at a time, causing severe functional impairment as well as significant neurovegetative symptoms, then consideration should be given to using an SSRI first (see MDD treatment algorithm in Figure 6.1). Conversely, if ADHD appears to be the most severe of the disorders, pharmacotherapy for ADHD would be initiated first.

A depression feasibility study[34] found that the majority of children and adolescents diagnosed with comorbid ADHD and MDD can be treated successfully with stimulant medication. However, if a child experiences increased irritability after stimulant medication is prescribed, then the best course of action might be to treat the depression before the ADHD and then retry the stimulant medication after the depressive symptoms begin to remit. The consensus panel recommended making one change at a time when managing psychotropic medications so that effectiveness can be adequately evaluated. Of course, this recommendation is good clinical practice for treating any disorder. After a treatment plan is implemented, symptoms should be reassessed regularly. This is particularly important given the warnings of increased suicidality with SSRIs. If necessary, pharmacotherapy for the comorbid condition can be initiated after the effects of medication for the more severe disorder are optimized. Figure 17.2 summarizes an algorithm for the pharmacologic treatment of MDD co-occurring with ADHD.[13] Stage 1 consists of prescribing either a methylphenidate or an amphetamine preparation, whereas stage 1 of the MDD algorithm consists of prescribing an SSRI (see Figure 6.1).

Table 17.3 summarizes the most common medications and doses for treating ADHD. Although noradrenergic antidepressants (e.g., desipramine and bupropion) are generally effective in treating ADHD,[35] TCAs do not work in children with MDD, and no RCTs of bupropion in depressed children are available. Consequently, using SSRIs to treat depression with an added stimulant to treat ADHD is preferable to prescribing a noradrenergic antidepressant, although there are exceptions. Atomoxetine is a noradrenergic reuptake inhibitor that is superior to placebo in the treatment of

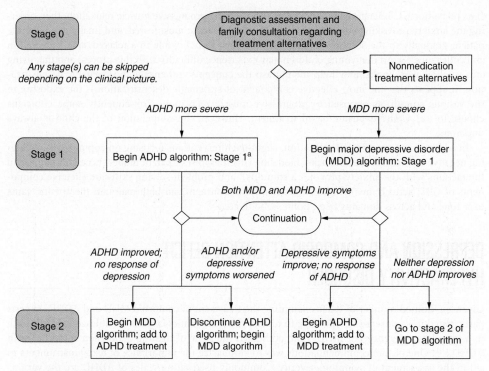

^aSee Pliszka, SR, Crismon ML, Hughes CW, et al. Texas Children's Medication Algorithm Project: revision of the algorithm for pharmacotherapy of attention-deficit/hyperactivity disorder. *J Am Acad Child Adolesc Psychiatry.* 2006;45:642–647.

■ **Figure 17.2 Texas Childhood Medication Algorithm Project (CMAP) for depression and ADHD.** (Reprinted from Hughes CW, Emslie GJ, Crismon ML, et al. Texas Children's Medication Algorithm Project: update from Texas Consensus Conference Panel on Medication Treatment of Childhood Major Depressive Disorder. *J Am Acad Child Adolesc Psychiatry.* 2007;46:667–686, with permission from the Texas Department of State Health Services.)

ADHD and has become increasingly popular.[36–38] Atomoxetine may be considered as the medication of choice for ADHD in persons with a substance abuse problem or in children who experience severe side effects from stimulants, such as mood lability or severe tics. Family opposition to the use of stimulants is also a factor.[39] Some report using low doses (0.5 to 1.0 mg/kg per day) of atomoxetine in combination with stimulants.[14] This is can be done when atomoxetine as well as stimulants fail to improve ADHD symptoms adequately or stimulants did not cover evening symptoms, even with long-acting forms. Atomoxetine is typically given in the afternoon to assist with evening behavior or to reduce "rebound" symptoms. It has fewer effects on appetite and sleep than stimulants, although it may produce nausea or sedation.

We would note here that in previous double-blind childhood depression studies where there was comorbid MDD/ADHD, it was not uncommon for ADHD symptoms to become worse as depression responded to treatment (probably because many ADHD symptoms were previously masked by the severity of the depression). This emphasizes the importance of identifying comorbid disorders early in assessment, so the possible worsening of certain symptoms of the comorbid condition resulting from treating the depression (e.g., with an SSRI) is not mistaken for side effects of the SSRI or interpreted as "disinhibition" caused by the medication. The simple addition of a stimulant at this point (typically 6 to 8 weeks out) often results in an overall clinical improvement. An additional precautionary note is highlighted in a recent report from the NIMH-sponsored PATS study (Preschool ADHD Treatment Study) that preschoolers with three or more coexisting disorders are not likely to respond to methylphenidate no matter what dosage is used.[40] This is similar to the results of the Multimodal Treatment of ADHD (MTA) in school-age children where those with coexisting disorders were less likely to respond to ADHD treatment.[3,41,42]

As noted in Figure 17.2 nonmedication treatment alternatives should be considered when devising a treatment plan for children and adolescents with comorbid depression and ADHD. Oftentimes, nonmedication treatments are used in conjunction to pharmacotherapy, rather than in isolation. The American Academy of Child and Adolescent Psychiatry published Practice Parameters[33] that contain the following treatment guidelines for clinicians:

- Psychoeducation for patients, their parents, and their teachers (http://www.parentsmedguide.org/).
- Information about the disorder, treatment, legal rights within the public school system, and so on.
- Referring the patient's parents to a support group (e.g., http://www.chadd.org).
- Family-based interventions if family dysfunction is an area of clinical concern.
- Consulting with educators to ensure academic needs are being met.
- Acting as an advocate if needed within the public school system.
- Helping families identify appropriate academic environments (e.g., schools that provide a greater degree of structure).
- Implementing behavior modification for target behaviors in school and at home.
- Helping the patient and family generate ways in which structure can be maintained in the child's environment.
- Social skills group therapy.
- Parent training (emphasized the younger the child is).
- Vocational evaluation, counseling, and training for adolescents.

Although the preceding guidelines should be considered, practitioners should always develop treatment plans to suit the individual's needs.[43] For instance, a child diagnosed with ADHD, inattentive type, has different treatment needs than one who is diagnosed with ADHD, combined type, or hyperactive/impulsive. Moreover, there can be variability in the treatment needs of individuals diagnosed with the same subtype of ADHD depending on other factors (e.g., family functioning, the presence of other disorders, learning disabilities, etc.). For instance, parent training and behavioral modification techniques are more likely to be emphasized in a younger child,[44] whereas vocational evaluation and counseling is more likely to be a focus in adolescents.[45] Given the chronic nature of ADHD, it is also important for the practitioner to reevaluate and adjust treatment as the child grows older because some may be fortunate enough to grow out of the disorder. Although individual therapy is typically recommended for the treatment of depression, individual therapy was not effective for ADHD in two large trials sponsored by the National Institute of Mental Health.[3,42,46] However, clinicians may determine that individual therapy is clinically indicated for specific cases to address issues such as treatment compliance in adolescents, self-esteem, and interpersonal relationships.

The best therapies continue to be the behaviorally based ones. A number of different behavioral programs are available for the treatment of children with ADHD,[47,48] including preschoolers.[49] Other interventions focus on the parents and are manual based.[45,50] In them, the basic principles for managing children with ADHD are taught to parents over 10 to 20 sessions, comprising psychoeducation about ADHD, the basic principles for rewarding appropriate and discouraging inappropriate behaviors, home management programs with reward systems, daily report cards, and learning to anticipate situations in which ADHD symptoms are exacerbated. Interestingly, in many cases parents are found to have undiagnosed ADHD histories, and some continue to have the symptoms, making recognition of the problems in their own children more difficult and affecting interventions until the parent's ADHD is also addressed.[48,51] Other family issues (parental substance abuse, neglect, marital problems, or depression) also need to be addressed for effective intervention with the child.[47]

MOOD DISORDER COMORBID WITH AGGRESSION AND OTHER DISRUPTIVE BEHAVIOR DISORDERS

Some children and adolescents with MDD present with behavioral problems (e.g., aggressiveness, conduct disorder, or oppositional defiant disorder) that impair functioning with peers, school, and/or family, and may even involve legal action. A careful differential diagnosis of bipolar disorder is necessary if a child or adolescent presents with excessive irritable mood and aggressive behavior (one should consider using the Young Mania Rating Scale[52] and Overt Aggression Scale[53] as part of the assessment), particularly when the child does not appear to respond to traditional ADHD treatment. If a diagnosis of bipolar disorder is made, the treatment plan might include implementation of a recent medication algorithm for the treatment of childhood bipolar disorder.[54]

If a child or adolescent presents with symptoms of conduct disorder or oppositional defiant disorder, it is recommended that a thorough assessment be conducted to rule out the presence of these disorders and possible substance abuse to determine treatment needs. A recent study indicates that a large percentage of individuals in juvenile detention have a mental illness. In these cases, assessment should include a clinical interview with the parents as well as the patient because the latter may not be forthcoming with information or acknowledge many of the troubles they have gotten into.[33] Additionally, it can be useful to obtain rating scales from the parents and schoolteachers, such as the Conners Parent-Teacher Rating Scale, CBCL[33] and completion of the BASC (teacher and parent). Treatment should be multimodal and can include family interventions (e.g., parent training, family therapy), individual therapy (e.g., supportive, exploratory, CBT), and group therapy.

Few studies have compared the efficacy of specific psychosocial treatments for aggression, and they are basically nonexistent for aggression comorbid with depression. Psychosocial interventions have included contingency management programs,[55,56] systematic training of social skills, anger management, problem solving, and behavior therapy.[57] There is some support for parent training[57] and psychoeducation.[58] More work is clearly merited.

Continued assessment regarding dangerousness to self or others is necessary given the nature of disruptive behavior disorders, and steps should be taken to ensure the safety of the patient as well as others. The following is a summary of different treatment considerations published by the American Academy of Child and Adolescent Psychiatry and Schur et al.[59]

- Parent training
  - Establish consistency between parents and across situations in the application of appropriate rules/expectations, consequences, and positive reinforcement.
- Family therapy
- Individual psychotherapy (specific approaches depend on the patient's age, level of engagement in the treatment process, and processing style)
  - Behavioral approaches
  - Exploratory approaches
  - Psychosocial skill-building training
    - Anger management
    - Assertiveness
    - Social skills training
- Peer interventions (encourage and identify a positive peer network)
- Collaborate with school personnel and juvenile justice system (when applicable) to facilitate a cohesiveness in treatment.
- Contingency management programs (e.g., token economy)
- Refer the family to additional resources as needed (e.g., social services within the community, Planned Parenthood, Big Brother and Big Sister programs, Friends Outside etc.).
- Vocational and independent-living skills counseling/training to help the adolescent make a successful transition to responsible adulthood.

Pappadopulos et al.[60] have developed a flowchart for the use of antipsychotics for aggressive youth (TRAAY) that begins with assessment and systematic behavioral interventions preceding the use of medication. Their recommendations acknowledge that aggression is common in a wide range of psychiatric conditions and interventions are designed accordingly. Unfortunately, data from controlled trials are beginning to accumulate only now, and recommendations have been based mostly on open-label studies and case reports and should be considered preliminary. Consequently, one should proceed with caution when using the medications mentioned in Table 17.3 and recognize the limitations of psychosocial and behavior interventions. Another limitation is that data supporting the use of medications have been based on studies involving disorders other than those with aggression.[59]

The atypical antipsychotics are distinguished from typical antipsychotics by their reduced tendency to produce extrapyramidal symptoms. Some data suggest that the pharmacologic action of the atypicals on serotonergic and possibly dopaminergic neurotransmitters systems accounts for the ability to inhibit aggression. The severity of symptoms and the presence of other disorders drive the intervention selected. Treatment should be implemented within the least restrictive environment. However, if symptoms become severe enough to pose a serious safety threat, some form of hospitalization is recommended.[33,59]

Atypical antipsychotics can be prescribed to help manage severe aggression in youth with depression.[13] Figure 17.3 shows a treatment algorithm for such intervention. However, it is recommended that the specific guidelines for aggression intervention should be consulted as well when doing so.[59,60]

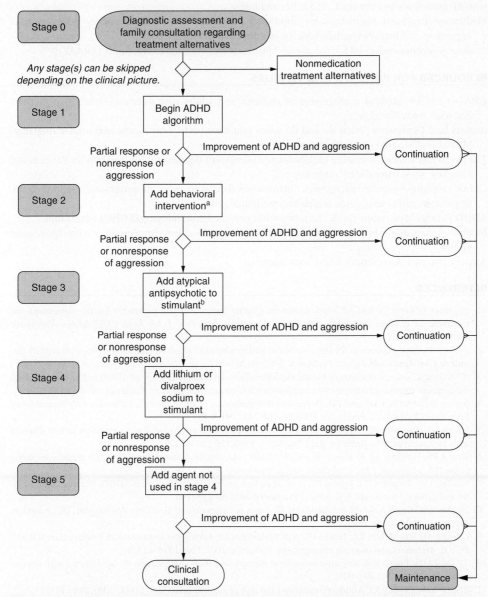

■ **Figure 17.3 Texas Childhood Medication Algorithm Project (CMAP) for depression with aggression.** (Reprinted from Pliszka, SR, Crismon ML, Hughes CW et al. Texas Children's Medication Algorithm Project: a revision of the algorithm for the pharmacotherapy of childhood attention-deficit/hyperactivity disorder. *J Am Acad Child Adolesc Psychiatry.* 2006;45:642–647, with permission from the Texas Department of State Health Services.)
[a]Evaluate adequacy of behavior treatment after inadequate response at any stage.
[b]If patient is an imminent threat to self or others, atypical antipsychotic may be started with behavioral treatment

The TRAAY guidelines do address the concern of how to manage aggressive symptoms in the context of depression along with other comorbid disorders. The two TRAAY articles provide important information on clinical management based on current clinical data and also regarding the potential misuse of antipsychotic agents for aggressive behavior. The importance of the recommendations is that they cross diagnostic boundaries and provide for a general approach to clinical management of aggression.

RESOURCES FOR PRACTITIONERS

AACAP guidelines (references 1, 2, 33, 61, and 62).

Medication treatment algorithms for childhood depression and ADHD, anxiety disorders, and aggression;[13,14] http://www.dshs.state.tx.us/mhprograms/cmappub.shtm.

Treatment recommendations for the use of Antipsychotics for Aggressive Youth (TRAAY)[59,60]

RESOURCES FOR PATIENTS AND FAMILIES

CHADD FACTS: Medical management of children and adults with attention-deficit hyperactivity disorder: www.chadd.org.

Anxiety and Depression: What do you do when you have both? http://www.adaa.org/GettingHelp? MFarchives/MontlyFeatures(september).asp.

The use of medication in treating childhood and adolescent depression: Information for Patients and Families: www.ParentsMedGuide.org.

CMAP website—psychoeducational: http://www.dshs.state.tx.us/mhprograms/cmappub.shtm; http://www.parentsmedguide.org/parentsmedguide.pdf.

ADHD Parents Medication Guide: http:/www.fda.gov/cder/drug/infopage/ADHD/default.htm.

Bipolar organization: http://www.ndmda.org/http://www.dbsalliance.org/site/PageServer?pagename =home.

Anxiety Disorder Association: http://www.adaa.org.

REFERENCES

1. Birmaher B, Brent D, AACAP Work Group on Quality Issues. Practice parameter for the assessment and treatment of children and adolescents with depressive disorders. *J Am Acad Child Adolesc Psychiatry.* 2007;46:1503–1526.
2. AACAP. Practice parameters for the assessment and treatment of children and adolescents with anxiety disorders. *J Am Acad Child Adolesc Psychiatry.* 2007;46:267–283.
3. MTA Group. National Institute of Mental Health Multimodal Treatment Study of ADHD follow-up: 24-month outcomes of treatment strategies for attention-deficit/hyperactivity disorder. *Pediatrics.* 2004;113:754–761.
4. Jensen JB, Burke N, Garfinkel BD. Depression and symptoms of attention deficit disorder with hyperactivity. *J Am Acad Child Adolesc Psychiatry.* 1988;27:742–747.
5. Jensen PS, Shervette RE, Xenakis SN, et al. Anxiety and depressive disorders in attention deficit disorder with hyperactivity: new findings. *Am J Psychiatry.* 1993;150:1203–1209.
6. Jensen PS, Hinshaw SP, Kraemer HC, et al. ADHD comorbidity findings from the MTA study: comparing comorbid subgroups. *J Am Acad Child Adolesc Psychiatry.* 2001;40:147–158.
7. Newcorn JH, Halperin JM, Jensen PS, et al. Symptom profiles in children with ADHD: effects of comorbidity and gender. *J Am Acad Child Adolesc Psychiatry.* 2001;40:137–146.
8. Hughes CW, Girgis A. *Child and Adolescent Measures of Diagnosis and Screening.* Washington, DC: American Psychiatric Publishing; 2008.
9. Cheung AH, Zuckerbrot RA, Jensen PS, et al. Guidelines for Adolescent Depression in Primary Care (GLAD-PC): II. Treatment and ongoing management. *Pediatrics.* 2007;120:e1314–e1326.
10. TEAM TADS. Fluoxetine, cognitive-behavioral therapy, and their combination for adolescents with depression. *JAMA.* 2005;292:807–820.
11. Jick H, Kaye JA, Jick SS. Antidepressants and the risk of suicidal behaviors. *JAMA.* 2004;292:338–343.
12. Pavuluri M, Birmaher B. A practical guide to using ratings of depression and anxiety in child psychiatric practice. *Curr Psychiatry Rep.* 2004;6:108–116.
13. Hughes CW, Emslie GJ, Crismon ML, et al. Texas Children's Medication Algorithm Project: update from Texas Consensus Conference Panel on Medication Treatment of Childhood Major Depressive Disorder. *J Am Acad Child Adolesc Psychiatry.* 2007;46:667–686.
14. Pliszka SR, Crismon ML, Hughes CW, et al. The Texas Children's Medication Algorithm Project: revision of the algorithm for pharmacotherapy of attention-deficit/hyperactivity disorder. *J Am Acad Child Adolesc Psychiatry.* 2006;45:642–657.

15. March JS, Biederman J, Wolkow R, et al. Sertraline in children and adolescents with obsessive-compulsive disorder. *JAMA*. 1998;280:1752–1756.
16. Birmaher B, Brent DA Work Group on Quality Issues. Practice parameters for the assessment and treatment of children and adolescents with depressive disorders. *J Am Acad Child Adolesc Psychiatry*. 1998;37:63S–83S.
17. Labellarte M, Ginsburg GS, Walkup J, et al. The treatment of anxiety disorders in children and adolescents. *Biol Psychiatry*. 1999;46:1567–1578.
18. Birmaher B, Axelson DA, Monk K, et al. Fluoxetine for the treatment of childhood anxiety disorder. *J Am Acad Child Adolesc Psychiatry*. 2003;42:415–423.
19. Walkup J, Labellarte M, Riddle MA, et al. Treatment of pediatric anxiety disorders: an open-label extension of the research units on pediatric psychopharmacology of anxiety study. *Adolesc Psychopharmacol*. 2002;12:175–188.
20. RUPP Group. Fluvoxamine for the treatment of anxiety disorders in children and adolescents. *N Engl J Med*. 2001;344:1279–1285.
21. Rynn MA, Siqueland L, Rickels K. Placebo-controlled trial of sertraline in the treatment of children with generalized anxiety disorder. *Am J Psychiatry*. 2001;158:2008–2014.
22. Wagner KD, Berard R, Sterin MB, et al. A multicenter, randomized, double-blind, placebo-controlled trial of paroxetine in children and adolescents with social anxiety disorder. *Arch Gen Psychiatry*. 2004;61:1153–1162.
23. Black B, Uhde TW. Treatment of elective mutism with fluoxetine: a double-blind, placebo-controlled study. *J Am Acad Child Adolesc Psychiatry*. 1994;33:1000–1006.
24. Greenhill LL. The use of psychotropic medication in preschoolers: indications, safety, and efficacy. *Can J Psychiatry*. 1998;43:576–580.
25. Riddle MA, Reeve EA, Yaryura-Tobia JA, et al. Fluvoxamine for children and adolescents with obsessive-compulsive disorder: a randomized, controlled, multicenter trial. *J Am Acad Child Adolesc Psychiatry*. 2001;40:222–229.
26. Riddle MA, Scahill L, King RA, et al. Double-blind, crossover trial of fluoxetine and placebo in children and adolescents with obsessive-compulsive disorder. *J Am Acad Child Adolesc Psychiatry*. 1992;31:1062–1069.
27. Renaud J, Birmaher B, Wassick SC, et al. Use of selective serotonin reuptake inhibitors for the treatment of childhood panic disorder. *J Am Acad Child Adolesc Psychiatry*. 1999;38:73–83.
28. Masi G, Toni C, Mucci M, et al. Paroxetine in child and adolescent outpatients with panic disorder. *J Child Adolesc Psychopharmacol*. 2001;11:151–157.
29. Hughes CW, Emslie GJ. *Treatment of Anxiety Disorders in Children and Adolescents*. Philadelphia: Williams and Wilkins; 1998.
30. Manassis K, Monga S. A therapeutic approach to children with adolescents with anxiety disorders and associated comorbid conditions. *J Am Acad Child Adolesc Psychiatry*. 2001;40:115–117.
31. Cartwright-Hatton HS, Roberts C, Chitsabesan P, et al. Systematic review of the efficacy of cognitive behavioral therapies for childhood and adolescent anxiety disorders. *Br J Clin Psychol*. 2004;43:421–436.
32. Compton SN, March JS, Brent DA, et al. Cognitive-behavioral psychotherapy for anxiety and depressive disorders in children and adolescents: an evidence-based medicine review. *J Am Acad Child Adolesc Psychiatry*. 2004;43:930–959.
33. AACAP. Practice parameter for the assessment and treatment of children and adolescents with attention-deficit/hyperactivity disorder. *J Am Acad Child Adolesc Psychiatry*. 2007;46:894–921.
34. Emslie GJ, Hughes CW, Crismon ML, et al. A feasibility study of the childhood depression medication algorithm: the Texas Children's Medication Algorithm Project (CMAP). *J Am Acad Child Adolesc Psychiatry*. 2004;43:1–9.
35. Daviss BW, Bentivoglio P, Racusin R, et al. Bupropion sustained release in adolescents with comorbid attention-deficit/hyperactivity disorder and depression. *J Am Acad Child Adolesc Psychiatry*. 2001;40:307–314.
36. Michelson D, Faries D, Wernicke J, et al. Atomoxetine in the treatment of children and adolescents with attention-deficit/hyperactivity disorder: a randomized, placebo-controlled, dose-response study. *Pediatrics*. 2001;108:1–9.
37. Michelson D, Allen AJ, Busner J, et al. Once-daily atomoxetine treatment for children and adolescents with attention deficit hyperactivity disorder: a randomized, placebo-controlled study. *Am J Psychiatry*. 2002;159:1896–1901.
38. Michelson D, Adler L, West SA, et al. Atomoxetine in adults with ADHD: two randomized, placebo-controlled studies. *Biol Psychiatry*. 2003;53:112–120.
39. Lopez MA, Toprac MG, Crismon ML, et al. A psychoeducational program for children with ADHD or depression and their families: results from the CMAP feasibility study. *Comm Ment Health J*. 2005;41:51–66.
40. Ghuman JK, Riddle MA, Vitiello B, et al. Comorbidity moderates response to methylphenidate in the Preschoolers with Attention-Deficit/Hyperactivity Disorder Treatment Study (PATS). *J Child Adolesc Psychopharmacol*. 2007;17:563–580.
41. Greenhill LL, Kollins SH, Abikoff HB. Efficacy and safety of immediate-release methylphenidate treatment for preschoolers with ADHD. *J Am Acad Child Adolesc Psychiatry*. 2006;45:1284–1293.

42. MTA. 14-month randomized clinical trial of treatment strategies for children with attention deficit hyperactivity disorder. *Arch Gen Psychiatry.* 1999;56:1073–1086.
43. Satterfield JH, Satterfield BT, Schell AM. Therapeutic interventions to prevent delinquency in hyperactive boys. *J Am Acad Child Adolesc Psychiatry.* 1987;26:56–64.
44. Tamm L, Swanson JM, Lerner MA, et al. Intervention for preschoolers at risk for attention-deficit/hyperactivity disorder (ADHD): service before diagnosis. *Clin Neurosci Res.* 2005;5:247–253.
45. Cunningham CE, Bremmer R, Secord M. *COPE: The Community Parent Education Program. A School-Based Family Systems Oriented Workshop for Parent of Children with Disruptive Behavior Disorders.* Hamilton, ON, Canada: COPE Works; 1997.
46. Kollins SH, Greenhill LL, Swanson JM. Rationale, design, and methods of the Preschool ADHD Treatment Study PATS. *J Am Acad Child Adolesc Psychiatry.* 2006;45:1275–1283.
47. Chronis AM, Chacko A, Fabiano GA, et al. Enhancements to the behavioral parent training paradigm for families of children with ADHD: review and future directions. *Clin Child Fam Psychol Rev.* 2004;7:1–27.
48. Sonuga-Burke EJ, Daley D, Thompson M. Does maternal ADHD reduce the effectiveness of parent training for preschool children's ADHD? *J Am Acad Child Adolesc Psychiatry.* 2002;41:696–702.
49. Kern L, DuPaul GJ, Robert J, et al. Multisetting assessment-based intervention for young children at risk for attention deficit hyperactivity disorder: initial effects on academic and behavioral functioning. *School Psychol Rev.* 2007;36:237–255.
50. Barkley RA. *Defiant Children: A Clinician's Manual for Assessment and Parent Training.* New York: Guilford Press; 1997.
51. Sonuga-Burke EJ, Thompson M, Daley D, et al. Parent training for attention deficit/hyperactivity disorder: is it as effective when delivered as routine rather than as specialist care? *Br J Clin Psychol.* 2004;43:449–457.
52. Young RC, Biggs JT, Ziegler VE, et al. A rating scale for mania: reliability, validity and sensitivity. *Br J Psychiatry.* 1978;133:429–433.
53. Yudofsky SC, Kopecky HJ, Kunik M, et al. The Overt Agitation Severity Scale for the Objective Rating of Agitation. *J Neuropsychiatry Clin Neurosci.* 1997;9:541–548.
54. Kowatch RA, Fristad M, Birmaher B, et al. Treatment guidelines for children and adolescents with bipolar disorder: child psychiatric workgroup on bipolar disorder. *J Am Acad Child Adolesc Psychiatry.* 2005;44: 213–235.
55. Pelham WE, Fabiano GA. Behavior modification. *Child Adolesc Psychiatr Clin N Am.* 2000;9:671–688.
56. Foxx RM. A comprehensive treatment program for inpatient adolescents. *Behav Intervent.* 1998;13:67–77.
57. Kazdin AE, Kendall PC. Current progress and future plans for developing effective treatments: comments and perspectives. *J Clin Child Psychol.* 1998;27:217–226.
58. Brestan EV, Eyber SM. Effective psychosocial treatments of conduct-disordered children and adolescents. *J Clin Child Psychol.* 1998;27:180–189.
59. Schur SB, Sikich L, Findling RL, et al. Treatment recommendations for the use of antipsychotics for aggressive youth (TRAAY). Part I. A review. *J Am Acad Child Adolesc Psychiatry.* 2003;42:132–144.
60. Pappadopulos E, Macintyre JC, Crismon ML, et al. Treatment recommendations for the use of antipsychotics for aggressive youth (TRAAY) II. *J Am Acad Child Adolesc Psychiatry.* 2003;42:145–161.
61. AACAP. Summary of the practice parameters for the assessment and treatment of children and adolescents with posttraumatic stress disorder. *J Am Acad Child Adolesc Psychiatry.* 1998;37:997–1001.
62. AACAP. Practice parameters for the assessment and treatment of children, adolescents, and adults with conduct disorder. *J Am Acad Child Adolesc Psychiatry.* 1997;36:122S–139S.

Managing Adolescents With Comorbid Depression and Substance Abuse

BENJAMIN I. GOLDSTEIN

KEY POINTS

Assessment and Monitoring

- Evaluate depression and other comorbidities as suggested in Chapters 3 and 17.
- Collect information from multiple sources, including the adolescent, parents, and school.
- Learn as much as possible about the adolescent's world (including family and peer influences), in an attempt to answer the question "Why does he or she continue to use?"
- Collect laboratory specimens such as urine drug screens (UDS) regularly. Know in advance whom you will tell, under what circumstances, and how you will use the information.
- Know when to refer.

Risk Behaviors

- Because of the increased risk posed by comorbid substance use disorders (SUDs), implement a safety plan at the first in-person contact with the adolescent, and maintain increased vigilance for suicidality during follow-up.
- Ascertain historical details regarding legal problems and history of violence, and maintain increased vigilance for violence and legal problems during follow-up.
- Provide or arrange for detailed education regarding safe-sex, sexually transmitted diseases (STDs), including HIV, and contraception.
- Help adolescents access appropriate resources, including condoms, oral contraception, pregnancy testing, and STD screening as indicated.
- Prioritize getting parents "on board" with these efforts.
- Educate the adolescent regarding the synergistic impact of depression and substance use on these risks.

Treatment

- Reframe "self-medication:" Drugs and alcohol are not acceptable "treatments" for depression.
- Deliver integrated rather than sequential treatment; don't wait for abstinence before starting antidepressant treatment.
- Antidepressants such as fluoxetine may be effective for reducing depressive symptoms, but their impact on substance use is likely to be modest.
- Medications to reduce substance use should be used judiciously; although little is known about these medications, untreated SUD confers significant health risks in its own right.
- Manual-based therapies should be considered; those focusing on family therapy, motivation-enhancement, and cognitive behavioral therapy (CBT) are publicly available.
- Significant family involvement in treatment should be sought, even if an option other than family therapy is selected.

Introduction

Findings from community samples suggest that the prevalence of mood disorders increases significantly with increasing substance use, from 5% of youth with no life-time substance use to approximately five times this rate among youth who use alcohol weekly or who use illicit substances even annually.[1] Similarly, depression is associated with increased risk of substance use. The prevalence of significant substance use among depressed adolescents in the community is 20% compared with 5% among nondepressed adolescents.[2] These disorders have a mutually exacerbating impact, both in terms of decreased treatment response and increased relapse and recurrence, and in terms of multiple hazardous consequences. For example, youth with comorbid depression and SUDs (i.e., abuse or dependence of alcohol or drugs) are at a markedly elevated risk of suicide and suicidal behaviors, legal difficulties, familial disruption, STDs and unplanned pregnancy, medication nonadherence, and academic difficulties.

Fortunately, recent years have seen a surge in research on this topic and there are now several evidence-based options for assessment, psychosocial interventions, and pharmacotherapy. Historically, clinicians treating youth with depression have often deferred antidepressant treatment when presented with an actively substance-using patient. The extant literature suggests that an integrated, parallel treatment process is optimal. The question remains, however, as to what practicing clinicians can do if they do not have specific training in addictions. Granted, there are certain circumstances in which specialized addiction services are warranted. For example, an adolescent who is using cocaine or heroin daily and who is not interested in engaging in treatment is probably not appropriate for a general psychiatry or depression clinic, or an adolescent medicine clinic for that matter. Indeed, a discussion of the management of intoxication or withdrawal syndromes is beyond the scope of this chapter. However, most depressed youth with comorbid SUD are not cocaine or heroin dependent. Most youth with SUD do not demonstrate the same level of physical health compromise that is frequently seen in adults. Most use cannabis or alcohol, and they tend to meet criteria for abuse or dependence more quickly and at lower frequencies and amounts of consumption than adults with SUD. What does this imply? A substantial proportion of youth with comorbid depression and SUD can be safely managed in clinical settings that do not specialize in SUD, provided certain modifications are made to incorporate a specific focus on SUD in assessment and treatment. The central aim of this chapter is to provide information regarding how to incorporate such an integrated perspective and to provide a starting point from which to acquire sufficient knowledge and confidence to maintain an integrated clinical practice.

ASSESSMENT AND MONITORING

The following section focuses specifically on substance use and SUD. See previous chapters for information regarding evaluation of depression (see Chapter 3) and of comorbidities other than SUD (see Chapter 17).

GATHER INFORMATION FROM MULTIPLE INFORMANTS

An important consideration in the assessment and monitoring of substance use among adolescents is to ascertain information from multiple sources. Information can be obtained from the adolescent via direct interview and self-report instruments. Collateral information should be obtained from parents or caregivers. School reports can be helpful because they may reflect inconsistency, repeated absences, and other behaviors that may raise suspicion of substance use. Mental status examination can help identify signs of acute intoxication or withdrawal. Finally, urine toxicology provides an invaluable source of objective information. Although adolescents do not always reliably report their substance use, adolescent self-report is an important source of information that can be maximized when confidentiality is maintained. Exercising an appropriate level of confidentiality during the assessment and treatment of SUD is part of the minimal standard of care.[3] Therefore, it is important to clarify with the parent and adolescent precisely what information the clinician is obliged to share with parents or others. Generally, breaches of confidentiality may be indicated when there is a threat to the health or safety of the adolescent or others. Parents are unaware of their adolescent's substance use approximately 50% of the time, and parent interview correctly identifies only about 25% of cases of adolescent SUD.[4] The yield from parent interview may depend on the age of the adolescent and degree of substance use. For example, parent reports may help identify substance *use* among early adolescents (12 to 13 years of age), whereas history of substance use can be ascertained directly for the vast majority of older adolescents. Parent reports for older adolescents may be more helpful in determining diagnoses of SUD.[4]

BECOME FAMILIAR WITH THE SYMPTOMS OF SUD

Whereas most clinicians who work with depressed adolescents can reel off the symptoms of depression from memory, the diagnostic criteria for SUD are often less familiar. It is relatively common to decide that an adolescent has a SUD based on a clinical *gestalt*. The drawback of using this approach is that it serves as a barrier to the systematic assessment of symptoms, particularly those that may not necessarily be brought to clinical attention spontaneously. The following are helpful mnemonics for the *DSM-IV* criteria for substance abuse and dependence:[5]

Substance dependence is ADDICTD:

- Activities are given up or reduced (criterion 6)
- Dependence, physical: tolerance (criterion 1)
- Dependence, physical: withdrawal (criterion 2)
- Intrapersonal (Internal) consequences, physical or psychological (criterion 7)
- Can't Cut down or Control use (criterion 4)
- Time-consuming (criterion 5)
- Duration or amount of use is greater than intended (criterion 3)

Substance abuse is WILD:

- Work, school, or home role obligation failures (criterion 1)
- Interpersonal or social consequences (criterion 4)
- Legal problems (criterion 3)
- Dangerous use (criterion 2)

WHAT ABOUT SUBTHRESHOLD SUBSTANCE USE?

The term "diagnostic orphans" has been used to describe adolescents who meet less than full criteria for substance dependence but yet do not meet criteria for substance abuse. The assessment and treatment of these adolescents follows the same principles as for those with full-threshold SUD.

WHAT ABOUT INFREQUENT SUBSTANCE USE OR EXPERIMENTATION?

Clinicians often wonder how much substance use is "normative" for adolescents with depression. Data from adults suggest that even moderate alcohol use may be associated with negative outcomes among people with depression.[6] Moreover, even infrequent use of substances among adolescents is associated with increased suicidality.[7] Depressed adolescents, and at times parents, argue that occasional drinking is normal and social. Treating clinicians are often loath to promote abstinence because of reluctance around limiting the adolescent's social circle or hedonic activities, particularly if the adolescent is not a so-called problem drinker. However, much like drinking during pregnancy, there is no known "safe" amount of substances for youth with depression. Given the alternatives that exist for socializing and relaxation, abstinence from all psychoactive substances is likely the safest treatment goal.

FORMULATE BY GETTING THE DETAILS AND BECOMING AN EXPERT

It is important for the treating clinician to become an expert regarding adolescents' substance use:

- Are there particular internal triggers for use, such as boredom, sadness, anger, or anxiety?
- Are there external cues such as offers from others or lack of parental supervision?
- Do their peers smoke cigarettes? Drink? Use drugs?

- What strategies have helped in the past to diminish craving or avert use?
- What type of expectancies do they have regarding substance use?
- Where do they use, and with whom?
- What is their relationship with that person?
- How much do they typically use, and what is the most they will use?
- What is their substance of choice? Do they ever combine substances?
- Do they pay for it? If yes, with what money? If no, who provides it and why?
- What was going on at the time?
- Was it planned?
- What was their mood like before? After? Did any symptoms improve? Did any get worse? What about the next day?
- How did they function, sleep, take medication, converse, get along with family?
- Any cutting? Illegal behaviors? Unprotected sex?
- What are the positive and negative consequences of substance use according to the adolescent? What about the parent?
- Could the use have been prevented?

Clinicians should collect this information to formulate the adolescent's substance use as they would the adolescent's depression:

- What factors predispose the adolescent to substance use? Is there a family history of SUD?
- What precipitated substance use in general, and what are common precipitants for recurrent episodes of use?
- Are there perpetuating factors that make it difficult for the adolescent to abstain? Does a household member (parent, sibling) use substances? What about peers?
- What about protective factors that clinicians can draw on, such as interests in athletics or art, or prosocial activities or friendships that the adolescent has more recently neglected?

A comprehensive "assessment" of substance use can also have therapeutic value because it allows adolescents to see the objective association between all of these factors over time, and because it demonstrates to the adolescents that clinicians are interested in their overall health in a holistic way and want to know more about them as unique individuals rather than just another high-risk youth.

EVALUATE FOR BIPOLAR DISORDER AND OTHER COMORBIDITIES

Depression is commonly the presenting mood disturbance for youth with bipolar disorder. Therefore, as mentioned in Chapters 1 and 3, it is important to evaluate for family history of bipolar disorder as well as for previous symptoms or episodes of mania and hypomania in order to rule out bipolar disorder. More specific to this chapter is the fact that bipolar disorder carries the greatest risk of SUD of all axis I disorders, so the presence of SUD should increase the threshold of suspicion for bipolar disorder even further. This is important in light of the risk of treatment-emergent mania or cycle acceleration if antidepressants are used without mood stabilizers.

Comorbid conduct disorder is a potent risk factor for SUD also and should similarly raise the threshold of suspicion for SUD. Other comorbidities such as ADHD, anxiety disorders (particularly panic disorder), and eating disorders (particularly bulimia or binge-eating disorder), also raise the risk of SUD to varying degrees. Identification and management of these comorbidities, as outlined in Chapter 17, is of central importance because they perpetuate substance use if left untreated.

USE STANDARDIZED QUESTIONNAIRES

Many instruments may be used to assess and quantify substance use and SUD. The following are examples of instruments that are relatively straightforward and provide important information regarding quantity, frequency, and consequences of substance use. Some are used to screen for substance problems, and others are used to monitor changes in substance problems, but all can be helpful to the clinician by highlighting important domains to assess.

- *Adolescent Obsessive-Compulsive Drinking Scale* (A-OCDS):[8] The A-OCDS is a 14-item self-report instrument that examines the frequency of thoughts about drinking, efforts made to resist those thoughts, distress caused by the thoughts, and frequency and intensity of drinking. It changes with treatment and therefore can be used to monitor response, as well as in the prediction of relapse.

- *Alcohol Use Disorders Identification Test* (AUDIT):[9] The AUDIT is a 10-item multiple-choice questionnaire that measures alcohol consumption, drinking-related behavior, and alcohol-related problems. Items are scored from 0 to 4 for a maximum possible score of 40, and scores of ≥8 are highly suggestive of problematic alcohol consumption.
- *CRAFFT*:[10] CRAFFT is a mnemonic for a general screen for substance problems. A score of ≥2 on the CRAFFT is suggestive of problematic substance use.

Ask the adolescent the following questions:

Car: Have you ever ridden in a *Car* driven by someone who was "high" or had been using alcohol or drugs?
Relax: Do you ever use alcohol or drugs to *Relax*, feel better about yourself or fit in?
Alone: Do you ever use alcohol or drugs while you are by yourself, *Alone*?
Forget: Do you ever *Forget* things you did while using alcohol or drugs?
Friends: Do your *Family* or *Friends* ever tell you that you should cut down on your drinking or drug use?
Trouble: Have you ever gotten in *Trouble* while you were using alcohol or drugs?

- *Drug Use Screening Inventory* (DUSI):[11] The DUSI is a self-administered questionnaire that quantifies drug use, examines insight into the presence of substance problems, and assesses the severity of substance-related problems in multiple domains. The DUSI quantifies severity of involvement with drugs and alcohol and commonly-associated health, psychiatric, and psychosocial problems. Domains that are assessed include social, familial, academic, and recreational functioning. The DUSI yields severity scores for each domain, and for overall problems, reflecting severity of disturbance from 0% to 100%.
- *Timeline Follow-Back* (TLFB):[12] The TLFB is a standardized calendar-style method of obtaining information on day-to-day substance use. Adolescents are provided with "memory aid" prompts around important dates such as holidays and birthdays. Other techniques include asking about days of complete abstinence and days of heavy use, and establishing a range of use by employing an exaggeration technique to help the adolescent identify quantities of use. The TLFB may offer specific advantages when quantifying substance use among adolescents with depression. Using a calendar method linked to significant events affords an opportunity to examine the temporal association between negative life events and substance use. For example, depressed adolescents with SUD may find that cannabis use in fact precedes self-injurious behavior or suicide attempts, or that interpersonal difficulties often stem from drinking alcohol rather than alcohol being a self-medication for the distress associated with such difficulties. The degree to which this instrument can be therapeutic as well as quantitative depends in part on the extent of the details that are obtained regarding the precipitants and context of substance use.

COLLECT LABORATORY SPECIMENS

Among psychiatric illnesses, SUD offers the advantage of having objective biologic tests. Specimens include hair samples and urinary drug screens (UDS) (drugs), liver enzymes (alcohol), and exhaled carbon monoxide (cigarettes). However, many youth with SUD do not have the same pattern of use as adults, and they may suffer consequences of substance use at lower frequencies and amounts of consumption. Indeed, although markers such as carbohydrate-deficient transferrin (CDT) and gamma-glutamyltransferase (GGT) may be sufficiently sensitive and specific in the detection of heavy alcohol consumption among adults, they may be less helpful in identifying adolescents with alcohol dependence who often demonstrate patterns of intermittent binge drinking. Although CDT and GGT are not generally considered part of the standard of care for adolescent SUDs, it is important to monitor hepatotoxicity in youth with heavy or chronic alcohol consumption.

In contrast to CDT and GGT, a qualitative UDS is part of the minimal standard of care for SUD.[3] Current practice parameters state that toxicology "should be a routine part of the formal evaluation and ongoing assessment of substance use both during and after treatment." It is important to consider several factors in advance of obtaining a UDS:

- Has the adolescent knowingly consented to the UDS?
- Has the decision to request a UDS been unduly influenced by parental suspicion, or was it reached after taking into consideration the entire clinical picture?
- Who will be informed of the results?
- How will the process of reporting the results transpire? For example, will adolescents be given an opportunity to divulge their substance use prior to the results being reported?
- How will the information be used if the UDS is positive versus negative?

It is important to bear in mind that substances such as amphetamines, cocaine, and opiates are not likely to be detectable in urine after 1 to 4 days. Although cannabis is often considered detectable 3 to 4 weeks after the most recent use, this estimate can be shorter if use is infrequent and quantity is low. UDS remains an important tool because although a negative test does not always rule out cannabis use, false-positive tests are rare.

The availability of these laboratory tests does not obviate the need for careful screening via interview and self-report, but they are an important tool in the assessment and monitoring of substance use. Moreover, use of UDS increases the reliability of the adolescent's self-reported substance use, which can have therapeutic value in itself. One approach to requesting UDS is to tell adolescents that it is likely to be positive if they have used cannabis in the past month. If the adolescent endorses substance use, the clinician may not wish to obtain a UDS. Another common clinical and research practice is to consider a refused UDS as equivalent to a positive UDS. See the National Institute of Drug Abuse (NIDA) and Substance Abuse and Mental Health Services Administration (SAMHSA) websites, provided in the resources section, for further details regarding laboratory specimens. A specific link is provided to the NIDA monograph on UDS.

KNOW WHEN TO REFER

The American Academy of Child and Adolescent Psychiatry (AACAP) has outlined a level-of-care utilization system to help clinicians determine in a standardized way which patients can safely be managed as regular outpatients and which require higher levels of care.[13] Current practice parameters advise that adolescents with SUD should be treated in the least restrictive setting that is safe and effective.[3] Several factors influence the choice of treatment setting:

- Is the adolescent safe, and able to care for himself or herself?
- Is the adolescent and family motivated and willing to cooperate with treatment?
- Does the adolescent's need for structure and limit setting exceed that of the least restrictive environment?
- Are there psychiatric or medical comorbidities?
- Are different treatment settings available?
- Does the adolescent or family have a preference regarding a particular setting?
- Have attempts at treatment in less restrictive settings (lower levels of care) been unsatisfactory?

An example of an adolescent who would require a higher level of care or a more restrictive setting would be a patient with diabetes with polysubstance dependence who has few prosocial supports and has resisted efforts to engage in treatment for his substance use. An example of an adolescent who could be appropriately treated as an outpatient is a physically healthy patient with cannabis abuse whose family supports substance-focused treatment and who does not think she needs to quit but is willing to engage in treatment that focuses on her substance use. When in doubt about referral, it is best to seek an opinion from an addiction specialist.

RISK BEHAVIORS

SUICIDALITY

Suicidal behavior is a major concern in the treatment of depressed adolescents and discussed in detail in Chapter 15. Substance use is a major additional risk factor for suicidality.[14] Brent and colleagues found that whereas SUD alone confers a 3-fold increase in the risk of suicide, the combination of a mood disorder and SUD increased risk 17-fold.[15] Even among adolescents with a previous history of suicide attempt, SUDs are associated with a 3- to 4-fold greater risk of a repeat attempt.[16] Furthermore, the association between alcohol, drugs, and suicidality among adolescents may not be restricted to those with SUDs because even infrequent use of alcohol (≥ 6 times in past year) and drugs (≥ 1 time in past year) distinguishes adolescents with, versus without, a history of suicidal ideation and attempts.[7] In light of the fact that adolescents with depression and SUD are at exceedingly high risk of attempted and completed suicide, it is important to prioritize safety plans and other strategies (discussed in Chapter 15) at the earliest possible opportunity, generally at the time of first in-person contact with the patient.

VIOLENCE AND LEGAL PROBLEMS

Recent findings from the Great Smoky Mountains Study indicate that comorbid depression and SUD in childhood confers a 12.6-fold increased risk of severe or violent criminal offenses in adolescence/adulthood.[17] In comparison, depression alone and SUD alone increase risk 2.3-fold and 3.5-fold, respectively. Approximately 50% of incarcerated youth with depression have comorbid SUD.[18] In addition, legal problems themselves are a risk factor for suicide among youth. For these reasons it is important to collect a careful history of violence and legal problems. Most clinicians routinely screen for history of arrests or incarceration. In addition to these factors, clinicians should ask about any contacts with police—even those that do not result in arrest or those that were precipitated by peers' behavior. Similar to suicidality, clinicians should maintain increased vigilance regarding risk of violence toward others. This includes routinely asking about fights, destruction of property, or threats of violence.

SEXUAL RISK BEHAVIORS

Adolescents with comorbid depression and SUD are at markedly increased risk of unplanned pregnancy, dating violence, and STDs including HIV. SUDs and mood disorders are each associated with at least a twofold increase in the risk of premarital teenage parenthood.[19] Unplanned sex while intoxicated significantly predicts multiple sexual partners and inconsistent condom use among adolescents.[20] Depressive symptoms among boys are associated with increased risk of condom nonuse, and the association between depressive symptoms and STD may be mediated by substance use.[21] Comprehensive health care of these adolescents should therefore integrate assessment and management of sexual attitudes and behaviors.

Unfortunately, treatment of SUDs that does not integrate a specific focus on HIV risk behaviors has little impact on these behaviors.[22] Fortunately, even brief targeted interventions hold promise. Thurstone and colleagues examined the impact of a one-session HIV intervention on safe sex-related attitudes and behaviors among adolescents enrolled in a 16-session CBT intervention for SUD.[23] The intervention focused on three areas: (1) knowledge regarding HIV transmission, prevention, and treatment; (2) potential dangers having sex while intoxicated; and (3) information, thoughts, and behaviors related to condom use. Barriers to condom use are explored and addressed. Instances of condom use are queried to provide an opportunity for positive reinforcement. Finally, instances of unprotected sex are discussed to stimulate discussion around strategies to increase safe-sex practices including condom use. Participants demonstrated significantly improved knowledge regarding HIV and beliefs regarding condom use, and there was a trend toward improvement in the intention to carry condoms and in the actual obtaining of condoms. The importance of educating adolescents regarding safe sex is further underscored by recent findings that the salience of thoughts regarding preventing pregnancy and/or HIV/AIDS significantly predicts condom use among adolescents even in situations where they are using substances.[24]

In addition to addressing adolescents' knowledge and behavior, it is important to get parents "on board." Many adolescents refuse to tell their parents that they are sexually active for fear—whether reasonably or unreasonably—that their parents will be angry. Whereas condoms are readily available, it can be more challenging to obtain oral contraception without parents knowing. Therefore it should be a clinical imperative to help adolescents broach this topic with their parents in a way that balances the adolescent's autonomy with concerns about unplanned pregnancy. Because sexual activity in and of itself does not generally constitute grounds for breaching confidentiality, the adolescent usually has to be on board with getting her parents on board. Finally, because many adolescents will have already participated in high-risk behaviors, it is important to consider testing sexually active adolescents for pregnancy and for STDs.

TREATMENT

OVERALL GOALS

All the treatment principles discussed in the other chapters of this book apply to youth with SUD as well. In addition to the overarching goals when treating adolescents with depression in general, the following are specific goals when dealing with depressed adolescents with SUD:

1. *Reduce* the frequency and amount of the adolescent's *substance use.*
2. *Prevent* or minimize *negative outcomes* that are related to substance use, including medication nonadherence, legal difficulties, injuries, accidents, suicide attempts, negative sexual outcomes (unwanted pregnancy, STDs, sexual assault).
3. *Promote "substance-free" homes*, and facilitate the process of minimizing substance use in the family members of adolescents with depression.

REFRAME SUBSTANCE USE AS A HEALTH-COMPROMISING BEHAVIOR

A common obstacle in the treatment of adolescents with comorbid depression and SUD is the concept of *self-medication*, a frequent explanation for why adolescents use substances that has ample face validity. The thought is that the adolescent is using substances to calm anxiety, improve mood, help with sleep, or reduce irritability. There will be times when clinicians may be inclined to subscribe to the adolescent's view that using drugs or alcohol is helping *improve* symptoms and that reduced substance use will *worsen* symptoms. There is no doubt that alcohol does have short-term anxiety relieving, sedating, or mood-elevating properties, and some observe the same for cannabis. However, no evidence indicates that illicit substances or alcohol help these problems in the long run, and plenty of evidence exists that shows they worsen the course of depression. Moreover, substance use interferes with the treatment of depression, both by direct physiologic action (e.g., alcohol disrupts sleep architecture and impacts multiple neurotransmitter systems) and by decreased medication adherence. As clinicians, we need not take a stance against substance use in depression because of moral or religious beliefs or because we do not believe that substances temporarily alleviate aversive mood states. Rather, we should be against substance use by depressed adolescents because of the substantial evidence that substance use is associated with outcomes such as attempted and completed suicide, unplanned pregnancy, STDs, and legal problems, all of which leads us to conclude that the risk/benefit ratio of using substances as self-medication is unacceptably poor. For this reason it is critical to be reminded of the central and unequivocal goal of reducing—ideally eliminating—substance use.

PHARMACOLOGIC TREATMENT

Note: Many of the medications discussed are not approved by the Food and Drug Administration for use with adolescents and are thus "off-label." The following is a selective review of the current literature and does not comprise a formal recommendation or advice regarding treatment.

Until recently, it was common to defer pharmacologic treatment of depression until the patient had "taken care of" their substance problem, and this was in part because of studies showing that depression among adult alcoholics frequently resolved with a few weeks of detoxification. However, depression among adolescents with SUD usually precedes SUD, does not usually resolve with detoxification, decreases response to the treatment of SUD, and increases the risk of SUD relapse. Therefore, integrated parallel treatment of SUD and depression is the current standard of care.[3]

ANTIDEPRESSANTS AND LITHIUM

A meta-analysis regarding treatment of depression among adults with SUD analyzed data from 14 high-quality placebo-controlled trials that included 848 patients.[25] As a whole, these medications had a moderate effect size (0.38) in terms of depression. Although antidepressants may reduce the quantity of substance use, they yield low rates of abstinence. The authors concluded that antidepressants are "not a stand-alone treatment, and concurrent therapy directly targeting the addiction is also indicated." Several studies of antidepressants for SUD (including nicotine dependence) among youth have been conducted: Fluoxetine and bupropion are the best studied.

Fluoxetine

An open study of fluoxetine 20mg/day and supportive psychotherapy for 13 adolescents with major depression and alcohol use disorder showed reductions in both alcohol consumption and depression symptoms.[26] Subsequently, Riggs and colleagues randomized 126 adolescents with major depression, conduct disorder, and SUD to 16 weeks of either fluoxetine 20 mg/day or placebo, in addition to CBT.[27] Fluoxetine showed a significant and large advantage over placebo in terms of depression symptoms but not in terms of response determined by clinical global impression. Self-reported substance use decreased by an average of 4.31 days per month, and there was a significant decline in conduct disorder symptoms, however, there were no between-group differences on these factors. Surprisingly, the proportion of substance-free weekly UDS was greater in the placebo group than in the fluoxetine group. However, this study found an association between remission from depression and changes in substance use; participants whose depression had remitted, independent of treatment group, showed a greater proportion of negative urine screens and greater reduction in self-reported days of drug use in the past month. In contrast, there was no significant difference in reduction of conduct disorder symptoms among subjects who did or did not remit from depression. Of note, four participants in the fluoxetine group experienced treatment-emergent suicidality compared to one in the placebo group.

Not all the findings regarding fluoxetine are positive. Findling and colleagues randomized 18 adolescents to fluoxetine 10 mg/day and 16 to placebo.[28] The fluoxetine dose could be increased to 20 mg after 4 weeks if indicated. The study was stopped prematurely after interim analyses showed no significant between-group differences in any of the study outcomes, including rates of positive UDS, depressive symptoms, global illness severity, global improvement, or functioning. One participant in each group was discontinued because of suicidal ideation.

Bupropion

A small naturalistic study followed 14 adolescents with SUD, ADHD, and a mood disorder who were treated with bupropion SR started at 100 mg/day and titrated to a maximum of 400 mg/day.[29] The mean daily dose was 315 mg in divided doses. Significant reductions in symptoms were observed at 6-month follow-up: 39% reduction in Drug Use Screening Inventory scores, 43% reduction in ADHD symptoms, and 76% reduction in depression symptoms. Global severity of both SUD and depression decreased significantly as well. Thirteen of the 14 participants completed the 6-month follow-up, and no significant adverse events were noted.

Sertraline

A pilot placebo-controlled study of sertraline (N = 5) versus placebo (N = 5) added to group CBT found no significant between-group differences in either depression or drinking outcome measures.[30]

Lithium

Geller and colleagues examined the efficacy of lithium for 25 adolescent outpatients with bipolar disorder (N = 17) or major depression with predictors of future bipolarity (N = 8).[31] Participants were assigned to 6 weeks of treatment, with 4 weeks at maintenance lithium levels of 0.9 to 1.3 mEq/L, or to 6 weeks of placebo. Subjects receiving lithium were significantly more likely to have negative UDS. Children's Global Assessment Scale (CGAS) scores were significantly improved among subjects in the lithium group as compared with those in the placebo group. Using intent-to-treat analyses, 46% of the active treatment group and 8% of the placebo group met the categorical response criterion of CGAS ≥65. Lithium was well tolerated in this group; only polyuria and polydipsia were significantly more common in the active treatment group.

PHARMACOTHERAPY SPECIFIC TO SUBSTANCE ABUSE DISORDER

Opinions vary regarding the use of medication in the treatment of comorbid SUD among depressed adolescents. The following expert opinions about the use of medication such as naltrexone and disulfiram were rendered in a recent clinical case-conference article: "[T]here is insufficient evidence at this time to support use of these agents in the first-line treatment of alcohol use disorders in adolescents," and "this adolescent should be started on naltrexone."[32] Although differences in treatment strategies are common in medicine, they are especially prominent where there is a paucity of evidence, as is the case for SUD-specific pharmacotherapy among depressed adolescents. Unfortunately, many adolescents with SUD continue to have clinically significant substance use despite treatment with antidepressants, and it can be difficult to engage these adolescents in consistent psychosocial treatment. Therefore it is important to be aware of the evidence for anticraving and aversion treatments. It is also important to note that little is known about how adolescents with SUD tolerate and respond to these medications, and to date, no data are available regarding use of these agents for adolescents with comorbid depression and SUD. The AACAP practice parameters indicate that pharmacotherapy targeting craving and aversion is optional, is recommended for use in treatment-resistant SUD, and should be considered with caution, particularly among adolescents with psychiatric comorbidity such as depression.[3] For now, clinicians should consider the risk/benefit ratio for these medications on a case-by-case basis, taking into account factors such as comorbid medical illness, drug interactions, and patient reliability. Discussion of the management of acute intoxication, detoxification, or withdrawal is beyond the scope of this chapter.

Naltrexone

Naltrexone is an opiate antagonist approved by the FDA in the United States for the treatment of alcoholism in adults. It decreases the quantity and frequency of alcohol consumption and increases the time to relapse among adults with alcohol dependence. To date, only two case reports and an open-label pilot study have been reported for adolescents. Deas and colleagues treated five adolescent outpatients with alcohol dependence with naltrexone 50 mg/day.[33] Two participants experienced nausea, and their dose was reduced to 25 mg/day for 1 week. There was a significant reduction in drinks per drinking day that was observable within 1 week and in irresistibility, craving, and overall scores in the Adolescent Obsessive-Compulsive Drinking Scale. A larger-scale placebo-controlled study is underway.

Disulfiram

Disulfiram is an aversive agent, which results in a highly unpleasant reaction with the ingestion of even small amounts of alcohol; this reaction is caused by a buildup of acetaldehyde because of inhibition of its oxidation. In extreme cases, alcohol consumption in patients taking disulfiram can result in respiratory depression or cardiovascular collapse. In one study, 26 adolescents were randomized to treatment with disulfiram 200 mg/day or placebo for 90 days.[34] Continuous abstinence was significantly more common in the disulfiram group (54%) compared with the placebo group (15%), and mean cumulative duration of abstinence was significantly greater in the disulfiram group (69 days) compared with the placebo group (30 days). Specific data regarding side effects were not reported, however the authors noted that there were no between-group differences in side effects except for diarrhea.

Ondansetron

Ondansetron is a 5-HT3 antagonist that may be specifically effective for adults who experienced early onset of alcohol dependence. Dawes and colleagues conducted an 8-week open-label study of ondansetron (4μg/kg twice daily) in 12 adolescents with alcohol dependence.[35] There was a significant decrease in drinks per drinking day during treatment and a nonsignificant decrease in percentage of days abstinent (61% pretreatment versus 74% posttreatment). The most common side effect was somnolence (33%), which was of mild severity. The only other side effect experienced by more than one subject was change in appetite (17%). Adolescent Obsessive-Compulsive Drinking Scale irresistibility and total scores were significantly correlated with drinking indexes and decreased significantly during treatment.[36] Although not emphasized in these studies, it should be noted that participants also received weekly CBT with motivational enhancement delivered by postdoctoral-level therapists.

Acamprosate

Acamprosate is reported to inhibit GABA transmission and antagonize glutamatergic transmission, and it has shown promise in the treatment of alcohol dependence among adults. In one study, detoxified (≥5 days) adolescent inpatients with alcohol dependence were randomized to acamprosate (1332 mg/day; N = 13) or placebo (N = 13) for 90 days.[37] Continuous abstinence was significantly more common in the acamprosate group (54%) compared with the placebo group (15%), and mean cumulative duration of abstinence was significantly greater in the acamprosate group (80 days) compared with the placebo group (33 days). Specific data regarding side effects were not reported; however, the authors noted no between-group differences in side effects.

Benzodiazepines and Stimulants

The treatments reviewed thus far have minimal abuse potential. In contrast, benzodiazepines, often used in the treatment of insomnia or comorbid anxiety, have high abuse and diversion potential. In these situations, behavioral interventions or SSRIs are preferred. Similarly, the management of comorbid ADHD among youth with depression and SUD poses challenges. In this situation, nonstimulants such as atomoxetine or bupropion are considered the first-line options, followed by transdermal or extended-release stimulant formulations.[38] Other management strategies are outlined in Chapter 16.

PSYCHOSOCIAL INTERVENTIONS

In the past decade, considerable research has been conducted on psychosocial interventions for substance abuse, and several effective manual-based treatments are now available. Given the number of studies, it is beyond the scope of this chapter to review them in detail. Instead, this section describes the different modalities tested and presents findings from selected studies. Overlap in principles and techniques is the rule rather than the exception. Most studies include two or more of the following methods: family involvement, group sessions, psychoeducation, refusal skills, motivational enhancement, and contingency management. Therefore, it is difficult to say which of these techniques is the "active ingredient." An important finding from the 600-subject Cannabis Youth Treatment (CYT) study was that a five-session intervention combining CBT and motivational enhancement therapy fared no worse than a substantially more expensive and resource-heavy intervention that included 12-sessions of CBT and motivational enhancement therapy in addition to parent education sessions, case management, and home visits.[39] Indeed, each of the five interventions tested resulted in significant pre- and postimprovement in terms of number of days abstinent and percentage of adolescents in recovery. Taken together, the current literature suggests that psychosocial interventions are an important part of treatment for youth with depression and SUD. Although no single modality stands out in terms of efficacy, current practice parameters recommend that either family therapy or significant familial involvement in treatment should be part of the minimal standard of care for these youth.[3] One of the central benefits of the burgeoning research on this topic is that coherent comprehensive manuals are now publicly available from organizations such as NIDA and SAMHSA (links provided in the resources section).

FAMILY THERAPY

Psychosocial interventions that incorporate family therapy approaches have been the most widely and positively studied. In addition to research supporting the overall efficacy of family therapy, it appears that part of the impact of these interventions relates to improvement in family interactions.[40] Several types of family therapy have been evaluated, including multisystemic therapy, functional family therapy, and brief strategic family therapy. These therapies differ in the degree to which they incorporate cognitive behavioral, motivational, parent training, and social system perspectives. The family therapy evaluated in the CYT study was multidimensional family therapy, which focuses on competency building, reducing involvement with deviant peers, increasing prosocial activities, and improving skills related to affect regulation and problem solving. Parent-related goals include reducing distress and substance use, and bolstering social support and parenting skills. Multidimensional family therapy attempts to foster appropriate parental involvement in terms of supervision, organization, and emotional attachment, as well as addressing motivation and urges, risks and benefits of substance use, communication skills and problem-solving skills. Despite the lack of between-group differences in the CYT study, several previous studies had suggested that family therapy may be superior to other interventions for SUD.[40]

GROUP THERAPY

Group interventions are commonly used for adolescents with major depression, SUD, or both. Some have argued that there is an inherent risk of "deviancy training" in such groups, which predicts increased delinquency, substance use, and other antisocial outcomes. See articles that examine in depth the "pro"[41] and "con"[42] positions on this topic. Although discourse on this topic continues, so too does research that employs group therapy as one of the components of psychosocial treatment for youth. For example, studies of CBT (described later) often incorporate a group methodology. Similarly, three of the five interventions in the CYT study employed group components, and these interventions were neither better nor worse than the interventions that did not include such a component. Most therapist manuals include a discussion regarding techniques for managing and preventing troublesome participation, whether that takes the form of quiet protest or active disruption.

COGNITIVE BEHAVIORAL THERAPY

Several studies have examined CBT for adolescents with SUD, one on patients with comorbid major depression and SUD specifically.[43] In that study, following assessment of depression and SUD, therapists conducted a feedback and treatment contract interview with the adolescent and parents to review the results of the assessment and to set individualized goals. Adolescents entered "contracts" comprising an agreement to strive for abstinence from substances and to help other adolescents in the program to do the same. In addition, adolescents agreed to a no-suicide contract. Sessions consisted of twice weekly group therapy and weekly family therapy. Parents also attended monthly psychoeducational group meetings. UDS were collected before randomly selected group sessions. Finally, crisis intervention sessions or telephone contacts were completed on an as-needed basis. Several skills were targeted in the group sessions, including goal setting, problem solving, thinking about consequences, increasing pleasant activities, expressing emotions, learning to relax, responding assertively (e.g., substance refusal), recognizing and modifying automatic thoughts, learning facts regarding the prevalence and consequences of substance use, and relapse prevention. Family sessions focused on parental monitoring and application of appropriate consequences, and they offered the option of focusing on improved familial communication and problem solving, enhancing parent–adolescent attachment, increasing pleasant family activities, and modifying negative family beliefs. This study showed high retention and session attendance, as well as improvement in measures of substance use and mood.

Latimer and colleagues compared an integrated family and CBT treatment versus psychoeducation for adolescents with SUD and found that adolescents in the integrated treatment used significantly less alcohol and cannabis at follow-up.[44] The integrated treatment included 16 problem-focused family sessions and 32 group CBT sessions delivered twice weekly. The CBT sessions focused on identifying precipitating events for substance use, defining beliefs that mediate between these events and substance use, analyzing evidence for irrational beliefs, and generating alternative beliefs by way of homework assignments. This initial component attempted to establish an attitudinal or cognitive basis for abstinence. Subsequent sessions focused on problem identification, problem solving, and decision making. In addition to focusing on substance use, CBT skills were also applied to the prevention of STDs and toward maximizing protective factors such as prosocial activities and peer networks. Ten of the CBT sessions were dedicated to the development of learning strategies (e.g., test taking, note taking, essay writing), with the rationale that academic success is a central protective factor against substance use.

It is important to note that even group CBT that does not target substance use can effectively reduce depressive symptoms among depressed youth with SUD, albeit more slowly than among youth without SUD.[45] However, the impact of such treatments on severity of substance use has not been reported.

MOTIVATIONAL INTERVIEWING/ENHANCEMENT

Motivational interviewing (MI) principles are at the core of the motivational enhancement therapy intervention used in the CYT study. The strategies of MI are summarized in Table 5.1.[46] Even practitioners with limited experience in psychosocial interventions can glean important approaches and skills from MI. For example, a central technique in MI is to always ask permission, even if only to talk about a topic. For example: "Can we talk about how smoking pot might be affecting your mood?" as opposed to "I am really concerned that your pot smoking is interfering with your depression treatment." Another technique is ongoing assessment of readiness to change. Readiness to change, and therefore to move toward action, is influenced by two central factors: *importance* and *confidence*, each of which should be assessed separately. For example, "How important is it for you to decrease your drinking? How confident are you that you can cut back?" The interviewer should ask the patient to scale importance and confidence from 1 to 10. Follow-up questions elicit in a non-judgmental fashion the reasons for the patient not yet having successfully reduced his alcohol use and what conditions would lead to increased prioritization of change: "Why are you at 2 and not at 8? What would need to happen for you to get to 8?"

The process of information exchange is central in MI. The exchange should be a two-way process that encourages thoughtful participation from the adolescent but integrates psychoeducation simultaneously. For example, the therapist elicits the adolescent's thoughts: "Do you think your drinking might be putting you at risk?" The adolescent answers: "Not really, I mean, lots of my friends get wasted on weekends, it's just part of being a teenager." The therapist's response provides the adolescent with clear information, and the adolescent's perspective on this information is elicited: "Studies show that teens that have depression and use substances have a much higher risk of suicidality than those who don't use substances. How does knowing that affect your opinion? What does this mean for your future?" In deciding what information to provide, practitioners should ask adolescents what they know about substance use and what additional information they would most like to know about it. This style contrasts with the traditional unilateral information giving by simultaneously providing information and an assessment of the implications and importance of those facts.

CONCLUSION

The information and management principles reviewed in this chapter focus on the relatively common scenario of problematic substance use among adolescents with depression. Some of the information covered, such as use of fluoxetine or CBT, is familiar to most professionals working with depressed youth. In contrast, other principles, such as using UDS to corroborate the adolescent's self-report, may seem foreign. As professionals working in the field of mental health, we are accustomed to accepting subjective experience and self-report at face value, and many are initially reluctant to employ a strategy other than simply "trusting" the patient. In fact, we do trust adolescents even when we request UDS. We trust that they honestly believe that smoking pot makes them feel better. We trust that they really think they can manage without the birth control pill. We also trust parents when they tell us this is the adolescent's problem and that they feel blamed when we refer them for family therapy. We trust that adolescents and their families are using the best strategies they can think of to have their needs met. But we also trust statistics, and we know that part of our role as professionals is to ascertain objectively and carefully the risks faced by adolescents and help them minimize those risks, even if it means having to hold our ground against internal or external accusations of acting like police officers, even if it means repeatedly broaching delicate topics such as suicide, violence, and safe sex. It is incumbent on us to try to engage these sometimes resistant, often challenging, always rewarding patients. The first step toward engaging these adolescents is having the confidence that we have the knowledge and skills to help them. Ideally this chapter will provide an impetus toward attaining that confidence.

RESOURCES FOR PATIENTS AND FAMILIES

"NIDA for Teens": http://teens.drugabuse.gov/. This website is geared toward adolescents, parents, and teachers, and it includes peer-driven messages regarding the dangers of substance use.

Parent- and adolescent-friendly website with reliable information: www.abovetheinfluence.com. Part of a national youth antidrug media campaign by the Office of National Drug Control Policy.

RESOURCES FOR PROFESSIONALS

References 3, 23, 32, 38, 39, 43, and 46.

The following websites provide access to publicly available manuals, assessment tools, and general information. They are user friendly, and each provides multiple links to other resources and organizations.

www.nida.nih.gov: main website for NIDA.

www.samhsa.gov: main website for SAMHSA.

www.drugabuse.gov/pdf/monographs/73.pdf: NIDA monograph regarding urine drug screening.

www.fmhi.usf.edu/samhsa/: a directory of web-based training resources for mental health and substance abuse professionals working with children and adolescents.

http://kap.samhsa.gov/products/manuals/cyt/: manuals from the CYT can be downloaded from this website or by contacting the SAMHSA at 1-800-729-6686.

www.motivationalinterviewing.org: a good starting point for clinicians interested in developing their motivational interviewing skills.

http://www.who.int/substance_abuse/publications/alcohol/en/print.html: free access to AUDIT, the Alcohol Use Disorders Identification Test: Guidelines for Use in Primary Care, 2nd ed., 2001. There is also a version in Spanish.

REFERENCES

1. Kandel DB, Johnson JG, Bird HR, et al. Psychiatric disorders associated with substance use among children and adolescents: findings from the Methods for the Epidemiology of Child and Adolescent Mental Disorders (MECA) Study. *J Abnormal Child Psychol.* 1997;25:121–132.
2. Lewinsohn PM, Hops H, Roberts RE, et al. Adolescent psychopathology: I. Prevalence and incidence of depression and other DSM-III-R disorders in high school students. *J Abnorm Psychol.* 1993;102:133–144.
3. Bukstein OG, Bernet W, Arnold V, et al. Work Group on Quality I: Practice parameter for the assessment and treatment of children and adolescents with substance use disorders. *J Am Acad Child Adolesc Psychiatry.* 2005;44:609–621.
4. Fisher SL, Bucholz KK, Reich W, et al. Teenagers are right—parents do not know much: an analysis of adolescent-parent agreement on reports of adolescent substance use, abuse, and dependence. *Alcohol Clin Exp Res.* 2006;30:1699–1710.
5. Bogenschutz MP, Quinn DK. Acronyms for substance use disorders. *J Clin Psychiatry.* 2001;62:474–475.
6. Worthington J, Fava M, Agustin C, et al. Consumption of alcohol, nicotine, and caffeine among depressed outpatients. Relationship with response to treatment. *Psychosomatics.* 1996;37:518–522.
7. Wu P, Hoven CW, Liu X, et al. Substance use, suicidal ideation and attempts in children and adolescents. *Suicide Life Threat Behav.* 2004;34:408–420.
8. Deas D, Roberts JS, Randall CL, et al. Confirmatory analysis of the adolescent obsessive compulsive drinking scale (A-OCDS): a measure of "craving" and problem drinking in adolescents/young adults. *J Natl Med Assoc.* 2002;94:879–887.
9. Saunders JB, Aasland OG, Babor TF, et al. Development of the Alcohol Use Disorders Identification Test (AUDIT): WHO Collaborative Project on Early Detection of Persons with Harmful Alcohol Consumption—II. *Addiction.* 1993;88:791–804.
10. Knight JR, Sherritt L, Shrier LA, et al. Validity of the CRAFFT substance abuse screening test among adolescent clinic patients. *Arch Pediatr Adolesc Med.* 2002;156:607–614.
11. Tarter RE. Evaluation and treatment of adolescent substance abuse: a decision tree method. *Am J Drug Alcohol Abuse.* 1990;16:1–46.

12. Sobell L, Sobell M. Timeline follow-back: a technique for assessing self-reported alcohol consumption. In: Litten R, Allen J, eds. *Measuring Alcohol Consumption: Psychosocial and Biochemical Methods.* Totowa, NJ: Humana Press; 1992:41–72.

13. American Academy of Child and Adolescent Psychiatry. *Child and Adolescent Level of Care Utilization System (CALOCUS) for Psychiatric and Addiction Services.* Washington, DC: American Academy of Child and Adolescent Psychiatry; 2001.

14. Levy JC, Deykin EY. Suicidality, depression, and substance abuse in adolescence. *Am J Psychiatry.* 1989; 146:1462–1467.

15. Brent DA, Perper JA, Moritz G, et al. Psychiatric risk factors for adolescent suicide: a case-control study. *J Am Acad Child Adolesc Psychiatry.* 1993;32:521–529.

16.. Esposito-Smythers C, Spirito A. Adolescent substance use and suicidal behavior: a review with implications for treatment research. *Alcohol Clin Exper Res.* 2004;28(5 suppl):77S–88S.

17. Copeland WE, Miller-Johnson S, Keeler G, et al. Childhood psychiatric disorders and young adult crime: a prospective, population-based study. *Am J Psychiatry.* 2007;164:1668–1675.

18. Domalanta DD, Risser WL, Roberts RE, et al. Prevalence of depression and other psychiatric disorders among incarcerated youths. *J Am Acad Child Adolesc Psychiatry.* 2003;42:477–484.

19. Kessler RC, Berglund PA, Foster CL, et al. Social consequences of psychiatric disorders, II: Teenage parenthood. *Am J Psychiatry.* 1997;154:1405–1411.

20. Poulin C, Graham L. The association between substance use, unplanned sexual intercourse, and other sexual behaviours among adolescent students. *Addiction.* 2001;96:607–621.

21. Shrier LA, Harris SK, Sternberg M, et al. Associations of depression, self-esteem, and substance use with sexual risk among adolescents. *Prevent Med.* 2001;33:179–189.

22. Jainchill N, Yagelka J, Hawke J, et al. Adolescent admissions to residential drug treatment: HIV risk behaviors pre- and posttreatment. *Psychol Addict Behav.* 1999;13:163–173.

23. Thurstone C, Riggs PD, Klein C, et al. A one-session human immunodeficiency virus risk-reduction intervention in adolescents with psychiatric and substance use disorders. *J Am Acad Child Adolesc Psychiatry.* 2007;46:1179–1186.

24. Bailey SL, Gao W, Clark DB. Diary study of substance use and unsafe sex among adolescents with substance use disorders. *J Adolesc Health.* 2006;38:297.e13–297.e20.

25. Nunes EV, Levin FR. Treatment of depression in patients with alcohol or other drug dependence: a meta-analysis. *JAMA.* 2004;291:1887–1896.

26. Cornelius JR, Bukstein OG, Birmaher B, et al. Fluoxetine in adolescents with major depression and an alcohol use disorder: an open-label trial. *Addict Behav.* 2001;26:735–739.

27. Riggs PD, Mikulich-Gilbertson SK, Davies RD, et al. A randomized controlled trial of fluoxetine and cognitive behavioral therapy in adolescents with major depression, behavior problems, and substance use disorders. *Arch Pediatr Adolesc Med.* 2007;161:1026–1034.

28. Findling RL, McNamara NK, Stansbrey RJ, et al. Fluoxetine versus placebo treatment of depression and co-morbid substance use. Annual meeting of the American Academy of Child and Adolescent Psychiatry, Boston, 2007.

29. Solhkhah R, Wilens TE, Daly J, et al. Bupropion SR for the treatment of substance-abusing outpatient adolescents with attention-deficit/hyperactivity disorder and mood disorders. *J Child Adolesc Psychopharmacol.* 2005;15:777–786.

30. Deas D, Randall CL, Roberts JS, et al. A double-blind, placebo-controlled trial of sertraline in depressed adolescent alcoholics: a pilot study. *Human Psychopharmacol.* 2000;15:461–469.

31. Geller B, Cooper TB, Sun K, et al. Double-blind and placebo-controlled study of lithium for adolescent bipolar disorders with secondary substance dependency. *J Am Acad Child Adolesc Psychiatry.* 1998;37:171–178.

32. Kratochvil CJ, Kazura A, Deas D, et al. Pharmacological management of a teen with significant alcohol use and depression. *J Am Acad Child Adolesc Psychiatry.* 2006;45:1011–1015.

33. Deas D, May MPHK, Randall C, et al. Naltrexone treatment of adolescent alcoholics: an open-label pilot study. *J Child Adolesc Psychopharmacol.* 2005;15:723–728.

34. Niederhofer H, Staffen W. Comparison of disulfiram and placebo in treatment of alcohol dependence of adolescents. *Drug Alcohol Rev.* 2003;22:295–297.

35. Dawes MA, Johnson BA, Ait-Daoud N, et al. A prospective, open-label trial of ondansetron in adolescents with alcohol dependence. *Addict Behav.* 2005;30:1077–1085.

36. Dawes MA, Johnson BA, Ma JZ, et al. Reductions in and relations between "craving" and drinking in a prospective, open-label trial of ondansetron in adolescents with alcohol dependence. *Addict Behav.* 2005; 30:1630–1637.

37. Niederhofer H, Staffen W. Acamprosate and its efficacy in treating alcohol dependent adolescents. *Eur Child Adolesc Psychiatry.* 2003;12:144–148.

38. Kratochvil CJ, Wilens TE, Upadhyaya H. Pharmacological management of a youth with ADHD, marijuana use, and mood symptoms. *J Am Acad Child Adolesc Psychiatry.* 2006;45:1138–1141.

39. Dennis M, Godley SH, Diamond G, et al. The Cannabis Youth Treatment (CYT) Study: main findings from two randomized trials. *J Subst Abuse Treat.* 2004;27:197–213.

40. Liddle HA. Family-based therapies for adolescent alcohol and drug use: research contributions and future research needs. *Addiction.* 2004;99(suppl 2):76–92.

41. Dishion TJ, McCord J, Poulin F. When interventions harm. Peer groups and problem behavior. *Am Psychol.* 1999;54:755–764.

42. Kaminer Y. Challenges and opportunities of group therapy for adolescent substance abuse: a critical review. *Addict Behav.* 2005;30:1765–1774.

43. Curry JF, Wells KC, Lochman JE, et al. Cognitive-behavioral intervention for depressed, substance-abusing adolescents: development and pilot testing. *J Am Acad Child Adolesc Psychiatry.* 2003;42:656–665.

44. Latimer WW, Winters KC, D'Zurilla T, et al. Integrated family and cognitive-behavioral therapy for adolescent substance abusers: a stage I efficacy study. *Drug Alcohol Depend.* 2003;71:303–317.

45. Rohde P, Clarke GN, Lewinsohn PM, et al. Impact of comorbidity on a cognitive-behavioral group treatment for adolescent depression. *J Am Acad Child Adolesc Psychiatry.* 2001;40:795–802.

46. Miller WR, Rollnick S. *Motivational Interviewing: Preparing People for Change.* 2nd ed. New York: Guilford Press; 2002.

Managing Adolescent Depression in Primary Care[a]

AMY H. CHEUNG AND RACHEL A. ZUCKERBROT

KEY POINTS

- Depression in children and adolescents frequently presents in the primary care setting.
- Very little research evidence is available to guide the identification and management of depression in children and adolescents in primary care settings. Clinical guidelines are mainly based on evidence extrapolated from child and adolescent depression research in other settings and on expert opinion.
- Regular surveillance for depressive symptoms in children and adolescents at high risk for depression is recommended and feasible in primary care settings.
- Several screening tools are available for use for free, including the Mood and Feelings Questionnaire, Columbia Depression Scale, and the Kutcher Adolescent Depression Scale.
- If a diagnosis of depression is suspected, the primary care professional should complete a full assessment and begin initial management (e.g., psychoeducation) even if a referral is to be made to mental health services.
- Safety planning regarding suicidality and self-harm is critical in all patients diagnosed with depression and should be done by the primary care professional.
- Patients with mild depression may be adequately managed with active monitoring and supportive counseling.
- Patients with moderate to severe depression should be treated with either medication or psychotherapy, or both, or referred for mental health services.
- Primary care professionals should continue to monitor patients with depression even if they have been referred for mental health services to ensure coordination of care.

Introduction

Adolescent depression is a disorder that commonly presents in primary care. Rates of depressive disorders in this setting have been estimated to be as high as 27%.[1] In many regions, primary care not only provides the first contact for adolescents with depression but, in underserviced areas, primary care professionals may be the only services available. Despite the large proportion of depressed adolescents who receive care from their primary care professionals, depression is often underidentified and inappropriately managed in primary care settings.[1]

Barriers to the identification and management of depression in teens involve issues related to the clinician, the parents, and the patients themselves. Clinicians cite as key barriers their lack of mental health training as well as inadequate mental health support. The symptoms of depression may also be a

[a]The authors have adapted this chapter from their contributions to a forthcoming book tentatively titled *Assessment and Treatment of Pediatric Depression: State of the Science; Best Practices* (Peter S. Jensen, MD, Amy Cheung, MD, Ruth Stein, MD, and Rachel A Zuckerbrot, MD, eds.), to be published by the Civic Research Institute. All rights reserved.

deterrent, with teens often presenting with irritability rather than sadness as a significant symptom. Furthermore, adolescents with depression may first present with somatic complaints such as headaches, stomachaches, and fatigue rather than the classic depressive symptoms (see Chapters 1 and 3).

Parents often do not know that their teens are depressed. Sometimes this is because they attribute the depressive symptoms to normal teenage angst. In addition, because depression is an internalizing disorder and teens do not often share their emotions with their parents, it is understandable that parents may often not be aware of depressive symptoms. Patients themselves may be resistant to sharing their emotions with their parents or primary care professionals because of stigma or lack of information about depressive symptoms. *Parent* in this chapter is used to mean parents, caregivers, and guardians.

SCREENING IN PRIMARY CARE SETTINGS

Teens do not usually announce they are depressed, even when asked general questions such as "how are you feeling?" To inquire about depressive symptoms (including suicidality), primary care professionals need to ask specifically about symptoms. Previous research demonstrates that inquiring about depression in a routine, systematic fashion, such as through the administration of a questionnaire, elicits more positive responses than asking those questions as part of a mnemonic-guided interview.[2] This is in keeping with studies showing that for personal information, such as sexual activity and substance abuse, teens tend to be more honest on a computer-based questionnaire than when asked in a face-to-face interview. A recent study conducted in large pediatric practices found that the incorporation of depression screening increased patient and parent satisfaction with the practice.[3] The study found that paper-based screens actually improved communication between the doctor and the patient, and the written responses helped the pediatrician focus the interview.

Although screening may be acceptable and feasible in primary care settings, little research supports the idea that screening on its own improves outcomes for adolescents with depression. Furthermore, there is still much debate about the comparative usefulness of universal screening (e.g., every teen presenting to a primary care setting would be screened) versus targeted screening of teens who are at high risk for depression.[2] The latter approach has generally been endorsed because of (1) the lack of research evidence to support universal screening, and (2) the cost of universal screening when the yield may be low. Therefore, targeted screening of teens at high risk of depression may be more reasonable in primary care settings.

Risk factors for depression were highlighted in previous chapters (e.g., Chapter 2) and include (1) family history of depression, (2) past history of sexual or physical abuse, (3) history of trauma or family conflict, (4) history of previous depressive symptoms, suicide attempts, or (5) history of other common comorbid illnesses such as anxiety disorders, attention deficit hyperactivity disorder (ADHD), substance use, and chronic medical conditions.

The implementation of a depression screen in primary care settings can be challenging; Table 19.1 summarizes the steps involved. The first stage is to convince office staff that depression screening is an important component of routine clinical care. This may be best accomplished through office meetings with the other providers to discuss the benefits of depression screening. Another point of meeting with the office staff is to get their help in designing a screening protocol that will work smoothly and efficiently. The input and expertise of office personnel can help design the most efficient system. Although it is helpful to pilot-test a screening procedure, it is also important not to pilot anything until as many of the problems are worked out in advance as possible.

TABLE 19.1 KEY PROCESSES FOR ESTABLISHING A SCREEN IN YOUR PRACTICE

1. Convince office staff that depression screening is an important part of routine care.
2. Establish the most efficient and acceptable way to incorporate screening into visits including (a) when screens will be handed out, (b) who will hand out the screens, (c) who will score the screens, and (d) who will be screened (e.g., high-risk youth only or every teen in a certain age range).
3. Choose method to notify parents and patients of the screening procedure.
4. Choose a screen (see Appendix 19.1 and Chapter 3 for examples).
5. Do a pilot run.

The staff will need to decide several issues. First, screening instruments should ideally be given to both parents and adolescents. However, this may not be feasible in primary care settings either because of staffing problems or because the teens may not present with their parents. In such situations, the adolescent alone should complete the screen. Ideally, primary care professionals should try to also obtain information from the family and other sources (e.g., teachers).

Second, the choice of the depression screen is critical. Unfortunately, not many well-tested screens for adolescents exist in the public domain. A depression screen should be chosen based on factors such as cost, length, ease of scoring, existence of translations into other languages, and acceptability to the adolescent and parent. In addition, instruments that ask specifically about suicide are very important with the adolescent population; not all screens include a suicide question. Perhaps the best validated screen in primary care settings is the Beck Depression Inventory (BDI).[4] However, it is not free. Furthermore, for younger patients or those with reading problems, the BDI may be too difficult. The Mood and Feelings Questionnaire (MFQ)[5] may be a better alternative: It is not copyrighted; it covers similar content to the BDI; unlike the BDI, it has a parent version; and it has been validated for children and adolescents. The Columbia Depression Screen (parent and child versions)[3] and the Kutcher Adolescent Depression Scale (KADS)[6] are free for use with permission (see Table 3.6). The KADS is included in Appendix 19.1.

Third, although screening at health maintenance visits fits in well with recommended guidelines, studies indicate that many cases are missed when psychosocial screening is not also done at the urgent-care visits. Depressed adolescents may not come for annual examinations but may present with headaches, stomachaches, or pelvic pain during urgent-care visits. Therefore, it may be necessary to conduct depression screens in teens during urgent-care visits.

Fourth, parents should be informed about what will be happening with their child at visits and told that practice screens do not interfere with the teen's confidentiality. Depending on the practice, primary care professionals may want to (1) mail letters to the parents when patients reach the age of screening to inform them about the process, (2) give letters when they arrive in the waiting room, or (3) post information in the waiting room. The adolescent will usually be best informed on the day of the appointment. A cover sheet attached to the screen outlining similar information to that contained in the parent letter usually works well. It is important to explain if and how the information will be shared with the teen's parent. It is also critical to encourage honesty.

Finally, which office staff member presents the screen to eligible adolescents also needs to be determined based on the structure of each practice. In some practices, the receptionist can hand out the screens and pertinent information sheets. However, this process will not work if the receptionist does not know which teens are eligible. The screens may also be administered by nurses or medical technicians who normally weigh the child or take vital signs. This allows a person more knowledgeable about the patient to hand out the screen. In addition, this may give the child the opportunity to complete the screen in the examination room, more private than the waiting room. In computerized offices, parents and adolescents may complete the screens either online before their visit, at kiosks in the waiting room, or on computer tablets. In addition to providing the screen, an office staff must also score the screen (unless a computer program does it). In most practices, this is generally done by the staff who handed out the screen. Many offices prefer primary care professionals to do the scoring because this enables him or her to become aware of which questions were positive and not merely glance at a total score. In fact, screens may be most useful to clinicians because they provide information that can focus their interview. The screen may be incorporated into the interview and thus give the primary care professional the opportunity to probe regarding positive answers and comment or affirm the negative responses. The best way to use screens is as a starting point to open up the topic and to follow up when the screens suggest that follow-up is needed. However, many clinicians feel uncomfortable with behavioral health issues and prefer to use the screens in a more algorithmic manner. In that case, cutoff scores must be chosen and are generally available for well-validated screens such as the MFQ, KADS, and the Columbia Depression Screen. That is, follow-up or referral will be needed when a certain score is reached.

ESTABLISHING PROCEDURES FOR A SUICIDAL ADOLESCENT

If screening is successful, primary care professionals are very likely to identify suicidal adolescents. Therefore, it is important for each practice to have developed emergency procedures to deal with these situations. This includes understanding what legal obligations (based on your local laws) are in effect to inform the parents and the authorities, resources that are available in the community to handle such crises (e.g., local emergency department, crisis services), and safety planning with the adolescent and, if appropriate, with parents. Appendix 19.2 presents a sample of safety measures that can be taken to minimize risk. Appendix 19.3 shows a handout about suicide for parents and adolescents.

ASSESSMENT AND DIAGNOSIS

Once the primary care professional recognizes a teen may be depressed either through the use of a screen or based on chief complaint, follow-up is a critical next step. It is important to remember that a positive screen does not always necessitate referral or treatment but does always require follow-up. It must also be kept in mind that a positive screen may be related to mental health issues other than depression. In addition, a person who does not have a diagnosis of depression may still be at risk for suicide.

Assessment and diagnostic procedures in the primary care setting vary greatly based on the comfort, knowledge and skills of clinicians. Some clinicians choose to refer all youth with any suspicion of depression or suicidality, others make the diagnosis but refer for treatment, and still others follow mild cases but refer severe or complicated ones. In addition, many geographic areas do not have access to child and adolescent mental health services, so primary care professionals need to manage patients despite their trepidation. A detailed description of assessment is presented in Chapter 3. To avoid repetition, we only discuss in this section issues particularly relevant to assessment in primary care settings.

A critical component of the evaluation of depression is conducting two separate interviews: one with the adolescent and one with the parent. Primary care professionals who treat younger children are accustomed to asking questions with the parent and child together. When treating adolescents, it is preferable to interview the adolescent privately; however, it is also important to have private interview time for the parent. Parents can provide information to guide the primary care professional or to confirm the diagnosis. Even if parents do not know that their teen is depressed, they may give details about their child's functioning ("he is up all night" or "she quit the team"). It needs to be kept in mind also that parents may fear their teen's wrath if they reveal "embarrassing" events. Finally, they may be uncomfortable discussing their personal or family history of depression or other mental health issues in front of their teen, information that could be relevant to a complete assessment.

Evaluation for major depressive disorder (MDD) covers all alternative diagnoses (for an algorithm for diagnosis, see Figure 1.1). Adolescents who do not meet the full criteria of MDD may still be quite impaired and in need of help (see Chapters 1 and 3 for criteria for MDD and subtypes). The key symptoms of depression that primary care professionals should inquire about are sadness/irritability, loss of interest, increased guilt, low energy and concentration, appetite changes, psychomotor agitation/retardation, and suicidality (see also Figure 1.1). The primary care professional may also classify them as having mild, moderate, or severe depression. Table 3.3 can assist in defining the severity of a depressive episode. In general, patients with mild depression present with fewer depressive symptoms than those with moderate and severe depression and are less impaired in their functioning. Also, patients with comorbid illness, psychosis, or suicidality are considered to have moderate or severe depression regardless of the number of symptoms. A large proportion of patients in primary care settings present with mild depression.

Along with depressive symptoms, the primary care professional also needs to do a complete history, including past history of mental illness (e.g., previous depressions, treatments, trauma, and abuse history), past medical history, and family psychiatric history. Clinicians must remember that patients and families may not understand the information being elicited. Therefore, asking about "psychiatric history" should be avoided. Instead, the primary care professional should be specific about *history of depressive symptoms, anxiety or worries, other emotional problems, drug or alcohol problems, suicide, and hospitalizations* both in the patient and in the immediate and extended family. Because many mental illnesses are partially inherited, this information may help with the diagnosis. The family history may also be helpful for treatment planning. For example, if an adolescent's mother responded poorly to antidepressants, the patient may be reluctant to start medication as first-line treatment. Finally, the primary care professional should inquire about comorbid conditions such

TABLE 19.2 TIPS FOR ASSESSING SUICIDALITY IN PRIMARY CARE

- Remember that thoughts about death or dying is a common symptom of depression and that many teens think about suicide but far fewer have attempted or will attempt suicide.
- You need to ask direct questions to assess for suicide risk. Remember that talking about suicide does not promote suicide in your patients.
- Introduce the topic gradually:
  - Start with "Sometimes when teens feel sad or bad about themselves, they sometimes wish they were never born. Has that thought ever crossed your mind?"
  - If the response is positive, progress to ask if, given the difficulties they have been experiencing, they ever thought that they would be better off dead.
  - Again, if the response is positive, ask if patients have ever hurt themselves or attempted to kill themselves before, and if they have future plans to kill themselves.
- Keep in mind that depressed teens who are using substances like alcohol are at increased risk of self-harm.
- For teens who have attempted suicide previously or who have self-harmed (without a wish to die, such as cutting), you may notice scars or fresh wounds on your physical examination.

as attention deficit hyperactivity disorder and anxiety disorders. The presence of comorbid disorders may complicate the diagnosis and treatment. For example, an adolescent with depression and anxiety may be missing school because of low motivation from the depression and avoidance because of the anxiety disorder. Therefore, even if the depression improves with treatment, attendance may still be an issue if the anxiety disorder is not addressed.

Impairment must be present to make a diagnosis of a mental "disorder," including depression. Therefore, one must assess a patient's overall functioning in different areas including school (e.g., grades), home (e.g., conflict with family), and peers (e.g., spending time with friends). These questions may be helpful to evaluate functioning:

- School: "How is John doing in school? Have his grades changed lately?"
- Home: "How is life at home? Does your mood affect your relationships with your family?"
- Peers: "Do you have good friends with whom you can talk? Has your mood affected your ability to maintain your friendships?"

If clinicians are unable to perform a complete assessment, evaluation of the potentially depressed child must at least include a determination of risk of harm, either from self-inflicted injury or from impaired judgment. The primary care professional must therefore always assess for suicidal and homicidal ideation, self-injurious behavior, altered mental state, substance use, and access to firearms. Table 19.2 lists some tips to evaluate suicidality.

Finally, clinicians must assess for medical conditions that can mimic symptoms of depression, including mononucleosis and other viral conditions, malignancies, anemia, and hypothyroidism (see Table 1.4 for a more complete list). Many clinicians order thyroid function tests to rule out depression, but routine testing is not always considered necessary; rather, the standard of care dictates that clinicians assess for a thyroid disorder as part of their evaluation and choose laboratory tests as needed to help with that evaluation. A targeted physical examination, based on the history, is also important.

INITIAL MANAGEMENT

Whether primary care professionals decide to manage a depressed adolescent in their practice or refer for mental health support, patients and families alike expect some initial management. Sometimes this is done as a bridge before mental health services are available; other times, it may be the preference of the patient and family.

Initial management includes education for the patient and family about depression, including symptomatology and treatment options, and safety planning. Education is a critical part of initial management, especially given the stigma and lack of knowledge about mental illness in the general population. Many advocacy and professional groups have developed handouts for families that are easily accessible either by mail or through the Internet; some of these are listed in the resources section at the end of the chapter. Appendix 19.4 list topics about depression that can be discussed with families and patients, Appendix 19.5 lists frequently asked questions about the treatment of depression.

Safety planning is also a critical aspect of the initial management of all cases. Primary care professionals should formalize a procedure for their practices to (1) make plans to ensure the safety of adolescents at risk for suicide, and (2) provide information to patients and families regarding safety in the home (see Appendix 19.4).

MANAGEMENT OF MILD DEPRESSIVE SYMPTOMS

Definitions of severity of depressive episodes can be found in Chapter 3 (see Table 3.3). Based on the limited literature available and expert consensus,[7–10] mild depressive symptoms can be managed initially with active monitoring and support. The primary care professional may also provide regular counseling and support to the patient.

ACTIVE MONITORING

Immediate treatment of a new-onset mild to moderate depressive episode may not always be indicated.[7–10] *Active monitoring* might be a better option than *watchfully waiting* to see if depressed adolescents improve. *Active monitoring* emphasizes what primary care professionals can do before initiating psychotherapeutic or pharmacologic treatment, such as:

- Scheduling frequent visits
- Prescribing regular exercise and leisure activities
- Recommending a peer support group
- Reviewing self-management goals
- Following patients up via telephone
- Providing patients and families with educational materials (see Appendix 19.6).

Note that although active monitoring does not have to be continued indefinitely, it should be continued even after individuals improve. If the patient's depression fails to improve or worsens after a predetermined amount of time, an evidence-based treatment is indicated (see also Chapter 4).

MANAGEMENT OF MODERATE AND SEVERE DEPRESSION

TREATMENT WITH PSYCHOTHERAPY

With the ongoing controversy regarding the use of antidepressants in adolescent depression, there has been a renewed interest in the use of evidence-based psychotherapies. This interest is particularly relevant to primary care professionals because psychotherapy is frequently the treatment preferred by patients (and their families) with mild to moderate depression. These patients are also the most likely to present in primary care settings. A substantive evidence base is now available for the efficacy of some forms of psychotherapy, specifically cognitive behavioral therapy (CBT) (see Chapter 8) and interpersonal therapy for adolescents (IPT-A) (see Chapter 9), as well as for combined CBT and fluoxetine.[11] However, a substantial gap in knowledge and research evidence remains regarding the use of these therapies in primary care settings.[8,12,13]

A major factor in determining the type of treatment is patient and family preference. Research shows that patient expectations of treatment benefit are closely linked to positive treatment outcomes.[14,15] However, determining patient preference may not be straightforward. Table 19.3 highlights points for discussion when determining patient preference; these same points can be discussed with parents. Specific advantages of psychotherapy are as follows:

- Psychotherapy does not cause physiologic side effects.
- Psychotherapy should teach patients coping skills to help them deal more effectively with their current and future life situation, whereas medication therapy alone does not.

TABLE 19.3 KEY POINTS FOR DISCUSSION ON DETERMINING PATIENT PREFERENCE

1. Ask patients to describe how they view their illness.
2. Share your own view of their illness.
3. Identify key differences between these two views.
4. Explain alternative treatments, including costs and benefits and advantages and disadvantages in their particular situation.
   - Indications/contraindications they have for particular therapies
   - Number of visits required? (more with psychotherapy)
   - Providers used? (psychotherapist vs. primary care physician and care manager)
   - Costs and side effects of medications
   - Restrictions imposed by insurance plan
5. Review the key points of your discussion, especially information on alternative treatments.
6. After reviewing the options, ask patients to identify the treatment they prefer.

Reproduced from Asarnow JR, Carlson G, Schuster M, et al. *Youth Partners in Care: Clinician Guide to Depression Assessment and Management Among Youth in Primary Care Settings.* Santa Monica, Calif: RAND; 1999 (adapted from Rubenstein LV, Unutzer J, Miranda J, et al. *Partners in Care: Clinician Guide to Depression Assessment and Management in Primary Care Settings.* Los Angeles, Calif.: UCLA School of Medicine; 1996). Copyright Youth Partners in Care, 1999.

- Many patients are looking for help with current real life problems, which is a major focus of therapy. To the extent that these problems are not caused entirely by the depression, they may not be susceptible to improve with "just a pill."
- Teaching patients the skills for coping with depression and life stresses may have more enduring benefits than medication alone, and accomplishing this may require psychotherapy (teaching coping skills is also useful for mild depression).[12]

Other factors also affect the choice of therapy during the acute phase of treatment. Table 19.4 presents a guide to help clinicians determine the optimal treatment. Critical issues that need to be assessed include the following:

- Severity of depression
- The presence of life stress
- Prior psychiatric history and prior history of treatment
- Comorbid conditions
- Logistic and geographic availability of treatment options
- The psychological mindedness of the patient
- Patient and family preference

TABLE 19.4 INDICATIONS FOR TYPES OF TREATMENT

Antidepressants	Psychotherapy
- Patient preference - Severe symptoms that are vegetative (sleeplessness, trouble concentrating, poor oral intake, constipation, psychomotor retardation, psychomotor agitation, disheveled appearance) - Prior history of multiple (>2) depressions - Family history of multiple depressions - Prior positive response to antidepressants - Not interested in thinking about problems - No response to 6–8 wk of psychotherapy - Unable to afford/get to regular sessions	- Patient preference - Severe life stress (e.g., significant psychological or social problems, functional disability problems that have causes other than depression itself) - Medications relatively contraindicated (pregnancy, breastfeeding, drug abuse, interactions with other medications) - Prior positive response to psychotherapy

Modified with permission from Asarnow JR, Carlson G, Schuster M, et al. *Youth Partners in Care: Clinician Guide to Depression Assessment and Management Among Youth in Primary Care Settings.* Santa Monica, Calif: RAND; 1999 (adapted from Rubenstein LV, Unutzer J, Miranda J, et al. *Partners in Care: Clinician Guide to Depression Assessment and Management in Primary Care Settings.* Los Angeles, Calif.: UCLA School of Medicine; 1996). Copyright Youth Partners in Care, 1999.

Once the primary care professional and the patient and family have agreed to psychotherapy treatment, there is the further step of deciding whether a patient would be more suited to CBT, IPT-A, or some other approach, taking into account that access to these therapies is likely to be limited. However, should the primary care professional have these options available, patient preference is a key factor. In general, CBT is more structured than IPT-A and focuses on thought and behavioral patterns associated with depression, whereas IPT focuses on interpersonal relationships. Furthermore, cognitive impairments, including learning disabilities, low IQ, and poor motivation, may significantly affect an adolescent's ability to benefit from CBT.

LOCATING APPROPRIATE RESOURCES IN THE COMMUNITY

Primary care professionals caring for depressed adolescents often rely on mental health providers in their local communities to deliver psychotherapy. How does a primary care professional determine which therapist is the most appropriate? A competent provider should not only be familiar with evidence-based therapies but also be adept at working with adolescents and their families. Regardless of the type of therapy, the fit between adolescent and therapist is critical; the adolescent should feel comfortable and motivated to work with the therapist. Other therapies often offered to address depressive symptoms include the following:

- Supportive therapy
- Counseling
- Family therapy (see Chapter 10)
- Psychodynamic psychotherapy (see Chapter 11)
- Eclectic (mixture of any of the modalities just listed along with CBT or IPT principles)

Although these therapies may yield benefits for some youth, they have not been evaluated in a vigorous scientific manner at this point. This is in contrast to CBT and IPT-A where evidence supports their value as stand-alone treatments for adolescents with mild to moderate depression.

After locating an appropriate therapist, a referral can be made. At that time, the primary care professional should obtain consent from the patient and family to ensure open communication between the mental health and primary care clinicians. Primary care professionals should also schedule follow-up appointments with the adolescent to ascertain whether the adolescent has linked successfully to the therapy, has been attending regularly, and whether the therapy is helpful. If not, the primary care professional should assess and address possible barriers to therapy attendance (e.g., stigma, transportation, level of motivation, time, parent burden, etc.). Motivational enhancement strategies and psychoeducation with the youth and family might be useful for facilitating this linkage. For some youth, school-based services may be preferable because of their easier accessibility. If depressive symptoms are not improving at the follow-up visit, primary care professionals should refer back to established treatment algorithms such as the GLAD PC (www.gladpc.org), Youth Partners in Care,[12] or Texas Medication Algorithms (see Figure 6.1) to determine the next treatment option. It is important to remember that most depressions resolve with time. If a youth fails to respond fully or partially to a course of treatment, mental health consultation should be considered to reevaluate the diagnosis, assess potential complicating factors, and identify the optimal next step in treatment.

TREATMENT WITH ANTIDEPRESSANTS

Detailed data on the pharmacology, effectiveness and unwanted effects of antidepressants are presented in Chapters 6 and 14. In brief, evaluation of antidepressants used to treat adult depression, such as the tricyclic antidepressants (TCAs), showed these medications to be no more efficacious in youth than placebo. Furthermore, they caused significant side effects in children and adolescents, such as cardiotoxicity, and there was a high risk of lethal overdose. With the introduction of selective serotonin reuptake inhibitors (SSRIs) in the 1990s—with a safer side-effect profile—the SSRIs began to be used to treat depressed adolescents. However, use of SSRIs in this population has come under scrutiny in recent years owing to concerns regarding their safety. In particular, the Food and Drug Administration (FDA) has issued black box warnings on all classes of antidepressants. Although clinical trial data suggest that adolescents treated with antidepressants are slightly more likely to experience suicidality compared with those on placebo, epidemiologic data suggest the use of antidepressants decreases the rate of completed suicide in youth. Therefore, antidepressants are likely to be beneficial to many and harmful to a few. The FDA warning is a reminder to patients, families, and providers to be vigilant about the possible adverse effects associated with these medications.[16]

In deciding whether to use medication, other factors also come into consideration. For example, availability and accessibility of practitioners to deliver psychotherapeutic treatments may be limited, or adolescents may not wish to participate in "talk therapy." It is important to obtain a family history of response to antidepressants because this may help in the selection of medication. Past suicidal ideation and behavior will impact on frequency of monitoring and may be an indication of the need to start medication sooner rather than later. It is of note that current suicidal behavior or high suicide risk requires emergency psychiatric assessment but is not an indication to begin outpatient pharmacotherapy. Antidepressant medication should be initiated in cases of severe depression, if the patient prefers medication, or if other treatment options are not available. In all cases, patients and families must agree to careful monitoring and follow-up. According to the 2004 FDA warning this should be at least weekly during the first month and biweekly thereafter, to monitor carefully for suicidality as well as other side effects such as akathisia, irritability, sleep disruption, increased agitation, and induction of mania or mixed states (http://www.fda.gov/cder/drug/antidepressants/default.htm). Face-to-face weekly follow-up may sometimes be difficult in primary care settings. In these cases, the parameters of the American Academy of Child and Adolescent Psychiatry (AACAP)[9] recommend that evaluations should be briefly carried out by telephone. It is of note that there are no data to suggest that the monitoring schedule proposed by the FDA or telephone calls have an impact on the risk of suicide.[9] In practice, the decision to treat should be based on a discussion of the risks and benefits, necessary for informed consent (see Chapter 4).

OTHER CONSIDERATIONS WHEN USING ANTIDEPRESSANT MEDICATIONS

SSRIs are generally well tolerated and have a relatively safe profile, although they may have drug interactions with both prescription and nonprescription medications (these issues are discussed in detail in Chapter 14). Thus it is critical for primary care professionals to know all the medications their patients are taking. In adolescents, a specific and detailed history must be taken. This can be problematic because some adolescents may not consider some medications or substances relevant to this history. Furthermore, teens may be concerned about disclosing drug use, particularly if the primary care professional cares for the whole family or parents accompany the adolescent to appointments.

ALCOHOL

Although there is no direct interaction between antidepressants and alcohol, there are issues of which primary care professionals should be aware. First, alcohol is a mood-depressant if used long term. Consuming alcohol while being treated with antidepressants is similar to putting out a fire and throwing gasoline on it. If a patient has only experienced depression while using alcohol long term, it will be difficult to ascertain benefit from treatment with antidepressants. Antidepressants can also decrease alcohol tolerance. Patients may notice that before starting treatment they did not feel the effects of alcohol as readily. In another words, a patient may feel intoxicated or pass out on smaller amounts of alcohol even if tolerance was higher before starting antidepressant medication. Alcohol can also interfere with the sleep cycle. Therefore, patients should be informed about this if they already have insomnia as a part of their depression. Chapter 18 provides information about managing depressed adolescents who abuse substances.

OVER-THE-COUNTER MEDICATIONS

In general, over-the-counter medications that cause sedation may increase this side effect of most antidepressants. The most common are sleep medications (e.g., Nytol), antiemetics such as Gravol, and antihistamines (e.g., Claritin, Benadryl). Antihistamines may also lead to increased risk of cardiac side effects when used with antidepressants. Certain cold medications can cause adverse effects when used in combination with antidepressants (see Chapter 14 and the Resources for Professionals section).

HERBAL REMEDIES

Any herbal remedies (discussed in Chapter 12) that increase serotonin in the brain may lead to an increased risk of serotonin syndrome. The most common is St. John's wort. Serotonin syndrome is rare, but clinicians should inform patients and their families about the signs and symptoms and that it can be severe enough to result in death. Patients with this syndrome may present with restlessness, tremor, diarrhea, agitation, anxiety, and confusion. As the syndrome progresses, it can lead to blood pressure changes, sweating, and dyspnea. Grapefruit or grapefruit juice can also influence the levels of specific antidepressants.

PRESCRIPTION MEDICATIONS

Once again, the risk of serotonin syndrome needs to be assessed when combining antidepressants with other prescription medications. An example is sumatriptan, used to treat migraine. Because sumatriptan is usually taken on an as-needed basis, it is common for adolescents to forget to mention this to the treating physician. Clinicians should be cautious when combining antidepressants. The most common interactions are with the following combinations: SSRI with another SSRI, SSRI with a monoamine oxidase inhibitor (MAOI), or SSRI with mirtazapine or venlafaxine.

SSRIs are nearly all metabolized in the liver via the cytochrome P450 (CYP) system (see Chapter 14). The SSRI can have an inhibitory effect on this system, causing changes in the blood levels of other drugs metabolized by the same system, as is the case with many psychiatric medications. Therefore, caution should be used when combining SSRIs with other psychiatric medications. An example is the risk of cardiac effects when combining tricyclic antidepressants with SSRIs. Finally, all antidepressants (with the exception of bupropion which has a greater risk) have a small risk of lowering the seizure threshold. Therefore, patients with a history of seizures should be advised accordingly.

STREET DRUGS

Although there are no specific interactions between commonly used street drugs and antidepressants, there are effects of drug use that can mimic symptoms of depression. For example, a common effect of marijuana use is amotivation. Clinicians need to be aware of the amount of marijuana use to better assess the impact of the depression on motivation and the ability to function academically. Other considerations include the use of stimulants or cocaine, which may mimic the symptoms of mania. In some cases, the effects of stimulants or cocaine use may be mistakenly attributed to treatment with antidepressants.

CONCLUSIONS

Adolescent depression commonly presents in the primary care setting. Although it is often difficult for primary care professionals to manage these cases successfully on their own, emerging evidence indicates that this is not only possible but also urgently needed to address the unmet mental health needs of adolescents. More importantly, a number of guides and tools are available to help primary care professionals to take on this task. Examples include the National Institute of Clinical Excellence Guidelines from the United Kingdom,[10] the AACAP parameters,[9] and the GLAD PC toolkit (see "Resources for Patients and Families" at end of chapter. All are available for use by primary care professionals via the Internet.

RESOURCES FOR PRACTITIONERS

Information on the management of adolescent depression in the primary care setting available from the Guidelines for Adolescent Depression in Primary Care (GLAD PC): www.gladpc.org.

Information on prescribing medications available from the Texas Medication Algorithm Project (TMAP): http://www.dshs.state.tx.us/mhprograms/mddpage.shtm.

American Academy of Child and Adolescent Psychiatry (AACAP) Practice Parameters on Depressive Disorders in Children and Adolescents available at http://www.aacap.org/galleries/PracticeParameters/InPress_2007_DepressiveDisorders.pdf.

Database of drug interactions mediated by cytochrome P450 maintained by Indiana University School of Medicine available at http://medicine.iupui.edu/flockhart/table.htm.

RESOURCES FOR PATIENTS AND FAMILIES

Families and patients can find information on depression and where to obtain support on the Depression and Bipolar Support Alliance website: http://www.dbsalliance.org/site/PageServer?pagename=home.

Patient and family guides on depression available from the Families for Depression Awareness website: http://www.familyaware.org/parentandteenguide.php.

Information on medications available from the Texas Medication Algorithm Project (TMAP): http://www.dshs.state.tx.us/mhprograms/CMAPmddED.shtm.

Information on adolescent depression in the primary care setting available from the Guidelines for Adolescent Depression in Primary Care (GLAD PC) website: www.gladpc.org.

Information on depression, medications, and suicide available from the American Academy of Child and Adolescent Psychiatry (AACAP) website (Facts for Families): http://www.aacap.org/cs/root/facts_for_families/facts_for_families.

REFERENCES

1. Kramer T, Garralda ME. Psychiatric disorders in adolescents in primary care. *Br J Psychiatry*. 1998;173:508–513.
2. Zuckerbrot RA, Jensen PS. Improving recognition of adolescent depression in primary care. *Arch Pediatr Adolesc Med*. 2006;160:694–704.
3. Zuckerbrot RA, Maxon L, Pagar D, et al. Adolescent depression screening in primary care: feasibility and acceptability. *Pediatrics*. 2007;119:101–108.
4. Beck AT, Steer RA. *Manual for the Beck Depression Inventory*. San Antonio, Tex: The Psychological Corporation; 1987.
5. Angold A, Costello EJ, Messer SC, et al. The development of a short questionnaire for use in epidemiological studies of depression in children and adolescents. *Int J Meth Psychiatr Res*. 1995;5:237–249.
6. Brooks SJ, Kutcher S. Diagnosis and measurement of adolescent depression: a review of commonly utilized instruments. *J Child Adolesc Psychopharmacol*. 2001;11:341–376.
7. Zuckerbrot RA, Cheung A, Jensen PS, et al. Guidelines for adolescent depression in primary care—GLAD PC—Part I. *Pediatrics*. 2007;120:e1299–e1312.
8. Cheung A, Zuckerbrot RA, Jensen PS, et al. Guidelines for adolescent depression in primary care—GLAD PC—Part II. *Pediatrics*. 2007;120:e1313–e1326.
9. Birmaher B, Brent D, AACAP Work Group on Quality Issues. Practice parameter for the assessment and treatment of children and adolescents with depressive disorders. *J Am Acad Child Adolesc Psychiatry*. 2007;46:1503–1526.
10. National Institute for Health and Clinical Excellence. *Depression in Children and Young People: Identification and Management in Primary, Community and Secondary Care*. National Clinical Practice Guideline No. 28. Leicester, UK: The British Psychological Society; 2005.
11. March J, Silva S, Petrycki S, et al. Fluoxetine, cognitive-behavioral therapy, and their combination for adolescents with depression: treatment for adolescents with depression study (TADS) randomized controlled trial. *JAMA*. 2004;292:807–820.
12. Asarnow JR, Jaycox LH, Duan N, et al. Effectiveness of a quality improvement intervention for adolescent depression in primary care clinics: a randomized controlled trial. *JAMA*. 2005;293:311–319.
13. Clarke G, Debar L, Lynch F, et al. A randomized effectiveness trial of brief cognitive-behavioral therapy for depressed adolescents receiving antidepressant medication. *J Am Acad Child Adolesc Psychiatry*. 2005;44:888–898.
14. Myers SS, Phillips RS, Davis RB, et al. Patient expectations as predictors of outcome in patients with acute low back pain. *J Gen Int Med*. 2008;23:148–153.
15. Aikens JE, Nease DE Jr, Nau DP, et al. Adherence to maintenance-phase antidepressant medication as a function of patient beliefs about medication. *Ann Fam Med*. 2005;3:23–30.
16. Cheung AH, Emslie GJ, Mayes TL. Review of the efficacy and safety of antidepressants in youth depression. *J Child Psychol Psychiatry*. 2005;46:735–754.

6-Item Kutcher Adolescent Depression Scale

6-ITEM Kutcher Adolescent Depression Scale: KADS

NAME :_____   DATE :_____

OVER THE LAST WEEK, HOW HAVE YOU BEEN "ON AVERAGE" OR "USUALLY"
REGARDING THE FOLLOWING:

1. Low mood, sadness, feeling blah or down, depressed, just can't be bothered.

    ☐   ☐   ☐   ☐
    0 – Hardly Ever   1 – Much of the time   2 – Most of the time   3 – All of the time

2. Feelings of worthlessness, hopelessness, letting people down, not being a good person.

    ☐   ☐   ☐   ☐
    0 – Hardly Ever   1 – Much of the time   2 – Most of the time   3 – All of the time

3. Feeling tired, feeling fatigued, low in energy, hard to get motivated, have to push to get things done, want to rest or lie down a lot.

    ☐   ☐   ☐   ☐
    0 – Hardly Ever   1 – Much of the time   2 – Most of the time   3 – All of the time

4. Feeling that life is not very much fun, not feeling good when usually (before getting sick) would feel good, not getting as much pleasure from fun things as usual (before getting sick).

    ☐   ☐   ☐   ☐
    0 – Hardly Ever   1 – Much of the time   2 – Most of the time   3 – All of the time

5. Feeling worried, nervous, panicky, tense, keyed up, anxious.

    ☐   ☐   ☐   ☐
    0 – Hardly Ever   1 – Much of the time   2 – Most of the time   3 – All of the time

6. Thoughts, plans, or actions about suicide or self-harm.

    ☐   ☐   ☐   ☐
    0 – Hardly Ever   1 – Much of the time   2 – Most of the time   3 – All of the time

SCORE TOTAL : _____

6-item KADS scoring:
Each item should be scored as 0, 1, 2, or 3. Add all 6 item scores to form a single Total Score.

Interpretation of total scores:
Total scores at or above 6 suggest "possible depression" (and a need for more thorough assessment). Total scores below 6 indicate is "probable not depressed".

Reference: LeBlanc JC, Almudevar A, Brooks SJ, et al. Screening for adolescent depression: comparison of the Kutcher Adolescent Depression Scale with the Beck Depression Inventory. *J Child Adolesc Psychopharmacol.* 2002;2(2):113–126.

Self-report instruments commonly used to assess depression in adolescents have limited or unknown reliability and validity in this age group. We describe a new self-report scale, the Kutcher Adolescent Depression Scale (KADS), designed specifically to diagnose and assess the severity of adolescent depression. This report compares the diagnostic validity of the full 16-item instrument, brief versions of it, and the Beck Depression Inventory (BDI) against the criteria for major depressive episode (MDE) from the Mini International Neuropsychiatric Interview (MINI). Some 309 of 1,712 grade 7 to grade 12 students who completed the BDI had scores that exceeded 15. All were invited for further assessment, of whom 161 agreed to assessment by the KADS, the BDI again, and a MINI diagnostic interview for MDE. Receiver operating characteristic (ROC) curve analysis was used to determine which KADS items best identified subjects experiencing an MDE.

Further ROC curve analyses established that the overall diagnostic ability of a six-item subscale of the KADS was at least as good as that of the BDI and was better than that of the full-length KADS. Used with a cut-off score of 6, the six-item KADS achieved sensitivity and specificity rates of 92% and 71%, respectively—a combination not achieved by other self-report instruments. The six-item KADS may prove to be an efficient and effective means of ruling out MDE in adolescents.

Reprinted with permission from Brooks SJ, Kutcher S. Diagnosis and measurement of adolescent depression: A review of commonly utilized instruments. *J Child Adolesc Psychopharmacol.* 2001;11:341–376. Also available at http://www.cprf.ca/newsite/admin/uploads/docs/6KADS.pdf.

Ways to Help Prevent Suicide in Depressed Adolescents

1. *Encourage adolescents and parents to make their homes safe.* In teens ages 10 to 19, the most common method of suicide is by firearm, followed closely by suffocation (mostly hanging) and poisoning. All guns and other weapons should be removed from the house, or at least locked up. Other potentially harmful items such as ropes, cords, sharp knives, alcohol and other drugs, and poisons should also be removed.
2. *Ask about suicide.* Providers and parents should ask regularly about thoughts of suicide. Providers should remind parents that making these inquiries will not promote the idea of suicide.
3. *Watch for suicidal behavior.* Behaviors to watch for in children and teens include:
   - Expressing self-destructive thoughts
   - Drawing morbid or death-related pictures
   - Using death as a theme during play in young children
   - Listening to music that centers around death
   - Playing video games that have a self-destructive theme
   - Reading books or other publications that focus on death
   - Watching television programs that center around death
   - Visiting Internet sites that contain death-related content
   - Giving away possessions.
4. *Watch for signs of drinking.* If a child has depression, feels suicidal, and drinks a lot of alcohol, the person is more likely to take his or her life. Parents are usually unaware that their child is drinking. If your child is drinking, you need to discuss this with your child and the clinician.
5. *Develop a suicide emergency plan.* Work with patients and parents to decide how do proceed if a child feels suicidal. It is important to be specific and provide adolescents with accurate names, phone numbers, and addresses.

Adapted with permission from materials prepared by Families for Depression Awareness. www.familyaware.org

Example of Information Handout for Adolescents and Parents

Suicide: What Should I Know?

Why am I having these thoughts?

Many young people with depression think about hurting or killing themselves at some time. In fact, thoughts about death and dying are one of the symptoms of depression. Just like depression is treatable if you recognize it and get help, these feelings and thoughts can be treated and you can feel better. But it is up to you to let people know when you are feeling very depressed or out of control, and it is up to you to let people help you through this time.

What are the warning signs?

Learn to recognize your own warning signs. Everybody is different, and the things you notice when you begin to feel very depressed may be different from those other people report. Here is a list of some things that may signal a problem:

- Feeling very hopeless, like nothing will ever get better
- Not wanting to be around friends or family or take part in fun activities
- Not caring about anything anymore, like school or how you look
- Drinking or using drugs
- Doing risky things, such as driving recklessly or getting into fights
- Having lots of thoughts or dreams about death and dying
- Having a lot of stress or life changes that seem hard to handle
- Feeling like you have a little more energy than usual

What can I do?

If you feel like things are getting out of control, you need to let someone know. Talk to your parents, your doctor, teacher, counselor, or a good friend! Don't keep these feelings inside. There are things you can do to help yourself get through these tough times. Don't be afraid to ask others to help you do these things as well.

- Keep your doctor or counselor informed about symptoms. Get symptoms treated early before they become worse.
- Keep in regular contact with someone on your treatment team. Set up a weekly (or even daily) time to check in with them and let them know how you are doing.
- Do what you can to reduce stresses. Learn what stressors are likely to really bother you and try to manage those first.
- Avoid alcohol and drugs. They may make you feel better temporarily, but they will eventually make your depression and suicidal feelings worse.
- Let your parents have responsibility for giving you your medications and keeping all medications in a safe place.
- Develop a plan with others about what you will do if you feel suicidal. Carry phone numbers of people you can contact and who will stay with you until you are safe.
- Always try to find something to look forward to.

Suicide is a serious subject. Although it can be difficult, talking about it is an important step to getting better. By letting people know when you are thinking about death or hurting yourself, you can begin to get the help you need.

PEOPLE CAN AND DO GET BETTER!

What to Discuss with Adolescents and Parents about Depression

Etiology
- Depression probably results from an innate predisposition coupled with recent stressors.

Importance of Recognizing Symptoms
- Poor concentration, loss of pleasure in activities, and fatigue can affect school attendance and academic functioning.
- Being irritable, short-tempered, and hard to please (all of which may be the result of depression) make peer and family relationships more difficult.
- Feelings of worthlessness can affect self-confidence, which in turn can affect schoolwork, extracurricular activities, and self esteem.
- In the context of other depressive symptoms, aches and pains for which there are no medical causes may be explained.

Expected Course of Disorder
- Treated depression will likely result in return to regular functioning in weeks or months. Without treatment, depression may last many months or years and is likely to recur.

Risk of Suicide
- Depressed patients are at an increased risk for suicide. In order to minimize the risks of a suicide attempt, it is important for parents to remove firearms, razors, drugs, etc., from the house. It is also important to keep in mind that asking about suicidal thoughts is a crucial part of identifying a potentially dangerous plan. Asking about suicide may help prevent—not promote—suicide.

Treatment Options
- Be clear about which specific treatments you can offer and which will require referral elsewhere.

If cognitive behavioral therapy (CBT) is going to be used, discuss the following:

- The principle of CBT is that thoughts influence behaviors and feelings, and vice versa. Treatment targets patients' thoughts and behaviors to improve their mood.
- Essential elements of CBT include increasing pleasurable activities (behavioral activation), reducing negative thoughts (cognitive restructuring), and improving assertiveness and problem-solving skills to reduce feelings of helplessness.

If interpersonal therapy for adolescents (IPT-A) is going to be used, discuss the following:

- The principle of IPT-A is that interpersonal problems may cause or exacerbate depression and that depression, in turn, may exacerbate interpersonal problems. Treatment will target patients' interpersonal problems to improve both interpersonal functioning and their mood.
- Essential elements of IPT-A include identifying an interpersonal problem area, improving interpersonal problem-solving skills, and modifying communication patterns.
- IPT-A is for children aged 12 and older; there is no evidence of efficacy for children under 12.

If medication is going to be used, discuss the following:

- The medications we recommend (first-line treatments) are safe, and dangerous side effects are rare.
- Common side effects are GI disturbances, changes in appetite, sleep disturbance, and sexual dysfunction.
- If your child develops a rash, contact the doctor immediately.
- If your child becomes agitated, silly, speaks too fast, seems over-energetic, and does with less sleep, stop the medication and call the doctor immediately.
- It is important to supervise medication administration; if your child has threatened or attempted suicide, keep medication in a secure location.
- Likely duration of medication treatment (6 months to 1 year after symptoms improve and sometimes longer).
- Medication, usually a selective serotonin reuptake inhibitor (SSRI), should be initiated concurrent with therapy if your child has severe symptoms or functional impairment, or is at risk for suicide.
- Medication should be stopped gradually under doctor's supervision due to the possibility of withdrawal symptoms (e.g., recurrence of depression, drowsiness, nausea, lethargy, headache, dizziness).
- There are limited scientific data and extensive clinical data to show that medication treatment for depression in children and teens is safe and effective.

Adapted with permission from the *Columbia Treatment Guidelines. Depressive Disorders*. Version 2. New York: Columbia University, Department of Child and Adolescent Psychiatry; 2002.

Frequently Asked Questions About Treatment of Depression

Q: **How will I know if my treatment for depression is working?**

A: As people recover from depression, the first symptoms that usually improve are problems with sleeping and loss of appetite (or excessive appetite). After that, energy and interest in activities improve, as do the ability to think clearly and to function more productively. The last symptom to improve is the feeling of being depressed and discouraged, which can happen many weeks after treatment has begun. Although this same sequence of improvements may not be what everyone goes through, it is common.

You may be the last to recognize when the treatment is helping. Although others may see you getting better and while you may notice that you are able to function better, you may continue to feel depressed. This lingering feeling of depression may interfere with your ability to believe you are getting better, so it is important to stick with your treatment even when you have doubts about its effectiveness.

Q: **Is there a difference in the way medications and psychotherapy work in the treatment of depression?**

A: Psychotherapy is a series of private talks with a therapist where you discuss the feelings, thoughts and behavior that cause difficulty. The goal of psychotherapy is to help you understand and master your problems so you can function better. Psychotherapy can help with the symptoms of depression, such as feelings of guilt and worthlessness, sadness, anger, doubt and indecision. Depression often is related to experiences or problems you have in your relationships with important people such as family, lovers, and friends. Through psychotherapy, you can examine and improve these relationships, or grieve and move beyond those that have been lost.

Antidepressant medications also help treat the psychological symptoms of depression, such as guilt, hopelessness, and anxiety. They are particularly effective in treating the neurovegetative symptoms of depression. *Neurovegetative* is a medical term referring to the physical symptoms commonly seen in depression, such as the loss of appetite (or excessive appetite), difficulty concentrating, feeling very nervous, or being unable to sit still.

Q: **What do I do if I think the treatment I am receiving is not helping?**

A: First, compare your perception of how the treatment is working with others who see you regularly and whom you trust. As mentioned in a previous answer, you may not feel better even though you are getting better. If others agree that progress is not occurring, however, don't keep quiet about it. Talk to your psychiatrist, your primary care physician, or your therapist.

Open, direct communication is essential for treatment, and it needs to flow in both directions—from patient to doctor and vice versa. A good doctor will want to hear from you and will value your concerns. Anyone who dismisses what you say may not be worth working with.

Ask your doctor why progress is not occurring. Ask how else you might be helped. For example, are there other treatments that could be considered?

You should also feel free to ask your doctor for a second opinion about your treatment. This means you or your doctor ask another medical professional to review your care and make suggestions to improve it. Getting a second opinion is common in medical practice. It can offer a fresh perspective and the opportunity to change or enhance your treatment. In general, a doctor welcomes a second opinion, and if he or she doesn't, you may not be working with the right doctor.

Last and not least, don't give up. Depression is a very treatable illness. Although some people respond to treatment in a month or two, others take longer. The statistics are encouraging: As many as 85 percent of people respond to appropriate treatment.

Q: **Why do I need to keep taking antidepressant medications after I feel better?**
A: You've heard medical doctors say you need to continue taking an antibiotic for as many days as prescribed—even if you feel better sooner. The same is true for antidepressants, although you have to take them longer.

Antidepressant medications treat your symptoms, making you feel better, but the illness continues. The medication is needed to control the illness until full recovery is achieved. If this is your first episode of depression, don't be surprised if your doctor says you need to take the medicine for six to nine months after you start feeling better. This is how long it takes the medicine to protect you against the depressive illness, which continues to cause imbalances in your brain chemistry and nerve cells. For someone who has suffered from more than one episode of depression, medication and psychotherapy may be necessary for longer periods of time.

Studies have shown the combination of psychotherapy and medication often is more effective than either treatment alone.

Once you begin feeling better, your doctor will focus treatment on helping you avoid a relapse, which is why he or she asks you to continue taking the medication. However, if you and your doctor decide to stop the medication, studies have shown the importance of stopping gradually. Abrupt discontinuation of antidepressant medications can increase the risk of a relapse.

Adapted from http://www.medem.com/MedLB/article_detaillb.cfm?article_ID=ZZZEDCIU2KC&sub_cat=128.

Family Support Action Plan

What a Parent Can Do to Help Their Child/Adolescent?

Family Support is a vital component in your child/adolescent's recovery from depression. It makes you a more engaged participant in your child's health care and helps rebuild your child/adolescent's confidence and sense of accomplishment. However, it can also be extremely difficult—after all, when your child/adolescent is depressed, s/he probably doesn't feel like accomplishing anything at all!

To help with Family Support, set goals to help you focus on your child/adolescent's recovery and recognize your child/adolescent's progress. Find things that have helped your child/adolescent in the past—identify goals that are simple and realistic and match your child/adolescent's natural "style" and personality. Work on only one goal at a time.

Adherence to Treatment Plan

Following through on health advice can be difficult when your child/adolescent is down. Your child/adolescent's success will depend on the severity of his/her symptoms, the presence of other health conditions, and your child/adolescent's comfort level in accepting your support. However, your child/adolescent's chances for recovery are excellent if you understand how you and your family naturally prefer to deal with your child/adolescent's health problems. Knowing what barriers are present will help you develop realistic health goals for your child/adolescent. ***Example goals:*** Remember to give your child/adolescent his/her medications. Participate in counseling. Help your child/adolescent keep appointments.

MY GOAL: _____

Relationships. It may be tempting for your child/adolescent to avoid contact with people when s/he is depressed, or to "shut out" concerned family and friends. Yet fulfilling relationships will be a significant part of your child/adolescent's recovery and long-term mental health. Understanding your child/adolescent's natural relational style for asking for and accepting help should guide the design of your Family Support plan. ***Example goals:*** Encourage your child/adolescent to talk with a friend every day. Attend scheduled social functions. Schedule times to talk and "just be" with your child/adolescent.

MY GOAL: _____

Nutrition and Exercise. Often, people who are depressed don't eat a balanced diet or get enough physical exercise—which can make them feel worse. Help your child/adolescent set goals to ensure good nutrition and regular exercise. ***Example goals:*** Encourage your child/adolescent to drink plenty of water. Eat fruits and vegetables. Avoid alcohol. Take a walk once a day. Go for a bike ride.

MY GOAL: _____

Spirituality and Pleasurable Activities. If spirituality has been an important part of your child/adolescent's life in the past, you should help to include it in your child/adolescent's current routine as well. Also, even though s/he may not feel as motivated, or get the same amount of pleasure as s/he used to, help him/her commit to a fun activity each day. ***Example goals:*** Recall a happy event. Do a hobby. Listen to music. Attend community or cultural events. Meditate. Worship. Do fun family activities. Take your child/adolescent to a fun place s/he wants to go.

MY GOAL: _____

Adapted with permission from Intermountain Healthcare.

Prevention of Depression and Early Intervention With Subclinical Depression

JUDY GARBER[a]

KEY POINTS

- The goal of prevention is to decrease the likelihood of depressive symptoms and disorders from occurring.
- The goal of early intervention with subclinical levels of depressive symptoms is to reduce these symptoms and keep them from developing into a full depressive episode.
- Prevention programs can target all members of a population (universal), those at greater risk (selective), or those already showing subclinical levels of depressive symptoms (indicated).
- Targeted (selective and indicated) programs have larger effect sizes than universal programs.
- The effects of depression prevention programs are small to moderate.
- The most effective prevention programs focus on cognitive restructuring, social problem solving, interpersonal communication skills, coping, and assertiveness training.
- Prevention programs typically are conducted with groups of children or adolescents in school or clinic settings.
- Guiding principles for depression prevention programs include keep it simple, keep it interesting, and make it relevant.

INTRODUCTION

WHY FOCUS ON PREVENTION?

Depression has a chronic, episodic course marked by considerable social and academic impairment, substance use problems, tobacco use, high-risk sexual behavior, physical health problems, and increased risk of suicide.[1-4] These sequelae account for a substantial proportion of the health care costs incurred by children and adolescents, and they are a significant economic and social burden to society.[5-6] Particularly relevant to prevention is the fact that depression is quite recurrent. The majority of individuals with early-onset depressions experience another episode in their adult life,[7-8] and most cases of recurrent adult depression have their initial onset during adolescence.[9] Therefore, childhood and adolescence are particularly critical and opportune developmental windows during which to prevent the onset and recurrence of depressive disorders and associated problems.

As described in detail in earlier chapters in this volume, efficacious psychosocial and pharmacologic treatments for adolescent depression exist, but such approaches only help about 65% of those treated, and only about 25% of depressed youth ever receive treatment.[10-11] Thus, despite potential benefits to individuals, society ultimately will be better off if depression can be prevented in the first place.[12] Therefore, prevention of depression, particularly among high-risk youth, may be more cost effective and safe as well as less distressing for individuals than waiting for the condition to appear and then trying to treat a full depressive episode.

[a] Judy Garber was supported in part by a grant (R01 MH64735) and an Independent Research Scientist Development Award (K02 MH66249) from the National Institute of Mental Health.

DEFINITIONS OF PREVENTION

Historically, types of prevention were categorized as primary, secondary, or tertiary.[13] Reducing the incidence of new cases of disorder in individuals who have not had the disorder was *primary prevention*, reducing the duration and severity of symptoms was *secondary prevention* (i.e., treatment), and reducing the recurrence of the disorder and its associated impairment in those who have already had it was *tertiary prevention* (maintenance).

The Institute of Medicine (IOM)[14] found this distinction to be too broad and instead introduced the classification of prevention programs into *universal, selective,* and *indicated,* based on the population groups to whom the interventions are directed. *Universal preventive interventions* are administered to all members of a population and do not select participants based on risk. *Selective preventions* are given to subgroups of a population whose risk is deemed to be above average (e.g., offspring of depressed parents). *Indicated preventive interventions* are provided to individuals who have detectable, subthreshold levels of signs or symptoms of the disorder but who do not currently meet diagnostic criteria for the disorder. Thus indicated prevention may be considered early intervention for subclinical depression.

Some studies have included both selective (e.g., offspring of depressed parents; family conflict) and indicated (i.e., subsyndromal depressive symptoms) samples to identify a particularly high-risk group.[15–18] Cuijpers[19] suggested that high-risk samples are likely to have greater statistical power to detect a prevention effect because of the increased probability of finding disorder in the no intervention group. However, given the etiologic complexity of mood disorders, no single risk factor is likely to identify all individuals who will develop the disorder, and not all individuals who develop the condition will have that particular risk factor. Therefore, it might make sense to provide the intervention to individuals who have multiple risk factors, although the cost of screening to find such a sample may be prohibitive, and the results might not generalize. Offord et al. provided a more extensive discussion of the advantages and disadvantages of the different types of preventive interventions.[20]

A distinction has been made between prevention and treatment.[21] Whereas a *prevention effect* is when there is little or no increase in symptoms in the intervention group relative to controls, a *treatment effect* is when a greater reduction in symptoms is found in the intervention group compared with controls. Most studies of depression prevention programs actually have found treatment rather than prevention effects.[22]

Mrazek and Haggerty[14] argued that the term *prevention* should be reserved for "interventions that occur before the initial onset of a disorder" (p. 23) and not recurrence. Interventions that occur subsequent to a diagnosis of depression have been considered treatment rather than prevention.[23] This distinction may simply be semantic, although both theory and empirical research suggest that different processes may underlie first versus subsequent depressive episodes,[24–25] and therefore different types of interventions may be needed to prevent them.

Interventions can be conceptualized along a continuum from *primary* prevention of the first onset of symptoms and disorder in a universal sample, to preventing onset in *selective* at risk samples, to *indicated* prevention aimed at keeping subsyndromal states from becoming a full disorder, to *prevention of recurrence* of new episodes among individuals who already have had an episode, to *treatment* of individuals experiencing a current depressive episode that includes a relapse prevention component and maintenance.[14] For an extensive discussion of the prevention of relapse and recurrence of depression in youth, see Kennard and colleagues.[26]

Are the essences of the interventions at these different points along the continuum the same, but in different doses, frequencies, and intensities, or rather are fundamentally different approaches to prevention and treatment needed? Thus far, there has been a tendency to start with existing treatments that have been efficacious in reducing symptoms in currently depressed adolescents—for example, cognitive behavior therapy (CBT), interpersonal psychotherapy (ITP)—and then translating them into prevention programs. Although a logical approach, it may not be the most efficient or effective strategy. Basic cognitive processes such as state-dependent learning and transfer of training may influence whether knowledge learned during a nondepressed state will generalize to the more affectively charged depressed state. Moreover, adolescents' motivation to participate and learn depression prevention strategies when they are euthymic should be addressed early in the intervention. No matter what the content of a prevention program, any intervention with youth should be guided by a few basic principles: *Keep it simple, keep it interesting, and make it relevant.* These likely are the nonspecifics that are necessary although probably not sufficient.

CAN DEPRESSION BE PREVENTED?

Qualitative[21,23,27–28] and quantitative[22,29–30] reviews of studies testing interventions to prevent depression in children and adolescents have concluded that (1) some targeted (i.e., selective, indicated) depression prevention programs are efficacious; (2) the effects generally have been small to moderate; and (3) the effects tend not to endure. Most studies have measured change in depressive symptoms, which may be more accurately considered early intervention. Far fewer studies have prevented the subsequent occurrence of depressive disorders, and none has yet shown that the first onset of a mood disorder can be prevented.

The Society for Prevention Research (SPR) set forth an overlapping set of standards of evidence by which programs can be judged to be efficacious, effective, and appropriate for dissemination.[31] SPR's Standards Committee recognized that effective programs and policies are a subset of efficacious interventions, and interventions that are ready for dissemination are a subset of effective programs and policies. Table 20.1 outlines these criteria.

Table 20.2 summarizes the evidence of the efficacy of specific intervention programs aimed at preventing depression in youth. Six aspects of depression prevention programs in youth are summarized: (1) effect of the program assessed at postintervention, (2) effect of the program assessed at follow-up of at least 3 months' duration, (3) replication of the program in at least two studies and replication by an independent research group, (4) whether diagnoses of depressive disorders were assessed, (5) sample size greater than 100 participants, and (6) whether some form of adherence/fidelity was assessed.

Clearly the *Penn Prevention Program* (PPP)[17,32] has been tested most extensively with universal, selective, and indicated samples, has shown both short- and long-term significant effects, and has been replicated multiple times and by independent researchers. Most studies of PPP have assessed depressive symptoms, although a few have included evaluations of depressive disorders. Samples sizes have been generally adequate, and evidence of satisfactory fidelity has been demonstrated.

The second most replicated depression program is the *Coping with Depression Course* developed by Clarke and colleagues.[33] Short-term efficacy was found when tested in a universal sample, and both short- and long-term efficacy have been found in selective and indicated samples. Significant effects have been replicated by independent researchers, depressive diagnoses have been assessed, sample sizes have been generally adequate, and adherence to the program protocol has been found.

The *Resourceful Adolescent Program* (RAP)[34–35] has been tested in large universal samples, found to be efficacious both at postintervention and follow-up, replicated by independent researchers, and

TABLE 20.1 STANDARDS OF EVIDENCE AS SET FORTH BY THE SOCIETY FOR PREVENTION RESEARCH[31]

Intervention Type	Criteria
Efficacy	• Tested in at least two controlled trials, preferably by different investigators • Involved representative samples from defined populations • Used psychometrically sound measures • Methodologically sound design (e.g., randomization; adequate power) • Data analyzed with rigorous statistical approaches • Showed consistent positive effects (without serious iatrogenic effects) • Reported at least one significant long-term follow-up
Effectiveness	• Meets all standards for efficacious interventions • Has manuals, appropriate training, and technical support available to allow third parties to adopt and implement the intervention with fidelity • Evaluated under real-world conditions in studies that include sound measurement of the level of implementation and engagement of the target audience (in both the intervention and control conditions) • Indicated the practical importance of intervention outcome effects • Clearly demonstrated to whom intervention findings can be generalized
Dissemination	• Meets all standards for efficacious and effective interventions • Provides evidence of the ability to "go to scale" • Presents clear cost information • Includes monitoring and evaluation tools so adopting agencies can evaluate how well the intervention works in their settings

TABLE 20.2 OUTCOMES OF DEPRESSION PREVENTION PROGRAMS IN CHILDREN AND ADOLESCENTS

Prevention Type	Program	Efficacy Post-test	Efficacy Follow-up	Replicate	Clinical Diagnoses	Power (N > 100)	Assess Fidelity	Program Focus/ Comments
	Penn Prevention Program	+	+	++	+	+	+	**Cognitive-Behavioral (CB) & Social Problem-solving**
Universal	Cardemil et al. (82-83)	+	+		–	+	+	significant effect for Latino, but not African American youth
	Chaplin et al. (52)	+	•		–	+	+	girls-only vs. coed groups
	Pattison & Lynd-Stevenson (84)	–	+		–	–	–	cognitive then social component vs. social then cognitive
	Quayle et al. (85)	+	+		–	–	–	Australian girls
	Gillham et al. (86)	+	–		–	+	+	significant intervention effect for 2 of 3 schools
Selective	Seligman et al. (57)	+	+		+	+	–	college students
Indicated	Jaycox et al. (17)	+	+		–	+	–	first test of PPP
	Gillham et al. (32)	+	+		–	–	–	2-year follow-up of Jaycox et al. sample
	Gillham et al. (81)	+	+		+	+	+	in primary care, moderated by gender and intervention fidelity
	Gillham et al. (87)	–	+		–	–	–	parent component
	Roberts et al. (88-89)	–	–		–	+	+	Australian children
	Yu & Seligman, (18)	+	+		–	+	–	Chinese children
	Coping with Depression Course							**CB Program**
Universal	Clarke et al. (90)	–	–	++	–	+	(+)	3- or 5-session universal programs not effective
	Horowitz et al. (45)	+	–		–	+	–	8-session universal program effective at post- but not at 6-mos.
Indicated	Clarke et al. (53)	+	–		–	+	–	45 minute sessions 3/week for 15 weeks

(continued)

TABLE 20.2 OUTCOMES OF DEPRESSION PREVENTION PROGRAMS IN CHILDREN AND ADOLESCENTS (CONTINUED)

Prevention Type	Program	Efficacy Post-test	Efficacy Follow-up	Replicate	Clinical Diagnoses	Power (N > 100)	Assess Fidelity	Program Focus/ Comments
Selective/ Indicated	Clarke et al. (15)	+	+		+	–	+	14-15 sessions; significantly reduced depressive disorders in at-risk youth
	Garber et al. (16)	+	●		+	+	+	4-site replication of Clarke et al. 2001
Indicated	Burton et al. (91)	+	+	++	–	+	–	4 sessions; all females
	Resourceful Adolescent Program	+	+		–	+	+	**CB & Interpersonal components**
Universal	Harnett & Dadds, (92)	–	–		–	+	(+)	significant for students both high and low in baseline symptoms
	Merry et al. (34)	+	+		–	+	(+)	
	Shochet et al. (35)	+	+		–	+	+	+ Parent component
	Problem-Solving for Life	+	–	–	–	+	–	**CB + Problem-Solving delivered by teachers**
Universal	Spence et al. (36, 38)	+	–		+	+	(+)	short- but not long-term effect
Universal + Indicated	Sheffield et al. (37)	–	–		+	+	(+)	combined indicated + universal no better than either alone
Universal	**Lars & Lisa**	+	+	–	–			**CB + Social Component**
	Pössel et al. (40, 65)					+	+	effects differed as a function of baseline symptoms (CES-D)
Selective	**Family Psycho-Education**	–	–	+	+	+	+	**Education & Family Communication**
	Beardslee et al. (69, 93-94)							improved communication; no group differences on depressive symptoms
Selective	**Family Bereavement Program**	+	+	–	+	+	+	**Parenting; Coping**
	Sandler et al. (70-71)							Children whose parent died

(continued)

TABLE 20.2 OUTCOMES OF DEPRESSION PREVENTION PROGRAMS IN CHILDREN AND ADOLESCENTS (CONTINUED)

Prevention Type	Program	Efficacy Post-test	Efficacy Follow-up	Replicate	Clinical Diagnoses	Power (N > 100)	Assess Fidelity	Program Focus/ Comments
Selective	*New Beginnings (divorce)* Wolchik et al. (73-75)	+	−	+	−	+	+	**Parenting; Coping** reduced internalizing in those with low mother-child relationship quality
Selective	*Educational Support Group* Gwynn & Brantley (72)	+	−	−	−	−	−	**Support** Children of divorce
Universal	*Interpersonal Psychotherapy, Adolescent Skills Training* Horowitz et al. (45)	+	+	+	+	+	−	**Interpersonal Communication** school-based IPT-AST vs. CBT vs. no intervention controls
Indicated	Young et al. (46)	+	+	−	+	−	−	sample mostly Hispanic females
Indicated	*Interpersonal Psychotherapy* Forsyth (66)	+	+	−	−	−	−	**Interpersonal** mostly female college students
Indicated	*Brief Cognitive-Behavioral* Stice et al. (44)	+	−	−	−	+	−	**CB** vs. waitlist, supportive-expressive, bibliotherapy, expressive writing, journaling
Indicated	*Cognitive-Behavioral* Peden et al. (43)	+	+	−	−	−	−	**CB** female college students
Selective	*Cognitive-Behavioral* Hyun et al. (41)	+	−	−	−	−	−	**CB** homeless, run away youth in a shelter; Korea
Universal	*Penn State Adolescent Study* Petersen et al. 1997 (39)	+	−	−	−	+	−	**Coping** Improved coping; significant effect for depressive sxs at post-test
Indicated	*Coping Skills* Lamb et al. (42)	+	−	−	−	−	−	**Coping** Coping skills rural high school students

(continued)

TABLE 20.2 OUTCOMES OF DEPRESSION PREVENTION PROGRAMS IN CHILDREN AND ADOLESCENTS (CONTINUED)

Prevention Type	Program	Efficacy Post-test	Efficacy Follow-up	Replicate	Clinical Diagnoses	Power (N > 100)	Assess Fidelity	Program Focus/ Comments
	Friends Program							**Reduce anxiety to prevent depression**
Universal	Lock & Barrett (63)	+	+	+	+	+	—	Significant prevention effect on depressive symptoms at 12, but Not at 24 or 36 months.
	Barrett et al. (95)	•	—	+	—	+	—	Follow-up of Lock & Barrett, 2003
	Lowry-Webster et al. (96-97)	+	+	+	+	+	—	significant effect at 12 months
	Stress Inoculation							**CB: Stress management**
Universal	Hains & Ellman (98)	+	—	—	—	—	—	Significant short-term effect for anxious subgroup
	CB + Interpersonal							**CB + Social**
Universal	Cecchini (99), Johnson (100)	—	—	—	—	—	—	Increased social skills; no effect on depression
	Mastery Learning Program							**School-based**
Universal	Kellam et al. (101)	—	—	—	—	+	—	Improved reading achievement not depressive symptoms
	Family-School Partnership (FSP)							**School-based**
Universal	Ialongo et al. (102)	—	—	—	—	+	—	Improved reading achievement not depressive symptoms

• not assessed in that study or not yet available; + = Yes; — = No; sxs = symptoms,
Post-test efficacy = significant effect of the intervention compared to control found at the immediate post-test assessment
Follow-up efficacy = significant effect of the intervention compared to control found at follow-up (at least 3 months)
Replicate = significant effect of the intervention has been replicated in at least two studies
++ = Replicated by at least two independent researchers
Clinical diagnoses = diagnoses of depressive disorders were assessed
Power (N >100) = the study had over 100 participants
Fidelity = the study assessed adherence to the intervention protocol; (+) = assessed fidelity with group leader report only

found to have satisfactory adherence. Given the large sample sizes, it is not surprising that diagnoses of depression have not been assessed.

The *Problem Solving for Life program* (PSFL),[36] which is administered by teachers, has been tested in large universal school samples. PSFL was found to have significant short-term effects in one study,[36] although this was not replicated,[37] and it has not shown significant long-term effects.[38]

In addition to the studies just cited, several other universal,[39,40] selective,[41] and indicated[42–44] depression prevention programs are cognitive behavioral and teach cognitive restructuring, problem solving, and coping. In general, these studies have found short-term efficacy at the postintervention evaluations, but only a few have shown long-term effects. These studies generally have not yet been replicated, and they have not assessed depressive diagnoses or the fidelity with which the interventions were delivered.

Recently, evidence of short-term efficacy of the *Interpersonal Psychotherapy—Adolescent Skills Training program* (IPT-AST) in both a large universal[45] and a small indicated[46] sample has been found. Young et al.[46] also showed that the significant effects endured through the 6-month follow-up, and they assessed depressive disorders as well as symptoms. There was a marginally significant trend for adolescents in the IPT-AST group (1/27 = 3.7%) to have fewer depressive diagnoses during the 6-month follow-up compared with controls (4/14 = 28.6%).

CONTEXT, STRUCTURE, AND CONTENT OF DEPRESSION PREVENTION PROGRAMS

Schools are an important context in which children and adolescents acquire new skills and spend a large proportion of their lives, and therefore, they are a logical location for implementing prevention programs. In a recent review of universal school-based interventions for the prevention of depression in children and adolescents, Spence and Shortt[47] used the standards set forth by SPR[31] as a benchmark to characterize school-based depression prevention programs. Their review included only studies that had some form of a control group, used well-recognized, reliable, and valid measures of depression, reported a minimum follow-up of 3 months, and focused on youth between 7 and 18 years of age. Consistent with the results of two recent meta-analyses of this literature,[22,30] Spence and Shortt concluded that there is not yet sufficient evidence of the effectiveness of universal school-based depression prevention programs to warrant their wide-scale implementation and dissemination at this time. Nevertheless, given the seriousness of the problem of depression, continued efforts at the development of universal programs aimed at its prevention are justified. Spence and Shortt[47] suggested that such programs may need to be more intensive and longer, with ongoing booster sessions, implemented by adequately trained and continuously supervised individuals, and focus on risk factors in the children's environment in addition to teaching individual skills.

Whereas universal programs tend to be delivered in schools, targeted (i.e., selective and indicated) programs are typically delivered in smaller groups in clinics, agencies, or after school. Few such programs have been tested in primary care settings, although see Stein and colleagues.[48] Interestingly, whereas targeted programs tend to be associated with greater levels of perceived stigma, participants evaluate them more positively.[49]

General features of effective interventions[50–51] applied to depression prevention programs would include the following:

- Education about depression: Describe the symptoms, causes, course, and prognosis.
- Normalization and destigmatization: Everyone experiences stress and distress at times; when should we be concerned about the condition?
- Provide a sense of hope: Depression is preventable and treatable.
- Enhance strengths and build skills (e.g., coping with stress, creating supportive social networks).
- Consider the larger context: The individual child is part of a family, peer group, school, neighborhood, and community. How might these different contexts contribute to the development and maintenance of depression, and how can they be used to facilitate prevention?
- Reassure parents that they are not to blame, but they can be part of the solution.

Overall, depression prevention programs are conducted in groups rather than individually. An advantage of a group format is that it allows participants to hear others' concerns, which helps normalize their experiences, and they learn how others have dealt with similar types of problems. A disadvantage is they do not allow sufficient time to address each individual's specific issues. Some groups have been single gender,[40,52] whereas others have included both males and females together.[15,34,36,53] A clear advantage of single versus mixed gender groups remains to be demonstrated. Groups have varied in size from as few as three to as many as an entire class (e.g., 30 students). The optimal group size for particular interventions has not yet been determined but is likely to be about eight.

These are the most common features of effective depression prevention programs:

- Psychoeducation about depression
- Cognitive-behavioral skills: cognitive restructuring and problem solving
- Interpersonal skills: communication, social problem solving, and assertiveness
- Coping with stress
- Some programs also have included a parenting component.

Whereas some interventions are primarily cognitive behavioral or interpersonally oriented, many have incorporated several of these different components. The best combination of techniques and the essential "active ingredients" are not yet known. Other approaches have not been studied with regard to the prevention of depression in youth including affect regulation, mindfulness, family-focused therapy, and a parenting program that is truly integrated into the intervention. Forehand and Compas[54] are currently testing a multifamily depression prevention program with at-risk offspring of depressed parents in which they specifically target coping and parenting. Preliminary analyses indicate promising effects.

COGNITIVE-BEHAVIORAL PROGRAMS

The majority of depression prevention programs administered to children and adolescents have been based on CBT principles.[55] CBT helps individuals identify, evaluate, and modify negative cognitions and develop coping and problem-solving skills (see Chapter 8). The most widely used cognitive-behavioral depression prevention program was developed at the University of Pennsylvania[17,32,56–58] and has been referred to as the Penn Prevention Program (PPP), the Penn Resiliency Program, and the Penn Optimism Program. This 12-session intervention was designed to target cognitive and behavioral risk factors, to promote resilience, and to prevent depressive symptoms in youth. PPP includes both a cognitive and a social problem-solving component. The cognitive component seeks to instill a flexible thinking style and teaches (1) the links between thoughts, feelings, and behaviors, (2) how to evaluate the accuracy of one's beliefs, and (3) how to generate less pessimistic and more realistic alternative thoughts through meta-cognition and cognitive restructuring. Additionally, the program teaches about appropriate distraction, relaxation, behavioral activation strategies (e.g., time management, antiprocrastination techniques), creative problem solving, information gathering, decision making, anticipating consequences, and graded task breakdown. The social problem-solving component teaches goal setting, perspective taking, active listening, assertiveness, negotiation, and generating and enacting appropriate strategies for solving interpersonal problems. Participants are trained to cope with family conflict and to use methods such as distancing from stress, distraction, and relaxation.

Clarke and colleagues[15,53] similarly have tested indicated samples of adolescents in a cognitive-behavioral prevention program, which was adapted from the Adolescent Coping with Depression Course.[33] In the first study,[53] the program consisted of three 45-minute sessions per week for 5 weeks. The intervention focused on identifying and challenging negative cognitions and developing coping skills. In a second study,[15] the program consisted of 15 1-hour sessions administered to adolescents exhibiting subclinical depressive symptoms who also had a parent with a history of depression. In this study the intervention taught cognitive restructuring skills, with a particular focus on negative cognitions related to having a depressed parent. The program also provided three parent information meetings to discuss the specific content of the sessions. A particular strength of these studies was their inclusion of clinical interviews, allowing the assessment of major depressive disorder in addition to self-reported depressive symptoms. The study by Clarke and colleagues[15] currently is being replicated in a multisite investigation at four different locations. Table 20.3 describes

TABLE 20.3 DESCRIPTION OF SESSIONS FROM THE PREVENTION OF DEPRESSION COURSE[15,16]

Session	Content
1	• Define depression; causes of depression • Introduce the "downward spiral;" relations among thoughts, feelings, and behaviors • Relation of stress and depression • Identify personal goals • Introduce the Mood Diary
2	• Identify negative thoughts • Keeping track of negative thoughts • Completing Mood Diaries
3	• What are common reactions to stress? Can these reactions be changed? • Define "activating event"—a situation or event that triggers negative thoughts • Identify and record activating events and negative thoughts • Positive statements
4	• Identify beliefs underlying negative thoughts ("tip of the iceberg") • Changing negative thoughts to more realistic thoughts • Generating counter-thoughts • Six helpful questions: a. Check it out. What is the evidence that my thought is accurate? b. What are some alternative explanations for the situation? c. What if it is true or somewhat true? What can I do? Will I still be okay? d. What are the odds that the "bad" thing I am thinking will actually happen? e. What would happen if I didn't believe this anymore? f. How useful is it for me to think this? Is this getting me what I want?
5	• Integrating the "A-B-C" method • Practice generating realistic counter-thoughts • Converting "nonpersonal" negative thoughts to personal thoughts
6	• What are the sources of our negative thinking? • Problem solving to deal with activating events that can stimulate negative thinking: a. Brainstorming b. Analysis of pros and cons c. Try and try again • How to deal with "activating events:" a. Don't respond or change how you respond b. Predict and prevent the activating event c. Change the activating event d. Accept the activating event and the consequences (emotions)
7	• Ways to interrupt negative thoughts: a. Thought stopping b. Worry time c. Balloon exercise • Using the "A-B-C" method in your life. Examples of real-world applications
8	• Anticipating and managing real-life stressors in the future; planning for emergencies • List anticipated major life stressors: a. Which events may trigger negative thoughts? b. Plan how to prevent and manage their negative effects c. Identify ways to maintain gains and manage future daily "hassles"
9–14	Monthly continuation sessions: • Review and further practice of cognitive restructuring • Review and further practice of problem solving • Relaxation training • Assertiveness training • Behavioral activation

the content of the eight weekly sessions used in this replication study.[16] Six monthly continuation sessions also were included.

The Problem Solving for Life program[36] is a universal intervention administered by teachers and involves eight weekly sessions, each lasting a class period (45 to 50 minutes). The curriculum integrates cognitive restructuring[55] and problem-solving skills training[59] through teaching about optimistic-thinking styles and a positive problem-solving orientation. Students learn to identify thoughts, feelings, and problem situations and the relations among these, as well as cognitive techniques to identify and challenge negative or irrational thoughts that may contribute to the development of negative affect and depressive symptoms. The second component focuses on the development of a positive orientation toward problem solving through the use of cognitive restructuring methods. Sheffield and colleagues[37] used the same program and added an indicated piece that also included cognitive-behavioral content relating to cognitive restructuring and problem-solving skills. The main difference was that the sessions were longer and it was administered in a small group format, which allowed more opportunity to teach interpersonal skills (e.g., assertion, conflict resolution, and negotiation) and self-reward.

The Resourceful Adolescent Program (RAP), tested in both Australia[35,60] and New Zealand[30] incorporates cognitive-behavioral and interpersonal therapy principles. RAP is an 11-session resilience building program conducted weekly during 40- to 50-minute class sessions in school. Sessions 1 to 7 follow CBT approaches.[53] Sessions 8 to 10 address interpersonal risk and protective factors in adolescent development.[61] The specific sessions are 1: establish rapport, 2: affirm existing strengths, 3 and 4: self-management and self-calming skills when faced with stress, 5 and 6: cognitive restructuring, 7: problem solving, 8: building and accessing social support networks, 9 and 10: discuss role transitions (e.g., moving toward greater independence while maintaining positive relationship with parents), perspective taking, and skills to promote harmony and avoid escalation of conflict, and 11: summary and termination. Shochet and colleagues[60] developed a Group Leader's Manual that describes each session and a complementary workbook for students.

The FRIENDS program[62,63] was developed primarily as an intervention to reduce anxiety. FRIENDS is an acronym for the different skills taught (F = feeling worried; R = relax and feel good; I = inner helpful thoughts; E = explore plans; N = nice work, reward yourself; D = don't forget to practice; and S = stay calm for life!). The program assists children in learning skills that help them cope with and manage anxiety and emotional distress through the application of learned coping and problem-solving skills. A few studies have shown that the program has a preventive effect on depressive symptoms as well as reducing anxiety.

Several of the cognitive-behavioral prevention programs also include an interpersonal component. For example, the PPP consists of both a cognitive component and a social problem-solving component.[17,32] In addition, others include a social skills training, assertiveness, or a social problem-solving component.[37,42,64-65] These components tend to be presented separately rather than being truly integrated into a combined cognitive-interpersonal approach.

INTERPERSONAL PROGRAMS

Although the majority of depression prevention programs have made cognitive-behavioral techniques the central component, some[46,66] have been based on interpersonal theories and therapies of depression such as interpersonal psychotherapy (IPT).[67] IPT targets several types of interpersonal problems hypothesized to be related to depression, including role transition, grief, interpersonal deficits, and interpersonal disputes. Clinical trials have shown that IPT adapted for adolescents (IPT-A)[61,68] is efficacious (see Chapter 9).

Given the promising results from studies of IPT-A for the treatment of depression in youth, Forsyth[66] developed and evaluated a four-session IPT-based, indicated depression prevention program for college students. The program discussed the relations among life events, role transitions, interpersonal problems, and depression. Moreover, it addressed role disputes, communication skills, and the four principal tasks of role transitions: giving up the old role; expressing guilt, anger, and loss; and acquiring new skills and developing new attachments and support groups.

Similarly, Young et al.[46] developed and tested an interpersonal psychotherapy-adolescent skills training group indicated prevention program based on IPT-A. The program consists of two individual sessions and eight weekly 90-minute group sessions targeting three types of interpersonal problems:

interpersonal role disputes, role transitions, and interpersonal deficits. The sessions focus on both psychoeducation and general interpersonal skill building. In the psychoeducation component, participants learn about prevention, depression, and the link between feelings and interpersonal interactions. The second component is aimed at developing interpersonal and communication skills.

FAMILY-FOCUSED PROGRAMS

Numerous parental and family risk factors are associated with depression in youth, including parental death, parental depression, marital conflict, and divorce (see Chapter 2). Several depression prevention programs have been developed to address these specific factors. Beardslee et al.[69] developed a selective prevention program targeting currently nonsymptomatic children (8 through 15 years of age) who had a parent with an affective disorder. The intervention consisted of six to ten sessions facilitated by a clinician that included individual meetings with both the children and parents, as well as a meeting with the entire family. The clinician-facilitated program used mostly psychoeducational techniques to increase understanding and communication within the family, and education about mood disorders, with an emphasis on connecting the information conveyed with the particular experiences of the family.

Sandler and colleagues[70-71] developed and tested the Family Bereavement Program (FBP) for children who had recently experienced the death of a parent. The 12-session FBP targeted positive parent–child exchanges and communication skills (e.g., effective listening and expression skills), emotional expression, mood-monitoring, planning of stable positive events (behavioral activation), handling negative events through emotion-focused and problem-focused coping, problem-solving skills, social skills, self-esteem enhancement, effective discipline practices, and cognitive reframing.

Several prevention programs have targeted children of divorced parents.[72-74] Gwynn and Brantley[72] tested an 8-week educational support group prevention program. Children were taught how to discuss divorce-related experiences and feelings with others, cope with visitation, and deal with conflicts involving siblings and parents, as well as problem-solving techniques.

Wolchik and colleagues[73] took an alternative approach to preventing problems in children of divorced parents. The divorced parent participated in a program called "New Beginnings" comprising ten group and two individual sessions. The program focused on the quality of the parent–child relationship by teaching listening skills, positive reinforcement of desired behaviors, and scheduling positive activities. In addition, the intervention taught anger management, listening skills, and discipline strategies, including clarifying expectations, being consistent, and monitoring misbehaviors and consequences. Improving contact with the noncustodial parent also was addressed by highlighting the importance of the father–child relationship and reducing obstacles to that contact. Finally, the intervention attempted to improve social support from other adults through the identification of potential resources, thereby extending the child's social network and available support for problem solving.

In a subsequent study, Wolchik and colleagues[74,75] developed a dual-component prevention program consisting of concurrent but separate interventions for both the mother and child. The 11-session child component focused on recognizing and labeling feelings, divorce information, problem solving, cognitive reframing, communication skills, and relaxation. The dual-component program was compared with an intervention targeting only the mother and a self-study condition consisting of the mother and child reading various age-appropriate self-help books on the topic of divorce.

EARLY INTERVENTION WITH SUBCLINICAL DEPRESSION

Individuals with subclinical depression clearly are at elevated risk of subsequently having a full major depressive episode[2-3] and therefore early intervention is warranted. Besides depression prevention studies with indicated samples,[5,32] few investigations have examined the efficacy of interventions specifically aimed at reducing subclinical depression in children and adolescents. Whereas the explicit goal of indicated prevention is to reduce the likelihood of a future depressive episode and may or may not reduce current subclinical symptoms, the aim of early intervention is to reduce the level of subthreshold depressive symptoms without necessarily preventing subsequent episodes. Interestingly, however, most indicated depression prevention programs in youth have been more like early intervention than prevention.[22]

Reviews of studies examining the efficacy of treatments for minor depression[76] or subclinical depression[77] have found a relative paucity of such investigations, and those that have been conducted have yielded small to moderate effect sizes. Oxman and Sengupta[76] suggested that nonspecific treatment factors common to the depression treatments and to active control conditions may be sufficiently potent to improve persons with minor depression. A meta-analytic review[77] in 2006 of eight studies of psychological treatments (i.e., some form of CBT) of subthreshold depression comprising 12 contrast groups with a total of 413 youth found a mean effect size of 0.55; 31 students needed to be screened to generate one positive outcome (see Table 4.1). Cuijpers and colleagues[77] concluded that psychological treatments have a significant moderate short-term effect on reducing subthreshold depression. The modest effect size may be partly owing to participants having started with subclinical symptom levels and therefore their scores did not have as far to decrease.

One logical setting to provide early intervention with subthreshold depression is in primary care. An interdisciplinary task force of experts developed Guidelines for Adolescent Depression in Primary Care (GLAD-PC)[78] to assist primary care clinicians in managing depression in youth 10 to 21 years of age. Relevant to the current discussion was their recommendation that primary care providers should consider a period (about 6 to 8 weeks) of active support and monitoring before recommending treatment (see Chapter 19).

Stein and colleagues[48] reviewed studies that examined the efficacy of psychosocial interventions delivered to adolescents by primary care physicians or their staff in a "real-world" primary care setting. They concluded there was some evidence that relatively simple primary care–based interventions can improve outcomes of adolescents with subclinical depression. For example, in a study of eight general practices in which 1,516 teens completed a variety of questionnaires including the Center for Epidemiologic Studies-Depression Scale (CES-D), Walker and colleagues[79] offered these youth an opportunity to receive general practice consultations to discuss health behavior concerns. Interested adolescents were randomly assigned to either a 20-minute consultation with a nurse aimed at improving self-efficacy for behavior change or to "standard care." Results indicated that among teens identified as having subthreshold levels of depressive symptoms (CES-D ≥16), those who received the consultation from the medical practice nurse had significantly lower CES-D scores compared with youth not receiving the consultation at the 3-month and 1-year follow-ups.

In the Youth Partners-in-Care study, Asarnow and colleagues[80] conducted one of the most carefully executed, controlled investigations to date in five health care organizations with 418 adolescent primary care patients. Youth with current depressive symptoms (i.e., CES-D ≥16) at baseline were randomly assigned to either "usual care" or a quality improvement intervention. In usual care, the primary care clinicians were provided with training and educational materials about depression evaluation and treatment. The quality improvement intervention included teams of experts at each site, as well as care managers who supported primary care clinicians with patient evaluation, education, evidence-based psychosocial treatment, medication when needed, and links to mental health services. Care managers, who had master's or doctoral degrees in mental health or nursing, followed patients up over the 6-month intervention period, coordinated care with the primary care clinician, and delivered the manualized CBT treatment. At the 6-month follow-up, adolescents in the quality improvement condition had significantly lower CES-D scores, a lower rate of severe depression, higher mental health–related quality of life, and greater satisfaction with mental health care. This study is the first to demonstrate that depression in adolescents can be improved in primary care office settings.

Finally, one study explicitly tested the effectiveness of a depression prevention program, the Penn Resiliency Program (PRP), when delivered by therapists in a primary care setting with 271 children 11–12 years of age.[81] Children with elevated depressive symptoms on the Children's Depression Inventory were randomized to PRP or usual care. Over the 2-year follow-up, the effect of PRP on depressive symptoms and explanatory style for negative events was moderated by sex, with girls benefiting more than boys. PRP significantly prevented depression, anxiety, and adjustment disorders (when combined) among high-symptom children. Not surprisingly, stronger effects were found when the intervention was delivered with high compared with low fidelity.

CONCLUSIONS

Overall, results of early interventions with adolescents experiencing subclinical depression show some promise, but many questions remain. For example, (1) to what extent is simple short-term support from a caring professional sufficient to reduce depressive symptoms? (2) How long do the effects last? (3) Are such interventions significantly better than "good" usual care? Primary care settings are a logical location for early identification and intervention with depressed youth, although adequately trained professionals often are not available. Despite the increasing pressure from government agencies for more widespread dissemination of depression prevention and early intervention programs, substantial questions remain as to whether or not the field is really ready.

As shown in Table 20.3, few depression prevention programs have found significant effects across time and across new investigators. Several studies have reported significant reductions in depressive symptoms, but far fewer have actually prevented the onset of depressive disorders. The fidelity with which the prevention programs have been implemented and the quality of the implementers often has not been assessed or linked to outcomes, despite the importance of this variable.[81]

Current depression prevention approaches emphasize building individual skills, but few address the larger context, including the quality of children's families, schools, neighborhoods, and community environments. What are the developmental, cultural, and gender differences that need to be considered when developing programs for preventing depression? Most depression prevention programs have emphasized cognitive-behavioral and/or interpersonal approaches, but little is understood about the developmental demands of such programs and when children are truly able to benefit from them. Moreover, to what extent do the skills (e.g., cognitive, coping, communication) taught in therapies with currently depressed individuals transfer when learned during a nondepressed state? How do we motivate children and adolescents to develop skills for changing depressive symptoms if they are not currently experiencing or have never had them?

Finally, what criteria should be used to determine if a preventive intervention has "worked"? The definition of "working" involves the size, duration, and specificity of the effect. Once an intervention has been found to be efficacious and effective,[31] we next need to understand how it worked, and for whom. Does the intervention produce change in the putative mediator(s), which in turn leads to change in depression? Equally important is to identify why a program did *not* work. Possible reasons for weak findings could be that the intervention was not designed or implemented well or with the "right" parameters regarding the number, length, and frequency of both acute and continuation sessions. Is the prevention program best implemented individually, in groups, families, or groups of families? What are the optimal characteristics of the group in terms of age, gender, and size? Who should deliver the intervention: professional clinicians, teachers, graduate students, peers?

For whom does the intervention work and for whom does it not work? By identifying significant moderators (e.g., sex, age, initial levels of depressive symptoms), we then can focus our efforts on the participant and design features (e.g., older, female, single gender groups, booster sessions) associated with the largest effect sizes. Equally as important, however, is to identify for whom the intervention was least effective (e.g., younger, male), determine possible reasons for the small effects with such individuals, and then modify or supplement the intervention to address these limitations.

Thus future studies of programs aimed at preventing depression in youth need to examine potential mediators and moderators, evaluate the fidelity and adherence of program implementation, assess participant attendance, compliance, and retention rates, conduct longer follow-up periods, and demonstrate that the effects are replicable. At this point, even the best studies have produced only small to moderate effect sizes, and the effects tend not to endure. In addition, studies of depression prevention programs for children and adolescents should test theoretically and empirically informed interventions, include no-intervention and active control groups, randomly assign participants to condition, use independent evaluators to do the assessments, measure both symptom and diagnostic outcomes specific to depression as well as comorbid disorders and levels of functional impairment, and conduct longer follow-up periods. Determining how and for whom an intervention works will allow us to disseminate it more efficiently and effectively to those most in need.

RESOURCES FOR PATIENTS AND FAMILIES

Coping with Stress, Greg Clarke, Ph.D.: Internet depression self-help site: www.feelbetter.org and www.jmir.org/2005/2/e16/.

Seligman MEP. *The Optimistic Child: A Revolutionary Program That Safeguards Children Against Depression and Builds Lifelong Resilience.* New York: Houghton Mifflin; 1995.

RESOURCES FOR PROFESSIONALS

References 21, 22, 26, 30, 35, 77, and 78.

Asarnow JR, Carlson G, Schuster M, et al. *Youth Partners in Care: Clinician Guide to Depression Assessment and Management Among Youth in Primary Care Settings.* Los Angeles, Calif: UCLA School of Medicine; 1999. Adapted from Rubenstein L, Unutzer J, Miranda J, et al. *Partners in Care: Clinician Guide to Depression Assessment and Management in Primary Care Settings.* Santa Monica, Calif: RAND; 1996.

Barrett PM, Lowry-Webster H, Turner C. *Friends for Children Group Leader Manual*—Edition II. Brisbane: Australian Academic Press; 2000.

Greenberg MT, Domitrovich C, Bumbarger B. The prevention of mental disorders in school-aged children: current state of the field. *Prevent Treat.* 2001;4:Article1. Retrieved March 1, 2002, from http://journals.apa.org/prevention/volume4/pre0040001a.html.

Merry SN. Prevention and early intervention for depression in young people—a practical possibility? *Curr Opin Psychiatry.* 2007;20:325–329.

"Coping with Stress," Greg Clarke, Ph.D.: depression self-help website: www.feelbetter.org and www.jmir.org/2005/2/e16/.

Penn Prevention Program: http://www.ppc.sas.upenn.edu/prpsum.htm; Jane Gillham, Ph.D., and Karen Reivich, Ph.D., co-directors; phone: 1-215-573–4128; fax: 1-215-746–6361; e-mail: info@pennproject.org.

Susan Spence, Department of Psychology, Division of Linguistics and Psychology, Macquarie University, NSW 2019, Australia; phone: +61 2 9850 8030; fax: +61 2 9850 9390; e-mail: sue.spence@mq.edu.au.

Therapy manuals for adolescent depression group treatment or prevention programs: www.kpchr.org/public/acwd/acwd.html

REFERENCES

1. Birmaher B, Ryan N, Williamson D, et al. Childhood and adolescent depression: a review of the past 10 years, Part I. *J Am Acad Child Adolesc Psychiatry.* 1996;35:1427–1439.
2. Fergusson DM, Horwood LJ, Ridder EM, et al. Subthreshold depression in adolescence and mental health outcomes in adulthood. *Arch Gen Psychiatry.* 2005;62:66–72.
3. Lewinsohn PM, Rohde P, Seeley JR, et al. Psychosocial characteristics of young adults who have experienced and recovered from major depressive disorder during adolescence. *J Abnorm Psychol.* 2003;112:353–363.
4. Pickles A, Rowe R, Simonoff E, et al. Child psychiatric symptoms and psychosocial impairment: relationship and prognostic significance. *Br J Psychiatry.* 2001;179:230–235.
5. Murray CJ, Lopez AD. *The Global Burden of Disease. A Comprehensive Assessment of Mortality and Disability from Diseases, Injuries, and Risk Factors in 1990 and Projected to 2020.* Cambridge: Harvard University Press; 1996.
6. World Health Organization. *World Health Report 2001. Mental Health: New Understanding, New Hope.* 2001. Retrieved from http://www.who. int/whr2001/2001/main/en/.
7. Birmaher B, Arbelaez C, Brent D. Course and outcome of child and adolescent major depressive disorder. *Child Adolesc Psychiatr Clin N Am.* 2002;11:619–637.
8. Weissman MM, Wolk S, Goldstein RB, et al. Depressed adolescents grown up. *JAMA.* 1999;281:1707–1713.
9. Kessler RC, Wai TC, Demler O, et al. Prevalence, severity, and comorbidity of 12-month DSM-IV disorders in the National Comorbidity Survey Replication. *Arch Gen Psychiatry.* 2005;62:617–627.
10. Hirschfeld R, Keller M, Panico S, et al. The National Depressive and Manic-Depressive Association consensus statement on the undertreatment of depression. *JAMA.* 1997;277:333–340.
11. Newman DL, Moffitt TE, Caspi A, et al. Psychiatric disorder in a birth cohort of young adults: prevalence, comorbidity, clinical significance, and new case incidence from ages 11 to 21. *J Consult Clin Psychol.* 1996;64:552–562.

12. Heller K. Coming of age of prevention science: comments on the 1994 National Institute of Mental Health–Institute of Medicine Prevention Reports. *Am Psychol.* 1996;51:1123–1127.

13. Caplan G. *Principles of Preventive Psychiatry.* New York: Basic Books; 1964.

14. Mrazek PJ, Haggerty RJ eds. *Reducing Risks for Mental Disorders: Frontiers for Preventive Intervention Research.* Washington, DC: National Academy Press, 1994.

15. Clarke GN, Hornbrook M, Lynch F, et al. A randomized trial of a group cognitive intervention for preventing depression in adolescent offspring of depressed parents. *Arch Gen Psychiatry.* 2001;58:1127–1134.

16. Garber J, Brent D, Clarke G, et al. Prevention of depression in at-risk adolescents: short-term outcome. Presented at the Child and Adolescent Depression Consortium, Pittsburgh, Pa, 2007.

17. Jaycox LH, Reivich KJ, Gillham J, et al. Prevention of depressive symptoms in school children. *Behav Res Ther.* 1994;32:801–816.

18. Yu DL, Seligman MEP. Preventing depressive symptoms in Chinese children. *Prevent Treat.* 2002;5, Article 9. Retrieved from http://journals.apa.org/prevention/volume5/pre0050009a.html.

19. Cuijpers P. Examining the effects of prevention programs on the incidence of new cases of mental disorders: the lack of statistical power. *Am J Psychiatry.* 2003;160:1385–1391.

20. Offord DR, Kraemer HC, Kazdin AE, et al. Lowering the burden of suffering from child psychiatric disorder: trade-offs among clinical, targeted, and universal interventions. *J Am Acad Child Adolesc Psychiatry.* 1998;37:686–694.

21. Gillham JE, Shatté AJ, Freres DR. Preventing depression: a review of cognitive-behavioral and family interventions. *App Prevent Psychol.* 2000;9:63–88.

22. Horowitz JL, Garber J. The prevention of depressive symptoms in children and adolescents: a meta-analytic review. *J Consult Clin Psychol.* 2006;74:401–415.

23. Sutton JM. Prevention of depression in youth: a qualitative review and future suggestions. *Clin Psychol Rev.* 2007;27:552–571.

24. Lewinsohn PM, Allen NB, Seeley JR, et al. First onset versus recurrence of depression: differential processes of psychosocial risk. *J Abnorm Psychol.* 1999;108:483–489.

25. Monroe SM, Harkness, KL. Life stress, the "kindling" hypothesis, and the recurrence of depression: considerations from a life stress perspective. *Psychol Rev.* 2005;112:417–445.

26. Kennard BD, Emslie GJ, Mayes TM, et al. Relapse and recurrence in pediatric depression. *Child Adolesc Psychiatr Clin N Am.* 2006;15:1057–1079.

27. Garber J, McCauley E. Prevention of depression and suicide in children and adolescents. In: Lewis M, ed. *Child and Adolescent Psychiatry: A Comprehensive Text.* 3rd ed. Baltimore: Williams & Wilkins, 2002:805–821.

28. Merry SN, Spence SH. Attempting to prevent depression in youth: a systematic review of the evidence. *Early Intervent Psychiatry.* 2007;1:128–137.

29. Jane-Llopis E, Hosman C, Jenkins R, et al. Predictors of efficacy in depression prevention programmes: meta-analysis. *Br J Psychiatry.* 2003;183:384–397.

30. Merry S, McDowell H, Hetrick S, et al. Psychological and/or educational interventions for the prevention of depression in children and adolescents. *Cochrane Database Syst Rev.* 2004;(1):CD0003380.

31. Flay BR, Biglan A, Boruch RF, et al. Standards of evidence: criteria for efficacy, effectiveness and dissemination. *Prevent Sci.* 2004;6:151–175.

32. Gillham JE, Reivich KJ, Jaycox LH, et al. Prevention of depressive symptoms in schoolchildren: two-year follow-up. *Psychol Sci.* 1995;6:343–351.

33. Clarke GN, Lewinsohn PM, Hops H. *Instructor's Manual for the Adolescent Coping with Depression Course.* Eugene, Ore: Castalia Press; 1990.

34. Merry SN, McDowell H, Wild CJ, et al. A randomized placebo controlled trial of a school-based depression prevention program. *J Am Acad Child Adolesc Psychiatry.* 2004;43:538–547.

35. Shochet I, Dadds M, Holland D, et al. The efficacy of a universal school-based program to prevent adolescent depression. *J Clin Child Psychol.* 2001;30:303–315.

36. Spence S, Sheffield JK, Donovan CL. Preventing adolescent depression: an evaluation of the Problem Solving for Life Program. *J Consult Clin Psychol.* 2003;71:3–13.

37. Sheffield JK, Spence SH, Rapee RM, et al. Evaluation of universal, indicated, and combined cognitive-behavioral approaches to the prevention of depression among adolescents. *J Consult Clin Psychol.* 2006;74:66–79.

38. Spence SH, Sheffield JK, Donovan CL. Long-term outcome of a school-based, universal approach to prevention of depression in adolescents. *J Consult Clin Psychol.* 2005;73:160–167.

39. Petersen AC, Leffert N, Graham B, et al. Promoting mental health during the transition into adolescence. In: Schulenberg J, Muggs JL, Hierrelmann AK, eds. *Health Risks and Developmental Transitions During Adolescence.* New York: Cambridge University Press; 1999:471–497.

40. Pössel P, Horn AB, Groen G, et al. School-based prevention of depressive symptoms in adolescents: a 6-month follow-up. *J Am Acad Child Adolesc Psychiatry.* 2004;43:1003–1010.

41. Hyun M-S, Cho Chung H-I, Lee Y-J. The effect of cognitive–behavioral group therapy on the self-esteem, depression, and self-efficacy of runaway adolescents in a shelter in South Korea. *App Nurs Res.* 2005;18:160–166.

42. Lamb JM, Puskar KR, Sereika M, et al. School-based intervention to promote coping in rural teens. *Am J Maternal Child Nurs.* 1998;23;187–194.

43. Peden AR, Rayens MK, Hall LA, et al. Preventing depression in high-risk college women: a report of an 18-month follow-up. *J Am College Health.* 2001;49:299–306.

44. Stice E, Burton E, Bearman SK, et al. Randomized trial of a brief depression prevention program: an elusive search for a psychosocial placebo control condition. *Behav Res Ther.* 2006;45:863–876.

45. Horowitz JL, Garber J, Ciesla JA, et al. Prevention of depressive symptoms in adolescents: a randomized trial of cognitive-behavioral and interpersonal prevention programs. *J Consult Clin Psychol.* 2007;75:693–706.

46. Young JF, Mufson L, Davies M. Efficacy of interpersonal psychotherapy-adolescent skills training: an indicated preventive intervention for depression. *J Child Psychol Psychiatry.* 2006;47:1254–1262.

47. Spence SH, Shortt AL. Can we justify the widespread dissemination of universal, school-based interventions for the prevention of depression among children and adolescents? *J Child Psychiatry Psychol.* 2007;48:526–542.

48. Stein REK, Zitner LE, Jensen PS. Interventions for adolescent depression in primary care. *Pediatrics.* 2006;118:669–682.

49. Rapee RM, Wignall, A, Sheffield J, et al. Adolescents' reactions to universal and indicated prevention programs for depression: perceived stigma and consumer satisfaction. *Prevent Sci.* 2006;7:167–177.

50. Greenberg MT. Current and future challenges in school-based prevention: the researcher perspective. *Prevent Sci.* 2004;5:5–13.

51. Maton KI, Schellenbach CJ, Leadbeater BJ, et al., eds. *Investing in Children, Youth, Families and Communities: Strength-Based Research and Policy.* Washington, DC: American Psychological Association; 2003.

52. Chaplin TM, Gillham JE, Reivich K, et al. Depression prevention for early adolescent girls: a pilot study of all-girls versus co-ed groups. *J Early Adolesc.* 2006;26:110–126.

53. Clarke GN, Hawkins W, Murphy M, et al. Targeted prevention of unipolar depressive disorder in an at-risk sample of high school adolescents: a randomized trial of a group cognitive intervention. *J Am Acad Child Adolesc Psychiatry.* 1995;34:312–321.

54. Forehand R, Compas B. A family cognitive behavioral prevention program for children of depressed parents. Presented at the Kansas Conference in Clinical Child and Adolescent Psychology: Translating Research Into Practice. Lawrence, Kan, 2008.

55. Beck AT, Rush AJ, Shaw BF, et al. *Cognitive Therapy of Depression.* New York: Guilford Press; 1979.

56. Reivich K. *The Prevention of Depressive Symptoms in Adolescents* [dissertation]. University of Pennsylvania, UMI No. 9627995; 1996.

57. Seligman MEP, Schulman P, DeRubeis RJ, et al. The prevention of depression and anxiety. *Prevent Treat.* 1999;2 (Electronic version, retrieved October 19, 2007, from http://journals.apa.org/prevention/volume2/pre0020008a.html).

58. Shatté AJ. *Prevention of Depressive Symptoms in Adolescents: Issues of Dissemination and Mechanisms of Change* [dissertation]. University of Pennsylvania, UMI No. 9713001; 1996.

59. D'Zurilla TJ, Nezu A. A study of the generation-of-alternatives process in social problem solving. *Cogn Ther Res.* 1980;4:67–72.

60. Shochet I, Holland D, Whitefield K. *Resourceful Adolescent Program (RAP): Group Leader's Manual.* Brisbane, Australia: Griffith University; 1997.

61. Mufson L, Moreau D, Weissman MM, et al. Modification of interpersonal psychotherapy with depressed adolescence (IPT-A): phase I and phase II studies. *J Am Acad Child Adolesc Psychiatry.* 1994;33:695–705.

62. Barrett PM. Interventions for child and youth anxiety disorders: involving parents, teachers, and peers. *Aust Educ Dev Psychol.* 1999;16:5–24.

63. Lock S, Barrett PM. A longitudinal study of developmental differences in universal preventive intervention for child anxiety. *Behav Change.* 2003;20:183–199.

64. Eggert LL, Thompson EA, Herting JR, et al. Reducing suicide potential among high-risk youth: tests of a school-based prevention program. *Suicide Life Threat Behav.* 1995;22:276–296.

65. Pössel P, Baldus C, Horn AB, et al. Influence of general self-efficacy on the effects of a school-based universal primary prevention program of depressive symptoms in adolescents: a randomized and controlled follow-up study. *J Child Psychol Psychiatry.* 2005;46:982–994.

66. Forsyth KM. *The Design and Implementation of a Depression Prevention Program.* University of Rhode Island. *Diss Abst Int.* 2000;61(12):6704B (UMI No. 9999536).

67. Weissman MM, Markowitz JC, Klerman GL. *A Comprehensive Guide to Interpersonal Psychotherapy.* New York: Basic Books; 2000.

68. Mufson L, Weissman MM, Moreau D, et al. Efficacy of interpersonal psychotherapy for depressed adolescents. *Arch Gen Psychiatry.* 1999;56:573–579.

69. Beardslee WR, Wright EJ, Salt P, et al. Examination of children's responses to two preventive intervention strategies over time. *J Am Acad Child Adolesc Psychiatry.* 1997;36:196–204.

70. Sandler IN, Ayers TS, Wolchik SA, et al. The Family Bereavement Program: efficacy evaluation of a theory-based prevention program for parentally bereaved children and adolescents. *J Consult Clin Psychol.* 2003;71:587–600.

71. Sandler IN, West SG, Baca L, et al. Linking empirically based theory and evaluation: the family bereavement program. *Am J Comm Psychol.* 1992;20:491–521.

72. Gwynn CA, Brantley HT. Effects of a divorce group intervention for elementary school children. *Psychol Schools.* 1987;24:161–164.

73. Wolchik SA, West SG, Westover S, et al. The children of divorce parenting intervention: outcome evaluation of an empirically based program. *Am J Commun Psychol.* 1993;21:293–331.

74. Wolchik SA, West SG, Sandler IN, et al. An experimental evalutation of theory-based mother and mother-child programs for children of divorce. *J Consult Clin Psychol.* 2000;68:843–856.

75. Wolchik SA, Sandler IN, Milsap RE, et al. Six-year follow-up of preventive interventions for children of divorce: a randomized controlled trial. *JAMA.* 2002;288:1874–1881.

76. Oxman TE, Sengupta A. Treatment of minor depression. *Am J Geriatr Psychiatry.* 2002;10:256–264.

77. Cuijpers P, Straten Av, Smits N, et al. Screening and early psychological intervention for depression in schools: systematic review and meta-analysis. *Eur Child Adolesc Psychiatry.* 2006;15:300–307.

78. Cheung A, Zuckerbrot RA, Jensen PS, et al. Guidelines for Adolescent Depression in Primary Care (GLAD-PC): II. Treatment and ongoing management. *Pediatrics.* 2007;120:e1313–e1326.

79. Walker Z, Townsend J, Oakley L, et al. Health promotion for adolescents in primary care: randomized controlled trial. *Br Med J.* 2002;325:524–529.

80. Asarnow JR, Jaycox LH, Duan N, et al. Effectiveness of a quality improvement intervention for adolescent depression in primary care clinics: a randomized controlled trial. *JAMA.* 2005,293:311–319.

81. Gillham JE, Hamilton J, Freres DR, et al. Preventing depression among early adolescents in the primary care setting: a randomized controlled study of the Penn Resiliency Program. *J Abnorm Child Psychol.* 2006;34: 203–219.

82. Cardemil EV, Reivich KJ, Seligman MEP. The prevention of depressive symptoms in low-income minority middle-school students. *Prevent Treat.* 2002;5:Article 8. Available at: http://journals.apa.org/prevention/volume5/pre0050008a.html.

83. Cardemil EV, Reivich KJ, Beevers CG, et al. The prevention of depressive symptoms in low-income minority children: two-year follow-up. *Behav Res Ther.* 2007;45:313–327.

84. Pattison C, Lynd-Stevenson RM. The prevention of depressive symptoms in children: immediate and long-term outcomes of a school-based program. *Behav. Change.* 2001;18:92–102.

85. Quayle D, Dzuirawiec S, Roberts C, et al. The effect of an optimism and life skills program on depressive symptoms in preadolescence. *Behav Change.* 2001;18:194–203.

86. Gillham JE, Reivich KJ, Freres DR, et al. School-based prevention of depressive symptoms: a randomized controlled study of the effectiveness and specificity of the Penn Resiliency Program. *J Consult Clin Psychol.* 2007;75:9–19.

87. Gillham JE, Reivich KJ, Freres DR, et al. School-based prevention of depression and anxiety symptoms in early adolescence: a pilot of a parent intervention component. *School Psychol Q.* 2006;21:323–348.

88. Roberts C, Kane R, Thomson H, et al. The prevention of depressive symptoms in rural school children: a randomized controlled trial. *J Consul Clin Psychol.* 2003;71:622–628.

89. Roberts C, Kane R, Bishop B, et al. The prevention of depressive symptoms in rural school children: a follow-up study. *Int J Ment Health Promotion.* 2004;6:4–16.

90. Clarke GN, Hawkins W, Murphy M, et al. School-based primary prevention of depressive symptomatology in adolescents: findings from two studies. *J Adolesc Res.* 1993;8:183–204.

91. Burton EM, Stice E, Bearman SK, et al. An experimental test of the affect-regulation theory of bulimic symptoms and substance use: a randomized trial. *Int J Eating Disord.* 2007;40:27–36.

92. Harnett PH, Dadds MR. Training school personnel to implement a universal school-based prevention of depression program under real world conditions. *J School Psychol.* 2004;42:343–357.

93. Beardslee WR, Gladstone TRG, Wright EJ, et al. A family-based approach to the prevention of depressive symptoms in children at risk: evidence of parental and child change. *Pediatrics.* 2003;112:119–131.

94. Beardslee WR, Wright EJ, Gladstone TRG, et al. Long-term effects from a randomized trial of two public health preventive interventions for parental depression. *J Fam Psychol.* 2007;21:703–713.

95. Barrett PM, Farrell LJ, Ollendick TH, et al. Long-term outcomes of an Australian universal prevention trial of anxiety and depression symptoms in children and youth: an evaluation of the Friends Program. *J Clin Child Adolesc Psychol.* 2006;35:403–411.

96. Lowry-Webster H, Barrett PM, Dadds MR. A universal prevention trial of anxiety and depressive symptomatology in childhood: preliminary data from an Australian study. *Behav Change.* 2001;18:36–50.

97. Lowry-Webster H, Barrett PM, Lock S. A universal prevention trial of anxiety symptomatology during childhood: results at one-year follow-up. *Behav Change.* 2003;20:25–43.

98. Hains AA, Ellman SW. Stress inoculation training as a preventive intervention for high school youths. *J Cogn Psychother.* 1994;8:219–232.

99. Cecchini TB. An interpersonal and cognitive-behavioral approach to childhood depression: a school-based primary prevention study. Utah State University, 1997. *Diss Abst Int.* 1997;58:12B (UMI No. 9820698).

100. Johnson NC. *A Follow-Up Study of a Primary Prevention Program Targeting Childhood Depression* [dissertation]. Utah State University, UMI No. 1402700; 2000.

101. Kellam SG, Rebok GW, Mayer LS, et al. Depressive symptoms over first grade and their response to a developmental epidemiologically based preventive trial aimed at improving achievement. *Dev Psychopathol.* 1994;6:463–481.

102. Ialongo NS, Werthamer L, Kellam SG, et al. Proximal impact of two first-grade preventive interventions on the early risk behaviors for later substance abuse, depression, and antisocial behavior. *Am J Community Psychol.* 1999;27:599–641.

Particular Issues
About Treatment
in Specific Groups

Treating Depression in Children and Adolescents With Chronic Physical Illness

ROBERTO ORTIZ-AGUAYO AND JOHN V. CAMPO

KEY POINTS

- Because of medical advances, the number of children living with chronic physical illness has risen, making this an increasingly important population to consider in caring for depressed youth. Children with chronic medical or neurologic illness are at increased risk to develop depressive disorders.
- The impact of depression on overall health and well-being is greatest when depression is comorbid with chronic physical disease. Physical disorders may increase the risk, cause, or perpetuate depression. Conversely, psychiatric disorder may negatively impact on the onset and course of physical disease.
- The possibility that a child's depressive symptoms may be caused, wholly or in part, by the comorbid physical disease should always be considered, and the current and past medical history should be carefully reviewed.
- Attributing depressive symptoms (e.g., fatigue, poor sleep, or appetite) exclusively to the chronic physical disease can be highly subjective and unreliable.
- Clinicians face numerous challenges in the evaluation and diagnosis of depression in chronically ill children. An integrative approach, with particular emphasis on the evaluation of changes in functioning from baseline and across domains, is recommended.
- Patients and families need to understand what is known about available treatments, including risks, benefits, financial costs, and commitment required in terms of time, effort, and overall family burden.
- Psychotherapeutic interventions are particularly appealing and often well received in the physically ill, where the use of antidepressant medications can pose challenges.
- Psychopharmacologic treatment is practically and culturally well suited to the management of depression in medical settings, yet it presents challenges given the increased likelihood of medication-related adverse events and pharmacodynamic and pharmacokinetic drug interactions. Accordingly, treatment must be individualized, carefully considering the risk of drug–disease and drug–drug interactions.
- Aspects to consider when selecting medication for depressed physically ill youth include safety, tolerability, efficacy, cost, and simplicity of administration, with safety the key issue.
- It is important to understand the patient's disease state and its pathophysiology. Physical illness can alter the absorption, distribution, metabolism, and elimination of medication, particularly when organ failure exists.
- Clinically relevant adverse effects of selective serotonin reuptake inhibitors (SSRIs) include platelet dysfunction associated with increased bleeding time and bruising. Although not problematic in healthy children, this is potentially risky in youth with clotting disorders, disorders of platelet function, and thrombocytopenia.
- SSRIs may increase the risk of gastrointestinal bleeding, primarily when used in combination with nonsteroidal anti-inflammatory drugs.
- Other classes of antidepressants may be used in cases of treatment-resistant depression when SSRIs are poorly tolerated or in the presence of other symptoms and disorders in association with depression that may warrant a different approach.

- Cardiac problems, particularly conduction abnormalities, pose special challenges. Psychoactive medications that prolong the QTc interval directly or indirectly need to be avoided when possible.
- Depression in diabetic patients is associated with worsening dietary and medication adherence, as well as poor metabolic control and higher usage costs.
- Functional pain symptoms are associated with depressive disorders across the lifespan, and antidepressants often play a role in pain management.

Introduction

Chronic illness has been defined as a medical condition that requires at least 6 months of continuous medical care and is associated with lifestyle changes.[1] Chronic physical disease is increasingly common in childhood. In the United States, approximately 10 to 20 million children live with a chronic illness,[2] with approximately 1% to 3% of children and adolescents suffering from significant functional impairment associated with a chronic physical health condition.[3] As a group, most chronic conditions have no specific cure but can be managed medically, and many are characterized by a variable course of symptoms, potential physical and psychosocial limitations, daily treatment regimes, and periods of acute exacerbation. Because advances in pediatric medicine, along with improved sanitation and social support services in industrialized countries, have led to high survival rates from previously fatal diseases, the number of children living with chronic physical illness has risen, making this an increasingly important population to consider in caring for depressed youth. Youth presenting somatic symptoms and disorders for which there is no clear medical explanation, such as irritable bowel syndrome and chronic fatigue, often meet criteria for a depressive disorder.[4,5]

Depressive disorders are chronic illnesses in their own right and carry significant disability. The World Health Organization has estimated depression to be the fourth leading cause of disease burden in 2000, and it is expected to become the second leading cause of global disease burden by 2020, behind heart disease; moreover, the impact of depression on overall health and well-being is greatest when depression is comorbid with chronic physical disease.[6] Rather than being *just another disorder* suffered by a physically ill child, the relationship between physical disease and depression is often complex and bidirectional.

Physical disorders can be an independent risk, etiologic, or perpetuating factor for depression, and some disorders such as migraine and the tendency to develop allergic diseases may share genetic vulnerability with depression.[7,8] Children with chronic physical illness have been found to be at greater risk of syndromal and subsyndromal depression in comparison with healthy peers, with risk being highest when the physical illness affects the central nervous system.[9–11] Disease-modifying relationships between depressive syndromes and chronic physical illness are many and, in the vast majority of cases and across disease categories, multifactorial.

Conversely, psychiatric disorders may negatively impact the onset and course of physical disease. First, depression may increase the likelihood of nonadherence to prescribed treatments[12,13] and interfere with a healthy lifestyle. Second, depression in physically ill youth is associated with greater health care usage and cost, less optimal medical outcomes, worsening metabolic markers of disease control, worsening functional impairment, lower scores in quality of life measures, and increased mortality.[14–17] Third, depression may also affect the physiology of the disease process itself.[16] For example, diabetic children are at elevated risk to develop depression,[18] which increases the risk of nonadherence to treatment, repeat hospitalization, and of disease-related complications such as diabetic retinopathy.[19] It follows that aggressively treating depressive illness in physically ill youth may not only relieve depression-related suffering and impairment but may also benefit the management of the comorbid physical disease.

Unfortunately, data on the treatment of depression in chronically ill children are limited, largely because randomized controlled trials (RCTs) have typically excluded physically ill youth. The aim of this chapter is to highlight what is currently known about the treatment of depression in children and adolescents with chronic physical illness and offering practical clinical guidance based on cumulative clinical experience, case reports and case series, and available studies. In the absence of data from systematic and representative RCTs, clinicians must weigh the evidence carefully and in the context of each individual case when making diagnostic and treatment decisions. Frank discussion of existing limitations to the evidence base with patients and families as well as with professional colleagues is imperative in the spirit of true informed consent and practice (see Chapter 4). *Child* and *children* are used to mean both children and adolescents unless specified otherwise.

ASSESSMENT AND DIAGNOSIS

As highlighted in Chapter 3 and other parts of this book, an accurate diagnosis should precede treatment and provide information about illness course, prognosis, and treatment, as well as facilitating clinical and research communication. Pediatric depressive disorders have been well validated as a diagnostic entity, and a diagnosis of depression in childhood has clear prognostic implications.[20] Given the complex relationship between depression and physical disease, a careful assessment is critical. The clinician must appreciate how physical disease and its treatment impact on mood, and remain alert to how mood and mood disorder may impact on chronic physical illness.

The differential diagnosis of depressive syndromes in children with chronic physical illness is broad and includes, but is not limited to, primary mood disorders (e.g., major depressive disorder, dysthymic disorder, bipolar disorder), transient reactions to stressors (e.g., adjustment disorders, bereavement), and mood disorders secondary to a general medical condition or its treatment (e.g., nutritional deficiency, left-sided stroke, tacrolimus, or steroid immunosuppression) (see also Table 1.4). Specific diagnostic criteria for each have been described in Chapters 1, 3, and elsewhere.[21,22] Depressive disorders are also frequently comorbid with other psychiatric disorders in physically ill youth, including anxiety disorders and posttraumatic stress disorder. In circumstances where there is considerable impairment, yet uncertainty about the specific diagnosis remains, it may be possible to identify circumscribed symptoms that are amenable to intervention.

Clinicians face numerous challenges in the evaluation and diagnosis of depression in chronically ill children. An integrative approach is recommended, with particular emphasis on the evaluation of *changes in functioning from baseline and across domains.* Consequently, clinicians working with chronically ill youth need to gather information from multiple sources and coordinate care with parents, other medical professionals, family, social agencies, schools, and relevant community systems. The taxing consequences of the child's chronic physical illness for the child and family should be assessed and relevant findings incorporated into treatment planning. Attention should be paid to peer interactions and developmental tasks that are disrupted by the illness, its timing, or its effects on physical appearance, sexual identity and development, and functional status. Individual, developmental, family, and cultural health beliefs and the quality of communication between the family, patient, and medical care providers should be assessed and included as relevant to the biopsychosocial formulation and as potential targets for intervention. Possible medicolegal issues and the role of health-care systems should also be explored. The possibility that the child's depressive symptoms may be explained, wholly or in part, by the comorbid physical disease should always be considered and the current and past medical history should be carefully reviewed. Current and recently prescribed medications should be determined, including the use of contraceptives, vitamins, dietary supplements, and herbal remedies. The clinician should consult the package insert, Internet resources, the pharmacy service, and the Medical Letter regarding potential psychiatric effects of current medications. It should be always kept in mind the possibility that a female patient may be pregnant. The possibility that a female patient may be pregnant should always be kept in mind.

Much has been written about the challenges associated with diagnosing depressive disorders in the physically ill, with both under- and overdiagnosis generating concern. Underrecognition reduces the number of youth capable of experiencing symptomatic relief and functional improvement, whereas overdiagnosis may be associated with the risk of stigmatizing a particular child or exposing him or her to needless or overly aggressive treatment. The risk of misattributing symptoms of the chronic physical disease (e.g., fatigue or poor sleep or appetite) to a mood disorder has been a topic of much discussion. Attributing a symptom such as fatigue to either the physical disease or to depression is highly subjective and thus notoriously unreliable. Similarly, dysphoria in the context of chronic physical illness must also be assessed, and a sympathetic adult can easily "explain away" associated emotional distress as situational and an adjustment to the existing physical health problem.

Although differentiating the consequences of traditional physical disease from depression is challenging, the existing social context and the stigma associated with a diagnosis of mental disorder and psychiatric treatment appear to mitigate the likelihood of reckless overdiagnosis of depression in chronically ill youth. Stigma can be a powerful and often subliminal motivation to consider subjective and somatic symptoms of depression as only a consequence of the physical disease and thus "nothing to be ashamed of." Well-meaning professionals may also wish to spare any additional "insult" to an already suffering child and family. It can thus be tempting for patients, families, and professionals to dismiss signs and symptoms of depression as a part of a "normal" or "justifiable" response to the underlying chronic illness. Biases in favor of or against the diagnosis of psychiatric disorder in the physically ill child have real consequences. Inadvertently creating a higher standard to diagnose depression in the physically ill results in underdiagnosis, and it places patients at further risk of physical and emotional decompensation owing to lack of treatment.

Because existing evidence suggests that most depressed children and adolescents are either unrecognized or inadequately treated, we recommend an inclusive approach to the diagnosis that considers all symptoms of depression elicited during examination as relevant regardless of whether physical illness could be responsible or not.[23] This approach requires clinicians to address all potential sources of the patient's subjective distress and impairment, and to initiate treatment based on a thoughtful evaluation of the risks and benefits in collaboration with the patient and family. Clinicians should carry out necessary laboratory investigations and request subspecialty consultation as guided by findings in the history and physical examination. Careful review of medications, with close attention to temporal relationships between psychiatric symptoms and the timing of medication initiation, discontinuation, and dosing change can be an invaluable part of the assessment. In our experience, by considering all symptoms of depression noted on examination to be relevant to the diagnosis of depression, the inclusive approach increases the sensitivity of clinicians to depression in the physically ill and is likely to be more reliable than one relying on the subjective judgment of clinicians in determining whether a particular symptom is "physical" or "mental."

TREATMENT

As described in earlier chapters, clinical research has documented the efficacy of several interventions for pediatric depression,[24] including psychotherapeutic treatments such as cognitive behavior therapy (CBT) (see Chapter 8) and interpersonal psychotherapy (IPT) (see Chapter 9), and pharmacologic treatment with antidepressants, most notably SSRIs[25,26] (see Chapter 6). Despite a lack of large RCTs addressing the treatment of depression in physically ill youth, there is no evidence that depressed youth with comorbid physical illness are less likely to respond to proven treatments than their physically healthy counterparts. It is somewhat reassuring that depressed adults with chronic physical illness appear to respond to treatment at levels comparable with those of healthy adults.[27] Consequently, active treatment consistent with the safe and effective management of depression in physically healthy children should be pursued in youth struggling with comorbid physical disease.

EDUCATION

It can be argued that the first and most important step in treatment involves creating informed consumers of care by a thoughtful discussion with the patient and family of assessment findings, diagnostic formulation, and their implications. Even in situations of relative uncertainty, patients and families benefit from working with the clinician to arrive at a shared working hypothesis regarding the patient's difficulties. Psychoeducation is included in treatment guidelines[25] and is critical to meaningful informed consent. Relevant issues to address include rationale for treatment and targets, potential benefits and risks of specific treatment alternatives, expected response, time to efficacy, and follow-up plans and expectations, including safety planning and criteria to seek emergency care. The clinician should also learn more about the child's physical health condition and its management because this understanding is critical to establishing credibility and delivering quality care.

Psychoeducation is especially important because patients and families are often unaware of the impact that depression can have on the course and management of the comorbid physical disorder (i.e., that depression can have negative implications for the child's physical health). Many pediatric professionals view depression solely as a *reaction* to the stress of living with an acute or chronic physical disorder and an analogue to grief associated with the loss of ideal physical health. Although there is no doubt that depressive disorders may be triggered by adverse life events, some individuals are especially vulnerable to develop depression in response to negative life events.[28] It is often helpful for patients and referring clinicians to understand that the diagnosis of a depressive disorder may reflect a vulnerability to suffer from depression on a chronic and recurrent basis, analogous to physical disorders such as asthma. Highlighting that the risk of recurrence is high can shed light on the seriousness of depression as a distinct entity regardless of the physical disease status.[20] Depression cannot be dismissed as a *onetime reactive event* in the life of a child with chronic physical illness. There is no reason to believe that depressed youth with chronic illness are any less at risk for negative outcomes and recurrence than those without comorbid physical disease. Evaluation of this understanding may prevent miscommunication and unrealistic expectations that could become obstacles to treatment or sources of distress to patients and caregivers. Psychoeducation, supportive management, and family and school involvement should remain important across each phase of the treatment.

Patients and families need to understand what is known about available treatments, which often involves sharing our uncertainty with regard to treatment of depression in the context of a comorbid physical disease. In addition to understanding the risks and benefits, potential interventions should also be understood with regard to their cost to the family, not only financially, but in terms of time, effort, and overall burden (see Chapter 4). Clinicians should seek out and respect patient and family preferences while providing the information necessary for an informed choice. In particular, clinicians need to be clear about harmful options and should not agree to such treatment regardless of patient and family preference.

NONSOMATIC TREATMENTS

Psychotherapeutic interventions (see Chapters 8 to 11) are particularly appealing and often well received in the physically ill,[29] where the use of antidepressant medications can pose special challenges (see later). Nevertheless, psychotherapeutic treatments present their own difficulties, with the most troublesome being the relative lack of access to qualified therapists. The time commitment necessary for travel and participation in regularly scheduled sessions can be burdensome to families already taxed by the demands of caring for a child with a chronic physical illness.

Several psychotherapeutic approaches have been described, most often anecdotally. Psychodynamic and family systems therapies have been helpful in exploring the patient's and the family's understanding of the illness and its prognosis, health beliefs, treatment and adherence, and relationships among family members and with professionals. Although without empirical support, play therapy interventions have been suggested as ways to offer developmentally sound access to emotional information in younger children and assist with education about the illness, treatment, and associated stressors. Positive effects on coping and resiliency have been reported in association with construction of a narrative explanation of the child and family's illness experience.[30,31] Structured therapies such as IPT have been applied to adjustment to the psychosocial challenges imposed by the illness process.[32] Similarly, CBT focuses on the structured development of critical analysis skills, restructuring of maladaptive thought patterns, improvement of social and problem-solving skills, and the promotion of active coping.[25] A small study of children suffering from depression and inflammatory bowel disease documented improvements in measures of depression, global adjustment, and physical functioning with CBT.[33] Another small trial found CBT to be superior to treatment as usual for youth with inflammatory bowel disease and subsyndromal depression.[34] Although relatively small, these studies show that chronic physical illness need not preclude the efficacy of CBT.

Other psychotherapeutic interventions have been used but have not been specifically tested in the management of depression per se. These include target-specific behavioral plans to improve adherence and extinguish maladaptive behaviors,[35] self-management strategies such as relaxation training; guided imagery; biofeedback; and hypnosis, and distraction approaches using video games.[36] Group therapy and the use of social service and community support resources may be invaluable to patients and families by encouraging the development of support networks, ongoing learning and coping through modeling and sharing of experiences, and by providing access to resources (e.g., financial, legal-advocacy, respite, medical foster care).

SOMATIC TREATMENTS

GENERAL CONSIDERATIONS

Psychopharmacologic treatment is practically and culturally well suited to the management of depression in medical settings, yet it presents special challenges given the increased likelihood of medication-related adverse events and both pharmacodynamic and pharmacokinetic drug interactions (see Chapter 14). Clinicians, patients, and families must realize that risk is more difficult to gauge when psychoactive medications are used in physically ill children. Because RCTs of antidepressants in physically ill children are lacking, such treatment is largely presumptive and frequently off-label (see Chapter 4). Accordingly, treatment must be individualized, carefully considering the risk of drug–disease and drug–drug interactions, and reviewing prescribing information in light of the patient's physical illness and other medications. Table 21.1 lists a number of simple generic measures that can reduce the likelihood of medication-related adverse events. First, the lowest effective dose of medication should be used. Second, a practice of initiating medication at a low dose and titrating upward gradually is wise. Third, polypharmacy should be avoided whenever possible and the possibility of drug–drug interactions should be carefully considered if medications must be combined. Finally, the clinician should use existing knowledge to reduce the risk of adverse effects in vulnerable populations (e.g., choosing the antidepressant least likely to lower seizure threshold for a child with epilepsy).[37]

The issues in selecting medication for depressed physically ill youth have been summarized by Preskorn[38] and include safety, tolerability, efficacy, cost, and simplicity of administration, with *safety* the key issue. Because pediatric studies of antidepressants have typically been conducted with children and adolescents who are otherwise physically well, the risks associated with treating a child with a specific chronic physical disease and a particular constellation of medical treatments are generally unknown. One way of quantifying the relative safety and tolerability of a drug is by using the therapeutic index, which refers to the ratio of the median dose that produces toxic or untoward effects to that necessary to achieve the desired effect. High-risk situations can develop when using a psychoactive medication with a relatively narrow therapeutic index in a vulnerable child (e.g., lithium carbonate in a child with renal failure) or when a psychoactive medication is prescribed to a patient taking another drug with a narrow therapeutic index (e.g., transplant patient taking tacrolimus who is prescribed fluvoxamine, an SSRI that inhibits the cytochrome P450 enzyme critical to its metabolism).

An understanding of the pharmacodynamic and pharmacokinetic properties of medications is especially useful, not only in considering the safety of a particular psychoactive drug in a specific medical context, but also in thinking through other critical features related to medication choice such as tolerability and rapidity of onset. Such knowledge can provide some guidance despite the uncertainty associated with prescribing treatments that have not been studied scientifically in the population of interest. A detailed discussion of pharmacodynamics, pharmacokinetics, and the role of the cytochrome P450 enzyme system is presented in Chapter 14 and is not repeated here; state-of-the-art psychopharmacologic practice requires this knowledge be applied to individual clinical circumstances.[39] Given that pharmacodynamics are relatively fixed in terms of the biologic properties of the agent and the host, the clinician must manipulate either dose or aspects of pharmacokinetics to adjust

TABLE 21.1 MINIMIZING PSYCHOACTIVE MEDICATION ADVERSE EFFECTS IN PHYSICALLY ILL YOUTH

1. Review and document current and recent medications.
2. Understand the pharmacodynamic and pharmacokinetic profiles of each medication.
3. Use the lowest effective dose: Be patient.
4. Be judicious when titrating dose: "Start low and go slow."
5. Avoid polypharmacy when possible.
6. Cross-reference each medication to predict possible drug–drug interactions.
7. Know the patient and consider medication choice in light of existing physical disease.
8. Make use of pharmacogenetic information when available.

the concentration of drug at relevant sites of action over the course of treatment. Similarly, a medication's *tolerability* and *efficacy* can be influenced by both pharmacodynamic and pharmacokinetic factors. Psychoactive medications typically have more than one site of action, and the potential for adverse effects is generally proportional to the number of sites of action for a particular drug. Accordingly, drugs with multiple sites of action, such as tricyclic antidepressants, may be more difficult to manage in the physically ill child. The importance of *simplicity* in choosing a psychoactive medication for a physically ill child cannot be ignored because these children often struggle with complicated medical regimens daily, and adherence can be a real challenge.

It is equally important to understand the patient's disease state and its pathophysiology. Physical illness can alter the absorption, distribution, metabolism, and elimination of medication relative to the healthy state. This is particularly relevant when dealing with organ failure. Diseases that limit the absorptive surface of the gastrointestinal tract or that affect gut motility can interfere with drug absorption, as can certain foods or other medications taken concurrently. A drug's volume of distribution can be altered in dehydration, in edematous states such as congestive heart failure, or in circumstances that affect drug-protein binding, including hepatic disease, malnutrition, and protein-wasting states such as nephrosis. Drug clearance can be decreased in congestive heart failure because of reductions in renal or hepatic perfusion, and volume of distribution may be affected by fluid retention or diuretic treatment.

Because most psychoactive medications, and virtually all the antidepressants, are primarily metabolized in the liver, hepatic disease can be disconcerting for the pharmacologist. In patients with liver failure, it is wise to initially reduce the dose by 25% to 50%, and then titrate the dose according to clinical response and adverse effects.[23,24] Drug excretion may be compromised in both hepatic and renal failure. Renal disease is typically less of a hindrance because renal excretion is not especially relevant for most psychoactive agents; the most notable exception is lithium. Renal failure can nevertheless influence the excretion of bupropion, paroxetine, venlafaxine, and some tricyclic antidepressants, and it may warrant dosage adjustment. Medical interventions such as dialysis or plasmapheresis can also alter drug pharmacokinetics and availability and deserve attention.

SELECTIVE SEROTONIN REUPTAKE INHIBITORS

As described in Chapters 6 and 13, SSRIs are considered the first line of pharmacologic treatment for pediatric depression.[25] From the clinician's perspective, SSRIs share a similar safety and side-effect profile. Patient-specific choice of agent can be guided by factors such as past treatment history, administration route and schedule, side-effect profile, and potential interactions with current medications, with most of the latter mediated via the cytochrome P450 enzyme system.[23,40]

Adverse effects of SSRIs are often related to dose initiation and adjustment, and they usually are self-limiting. Density of 5HT receptors in the gastrointestinal tract makes this system particularly sensitive to SSRI-related side effects, including nausea, vomiting, dyspepsia, and changes in bowel habits. Central nervous system side effects include headache, insomnia, dizziness, daytime sedation, apathy, amotivation, and occasional extrapyramidal side effects such as tremor or akathisia.[40] Other common side effects include sexual dysfunction, weight gain, and hyperhidrosis. Clinically relevant adverse effects of SSRIs include platelet dysfunction associated with increased bleeding time and bruising. Although typically not problematic in healthy children, this is potentially risky in youth with clotting disorders, disorders of platelet function, and thrombocytopenia. Unfortunately, evidence-based guidelines about whether and how to proceed with SSRI treatment in a patient with one of these disorders are not available. There is weak evidence from epidemiologic data that the use of SSRIs may be associated with a small risk of gastrointestinal bleeding, primarily when used in combination with nonsteroidal anti-inflammatory drugs.[41] Although rare, severe or life-threatening side effects include the syndrome of inappropriate antidiuretic hormone, manic activation, suicidality, and the serotonin syndrome.[40,42]

Serotonin toxicity can develop across a spectrum, from mild adverse effects to the serotonin syndrome (see also Chapter 14). Symptoms include altered mental status (e.g., agitation, excitement, restlessness, confusion, and hallucinations), neuromuscular hyperactivity (e.g., tremor, myoclonus, hyperreflexia), and autonomic instability (fever, sweating, tachycardia, rapid changes in blood pressure), as well as loss of coordination, nausea, vomiting, and diarrhea. Serotonin syndrome associated with SSRI use is relatively unusual, developing most often when an SSRI is combined with another drug that affects serotonin metabolism such as dextromethorphan, the narcotic meperidine, monoamine oxidase inhibitors (MAOIs), other serotonergic antidepressants, buspirone, and serotonin precursors such as tryptophan.[37] Because triptan antimigraine drugs, such as sumatriptan, are serotonin receptor agonists, caution is suggested before prescribing these medications in combination with SSRIs or other serotonergic antidepressants. The risk of serotonin toxicity is difficult to quantify, so clinicians should discuss this with patients and families and balance the risks and benefits of combining potentially problematic agents.

OTHER ANTIDEPRESSANTS

As already highlighted, SSRIs are the best studied antidepressants for use in children and adolescents, but other classes of antidepressants may be used in pediatric settings. This is most likely to occur with cases of treatment-resistant depression, when SSRIs are poorly tolerated, or in the presence of other symptoms or disorders in association with depression that may warrant a novel approach. Serotonin norepinephrine reuptake inhibitors (SNRIs) include *venlafaxine* and *duloxetine* and are agents that inhibit the presynaptic reuptake of norepinephrine, serotonin, and, to a lesser extent, dopamine. Venlafaxine is currently approved in the United States for the treatment of major depressive disorder in adults. Venlafaxine was recently studied as a treatment for depressed adolescents who had failed treatment with an SSRI, but it offered no special benefit over switching to a different SSRI, with the added risk of elevation in blood pressure and heart rate.[43] Also, the drug's short half-life may be responsible for a tendency to experience discontinuation symptoms after missed doses or dose reductions.[44] Duloxetine is another SNRI approved in the United States for the treatment of major depressive disorder, generalized anxiety disorder, and diabetic neuropathic pain in adults, and for treatment of stress-related urinary incontinence in other countries. Other drugs in this class are currently only marketed outside of the United States (e.g., milnacipran) or are in different stages of development (e.g. bicifadine, desvenlafaxine).

Mirtazapine is a novel antidepressant with a unique pharmacodynamic signature and little impact on the P450 enzyme system. The drug presumably boosts both serotonin and norepinephrine by blocking presynaptic α_2 adrenergic receptors, and also blocks HT2A, HT2C, HT3 serotonin receptors, and H1 histamine receptors. Its tendency to increase appetite and cause weight gain may be exploited in the treatment of depressed youth with anorexia owing to physical disease, and its sedating properties can be useful in patients with insomnia. Mirtazapine's ability to block the serotonin HT_3 receptor make it worthy of consideration in depressed patients struggling with nausea and gastrointestinal discomfort.

Bupropion is presumed to exert its mechanism of action by inhibiting presynaptic norepinephrine and dopaminergic reuptake, and it is an inhibitor of CYP2D6.[45] It should be used with caution in patients taking dopaminergic drugs such as levodopa or amantadine. It is generally considered to be energizing and therefore of potential benefit in patients with melancholic features, apathy, or fatigue. Its dopaminergic actions may also be of use in treating symptoms of inattention and cognitive slowing. Particular caution is warranted when administering bupropion to patients with epilepsy and bulimia nervosa because of an increased risk of lowering seizure threshold. In adults, bupropion has a lower risk of manic activation in patients with bipolar depression when compared with venlafaxine but not when compared with other SSRIs such as sertraline[46] or paroxetine.[47] Such comparative studies are not currently available in children.

Based on adult data, some clinicians have favored the use of *tricyclic antidepressants* (TCAs) for children with pain syndromes,[42,48] but their use in patients with comorbid depression is difficult to justify given that existing research has not found TCAs to be superior to placebo in the treatment of pediatric depression. Their use in physically ill children is complicated by effects on cardiac conduction, potential lethality in overdose, and rare reports of sudden death.[49] Heart rate, blood pressure, and electrocardiogram should be obtained at baseline and monitored during treatment if TCAs are used, particularly in the physically ill child.[50] TCAs should be avoided in youth with cardiac disease and conduction abnormalities.

Experience with MAOIs in pediatric depression is limited. The numerous potential side effects and necessary dietary and lifestyle restrictions are difficult to justify in all but the most severe cases of treatment refractory depression, and the complexities associated with their use make them undesirable as agents for children with comorbid physical illness. The potential for serious serotonin syndrome is great when MAOIs are combined with other serotonergic drugs.

TABLE 21.2 ADJUNCTIVE AGENTS

Agent	Target Symptoms	Potential Additional Advantage
Anticonvulsants	Bipolar disorder, treatment-resistant depression, aggression	Epilepsy, migraine prophylaxis
Antipsychotics	Bipolar disorder, treatment-resistant depression, aggression, psychosis	Acute and Intractable migraine, cyclic vomiting, nausea, tics
Benzodiazepines	Anxiety, agitation	Insomnia, procedural anxiety, nausea, muscular spasms, alcohol withdrawal, catatonia
Lithium	Bipolar disorder, treatment-resistant depression, aggression	Cluster headache prophylaxis, mobilization of neutrophils
Stimulants	Inattention, hyperactivity, impulsivity, treatment-resistant depression	Fatigue, adjunct to opiates in pain, compulsive eating/obesity, circadian rhythm dysregulation

OTHER AGENTS

Other psychopharmacologic agents are commonly used in depressed youth, who often suffer from a variety of comorbid psychiatric disorders, particularly anxiety. Selection is guided by factors including target symptoms, urgency of response, underlying pathology, and potential for drug–drug or drug–disease interactions. Table 21.2 lists a number of agents, target symptoms, and potential advantages.

Benzodiazepines are commonly used to treat comorbid anxiety or agitation in depressed youth. Benzodiazepines can suppress respiratory drive; this is more of an issue at higher doses, when used parenterally, or when combined with other drugs that also suppress respiratory drive.

Lamotrigine is a voltage-sensitive sodium channel antagonist that inhibits glutamate and aspartate release. It has been used as an anticonvulsant and mood stabilizer and, more recently, as a treatment for bipolar depression and neuropathic pain, as well as an adjunctive treatment for major depression. Its unique properties may be exploited in youth with comorbid epilepsy or chronic pain syndromes, but caution must be exercised given rare reports of sudden death, rare blood dyscrasias, and the risk of life threatening skin rash associated with Stevens-Johnson syndrome.

Lithium salts are commonly used in the treatment of bipolar disorder and as augmentation agents in treatment for refractory depression. Lithium is one of the few psychoactive drugs excreted virtually unchanged in the urine. It is subject to dialysis owing to its small molecular size. With careful blood-level monitoring, it can be administered as a single dose just after dialysis in patients with renal failure. Because of the drug's relatively narrow therapeutic index, close monitoring is particularly important. Lithium can also be associated with cardiac conduction abnormalities, arrhythmias, syncope, and T-wave flattening on electrocardiogram.[51] Dehydration poses a special risk to patients taking lithium because it reduces its volume of distribution and increases the serum level (all other things being equal). Edematous states increase the volume of distribution for lithium.[52] Lithium can produce nephrogenic diabetes insipidus at the level of the renal tubule and decrease renal concentration.[47] Caution is also warranted when lithium is prescribed to youth with cystic fibrosis, where the core genetic defect involves ion channels important to electrolyte transport.[53]

COMMON CLINICAL SCENARIOS

CARDIOVASCULAR DISEASE

Cardiac problems pose special challenges, particularly regarding the risk of conduction abnormalities. Congenital prolongation of the QTc is associated with higher risk of sudden death in its own right; the use of psychoactive medications that prolong the QTc directly or indirectly can prove catastrophic in these cases. Drugs of special concern include traditional antipsychotics and atypical antipsychotics; both classes are associated with lengthening of the QT interval and the development of multifocal ventricular tachycardia followed by ventricular fibrillation and sudden death. Other psychoactive medications that deserve special attention include stimulants, TCAs, and SNRIs. SSRIs are relatively benign drugs from the cardiovascular perspective but are associated with a very modest slowing of heart rate and, rarely, bradycardia.[54] TCAs are class I antiarrhythmics, influence conduction, increase heart rate, and blood pressure; they are associated with sudden death and are lethal in overdose.[49] SNRIs and bupropion are associated with increases in blood pressure and heart rate. Conduction abnormalities are also associated with the use of lithium, making electrocardiographic monitoring necessary when used in youth with cardiovascular disease.[51]

DIABETES

Elevated rates of psychiatric comorbidity are consistently found in diabetic youth compared with the physically well.[18,55] In adults, depression has been found to be an independent risk factor for type 2 diabetes mellitus, and depression in diabetic patients is associated with worsening dietary and medication adherence, as well as poor metabolic control and higher usage costs.[56] Treatment with SSRIs is associated with improved glycemic control in diabetic adults and may be associated with some risk of hypoglycemia during the initial phase of treatment.[57] The risk/benefit ratio seems to favor the use of SSRIs for the treatment of depression in diabetic patients.[58] TCAs and MAOIs are associated with carbohydrate craving and severe hypoglycemia, respectively. Atypical antipsychotics are problematic in the diabetic population given their association with increased appetite, weight gain, and deterioration of glycemic control.

Psychotherapeutic interventions are also worthy of consideration in this population. A pilot study by Channon and colleagues[59] showed a modest but sustained decrease in HbA1c levels as well as decreased fear of hypoglycemia in adolescents who underwent a course of motivational interviewing, suggesting promise for this intervention in the education and treatment of this challenging population.

PAIN

Pain is a complex sensory and emotional experience related to actual or potential tissue damage or described as representative of such damage.[60,61] Functional pain symptoms are associated with depressive disorders across the lifespan.[4,62] Depressive symptoms appear to mediate the course of pain symptoms in youth with chronic pain caused by juvenile rheumatoid arthritis[63] and are associated with functional disability.[64] Serotonergic systems are probably involved in centrally mediated pain modulation and are implicated in disorders commonly associated with depression such as irritable bowel syndrome, fibromyalgia, and migraine.[36] The experience of pain is subjective and may be influenced by a myriad of "nonphysiologic" factors such as cognitions, meanings, personality, cultural and family dynamics, and potential gains. Depression can influence the pain experience and the resultant disability. For example, it can be postulated that negative cognitions associated with depressive states may increase the perception of pain, sense of urgency, and disability. The anergia and anhedonia associated with depression can also impact the pain sufferer's ability to use distraction strategies or adhere to adjunctive treatments, such as physical therapy, therefore impairing recovery. Cumulative evidence points toward the need to screen for depression or other psychiatric symptoms during assessment and treatment of pain.

Ideally, the treatment of pain should be multimodal and may include pharmacologic and psychotherapeutic interventions with a focus on comfort and return of function.[48,60] Antidepressant treatment may reduce the need for ongoing use of analgesics. Antidepressants, anticonvulsants, stimulants, and antipsychotics have all been employed to this end. SSRIs can be of use, particularly in the setting of underlying depression and anxiety. Because serotonergic neurotransmission plays an important role in gut sensation in functional gastrointestinal disorders and in nausea, agents impacting on serotonin may be worthy of study in affected populations.

An open trial of the SSRI citalopram found it to be a promising treatment for youth with functional abdominal pain, and it noted concomitant improvements in ratings of anxiety, depressive, and other somatic symptoms.[4] RCTs are needed to explore the usefulness of SSRIs in this population. Clinical and anecdotal experience as well as data from adult studies[65,66] point to the potential benefit of SNRIs in the treatment of functional pain syndromes, but pediatric experience is quite limited.[67] SSRIs and SNRIs have also been used in the preventive treatment of migraine[68,69] with varying efficacy. TCAs have been extensively used in adults in the treatment of neuropathic and non-neuropathic pain. Neuropathic pain is a type of pain caused by dysfunction in the peripheral or central nervous system, and it is distinguished from nociceptive or non-neuropathic pain— essentially pain caused by stimulation of pain receptors, which is usually the result of tissue damage. Proposed mechanisms of action for the TCAs in pain include synergistic relationship with opiates as well as direct analgesic effects. Their poor effectiveness in child depression and lethality potential in overdose limit their use in pediatric pain patients. Anticonvulsants may be useful in neuropathic pain, and as previously mentioned, they can provide effective prophylaxis in migraine.

Behavior modification focusing on regulatory functions such as sleep and exercise[70,71] and cognitive-behavioral therapy have been found useful in the treatment of chronic migraines in adults.[72] Anecdotal evidence points toward their effectiveness as adjuvant treatment in young patients.

EPILEPSY

Children with epilepsy are at significant increased risk of comorbid psychiatric illness, including mood disorders,[73] with rates of psychopathology estimated at 37% to 77%.[74] Epileptic children with low cognitive functioning and family risk factors are at higher risk.[74] Epidemiologic studies have reported associations between epilepsy in children, depression[30,73,74] and suicidal ideation.[75] Children with epilepsy treated with phenobarbital experience higher rates of major depression and suicidal ideation than those treated with other antiepileptic agents.[76–78]

Using the lowest possible dose of psychoactive medication is recommended in pediatric epilepsy because drug-induced seizures are generally dose related. SSRIs are considered relatively safe in the treatment of depression and anxiety in children with epilepsy and the preferred first-line agents.[23,73,74] Some have questioned whether active treatment of depression in epileptic children may actually improve seizure control,[23] and fluoxetine is reported to have anticonvulsant properties.[79] Lithium is reported to lower seizure threshold. Among the atypical antipsychotic medications, the risk of seizures appears to be highest with clozapine, and chlorpromazine is regarded as having the highest risk among the traditional antipsychotics.[38] Tramadol (an atypical opioid analgesic) in combination with antidepressants increases the risk of seizures.

Although a discussion regarding all potential interactions with antiepileptic agents is beyond the scope of this chapter, factors to consider when choosing a psychotropic agent include whether the drug:

- Interferes with the pharmacodynamics or pharmacokinetics of prescribed antiepileptic medication.
- Is a γ-aminobutyric acid (GABA) antagonist—in general, low potential for GABA antagonism is desirable.
- Interferes with antiepileptic drug levels.
- Offers the capacity for slow titration because lowering of seizure threshold is usually a dose-related phenomenon.

PULMONARY DISEASE

Changes in blood oxygenation and level of carbon dioxide can affect pharmacokinetics via changes in serum pH. Benzodiazepines have the potential to induce respiratory depression and hypercabia (high levels of carbon dioxide in the circulating blood) in patients with pulmonary disease, but use in such patients suffering from severe anxiety must be balanced with the fact that reduction in anxiety may decrease the work of breathing, relax the patient, and sometimes aid in weaning patients from mechanical ventilation. Higher doses, concurrent use with opiates, and intravenous administration carry the greater risk; lorazepam is the preferred agent.

Although traditional antipsychotics are not free of respiratory effects, atypical antipsychotics may be used in the short-term management of anxiety in hospitalized patients. SSRIs and buspirone are generally preferred for the chronic management of anxiety in patients with pulmonary disease because these drugs are not associated with respiratory depression. Caution should be exercised in using TCAs in youth with asthma.

PREMENSTRUAL SYNDROME AND PREMENSTRUAL DYSPHORIC DISORDER

Premenstrual symptoms are extremely prevalent in females of reproductive age, with up to 90% reporting at least one emotional or physical symptom during the luteal phase of the menstrual cycle. A subset of approximately 10% present with a constellation of symptoms severe enough to meet criteria for premenstrual dysphoric disorder.[80] Various hormonal and nonhormonal pathophysiologic mechanisms have been proposed, and most likely the disorder represents a phenotypical endpoint to a myriad of genotypes and endogenous and environmental factors.

A variety of symptom criteria and definitions have been proposed for the diagnosis of premenstrual syndrome (PMS) or premenstrual dysphoric disorder,[81] including diagnostic criteria for further study in *DSM-IV*.[21] In *ICD-10*[22] it is listed as *premenstrual tension syndrome* in Chapter XIV, on the subject of diseases of the genitourinary system. To make this diagnosis, most experts agree that symptoms must be documented through several menstrual cycles, are severe enough to cause impairment, include at least one physical and one emotional symptom, occur during the luteal phase of the menstrual cycle, and are followed by marked improvement or resolution after ovulation. The diagnosis must be exclusive of other organic pathology or exacerbation of other psychiatric illness.

Assessment of patients who complain of premenstrual symptoms should include (1) a review of past medical and reproductive history; (2) physical examination—to rule out underlying conditions that may be exacerbated with menstrual changes such as endometriosis, infections, migraines, and other neurologic disorders; and (3) careful screening for underlying psychiatric disorders that may also show symptom exacerbations with menstrual changes. Patients should be encouraged to keep prospective records of symptoms for a few menstrual cycles and, if indicated, continue recording during treatment. Referral to experienced gynecology or endocrinology colleagues is recommended if underlying hormonal dysregulation is suspected or if specialized treatment is required.

Treatment is guided by the severity of symptoms and impairment. Mild to moderate symptoms can be managed with supportive measures including sleep hygiene, nutritional supplementation, moderate aerobic exercise, and judicious use of analgesics. Suppression of ovulation with oral contraceptives shows the best results on both mood and physical symptoms with use of longer hormonal dosing cycles (i.e., 24/4).[82,83] Adolescent patients who opt for the use of oral contraceptives should be counseled regarding the need for adequate exercise and nutritional intake, particularly calcium and vitamin D, to address increased risk of osteoporosis. SSRIs are effective in decreasing PMS symptoms within days of initiating treatment, and their use during the luteal phase (starting 1 to 2 weeks before anticipated menses and stopping following onset of menses) is proven effective and well tolerated; small studies have shown similar results in adolescents.[84] Judicious use of anxiolytics can target specific symptoms. Referral to specialized clinicians may be considered in cases without adequate response to first-line agents such as contraceptives, SSRIs, and supportive measures, although treatments such as gonadotropin-releasing hormone agonists or surgical interventions are generally not considered appropriate in adolescents.[84]

RESOURCES FOR PATIENTS AND PARENTS

National Alliance on Mental Illness: http://www.nami.org/
Familydoctor.org from the American Academy of Family Physicians: http://familydoctor.org/online/
    famdocen/home/common/mentalhealth.html
Parentmedguide.org

RESOURCES FOR PROFESSIONALS

American Academy of Psychosomatic Medicine: http://www.psychosomatic.org/
Academy of Psychosomatic Medicine (links and resources): http://www.apm.org/links.shtml

REFERENCES

1. LeBlanc LA, Goldsmith T, Patel DL. Behavioral aspects of chronic illness in children and adolescents. *Pediatr Clin N Am*. 2003;50:859–878.
2. American Academy of Pediatrics. Psychosocial risks of chronic health conditions in childhood and adolescence. Committee on Children with Disabilities and Committee on Psychosocial Aspects of Child and Family Health. *Pediatrics*. 1993;92:876–878.

3. Gortmaker SL, Walker DK, Weitzman M, et al. Chronic conditions, socioeconomic risks, and behavioral problems in children and adolescents. *Pediatrics*. 1990;85:267–276.
4. Campo JV, Perel J, Lucas A, et al. Citalopram treatment of pediatric recurrent abdominal pain and comorbid internalizing disorders: an exploratory study. *J Am Acad Child Adolesc Psychiatry*. 2004;43:1234–1242.
5. Liakopoulou-Kairis M, Alifieraki T, Protagora D, et al. Recurrent abdominal pain and headache—psychopathology, life events, and family functioning. *Eur Child Adolesc Psychiatry*. 2002;11:115–22.
6. Moussavi S, Chatterji S, Verdes E, et al. Depression, chronic diseases, and decrements in health: results from the World Health Surveys. *Lancet*. 2007;370:851–858.
7. Merikangas KR, Stevens DE. Comorbidity of migraine and psychiatric disorders. *Neurol Clin*. 1997;15:115–123.
8. Wamboldt MZ, Schmitz S, Mrazek D. Genetic association between atopy and behavioral symptoms in middle childhood. *J Child Psychol Psychiatry*. 1998;39:1007–1016.
9. Rutter M, Graham P, Yule W. *A Neuropsychiatric Study in Childhood*. Philadelphia: JB Lippincott; 1970.
10. Rutter M, Tizard J, Whitmore K. *Education, Health, and Behavior*. London: Longman; 1970.
11. McDaniel JS, Brown FW, Cole SA. Assessment of depression and grief reactions in the medically ill. In: Stodudemiere A, Fogel BS, Greenberg DB, eds. *Psychiatric Care of the Medical Patient*. Oxford, UK: Oxford University Press; 2000:149–164.
12. DiMatteo MR, Lepper HS, Croghan TW. Depression is a risk factor for noncompliance with medical treatment: meta-analysis of the effects of anxiety and depression on patient adherence. *Arch Intern Med*. 2000;160:2101–2107.
13. Garrison MM, Katon WJ, Richardson LP. The impact of psychiatric comorbidities on readmissions for diabetes in youth. *Diabetes Care*. 2005;28:2150–2154.
14. Strunk R. Deaths from asthma in childhood: patterns before and after professional intervention. *Pediatr Asthma Allergy Immunol*. 1987;1:5–13.
15. Lernmark B, Persson B, Fisher L, et al. Symptoms of depression are important to psychological adaptation and metabolic control in children with diabetes mellitus. *Diabetic Med*. 1999;16:14–22.
16. Dantzer C, Swendsen J, Maurice-Tison S, et al. Anxiety and depression in juvenile diabetes: a critical review. *Clin Psychol Rev*. 2003;23:787–800.
17. Katon WJ. Clinical and health service relationships between major depression, depressive symptoms, and general medical illness. *Biol Psychiatry*. 2003;54:216–226.
18. Kovacs M, Goldston D, Obrosky DS, et al. Psychiatric disorders in youths with IDDM: rates and risk factors. *Diabetes Care*. 1997;20:36–44.
19. Kovacs M, Mukerji P, Drash A, et al. Biomedical and psychiatric risk factors for retinopathy among children with IDDM. *Diabetes Care*. 1995;18:1592–1599.
20. Birmaher B, Ryan N, Williamson D, et al. Childhood and adolescent depression: a review of the past 10 years. Part I. *J Am Acad Child Adolesc Psychiatry*. 1996;35:1427–1439.
21. American Psychiatric Association. *Diagnostic and Statistical Manual of Mental Disorders, 4th edition (DSM-IV)*. Washington, DC: Author; 1994.
22. World Health Organization. *International Statistical Classification of Diseases and Health Related Problems ICD-10*. 2nd ed. Geneva: World Health Organization; 2004.
23. Campo JV, Perel JM. Pediatric psychopharmacology in the consultation-liaison setting. In: Rosenberg DR, Davanzo PA, Gershon S, eds. *Pharmacotherapy for Child and Adolescent Psychiatric Disorders*. 2nd ed. New York: Marcel Dekker; 2002:635–678.
24. Campo JV. Disorders primarily seen in general medical settings. In: Findling R, ed. *Clinical Manual of Child and Adolescent Psychopharmacology*. Arlington, Va: American Psychiatric Publishing; 2007.
25. Birmaher B, Brent D, AACAP Work Group on Quality Issues. Practice parameter for the assessment and treatment of children and adolescents with depressive disorders. *J Am Acad Child Adolesc Psychiatry*. 2007; 46:1503–1526.
26. Bridge JA, Iyengar S, Salary CB, et al. Clinical response and risk for reported suicidal ideation and suicide attempts in pediatric antidepressant treatment: a meta-analysis of randomized controlled trials. *JAMA*. 2007; 297:1683–1696.
27. Harpole LH, Williams JW Jr, Olsen MK, et al. Improving depression outcomes in older adults with comorbid medical illness. *Gen Hosp Psychiatry*. 2005;27:4–12.
28. Caspi A, Sugden K, Moffitt TE, et al. Influence of life stress on depression: moderation by a polymorphism in the 5-HTT gene. *Science*. 2003;301:386–389.
29. Asarnow JR, Jaycox LH, Duan N, et al. Effectiveness of a quality improvement intervention for adolescent depression in primary care clinics: a randomized controlled trial. *JAMA*. 2005;293:311–319.
30. Szigethy E, Whitton SW, Levy-Warren A, et al. Cognitive-behavioral therapy for depression in adolescents with inflammatory bowel disease: a pilot study. *J Am Acad Child Adolesc Psychiatry*. 2004;43:1469–1477.
31. Focht L, Beardslee WR. "Speech after long silence:" the use of narrative therapy in a preventive intervention for children of parents with affective disorder. *Fam Process*. 1996;35:407–422.
32. Markowitz JC, Kocsis JH, Fishman B, et al. Treatment of depressive symptoms in human immunodeficiency virus-positive patients. *Arch Gen Psychiatry*. 1998;55:452–457.

33. Szigethy EM, Whitton S, Levy-Warren A, et al. Depressive symptoms and inflammatory bowel disease in children and adolescents: a cross-sectional study. *J Pediatr Gastroenterol Nutr.* 2004;39:395–403.

34. Szigethy E, Kenney E, Carpenter J, et al. Cognitive-behavioral therapy for adolescents with inflammatory bowel disease and subsyndromal depression. *J Am Acad Child Adolesc Psychiatry.* 2007;46:1290–1298.

35. Shaw RJ, DeMaso DR. *Clinical Manual of Pediatric Psychosomatic Medicine: Mental Health Consultation with Physically Ill Children and Adolescents.* Arlington, VA: American Psychiatric Publishing; 2006:239.

36. Vasterling J, Jenkings RA, Tope DM, et al. Cognitive distraction and relaxation training for the control of side effects due to cancer chemotherapy. *J Behav Med.* 2003;16:65–80.

37. Haddad PM, Dursun SM. Neurological complications of psychiatric drugs: clinical features and management. *Hum Psychopharmacol.* 2008;23(suppl 1):15–26.

38. Preskorn SH. *Outpatient Management of Depression: A Guide for the Primary-Care Practitioner.* 2nd ed. West Islip, NY: Professional Communications; 1999.

39. Oesterheld JR, Flockhart DA. Pharmacokinetics II: cytochrome P450-mediated drug interactions. In: Martin A, Scahill L, Charney DS, et al., eds. *Pediatric Psychopharmacology: Principles and Practice.* New York: Oxford University Press; 2003:54–66.

40. Chiue S, Leonard HL. Antidepressants I: Selective serotonin reuptake inhibitors. In: Martin A, Scahill L, Charney DS, et al., eds. *Pediatric Psychopharmacology: Principles and Practice.* New York, NY: Oxford University Press; 2003:274–283.

41. Yuan Y, Tsoi K, Hunt RH. Selective serotonin reuptake inhibitors and risk of upper GI bleeding: confusion or confounding? *Am J Med.* 2006;119:719–727.

42. Stoddard FJ, Usher CT, Abrams AN. Psychopharmacology in pediatric critical care. *Child Adolesc Psychiatr Clin N Am.* 2006;15:611–655.

43. Brent D, Emslie G, Clarke G, et al. Switching to another SSRI or to venlafaxine with or without cognitive behavioral therapy for adolescents with SSRI-resistant depression: the TORDIA randomized controlled trial. *JAMA.* 2008;299:901–913.

44. Fava M, Mulroy R, Alpert J, et al. Emergence of adverse events following discontinuation of treatment with extended-release venlafaxine. *Am J Psychiatry.* 1997;154:1760–1762.

45. Stahl SM. *Essential Psychopharmacology: The Prescribers' Guide.* Cambridge, UK: Cambridge University Press; 2005:37–42.

46. Post RM, Altshuler LL, Leverich GS, et al. Mood switch in bipolar depression: comparison of adjunctive venlafaxine, bupropion, and sertraline. *Br J Psychiatry.* 2006;189:124–131.

47. Sachs GS, Nierenberg AA, Calibrese JR, et al. Effectiveness of adjunctive antidepressant treatment for bipolar depression. *N Engl J Med.* 2007;356:1711–1722.

48. Shaw RJ, DeMaso DR. *Clinical Manual of Pediatric Psychosomatic Medicine: Mental Health Consultation with Physically Ill Children and Adolescents.* Arlington, Va: American Psychiatric Publishing; 2006:169–203.

49. Geller B, Reising D, Leonard HL, et al. Critical review of tricyclic antidepressant use in children and adolescents. *J Am Acad Child Adolesc Psychiatry.* 1999;38:513–516.

50. Gundersen K, Geller B. Antidepressants II: tricyclic agents. In: Martin A, Scahill L, Charney DS, et al., eds. *Pediatric Psychopharmacology: Principles and Practice.* New York: Oxford University Press; 2003:284–294.

51. Dunner DL. Optimizing lithium treatment. *J Clin Psychiatry.* 2000;61(suppl 9):76–81.

52. Rubey RN. Lydiard RB. Pharmacological treatment of anxiety in the medically ill patient. *Semin Clin Neuropsychiatry.* 1999;4:133–147.

53. Brager NP, Campbell NR, Reisch H, et al. Reduced renal fractional excretion of lithium in cystic fibrosis. *Br J Clin Pharmacol.* 1996;41:157–159.

54. Settle EC Jr. Antidepressant drugs: disturbing and potentially dangerous adverse effects. *J Clin Psychiatry.* 1998;59(suppl 16):25–30, 40–42.

55. Davies S, Heyman I, Goodman R. A population survey of mental health problems in children with epilepsy. *Dev Med Child Neurol.* 2003;45:292–295.

56. Fenton WS, Stover ES. Mood disorders: cardiovascular and diabetes comorbidity. *Curr Opin Psychiatry.* 2006;19:421–427.

57. Carney C. Diabetes mellitus and major depressive disorder: an overview of prevalence, complication and treatment. *Depress Anxiety.* 1998;7:149–157.

58. Goodnick PJ, Henry JH, Buki VM. Treatment of depression in patients with diabetes mellitus. *J Clin Psychiatry.* 1995;56:128–135.

59. Channon S, Smith VJ, Gregory JW. A pilot study of motivational interviewing in adolescents with diabetes. *Arch Dis Child.* 2003;88:680–683.

60. McCulloch R, Collins JJ. Pain in children who have life-limiting conditions. *Child Adolesc Psychiatr Clin N Am.* 2006;15:657–682.

61. Basbaum AI, Jessell TM. The perception of pain. In: Kandel ER, Schwartz JH, Jessell TM, eds. *Principles of Neural Science.* 4th ed. New York: McGraw-Hill; 2000:472–491.

62. Kroenke K. Somatoform disorders and recent diagnostic controversies. *Psychiatr Clin N Am.* 2007;30:593–619.

63. Hoff AL, Palermo TM, Schluchter M, et al. Longitudinal relationships of depressive symptoms to pain intensity and functional disability among children with disease-related pain. *J Pediatr Psychol*. 2006;31: 1046–1056.

64. Kashikar-Zuck S, Goldschneider KR, Powers SW, et al. Depression and functional disability in chronic pediatric pain. *Clin J Pain*. 2001;17:341–349.

65. Kroenke K, Messina N, Benattia I, et al. Venlafaxine extended release in the short-term treatment of depressed and anxious primary care patients with multisomatoform disorder. *J Clin Psychiatry*. 2006;67:72–80.

66. Brannan SK, Mallinckrodt CH, Brown EB, et al. Duloxetine 60 mg once-daily in the treatment of painful physical symptoms in patients with major depressive disorder. *J Psychiatr Res*. 2005;39:43–53.

67. Desarkar P, Das A, Sinha VK. Duloxetine for childhood depression with pain and dissociative symptoms. *Eur Child Adolesc Psychiatry*. 2006;15:496–499.

68. Punay NC, Couch JR. Antidepressants in the treatment of migraine headache. *Curr Pain Headache Rep*. 2003;7:51–54.

69. Rapoport AM, Bigal ME. Preventive migraine therapy: what is new? *Neurol Sci*. 2004;25:S177–S185.

70. Calhoun AH, Ford S. Behavioral sleep modification may revert transformed migraine to episodic migraine. *Headache*. 2007;47:1178–1183.

71. Sandor PS, Afra J. Nonpharmacologic treatment of migraine. *Curr Pain Headache Rep*. 2005;9:202–205.

72. Kropp P, Gerber WD, Keinath-Specht A, et al. Behavioral treatment in migraine. Cognitive-behavioral therapy and blood-volume-pulse biofeedback: a cross-over study with a two-year follow-up. *Funct Neurol*. 1997;12:17–24.

73. Pellock JM. Understanding comorbidities affecting children with epilepsy. *Neurology*. 2004;62:S17–S23.

74. Plioplys S, Dunn DW, Caplan R. 10-year research update review: psychiatric problems in children with epilepsy. *J Am Acad Child Adolesc Psychiatry*. 2007;46:1389–1402.

75. Caplan R, Siddarth P, Gurbani S, et al. Depression and anxiety in pediatric epilepsy. *Epilepsia*. 2005;46:720–730.

76. Brent DA, Crumrine PA, Varma RR, et al. Phenobarbital treatment and major depressive disorder in children with epilepsy. *Pediatrics*. 1987;80:909–917.

77. Brent DA, Crumrine PK, Varma R, et al. Phenobarbital treatment and major depressive disorder in children with epilepsy: a naturalistic follow-up. *Pediatrics*. 1990;85:1086–1091.

78. Campbell JJ, McNamara ME. A case of phenobarbital behavioral toxicity presenting as a menstrually related mood disorder. *J Clin Psychiatry*. 1993;54:441.

79. Favale E, Rubino V, Mainardi P, et al. Anticonvulsant effect of fluoxetine in humans. *Neurology*. 1995;45: 1926–1927.

80. Mishell DR. Premenstrual disorders: epidemiology and disease burden. *Am J Manage Care*. 2005;11: S473–S479.

81. American College of Obstetrics and Gynecology. *Practice Bulletin: Premenstrual Syndrome*. Washington, DC: American College of Obstetrics and Gynecology; 2000:15.

82. Yonkers, KA, Brown C, Pearlstein TB, et al. Efficacy of a new low dose oral contraceptive with drospirenone in premenstrual dysphoric disorder. *Obstet Gynecol*. 2005;106:492–501.

83. Sillem M, Schneidereit R, Heithecker R, et al. Use of an oral contraceptive containing drospirenone in an extended regimen. *Eur J Contracep Reprod Health Care*. 2003;8:162–169.

84. Braverman PK. Premenstrual syndrome and premenstrual dysphoric disorder. *J Pediatr Adolesce Gynecol*. 2007;20:3–12.

Treating Depression in the Developmentally Disabled: Intellectual Disability and Pervasive Developmental Disorders[a]

BRUCE J. TONGE, MICHAEL GORDON, AND GLENN A. MELVIN

KEY POINTS

- Many depressed children and adolescents with mild intellectual disability (ID) are able to report on their internal world and, with prompting, able to describe depressive symptoms such as sadness, hopelessness, and suicidal thinking.
- The ability of children and adolescents with pervasive developmental disorders (PDD) to report depressive symptoms depends in part on their overall level of functioning, language skills, and cognitive ability.
- In youth with moderate to severe ID or moderate to severe PDD, observations of clinicians and caregivers are very important for making the diagnosis of depression.
- An understanding of the social factors, changes to the young person's environment, and possible intercurrent medical problems is critical in developing a treatment plan.
- There are no randomized control trials using antidepressant medication for the treatment of major depression in youth with ID or PDD.
- Based on evidence from open trials, case reports, and extrapolation of results from depressed nonintellectually disabled children, selective serotonin reuptake inhibitors (SSRIs) appear to be the antidepressants of choice for use in depressed youth with ID and PDD. The same can be said about psychosocial interventions, especially CBT and supportive therapy.
- Before beginning a pharmacologic treatment, clear target symptoms, a framework for monitoring response, and the duration of the medication trial should be established and possible side effects explained.
- Depressed youth with PDD appear to be more vulnerable to side effects of SSRIs, particularly agitation and disinhibition.
- When treating these youth, clinicians should begin with a low dose, increase the dose slowly, and monitor side effects carefully.

Introduction *This chapter considers the assessment and treatment of depression in young people with developmental disabilities; this term is used to mean both intellectual disability (ID) and pervasive developmental disorders (PDD). DSM-IV and ICD-10 use "mental retardation" to describe individuals with significantly low intellectual functioning, but we favor "intellectual disability," which is the preferred term by the National Association for the Dually Diagnosed in the United States and is increasingly used elsewhere, for example in the United Kingdom, Canada, and Australia.[1] Autism, Asperger disorder, and PDD not otherwise specified are referred to as*

[a]This chapter was supported by the research grants made available by NHMRC (Australia) 113844 and NIM/NIMH 61809–06.

pervasive developmental disorders (PDDs) or autism spectrum disorders. Although ID and PDD are considered separately in this chapter, there is a significant overlap, with approximately 75% of individuals with autistic spectrum disorders suffering from ID.[2]

Depression is a common and treatable condition that is underrecognized in developmentally disabled youth. However, there is limited knowledge on the typical symptoms of depression seen in this group, particularly in those with more profound disabilities, and on effective treatments. In children and adolescents with autism spectrum disorders, the overall level of depressive symptoms is generally high, peaking in early adolescence, and lessening to some extent in late adolescence.[3]

DEPRESSION AND INTELLECTUAL DISABILITY

ID is diagnosed in people whose standardized intelligence quotient (IQ) is less than two standard deviations below the mean (equivalent to an IQ of 70), who also show limitations in daily living skills, and with an onset before 18 years of age.[4] ID is classified into four categories based on IQ score: mild (IQ 50–55 to 70), moderate (IQ 35–40 to 50–55), severe (IQ 20–25 to 35–40), and profound (IQ < 20–25).[4]

PREVALENCE

Although it is possible to make a diagnosis of major depression and dysthymic disorder in people with ID, the boundary between major depression and subclinical depression is more difficult to define in those with severe and profound ID; it is easier to establish whether they suffer from depressive symptoms than whether the disorder is major depression or dysthymia.

In developed countries, the prevalence of ID from all causes is 1.5% to 2%.[3] In adults with ID, about 8% suffer from a depressive disorder.[5] There are no reliable studies on the prevalence of depressive illness in children with ID. However, prevalence of psychiatric symptoms overall has been estimated as 30% to 40%, three to four times the rate in children in general.[3]

ASSESSING DEPRESSION

The United Kingdom's Royal College of Psychiatrists has reviewed and modified the *ICD-10* diagnostic criteria to produce *The Diagnostic Criteria for Psychiatric Disorders for Use with Adults with Learning Disabilities/Mental Retardation (DC-LC)*.[6] The National Association for the Dually Diagnosed in the United States has produced the *Diagnostic Manual-Intellectual Disability (DM-ID)*, which includes evidence-based modifications to the *DSM-IV* criteria for use in persons with ID, including children.[1] These landmark publications provide guidance regarding the diagnosis of depressive disorders in young people with ID and highlight the limitations surrounding diagnosis in this population.

Symptoms of depression in youth with ID include depressed mood, observed sad or miserable facial expressions, crying and irritability, loss of interest in usual activities or usual stereotypical interests, and appetite and sleep disturbances.[7] Self-injury behaviors may become more common or pronounced during a depressive episode.[7] Reduced food intake or food refusal is reported to be a marker of depression in adults with severe and profound ID.[8] Slowed movements, impaired self-care, particularly if progressing onto catatonia, are suggestive of a psychotic depression. Also, negative automatic thoughts and hopelessness are reported as symptoms of depression in adults with mild ID.[9] Depression is associated also with a decline in daily living skills, social withdrawal, and adversely affects the quality of life of young persons with ID and their family.

In addition to the depressive symptoms, suicidal thoughts and suicide attempts are reported in adult patients with both mild and severe ID.[10] Suicidal thinking or deliberate self-harm should alert clinicians that patients may be suffering from a depressive disorder. Developmentally disabled adolescents are at increased risk of depression and suicide, and they commonly experience other risk factors associated with suicide, including difficulties coping with change, increased anxiety, being bullied, social isolation, and lack of understanding from the social support network.[11] As a young person with ID develops greater self-awareness during adolescence, the risk of self-harm may increase.

TABLE 22.1 SELECTED SCALES TO RATE DEPRESSIVE SYMPTOMS IN PEOPLE WITH INTELLECTUAL DISABILITY

Scale	Rater (Target Group)	Comments
The Intellectual Disability Mood Scale[12]	Self-report mood questionnaire (for adolescents with mild ID)	• 12 depressive key words or terms. • 5-point Likert scale. • Pictorial representation of buckets filled with increasing levels of liquid. Patients point to the bucket that most closely corresponds to their feelings. • Satisfactory psychometric properties. • In the public domain.
Checklist for Carers[13]	Parent screening questionnaire	• Simple one-page inventory developed for the assessment of depression in adults with intellectual disability. • Might be applicable to adolescents as a parent screening tool. • Depressive symptoms include depressed mood, depressed thinking, loss of interest, irritability, anxiety, impaired social interaction and communication, general functioning, appetite/weight, and sleep. • Available free from the author.
Mood and Anxiety Semi-Structured (MASS) interview[58]	Semistructured clinician interview of multiple informants	• Draws on *DSM-IV* symptomatology. • 35 symptoms based on behavioral descriptors. • Psychometric properties reported for adult psychiatric inpatients. • 30–60 minutes to complete.
Developmental Behaviour Checklist (DBC)[14,59]	Parent, caregiver, or teacher completed questionnaire	• Covering a broad range (96 symptoms) of psychopathology in youth with ID and PDD. • Disruptive, self-absorbed, communication, anxiety, and social relating subscales. A depression subscale is identified in the manual.

ID, intellectual disability; PDD, pervasive developmental disorder.

Clinicians need to gather information from others who know the young person well, including parents, caregivers, teachers, and respite workers, in addition to the direct examination of the young person. Daily mood charts or diaries completed by parents or caregivers recording information such as weight, appetite, self-harm episodes, and sleep patterns can also assist in diagnosis. Clinical evaluation should include standardized assessment tools. Several clinician, parent, caregiver, teacher, and self-rated instruments are available.[12–17] Table 22.1 summarizes some of those specifically developed for use in ID. Other scales devised for general use, such as Child Behavior Checklist, have also been used in patients with mild ID[15] (see Chapter 3).

Most self-report questionnaires for the measurement of mood in youth assume a level of self-awareness, social comprehension, and understanding of abstract ideas, such as moods and feelings, which is not present in most youth with PDD and moderate and severe ID. Adolescents with mild ID are able consistently to report on their mood in questionnaires used in the general population such as the Beck Depression Inventory.[9] As occurs in children and adolescents without developmental disabilities, there is often poor agreement between parent reports and reports by youth with mild ID.[16]

PARTICULAR ISSUES IN THE PRESENTATION AND DIAGNOSIS OF DEPRESSION

The literature refers to atypical manifestations of depressive symptoms in patients with ID when using modified criteria (e.g., reduced self-care, apparent loss of capacity to self-care), or when substituting symptoms (e.g., aggression or tantrums) for *DSM-IV* criteria.[18] It has been argued that other behaviors should be substituted for the traditional depressive symptoms in people with severe or profound cognitive impairment who have diminished capacity to report depressive symptoms. Davis et al.[17] described substituting *DSM-IV* criteria with symptoms based on observed behavior. In adults with ID, observer-reported tearfulness has been substituted for depressed mood; observer-reported marked reduction in social participation has been substituted for diminished interest or pleasure; significantly elevated challenging behaviors, aggression, and self-harm have been substituted for feelings of worthlessness or guilt.[17] However, this approach has been criticized for lacking a rationale on which the substitution is based.[18] In severe or profound ID, other authors have argued for substituting challenging behaviors (such as self-injury, aggression, and screaming) for depressive symptoms, allowing clinicians who have detected other depressive symptoms to make a diagnosis of depression.[19] The validity of these "depressive equivalents" has not been established.[20]

The *DC-LD* is a consensus document that combines modified depressive symptoms (e.g., social withdrawal, reduction in the quantity of speech/communication, reduction in self care) with standard *DSM-IV* criteria (loss of interest or pleasure).[6] *DC-LD* also allows for depressive episodes to be classified into categories of recurrent, in remission, with psychotic symptoms, and bipolar depression.[21]

Both adults and children with mild cognitive impairment are more likely to show depressive symptoms and to be diagnosed with major depression than those with severe ID.[22,23] The course of psychiatric symptoms also varies in youth depending on the level of cognitive impairment. For example, an 11-year follow-up study showed that overall psychiatric symptoms decreased over time, but youth with mild ID showed a larger reduction than those with severe or profound ID.[24] It is unclear, however, how this relates to depressive illness, not specifically considered in the study, which increases in frequency during adolescence.

Where there has been deterioration in overall functioning, diagnoses other than depression should also be considered, including anxiety, bipolar disorder, psychosis, and medical and neurologic conditions. Persons with very low IQ are often unable to express their complaints; they may look sad or tired as a result of a physical illness. Because anxiety is highly comorbid with depression, if the young person is reacting to environmental stressors—such as changes in routine, an illness (e.g., urinary tract infection, constipation), or unfamiliar caregivers—associated emotional or behavioral problems may be caused by anxiety rather than depression. Delusions related to worthlessness and guilt in the context of low mood are suggestive of a psychotic depression in young people with mild ID who are able to communicate these thoughts.

Known causes of ID, such as fragile X, Prader-Willi, Down, and Williams syndromes, are associated with specific behavioral phenotypes or clusters of symptoms.[25] Behavioral phenotypes are temperamental characteristics or psychiatric symptoms that are frequently seen in association with a genetic condition but are not a core diagnostic feature of this condition.[26] For instance, in Williams syndrome there are often marked levels of anxiety, significant hyperactivity, hyperacusis, and uninhibited social behavior.[26] Rates of psychopathology are relatively low in children with Down syndrome. Although they show more problems than children in the general population, these are predominantly externalizing (e.g., stubbornness, oppositionality, inattention).[27] Depression is rare in children with Down syndrome but increases in adults and may be mistaken for early dementia.

PSYCHOSOCIAL RISK FACTORS

IQ needs to be taken into account when considering psychosocial factors. For example, the capacity to evaluate and compare oneself with others is unlikely to exist in persons of very low IQ. Children and adolescents with mild or moderate ID are more prone to experience low self-esteem because they have greater difficulty negotiating the tasks of growing up. An important role for the clinician is helping parents and teachers to better understand the young person's competencies and emotional maturity and how this might not match their chronological age.

Many young people with ID experience temporary respite care from their parents; some may live in supported accommodation and a few in institutions. Inconsistent care can contribute to depression because supported accommodation staff are often poorly paid and inadequately trained. Children who are depressed or withdrawn are less likely to be attended to than those who display aggressive and disruptive behaviors. Children with developmental disabilities are also vulnerable and at risk of physical and sexual abuse from adults and peers while in care.

TREATMENT

Randomized controlled data for the treatment of depression in youth with ID are not available and unlikely to become so in the near future given the nature of this population and its low priority for research, policy, and funding. Thus clinical experience, evidence from random controlled trials (RCTs) in depressed youth without ID, and from depressed adults with ID need to be used as a guide. As always, treatment is based on a comprehensive diagnostic assessment (see Chapter 3).

INFORMED CONSENT

Consent to treatment, particularly to an invasive treatment, such as electroconvulsive therapy (ECT) poses particular problems in persons with ID (see also Chapter 4). As with any medical intervention, it is expected that age-appropriate information will be provided to the young person and caregivers, sufficient for them to understand the procedure, risks, benefits, and alternative treatments available. Youth with mild ID are usually competent to give consent. In the case of youth with moderate to severe ID, there is a need to assess their ability to comprehend the procedure. Where the young person is not of legal age or is not competent to give informed consent, consent should be obtained from parents or legal guardians. Where consent is obtained from a person on behalf of the child, there is a separate requirement of medical staff to explain the procedure to the young person directly. Every attempt should be made to reduce the stress for children and adolescents with ID undergoing hospitalization or an invasive procedure.

SUPPORTIVE MANAGEMENT

In adults with mild to moderate intellectual disability there are case studies and uncontrolled evidence that modified supportive psychotherapy may be a valuable option for the treatment of depression.[17] This encompasses education about depression, limited instruction on problem solving, and the opportunity to discuss depressive feelings.[17]

PSYCHOSOCIAL MANAGEMENT

Dealing with psychosocial issues is even more important in the developmentally disabled than in nondisabled youth. Clinicians need to identify and manage the many psychosocial factors that can contribute to the depression, including stresses associated with the transition to adolescence, exposure to psychosocial adversity such as bullying and criticism at school, and family dysfunction. Parental depression, impaired parent–child relationships, and family dysfunction also interact with depression in the child. Caring for children with ID that are showing challenging behaviors diminishes parental self-efficacy and results in reduced employment opportunities for the parents, with the associated hardships. There are emotional sequelae for these parents, often grieving over the loss of their child's potential. These children's diminished capacity to provide spontaneous, appropriate, reciprocal interaction with their parents can also impact negatively on the parent's mental state.

Compared with parents in the general community, parents of children with ID have higher rates of depressive symptoms—those with a child with autism and single parents the highest.[28] Many parents feel guilty over their child's disability, believing they are responsible and, as a consequence, can show driven, compulsive caregiving. Because genetic factors are implicated in about 14% of cases of mild ID and about 45% in moderate-profound ID,[29] a number of children with ID have parents who are also developmentally disabled and thus restricted in their parenting abilities. Parental depression has an effect on the emotional state of the child and may require treatment in its own right. Conversely, early intervention programs for children with PDD result in an improvement in maternal depression.[30] Parent education and skills training lead to continuing improvement in parental mental health and family well-being in parents of young children with autism.[31] Therefore, parent education, treatment of parent mental health problems, family support, and improvements in social and living conditions are likely to reduce risk factors, facilitate recovery, and prevent relapse.[31,32]

In the family, an assessment of the changes to the parental and siblings' relationships and roles brought about by having a developmentally disabled child needs to be contemplated. An understanding of how family time is apportioned, finding out if any members are overinvolved, redistributing family tasks, and developing an adaptive family routine can have a positive impact on the depressed youth with ID.[33] In thinking about factors causing or influencing the depression, it is important to consider also whether the current school meets the academic, relationship, and emotional needs of the intellectually disabled child.

COGNITIVE BEHAVIOR THERAPY

A range of cognitive behavior therapy (CBT) interventions are advocated based on their effectiveness in depressed youth without intellectual disability (see Chapter 8), including individual, group, parent, and family approaches.[34] There are case studies and some empirical evidence that CBT, appropriately modified, is effective for this population.[35,36] It may include relaxation exercises, modeling prosocial behavior, practicing positive self-statements, and creating rewarding school and social experiences.[36] Level of cognitive ability ought to be considered when contemplating CBT treatment. Intelligence has been associated with the ability to comprehend the concepts underlying CBT; most normal children 5 to 8 years of age are able to understand some of these concepts and able to engage in CBT.[37,38] The cognitive elements of CBT are unlikely to be useful with depressed youth with severe ID who lack sufficient communication and cognitive ability, but behavioral interventions such as pleasant events scheduling and rewarding achievement might be used and help to improve mood.[36]

OTHER PSYCHOTHERAPEUTIC APPROACHES

Family therapy has been used to manage children with intellectual disability, but specific use for depressive disorders or symptoms has not been reported.[39,40] Parent–child interaction therapy was shown to be superior to wait list in the management of disruptive behavior in young children with ID.[40] The efficacy of interpersonal psychotherapy for the treatment of depression in children with ID has not been investigated.

PHARMACOLOGIC MANAGEMENT

A detailed discussion of the medication treatment of major depression in youth without ID is given in Chapter 6 and is not repeated here. Suffice to say that there is empirical evidence that SSRIs, particularly fluoxetine, are effective for the acute treatment of youth with major depression.[41] There are no RCTs of pharmacologic treatments for youth with comorbid ID and major depression. Further, ID is frequently cited as an exclusion criterion. There are many obstacles to conducting pharmacologic treatment research in youth with ID related to (1) ethical considerations, including the challenge of obtaining informed consent, (2) lack of funding, and (3) methodological problems, such as sample composition owing to the heterogeneity of ID. Anecdotal evidence suggests that SSRIs are effective for the treatment of depressive symptoms and major depression in adults and adolescents with ID.[42] For example, paroxetine was reported to be useful in a small open-label study of adolescents with mild ID and major depression.[43] Use of antidepressants in youth with ID needs to take into consideration the general precautions, drug–drug interactions, and side effects described in Chapter 14. However, individuals with ID may require lower doses and be more sensitive to side effects such as agitation than their non-ID counterparts.[44]

The practicalities of prescribing and monitoring antidepressants are the same as those in non-ID youth, already described in Chapters 6 and 14, including a detailed explanation of the reasons for the recommendation, target symptoms, side effects (particularly agitation), duration, and monitoring (particularly of suicidality) to patient (when appropriate) and caregivers. However, assessment of unwanted effects in patients with severe or profound ID can be problematic.

Practitioners need to be aware that once medication is started it may be difficult to discontinue if it is only marginally effective because of pressure from caregivers who may mistakenly see the medication as helping. Using rating scales to measure change can facilitate this process.

OTHER SOMATIC TREATMENTS

There may be a role for the use of ECT in patients with ID who are at acute risk of serious self-harm, who are unable to take medications, where medications are contraindicated, or a series of other treatments have failed. ECT could also be considered for catatonic depression and psychotic depression with similar provisos as for non-ID youth (see Chapter 7).

DEPRESSION AND PERVASIVE DEVELOPMENTAL DISORDERS

Youth with PDD show higher levels of psychopathology than those with ID who do not have a comorbid PDD, including more depressive symptoms.[3] Autistic disorder manifests with a triad of symptoms: marked impairment of social functioning, communication, and stereotypical behaviors and restricted interests.[4] Young people with Asperger's disorder have impaired social interaction and restricted and stereotyped behavior and interests but show no delay in language and cognitive development. The diagnosis of PDD (NOS) or atypical autism is made when there are pervasive and severe social impairments and impaired communication skills or stereotyped behaviors that do not meet the full criteria for autism or Asperger's disorder because symptoms are insufficient in number or began after 3 years of age.[4] If a young person with autism shows intellectual abilities in the normal range, their autism is referred to as "high functioning."

Prevalence of autistic spectrum disorder is about 1 in 150 people; estimates of the prevalence of depressive symptoms in PDD range from 4.4% to 57.6%.[2] The wide range of estimates highlights the variability of symptoms and the difficulties making a diagnosis of depression in this group. Youth with autistic spectrum disorder have higher levels of psychopathology than other young people with ID.[3] Almost three quarters of children and adolescents with autism have comorbid psychopathology, most commonly disruptive behavior disorders, anxiety, and depression.[3] In one study of 100 children with Asperger's disorder, 3% had a diagnosis of a depressive disorder.[45]

PARTICULAR ISSUES IN DIAGNOSING MAJOR DEPRESSION

The number of impediments to diagnosing depression in youth with PDD include the following:

- The inability of the young person to monitor their internal world (although this may not be the case in some youth with Asperger's disorder).
- Difficulty expressing feelings.
- Overlap between depressive symptoms and core symptoms of PDD. For example, social withdrawal, change in sleep architecture, and appetite disturbance are common to both major depression and PDD.[7]
- Clinicians' and caregivers' ability to detect signs of depression.
- Associated low IQ in about 70% of the youth with PDD (thus the problems in diagnosing major depression described for youth with ID also apply to youth with PDD and low IQ).
- Impaired language skills is a core feature of youth with autism.

Anecdotal evidence suggests that onset of irritability may often be a manifestation of depression in youth with PDD. Conversely, irritability in response to social demands or environmental change can be mistaken for depression. It is our experience that parents—who are likely to experience stress and depression themselves—may be less able to identify these symptoms in their PDD child.

Suicidal thoughts and attempted suicide are issues in high functioning individuals with PDD and comorbid depressive disorder.[46] Increased awareness of the limitations that the PDD places on them, social isolation, the capacity for impulsive behavior, low frustration tolerance, propensity to be the victim of bullying, and difficulty sharing feelings with others are risk factors for suicidality in these youth.[2]

RISK FACTORS

The factors mentioned as contributing to the onset and persistence of depressive symptoms in youth with ID are also relevant to PDD. Youth with mild levels of ID and comorbid PDD, in particular Asperger's disorder, may be more at risk of developing depressive symptoms and depressive disorders than youth with PDD and moderate or severe intellectual disability.[47]

SPECIFIC ISSUES IN TREATMENT

Education

The recommendations made for children with ID also apply to those with PDD. The stress of managing a child with PDD for parents and caregivers is often profound. Parents usually struggle with the child's social and cognitive disability, may deny their child's impairments, and come to distrust the medical establishment. This is particularly true if diagnosis has been delayed by medical staff who may have reassured parents their child did not suffer with PDD. In the absence of curative medical treatments for PDD, parents may seek out and subject their children to unproven treatments. Ongoing education and support for the parents or caregivers are key components of any intervention.

Psychosocial Management

Interventions need to target the factors that may contribute to the onset or maintenance of depressive symptoms. These include improving social skills through social skills groups, involvement in appropriate extracurricular social groups (such as a support groups, scouts, guides), or mentoring programs. Where academic failure is contributing to depressive symptoms, enrollment in a school specializing in teaching children with autistic spectrum disorders or intellectual disability may be more appropriate than mainstream schooling. Alternatively, a tailored education program, remedial classes, and employment of a dedicated teaching aide should be considered. For older depressed adolescents, a program to assist their transition from school to sheltered employment may be helpful. Psychosocial interventions directed at parents can also be useful.[30] In older adolescents with high functioning autism or Asperger's disorder, supportive counseling should be considered to increase awareness of the differences from others, manage daily living tasks, discuss relationships, and help them work through their growing insight into the limitations of having a PDD.[2]

As is the case with the developmentally disabled, many youth with PDD have comorbid neurological illnesses such as epilepsy.[45] Medical conditions that have been overlooked or are not being monitored can affect the mental state of the young person with PDD. One of the roles of the clinician is to assess and treat the medical needs of these children, facilitate referral, and advocate for appropriate services.

Pharmacological Management

Although SSRIs are the most frequently prescribed psychotropic agents in people suffering with PDD,[48] only the atypical antipsychotic risperidone is approved for the treatment of irritability in autism by the Food and Drug Administration (FDA) (http://www.fda.gov/bbs/topics/news/2006/new01485.html). RCTs have demonstrated that 0.5 to 3.5 mg of risperidone daily is effective in the treatment of irritability (not necessarily owing to depression) in children and adolescents with PDD.[49,50] Although RCT data are lacking, other antipsychotic drugs may also be effective in treating irritability. Adverse effects of risperidone include sedation, weight gain, changes to sleep architecture, extrapyramidal symptoms, and hyperprolactinemia.[48] Before prescribing risperidone, a full physical examination should be conducted noting height and weight and the presence or absence of gynecomastia, galactorrhea, and extrapyramidal symptoms, as well as performing baseline liver function tests, blood count, glucose and triglycerides, and these should be monitored regularly during treatment given the risk of risperidone-induced obesity, dyslipidemia, and diabetes.[48]

Apart from RCT data for depressed youth in general, there is a paucity of evidence to guide the prescription of antidepressants in PDD. Depression is only one of a number of target symptoms identified for treatment—such as repetitive behaviors, emotional reactivity, obsessiveness, restricted range of interests, and emotional liability—in the few uncontrolled studies examining the use of antidepressants in people with PDD.[51] There are anecdotal and open-label studies showing that fluoxetine and citalopram are effective in depressed children and adolescents.[51-54] In young children with autism, response to fluoxetine was predicted in part by a family history of mood disorders.[51]

Common side effects of young people with PDD treated with SSRIs are insomnia, anxiety, incontinence, sedation, diarrhea, anorexia, disinhibition, hyperactivity, agitation, and activation.[48,53,55,56] Activation has been reported as occurring in up to a fifth of all PDD patients taking SSRIs, with younger patients being more at risk.[48] A case series suggests that extrapyramidal side effects are also more common in autistic children treated with SSRIs.[57] Because there are no predictors of who will develop side effects, a slow introduction tapering up to a moderate dose is recommended.[48] Given that serotonin syndrome is a life-threatening condition (see Chapters 14 and 21) and likely to be underrecognized in this population, clinicians should exercise particular care ascertaining what other medications—including alternative medicine remedies—the patient is taking (such as tramadol or other serotonergic agents) because the combination can cause serotonin syndrome.

RESOURCES FOR PATIENTS AND FAMILIES

The Autism Society of America has introductory information about autism that may be useful to parents and families: http://www.autism-society.org.

An Autism fact sheet is provided by the National Institute of Neurological Disorders and Stroke: http://www.ninds.nih.gov/disorders/autism/detail_autism.htm.

The U.S. Centers for Disease Control and Prevention has a resource for children with autism that includes links to websites that address mental health assistance and autism resources by state: http://www.cdc.gov/ncbddd/autism/resources/familyresources.htm.

Information and tips for parents and teachers of intellectually disabled (mentally retarded) children are presented by the U.S. National Dissemination Center for Children with Disabilities: http://www.nichcy.org/pubs/factshe/fs8txt.htm.

RESOURCES FOR PROFESSIONALS

The National Association for the Dually Diagnosed (NADD) is a resource for professionals working with individuals with intellectual and developmental disability and mental health problems: http://www.thenadd.org/.

The National Institute of Mental Health provides a detailed overview of autism spectrum disorders (pervasive developmental delay) appropriate for professionals: http://www.nimh.nih.gov/health/publications/autism/complete-publication.shtml#.

Medline Plus has an autism page with a broad range of links to sites that provide information about topics including diagnosis and symptoms, research, genetics, and treatment: http://www.nlm.nih.gov/medlineplus/autism.html.

Learning About Intellectual Disabilities and Health is a comprehensive English website about intellectual disability and health, a collaboration between the Down's Syndrome Association and the University of London: http://www.intellectualdisability.info/home.htm.

This site includes information on depression in adults with intellectual disability: http://www.intellectualdisability.info/mental_phys_health/depression_idhtm.htm.

REFERENCES

1. Fletcher R, Loschem E, Stavrakaki C, et al., eds. *Diagnostic Manual-Intellectual Disability*. New York: NADD Press; 2007.
2. Lainhart JE. Psychiatric problems in individuals with autism, their parents and siblings. *Int Rev Psychiatry*. 1999;11:278–298.
3. Tonge BJ, Einfeld SL. Psychopathology and intellectual disability: The Australian Child to Adult Longitudinal Study. In: Glidden L, ed. *International Review of Research in Mental Retardation*. New York: Academic Press; 2003:61–91.
4. American Psychiatric Association. *Diagnostic and Statistical Manual of Mental Disorders, 4th Edition, Text Revision*. Washington, DC: American Psychiatric Association; 2000.
5. White P, Chant D, Edwards N, et al. Prevalence of intellectual disability and comorbid mental illness in an Australian community sample. *Aust N Z J Psychiatry*. 2005;39:395–400.
6. Royal College of Psychiatrists. *DC-LD (Diagnostic Criteria for Psychiatric Disorders for Use with Adults with Learning Disabilities/Mental Retardation)*. London: Gaskell; 2001.
7. Stewart ME, Barnard L, Pearson J, et al. Presentation of depression in autism and Asperger's syndrome: a review. *Autism*. 2006;10:103–116.
8. Mayville SB, Matson JL, Laud RB, et al. The relationship between depression and feeding disorder symptoms among persons with severe and profound mental retardation. *J Dev Phys Disabil*. 2005;17:213–224.
9. Beck DC, Carlson GA, Russell AT, et al. Use of depression rating instruments in developmentally and educationally delayed adolescents. *J Am Acad Child Adolesc Psychiatry*. 1987;26:97–100.
10. Davis JP, Judd FK, Herrman H. Depression in adults with intellectual disability. 1: A review. *Aust N Z J Psychiatry*. 1997;31:232–242.
11. Saulnier C, Volkmar F. Mental health problems in people with autism and related disorders. In: Bouras N, Holt G, eds. *Psychiatric and Behavioural Disorders in Intellectual and Developmental Disabilities*. 2nd ed. Cambridge: Cambridge University Press; 2007:215–224.

12. Argus GR, Terry PC, Bramston P, et al. Measurement of mood in adolescents with intellectual disability. *Res Dev Disabil.* 2004;25:493–507.

13. Torr J. Checklist for carers [unpublished psychological inventory]; 2004. Available at: jennifer.torr@med. monash.edu.au.

14. Einfeld SL, Tonge BJ. The Developmental Behavior Checklist: The development and validation of an instrument to assess behavioral and emotional disturbance in children and adolescents with mental retardation. *J Autism Dev Disord.* 1995;25:81–98.

15. Achenbach TM, Rescorla LA. *Manual for ASEBA School-Age Forms & Profiles.* Burlington: University of Vermont, Research Center for Children, Youth, & Families; 2001.

16. Masi G, Brovedani P, Mucci M et al. Assessment of anxiety and depression in adolescents with mental retardation. *Child Psychiatry Hum Dev.* 2002;32:227–237.

17. McBride JA. Assessment and diagnosis of depression in people with intellectual disability. *J Intellect Disabil Res.* 2003;47:1–13.

18. Davis JP, Judd FK, Herrman H. Depression in adults with intellectual disability. 2: A pilot study. *Aust N Z J Psychiatry.* 1997;31:243–251.

19. Ross E, Oliver C. The assessment of mood in adults who have severe or profound mental retardation. *Clin Psychol Rev.* 2003;23:225–245.

20. Tsiouris JA, Mann R, Patti PJ, et al. Challenging behaviours should not be considered as depressive equivalents in individuals with intellectual disability. *J Intellect Disabil Res.* 2003;47:14–21.

21. Smiley E, Cooper S. Intellectual disabilities, depressive episode, diagnostic criteria and diagnostic criteria for psychiatric disorders for use with adults with learning disabilities/mental retardation (DC-LD). *J Intellect Disabil Res.* 2003;47:S62–S71.

22. Holden B, Gitlesen JP. The association between severity of intellectual disability and psychiatric symptomatology. *J Intellect Disabil Res.* 2004;48:556–562.

23. Dekker MC, Koot HM, Ende JVD, et al. Emotional and behavioral problems in children and adolescents with and without intellectual disability. *J Child Psychol Psychiatry.* 2002;43:1087–1098.

24. Einfeld SL, Piccinin AM, Mackinnon A, et al. Psychopathology in young people with intellectual disability. *JAMA.* 2006;296:1981–1989.

25. Tonge B. Psychiatric and behavior disorders among children and adolescents with intellectual disability. In: Gelder MG, Lopez-Ibor JJ, Andreasen N., eds. *New Oxford Textbook of Psychiatry.* New York, NY: Cambridge University Press. 2000; 1965–1972.

26. Einfeld SL. Intellectual handicap in contemporary psychiatry. *Aust N Z J Psychiatry.* 1997;31:452–456.

27. Dykens EM. Psychiatric and behavioral disorders in persons with Down syndrome. *Ment Retard Dev Disabil Res Rev.* 2007;13:272–278.

28. Olsson MB, Hwang CP. Depression in mothers and fathers of children with intellectual disability. *J Intellect Disabil Res.* 2001;45:535–543.

29. Raynham H, Gibbons J, Flint J, et al. The genetic basis for mental retardation. *Q J Med.* 1996;89:169–175.

30. McConachie H, Diggle T. Parental implemented early intervention for young children with autism spectrum disorder: a systematic review. *J Eval Clin Pract.* 2006;13:120–129.

31. Tonge B, Brereton A, Kiomall M, et al. Effects of parental mental health of an education and skills training program for parents of young children with autism: a randomised controlled trial. *J Am Acad Child Adolesc Psychiatry.* 2006;45:562–569.

32. Levitas A, Gilson SF. Predictable crises in the lives of persons with mental retardation. *Ment Health Aspects Dev Disabil.* 2001;4:89–100.

33. Schneider J, Wedgewood N, Llewellyn G, et al. Families challenged by and accommodating to the adolescent years. *J Intellect Disabil Res.* 2006;50:926–936.

34. Turk J. Children with developmental disabilities and their parents. In: Graham PJ, ed., *Cognitive Behavior Therapy for Children and Families.* Cambridge: Cambridge University Press; 2005:244–262.

35. Lindsay WR, Howells L, Pitcaithly D. Cognitive therapy for depression in individuals with intellectual disabilities. *Br J Med Psychol.* 1993;66:135–141.

36. Tonge B. The psychopathology of children with intellectual disabilities. In: Bouras N, Holt G, eds., *Psychiatric and Behavioral Disorders in Intellectual and Developmental Disabilities.* 2nd ed. Cambridge: Cambridge University Press; 2007:93–112.

37. Quakley S, Coker S, Palmer K, et al. Can children distinguish between thoughts and behaviours? *Behav Cogn Psychother.* 2003;31:159–168.

38. Doherr L, Reynolds S, Wetherly, et al. Young children's ability to engage in cognitive therapy tasks: associations with age and educational experience. *Behav Cogn Psychother.* 2005;33:201–215.

39. Lloyd H, Dallos R. Solution-focused brief therapy with families who have a child with intellectual disabilities: a description of the content of initial sessions and the processes. *Clin Child Psychol Psychiatry.* 2006; 11:367–386.

40. Bagner DM, Eyberg SM. Parent-child interaction therapy for disruptive behavior in children with mental retardation: a randomized control trial. *J Clin Child Adolesc Psychol.* 2007;36:418–429.

41. March JS, Silva S, Petrycki S, et al. Fluoxetine, cognitive-behavioral therapy, and their combination for adolescents with depression. *JAMA.* 2004;292:807–820.
42. Janowsky DS, Davis JM. Diagnosis and treatment of depression in patients with mental retardation. *Curr Psychiatry Rep.* 2005;7:421–428.
43. Masi G, Marcheschi M, Pfanner P. Paroxetine in depressed adolescents with intellectual disability: an open label study. *J Intellect Disabil Res.*1997;41:268–272.
44. Haw C, Stubbs J. A survey of off-label prescribing for inpatients with mild intellectual disability and mental illness. *J Intellect Disabil Res.* 2005;49:858–864.
45. Cederlund M, Gillberg C. One hundred males with Asperger syndrome: a clinical study of background and associated factors. *Dev Med Child Neurol.* 2004;46:652–660.
46. Fitzgerald M. Suicide and Asperger's syndrome. *Crisis.* 2007;28:1–3.
47. Ghaziuddin M, Ghaziuddin N, Greden J. Depression in persons with autism: implications for research and clinical care. *J Autism Dev Disord.* 2002;32:299–306.
48. McCraken JT. Safety issues with drug therapies for autism spectrum disorders. *J Clin Psychiatry.* 2005; 66:32–37.
49. Shea S, Turgay A, Carroll A, et al. Risperidone in the treatment of disruptive behavioral symptoms in children with autistic and other pervasive developmental disorders. *Pediatrics.* 2004;114:e634–e641.
50. McCraken JT, McGough J, Shah B, et al. Risperidone in children with autism and serious behavioral problems. *N Engl J Med.* 2002;347:314–321.
51. Delong GR, Ritch CR, Burch S. Fluoxetine response in children with autistic spectrum disorders: correlation with familial major affective disorder and intellectual achievement. *Dev Med Child Neurol.* 2002;44:652–659.
52. Ghaziuddin M, Tsai L, Ghaziuddin N. Fluoxetine in autism with depression. *J Am Acad Child Adolesc Psychiatry.* 1991;30:508–509.
53. Fatemi SH, Realmuto GM, Khan L, et al. Fluoxetine in treatment of adolescent patients with autism: a longitudinal open trial. *J Autism Dev Disord.* 1998;28:303–307.
54. Namerow LB, Thomas P, Bostic JQ, et al. Use of citalopram in pervasive developmental disorders. *Dev Behav Pediatr.* 2003;24:104–108.
55. Hollander E, Phillips A, Chaplin W, et al. A placebo controlled crossover trial of liquid fluoxetine on repetitive behaviors in childhood and adolescent autism. *Neuropsychopharmacology.* 2005;30:582–589.
56. Racusin R, Kovner-Kline K, King BH. Selective serotonin reuptake inhibitors in intellectual disability. *Ment Retard Dev Disabil Res Rev.* 1999;5:264–269.
57. Sokolski KN, Chicz-Demet A, Demet EM. Selective serotonin reuptake inhibitor-related extrapyramidal symptoms in autistic children: a case series. *J Child Adolesc Psychopharmacol.* 2004;14:143–147.
58. Charlot L, Deutsch C, Hunt A, et al. Validation of the mood and anxiety semi-structured (MASS) interview for patients with intellectual disabilities. *J Intellect Disabil Res.* 2007;51:821–834.
59. Einfeld SL, Tonge BJ. *Manual for the Developmental Behavior Checklist, 2nd ed.—Primary Carer Version (DBC-P) and Teacher Version (DBC-T).* Melbourne and Sydney: Monash University Centre for Developmental Psychiatry and Psychology and School of Psychiatry, University of New South Wales; 2002.

Depression in Immigrant and Minority Children and Youth

ANDRES J. PUMARIEGA, EUGENIO M. ROTHE, AND KENNETH M. ROGERS

KEY POINTS

- The United States and other developed Western countries are facing a rapidly changing demographic and cultural landscape, with their population becoming increasing multiracial and multicultural.
- Native, minority, and immigrant children and youth face many barriers to effective mental health care. These include population barriers (socioeconomic disparities, stigma, poor health education, lack of documentation), provider factors (deficits in cross-cultural knowledge and skills and attitudinal sensitivity), and systemic factors (services location and organization, lack of culturally competent services).
- Cultural groups' understanding of depression varies and influences their help-seeking behaviors. They often invoke spiritual, supernatural, sociological, and interpersonal explanatory models. Stigma is also high.
- Diagnosing depression in these children is challenging for clinicians. For example,
  - Somatization and anger are frequent.
  - Depressed individuals of Asian origin show heightened reactivity during depression; Whites show less.
  - Comorbidity is very common (anxiety, disruptive behavioral symptoms, substance abuse, posttraumatic stress disorder), particularly in disadvantaged groups.
- Drug pharmacokinetics and pharmacodynamics can vary according to ethnicity. For example, there is a large percentage of slow metabolizers among Asian children; as a result they often experience Western medicines as "too strong" and suffer more side effects.
- The diagnosis and treatment of immigrant and minority children must be contextual, addressing psychosocial and cultural needs, and consonant with their values and beliefs. This is facilitated by including key members of the extended family, such as grandmothers, and other "adopted" relatives.
- Clinicians need to be aware of variations in the expression of affect and behavior. For example,
  - Subdued expressiveness in Asian and American Indian children and adolescents.
  - Aversion of eye contact with adults in Asian, African Americans, or mainland Latino children and adolescents.
  - Feelings, particularly anger, are not to be expressed openly or verbally by Native Americans, whose culture emphasizes nonverbal communication.
- Use of alternative treatments is very high in these groups.
- Home-based or community-based alternatives to hospitalization usually result in better outcomes for these youth, whereas involuntary hospitalization tends to recreate past traumas of oppression and reduce access to natural supports from the ethnic minority community or church.
- Because depression is usually recurrent, the need for continuous treatment—not only when the child is in crisis—should be stressed.

Introduction
The United States faces a rapidly changing demographic and cultural landscape, with its population becoming increasing multiracial and multicultural. This is largely a result of three major factors: progressive aging and low birthrate of the European-origin population, lower mean ages and increasing birthrates in non-European minority groups, and a significant rise in immigration from developing countries, especially from Latin America and Asia. There will no longer be a numeric majority of Euro-Americans by 2050; this will happen before 2030 among children younger than 18 years and is already true among 6-year-olds.[1]

Such changes are occurring in European and other European-origin nations as a result of similar dynamics. Here the predominance of legal and illegal migrants is from Africa, the Middle East and Asia, frequently Muslims, and often escaping extreme poverty or civil strife.

These changes are highly significant for child mental health services. First, the acceptability of such services and their use are highly governed by cultural attitudes, beliefs, and practices. The current science base around diagnosis and treatments is derived from research primarily involving European-origin populations, so its validity for these emerging populations is questionable. At the same time, these populations face many challenges around mental illness and emotional disturbances, including lower access to treatment services and evidence-based treatments, and higher burdens of morbidity and mortality than Euro-Americans. In regard to depressive symptomatology and disorders, these challenges are exemplified by the rapidly rising rates of suicidality and suicide attempts among Latino and African American youth as compared with Euro-Americans, as highlighted by the most recent Youth Risk Behavior Survey.[2] As a result, cultural and racial factors relating to depressive symptomatology and disorders deserve closer attention and consideration.

EPIDEMIOLOGY AND RISK FACTORS

Whereas earlier studies showed lower rates of depressive disorders among African American youth compared with Whites,[3] more recent studies have found higher rates of depressive symptomatology and disorders among minority youth (including African American, Latino, and American Indian) compared with white youth.[4,5] These differences are further confounded by gender interactions, with depressive symptoms higher in African American versus white males but nearly equal between African American and white female children.[6] Suicide rates for minority youth have been lower historically, but these rates have increased substantially in recent years and now equal or surpass those for Whites. These changes have been most striking among African American males and Latino females, leading the U.S. Surgeon General to declare suicide among African American males an emerging public health issue.[7]

Latinos are the largest, fastest growing, and youngest minority population in the United States, with 39% of Latinos younger than 20 years compared with 29% for other ethnic groups.[1] Risk factors for depressive symptomatology and disorders and suicide among Latino youth are numerous and influenced by their cultural background and immigration status. Risks for certain morbidities associated with psychopathology, including substance abuse and suicidality, increase with exposure to Western cultural values and practices.[8–10] This increased risk may result from the loss of protective cultural values and beliefs (such as family support and taboos on substance use and suicide) and exposure to risk-enhancing factors (such as acculturation stressors, media exposure, and peer pressure). Many minority and immigrant youth also live in impoverished conditions, with limited family supports and exposed to increased levels of community violence, domestic violence, abuse, and neglect. These circumstances subject them to stressors and traumas associated with increased rates of depression and suicidal symptoms in all populations, but which are exacerbated by the stressors associated with acculturation and discrimination.[11]

Native populations (such as American Indians, Native Alaskans, aboriginal populations in Australia, New Zealand Maoris, and other Native Pacific Islanders) share many of the disadvantages of other minority groups, such as poverty and high incarceration rates, often magnified by the loss of their cultural identity through forced assimilation by the colonizing culture and feelings of dispossession. At the same time, these populations suffer from some of the highest suicide rates recorded. For example, American Indian youth in the United States have the highest suicide rate of all ethnic groups in the United States.[12-14] Australian aboriginal youth account for a high percentage of the increase of rural suicides over the last decade,[15] and suicidality in Sami adolescent youth in the Arctic Circle, although equal to dominant culture youth, is associated with divergence from traditional cultural norms.[16] Contributing factors for these increases include acculturation pressures, discrimination, gender role pressures, past traumas and losses, and poverty, in addition to mental illness.

European immigrants in the United States and immigrants of Islamic or Asian origin in Europe have demonstrated patterns similar to those seen in U.S. immigrant groups from developing countries with regard to increases in depressive and anxiety symptomatology in youth, with some studies showing higher rates than those found in dominant culture peers.[17-19] There are some generational differences in the increases of depressive symptoms by gender, with one study citing first-generation immigrant females and second-generation males being most affected.[20]

EVIDENCE FOR DISPARITIES

Minority and immigrant children and youth face a number of barriers to effective mental health care. These include population barriers (socioeconomic disparities, stigma, poor health education, lack of documentation), provider factors (deficits in cross-cultural knowledge and skills and attitudinal sensitivity), and systemic factors (services location and organization, lack of culturally competent services, etc.). These barriers result in increased mental health disparities among these populations. Minority youth often lack public or private insurance or reside in neighborhoods where services are rarely available. These issues are particularly acute among young children and among Latino youth.[21] Hispanic families underuse mental health services because of language and cultural barriers;[22] Asian Americans experience shame around mental illness.[23]

Significant evidence indicates that psychiatric disorders are frequently misdiagnosed among culturally diverse youth; various studies have found an overdiagnosis of conduct disorder and underdiagnosis of depressive disorders.[24-26] Misdiagnosis largely originates from difficulties that clinicians from majority and minority origins have in addressing cultural differences, including cognitive biases stemming from stereotyping, lack of systematic assessment, and lack of contextualization of information obtained in diagnostic assessments.[27] The majority of care for depression is provided by primary care physicians who may have relatively little experience with depression in children and adolescents and have added disincentives such as decreased reimbursement for identifying a mental health versus a somatic health problem.[28]

Effectiveness in addressing cultural factors is not only related to knowledge about the family's culture but also the clinician's ability to form a patient- and family-centered alliance in which the clinician respects the family's knowledge and unique perspectives on the child, avoids stereotyping, and empowers them to make treatment decisions. Cooper and colleagues[29] demonstrated that the failure to form such alliances contributes to significant barriers in assessment and subsequent use of health services by minority patients, whereas race-concordant clinician-patient pairs tended to prevent such misalliance.

All of these factors result in significant underuse of community mental health services by minority youth and their families. Zito and colleagues,[30] studying children 5 through 15 years old enrolled in the Maryland Medicaid system, found that white youth were 2.5 times more likely than African Americans to receive any type of psychotropic medication, and African Americans received fewer prescriptions and had fewer physician visits. These findings parallel those of Cuffe et al.[31] that African American youth receive significantly lower rates of treatment than Whites and stay in treatment half as long as white children. Latino children receive an average of half as many counseling sessions[32] and significantly fewer specialty mental health services and at a later age[33] than Whites and African Americans. Additionally, there are fewer psychiatrists (and even primary care physicians) practicing in inner-city and low-income areas where minority populations live.[34]

CULTURAL CHALLENGES TO DIAGNOSIS AND TREATMENT

Diagnosing depression in minority and immigrant children can be challenging to clinicians unfamiliar with these issues. Children from diverse populations can demonstrate different symptomatology than Euro-Americans. Somatization and anger, for example, are symptoms more frequently associated with depression in minority youth.[35,36] The degree of emotional reactivity can also vary during depression, with individuals of Asian origin showing heightened reactivity, whereas Whites show less.[37] Diagnosis is more challenging with depressed minority children owing to the frequent presence of comorbidities. For example, stresses associated to immigration, acculturation, discrimination, and community violence contribute not only to depression but also to comorbid anxiety, disruptive behavioral symptoms, substance abuse, and posttraumatic stress disorder.[38–40]

Kleinman[41] argues that culture shapes the way individuals not only express, but also the way they understand the symptoms of illness. Diverse cultural groups' understanding of depression can vary significantly and influence their help-seeking behavior, invoking spiritual, supernatural, sociological, and interpersonal explanatory models. For example, African Americans often conceptualize depressive symptoms as part of their experience of sociopolitical oppression.[42] Depressive symptoms can be even subsumed into culture-bound syndromes. For example, *susto,* a common culture-bound syndrome seen among mainland Latinos of Indian origin, involves acute anxiety followed by chronic depression; the explanatory model is one of a distressing experience causing the loss of the soul.[43] Such expressions often lead families to seek help from a spiritual healer rather than a mental health professional.

As with many people of lower socioeconomic status, individuals of immigrant and minority backgrounds tend to postpone seeking treatment until either the child's situation is fairly critical or the family is under significant distress from his or her symptoms. This may be partly related to their educational background, the multiple demands they face in their daily lives, and the perceived barriers to treatment, but also to cultural values that are more present focused and not as prevention oriented. At times, immigrant and minority families may even seek treatment under pressure from external authorities (such as school or child welfare officials), which starts treatment out on a less than amicable footing and on a more urgent basis, resulting in higher rates of involuntary commitment.[24] These same factors may also contribute to premature termination from treatment. These trends have significant implications for the effectiveness of treatment, which may have to be more intensive from the outset. Symptomatic improvement without remission owing to premature termination is associated with poor prognosis, more recurrences, and poorer outcomes.

STIGMA

Stigma is a major barrier to seeking mental health services in general, and cultural beliefs play a large role in the perpetuation of stigma. Many cultures have major negative associations with any type of mental health assistance, often equating it with serious psychopathology and social undesirability. The fear of double stigmatization (being culturally different as well as "crazy") also presents major barriers for these families and youth to accessing services.[44] Some of these attitudes may originate in negative experiences with the mental health system by minority populations in the United States (including oppression) and by immigrants in their home nations.[45]

Help-seeking behaviors are not just governed by explanatory models of illness, but also by reality factors such as daily needs and stresses on children and families, and by basic cultural values that influence attitudes about services. With immigrant and minority children and adolescents who suffer from depression, variables such as loss, abuse, neglect, poverty, and limited family and community supports abound. If not addressed, these tend to perpetuate and aggravate depression but also play a role in access to treatment and adherence.[46,47]

BIOLOGIC FACTORS

Biologic factors related to culture have risen in importance as we rely more on pharmacologic treatments for different mental disorders, including depression. Various genes control the metabolism of drugs through their effects on drug-metabolizing enzymes, receptor regulation, and transporters;

their polymorphisms are associated with different racial and ethnic populations. The field of ethnopharmacology focuses on interethnic differences in pharmacokinetics, how the drug affects the organism, and pharmacodynamics, how the drug affects the target organs. Drugs are usually metabolized in two phases: oxidation through the cytochrome P450 (CYP) enzymes (phase I), and conjugation through transferases (phase II). Polymorphisms in phase I are responsible for the differences in how members of different ethnic groups metabolize drugs leading to poor metabolizers (PMs), who have decreased enzyme activity, and extended metabolizers (EMs), who have increased enzyme activity. Many psychotropic drugs, including the antidepressants, are metabolized by CYP (2D6).[48] Enzymes, such as catechol-O-methyl transferase (COMT; metabolizing dopamine) and monoamine oxidase (MAO; metabolizing norepinephrine), are highly polymorphic and are increased among Asians. Receptors, such as the serotonin transporter, are genetically governed and also include racially related polymorphisms[49] (see Chapter 14 for more details).

Biologic systems are not static, and the expression of genes is also influenced by variables such as environment, age, gender, nutrients, various plants and foods, steroid hormones, and other chemicals. For example, grapefruit juice may increase serum concentrations of nefazodone, antivirals, and alprazolam by affecting CYP (3A4), and corn affects CPY (2D6), thus influencing antidepressant levels. These facts should be taken into account when treating adolescents of Caribbean origin (high citric diets) and of Mexican and Central American origin (high corn diets). When individuals migrate, they often leave behind the dietary habits of their countries of origin and metabolize similarly as members of the host country. For this reason, it is important to evaluate the individual's immigration and generational status and personal adherence to traditional practices.[48] Additional racial or ethnic sensitivities to pharmacotherapy need to be considered. For example, African Americans (and Caribbean Latinos with African heritage) experience extrapyramidal side effects more frequently than other groups because of metabolic differences. Asians are frequent users of traditional medicines, have a large percentage of slow metabolizers (SMs), often experience Western medicines as being "too strong," and show many side effects.[48]

APPLICATION OF THE CULTURAL COMPETENCE MODEL TO THE DIAGNOSIS AND TREATMENT OF DEPRESSION

Culturally competent clinicians are aware and accepting of cultural differences, and they are conscious of their own culture and the biases it may create. They strive to acquire knowledge about the populations they serve, modify clinical approaches to the needs of their diverse patients and families, and attempt to bridge understanding between traditional and mainstream cultures. Cultural competence also extends to systems of care that provide treatment to children and families of diverse backgrounds. These should (1) value and adapt to cultural, ethnic, and religious diversity; (2) understand and manage the dynamics of cultural differences; (3) institutionalize cultural knowledge through training and knowledge development; and (4) adapt policies and procedures to serve diverse families better, accounting for unique characteristics such as their socioeconomic status, level of acculturation, and experience with the service system.[50]

Language and communication are critical in obtaining accurate clinical information and establishing a therapeutic alliance, especially with family members. However, many immigrants (particularly recent immigrants and especially parents, but also at times children) are not fluent in the dominant language and may not be able to participate fully in the evaluation and treatment. Translation and interpretation are typically considered a menial or informal task rather than one central to the clinical process. This is reflected in the use of poorly staffed telephonic translation services, untrained translators, and even family members, particularly siblings or the child. This latter practice should be prohibited except in dire emergencies because of the adverse impact it has on children and on family relations. Interpreters should have proper training in both the skill of translation and in psychiatric terminology and services. They should understand the family's culture and address verbal, nonverbal, and implicit communications. Ideally, they should not only serve as linguistic interpreters, but also (by virtue of their knowledge of the culture) as cultural consultants; helping decipher not only verbal but also nonverbal communication, critical to the development of a therapeutic alliance. Similarly, rating instruments used should not only be translated to the language of the family member or child but also validated and normed for that given ethnic/racial population to obtain valid results. Rating instruments can also contain inherent biases in terms of unfamiliar terminology. Even Likert-type scales can have different culturally based response biases (for example, in some cultures there is a tendency to respond in the middle choices and not at the extremes). These can be controlled for by proper psychometric analysis, often not available if the scale has not been normed outside its country or population of origin[50] (see also Chapter 3).

The initial interview is critical to establish a strong therapeutic alliance and to obtain vital information about how culture influences the child and family's needs and understanding. It is important to open a dialogue with the patient and the family and ask questions about beliefs and attitudes about treatment. The clinician should explore the patient's and the family's concerns and empower them to make the most appropriate treatment choices, addressing the perceptions of power differentials with the clinician.

The clinician should inquire about barriers that may prevent the family from obtaining services for their depressed child. Hospitals are bureaucratic institutions and staffed by persons that can seem intimidating. They have long waiting periods, and the family is often not acquainted with the formality and nature of the psychiatric examination. Community clinics are generally more appropriate treatment settings for immigrant and minority children and families.[51] These should be located in places that minority families feel comfortable accessing and should be affiliated with institutions that are favorably viewed. Schools are one of the most influential institutions for minority and immigrant children, so interventions should also be directed at improving school experiences.[50]

The diagnosis and treatment must be contextual, addressing psychosocial and cultural needs and consonant with their values and beliefs. For example, this is facilitated by including key members of the extended family, such as grandmothers, in assessment and treatment. It also involves exploring family and cultural values, which can be done during the initial interview. It is important to inquire about the family's spiritual and religious beliefs and practices, family and gender roles, language preference, and language fluency of key family members (the latter serving as a proxy for level of acculturation).[50]

The clinician should assess the strengths and vulnerabilities of the depressed child or adolescent and of key family members, taking into account the danger of prematurely attaching labels. The clinician should be aware that sometimes minority and immigrant children perceive themselves differently from how the dominant culture perceives them, especially biracial children. The clinician should attend to variations in the expression of affect and behavior. For example, subdued expressiveness in Asian and American Indian children and adolescents or aversion of eye contact with adults in Asian, African Americans, or mainland Latino children and adolescents are signs of respect for elders. Native American culture emphasizes nonverbal communication—feelings, particularly anger, are not to be expressed openly or verbally. Clinicians who are unfamiliar with these cultural nuances could misinterpret them as signs of dysthymia or subclinical depression. However, African American and Hispanic children who show disruptive behaviors in the classroom may be depressed and seeking negative attention, but clinicians may miss underlying depressive symptoms.[21]

A history of the child's and family's migration experience should be an essential part of the diagnostic interview.[52] Many immigrant children have suffered prolonged and traumatic separations and reunifications from family members, social uprooting, and abrupt geographic relocations. For inner-city children, it is important to inquire about exposure to violence at home or in their community, including the death of peers, sequential losses of parenting figures, and abuse or punitive childrearing.[51]

Treatment of minority children must be contextual, addressing psychosocial and cultural needs as well as psychological and biologic ones. The clinician must evaluate and mobilize familial, neighborhood, and community resources, address contributing and sustaining environmental factors, and enhance strengths that the child and family bring to treatment. The clinician should support parents in the development of appropriate behavioral management skills consonant with their cultural values and beliefs. They must respect culturally established means of communication and family role functioning but also foster family flexibility in dealing with their bicultural offspring.[50]

Psychological interventions should be congruent with the values and beliefs of culturally diverse children and their families. Diverse children and families are more accepting of and responsive to therapeutic approaches with a practical problem-focused, here-and-now orientation. Clinicians must be realistic about the acceptability of therapeutic interventions that may not be consonant with the family's cultural values. At the same time, clinicians must advise families about parenting approaches that may be acceptable in their culture of origin but may be considered unacceptable or illegal in mainstream culture, such as the use of corporal punishment. Consultation from and collaboration with traditional healers (such as *curanderas, santeros,* shaman, and religious ministers or priests), including the use of rituals and ceremonies from the youth's culture, may be an important component of treatment for children from more traditional families. This helps prevent conflict between healing orientations that families may experience, and it can help develop traditional healers as potential collaborators. Referral to same-culture clinicians or culturally specific programs (e.g., community-based clinics oriented to specific cultural groups) is associated with improved attendance and adherence.[50]

A value-neutral approach, in which the clinician models openness to the diverse cultural influences on the child and judicious self-disclosure of similar experiences, are helpful techniques. Confidentiality in psychotherapy must be addressed so the clinician is not perceived as driving a wedge between the patient and his or her family, nor used by the patient to resist dealing with family issues. Home-based or community-based alternatives to hospitalization usually result in better outcomes for these children and youth; involuntary hospitalization tends to recreate past traumas of oppression. If at all possible, out-of-home placement should be accomplished with the cooperation of the family and youth. An interagency system of care approach is consistent with cultural competence because it uses community resources and empowers the child and family to a maximum extent.[50]

In addition to being mindful and addressing ethnopharmacologic issues, there are numerous interpersonal aspects of pharmacotherapy with minority children that require attention. These include proper informed consent and family collaboration, particularly with traditional family decision makers (typically outside of the nuclear family); demystification of medications (not only education on their mechanisms of action, but also addressing suspicions and myths); and empowerment of children and families to make medication choices and address power differentials with clinicians.[50]

Table 23.1 summarizes practical strategies for the diagnosis and treatment of depression in immigrant and minority youth.

TABLE 23.1 SUMMARY OF PRACTICAL STRATEGIES TO OPTIMIZE OUTCOMES OF YOUTH DEPRESSION AMONG MINORITY AND IMMIGRANT GROUPS

Evaluation

- Be prepared to spend more time with them than with mainstream patients.
- If possible, involve the extended family, particularly grandmothers, who play a key role in the upbringing of the children in many minority and immigrant groups.
- Ensure the patient and family can communicate well enough with you; if not, use an interpreter.
- Avoid using family members as interpreters; this practice can cause problems and misunderstandings.
- Before the appointment, become familiar with the ethnic, cultural, and race issue of your patient and family. If it is not possible, ask them about their beliefs and customs.
- Ensure you are not coming across as judgmental (e.g., about use of alternative treatments).
- Avoid questions that can be answered yes/no; people in other cultures are likely to answer "yes" out of respect or because they don't understand the question.

Diagnosing Depression

- Among others, Asian, African American, or Latino children and adolescents often avoid eye contact with adults in authority, which can be misinterpreted as despondency.
- Presentations with somatic complaints and anger are frequent.
- Depressed individuals of Asian origin show heightened reactivity during depression; Whites show less.
- Comorbid anxiety, disruptive behavioral symptoms, substance abuse, and posttraumatic stress disorder are common, particularly if they are disadvantaged. Hence depression should be excluded in youth presenting with those symptoms.
- Use rating scales in their mother tongue that have been validated with the population being served (there are now several available in most languages, such as the CDI, BDI, CBCL/YSR/TRF, and SDQ (see Chapter 3).

(continued)

TABLE 23.1 SUMMARY OF PRACTICAL STRATEGIES TO OPTIMIZE OUTCOMES OF YOUTH DEPRESSION AMONG MINORITY AND IMMIGRANT GROUPS (CONTINUED)

Treatment

- Discuss treatment options and risks carefully and ensure they are understood. If possible, provide also written information in their own language or websites where they can access that information (see "Resources for Patients and Families" at the end of the chapter).
- Explore the financial burden of treatment and do not prescribe treatments families can't afford.
- Explore families' and patients' own ideas about the etiology of the disorder. Politely and respectfully educate them about the etiology (being careful to avoid misinterpretations or blame), prognosis, and treatment of depression and work to bridge explanatory models from their culture to Western-oriented culture.
- Use interventions that are consonant with the cultural values and beliefs of the child's family and, if possible, have some evidence base with their ethnic/cultural group.
- If possible, choose treatments that can be delivered at home, in their local community, or by culturally sensitive practitioners or agencies.
- Avoid hospitalization if at all possible, particularly involuntary hospitalization.
- Allow parents to obtain appropriate consent from elders or culturally designated family decision makers before proceeding with treatment.
- Be aware that some racial groups are more sensitive to medications. If you don't know about the specific group, start with lower doses and build up dose slowly.
- Ascertain which alternative treatments patients may be taking and check whether they can interact with antidepressants (see Chapter 14).
- If necessary, seek help from a clinician who is knowledgeable in working with the particular cultural/ethnic group.
- Be open to collaboration with religious leaders (e.g., priest, imam) or traditional healer (e.g., shaman, *curandera*) if requested by the family.

EVIDENCE-BASED TREATMENTS FOR MINORITY AND IMMIGRANT CHILDREN AND YOUTH

A number of evidence-based interventions are gaining research support for use with minority and immigrant children and youth. Cognitive-behavioral and interpersonal psychotherapies have some research evidence with Latino and African American youth.[53–55] Interestingly, interpersonal psychotherapy was originally evaluated with a largely Latino sample[56] and was later shown to be more effective than cognitive-behavioral psychotherapy in a head-to-head trial,[57] lending some support to the importance of congruence between cultural values (*personalismo*, or interpersonal skills, in Latinos) and the effectiveness of psychotherapeutic interventions. School-based preventive interventions have also been used with diverse children and youth. Cardemil et al.[57] demonstrated the effectiveness of a school-based cognitive intervention for depression as far out as 2 years. Kataoka et al.[58] demonstrated the effectiveness of a school-based cognitive behavioral therapy for trauma-related depression or posttraumatic stress with Latino children and youth.

Some therapists have developed interventions that are specific for particular ethnic and racial groups, which have been evaluated for efficacy.[59,60] Group and family psychotherapy, particularly approaches that integrate cultural and ethnic identity themes, psychoeducation, and culturally consonant coping approaches, have also been reported as both well accepted and successful.[61]

There is little psychopharmacologic research with minority and immigrant children using double-blind placebo-controlled trials. The Treatment of Adolescent Depression Study (TADS)[62] had a 26 percent minority representation among its participants, and minority status was found not to be a moderator of acute outcome. However, no separate analysis on the effectiveness of the treatments examined has been published. There are problems around minority inclusion in research trials, and one of the unfortunate results of such lack of evidence is the significantly lower numbers of minority children and youth who receive treatment for depression.[63,64]

CONCLUSIONS

Work in the area of cultural competence in children's mental health continues to evolve and develop as the fields of business, education, health care, and human services become aware of its importance to the multicultural society in the United States. The surgeon general's supplement on mental health, culture, race, and ethnicity[7] has further outlined significant issues in ethnic/racial mental health disparities and the need for expanding research in this area. This report has complemented the federal initiative on health disparities, which involves the identification of inequalities not only in mental health status but also in physical health. Research in epidemiology and services examining mental health disparities for minority and underserved youth is also pointing the way toward the system of care reforms needed to improve the cultural competence of child mental health services.[7,50]

RESOURCES FOR PRACTITIONERS

References 7, 44, and 45.

Gaw AC, ed. *Culture, Ethnicity, and Mental Illness*. Washington, DC: American Psychiatric Press; 1993.

Pedro Ruiz, ed., *Ethnicity and Psychopharmacology*. Washington, DC: American Psychiatric Press; 2000.

Four Racial Ethnic Panels. *Cultural Competence Standards for Managed Mental Health Services for Four Underserved/Underrepresented Racial/Ethnic Groups*. Rockville, Md: Center for Mental Health Services, Substance Abuse and Mental Health Administration, U.S. Department of Health and Human Services; 1999.

The Spanish version of the Beck Depression Inventory (BDI) can be purchased at http://harcourtassessment.com/HAIWEB/Cultures/en-us/Productdetail.htm?Pid=015–8018–370&Mode=detail&Leaf=otherlanguage.

The Child Behavior Checklist/Youth Self-Report Form/Teacher Report Form (by Achenbach) are translated into multiple languages and validated with multiple populations and include depression scales and cross-references to broad *DSM* categories. They can be purchased at http://www.aseba.org/index.html.

The Strengths and Difficulties Questionnaire (SDQ) in different languages can be downloaded free of charge from http://www.sdqinfo.com/b3.html.

The Center for Epidemiological Studies-Depression (CES-D) scale has been translated into multiple languages and normed for adolescents and modified for children; public domain, multiple sources.

RESOURCES FOR PATIENTS AND FAMILIES

American Academy of Child and Adolescent Psychiatry Facts for Families; available in Spanish, German, Malaysian, Polish, Icelandic, and Arabic at http://www.aacap.org/cs/root/facts_for_families/facts_for_families.

Healthy Minds.org website, sponsored by the American Psychiatric Association, has many downloadable pamphlets relating to mental health of children and youth in diverse populations, at http://healthyminds.org/.

Information about depression, not specifically in children, in more than 20 languages (including uncommon ones such as Khemer, Farsi, Lao, Punjabi, and Somalian) can be found at http://www.beyondblue.org.au/index.aspx?link_id=102.

General information about depression in Spanish: http://depression-screening.org/espanol/espanol.htm.

REFERENCES

1. U.S. Census. Population Reports, 2000. Available at: www.census.gov/population/index.html.
2. Eaton D, Kann K, Kinchen S, et al. Youth risk behavior surveillance—United States, 2005. *Mortal Morbid Wkly Rep.* 2006;55(S S05):1–108.
3. Angold A, Erkanli A, Farmer E, et al. Psychiatric disorder, impairment, and service use in rural African-American and white youth. *Arch Gen Psychiatr.* 2002;59:893–901.
4. Roberts R, Roberts C, Chen Y. Ethnocultural differences in prevalence of adolescent depression. *Am J Community Psychol.* 1997;25:95–110.
5. Sen B. Adolescent propensity for depressed mood and help seeking: race and gender differences. *J Ment Health Policy Econ.* 2004;7:133–145.

6. Kistner J, David C, White B. Ethnic and sex differences in children's depressive symptoms: mediating effects of perceived and actual competence. *J Clin Child Adolesc Psychol.* 2003;32:341–350.

7. U.S. Office of the Surgeon General. *Mental Health: Race, Ethnicity, and Culture: A Supplement to the Surgeon General's Report on Mental Health.* Washington, DC: Substance Abuse and Mental Health Administration, U.S. Department of Health and Human Services; 2001.

8. Swanson J, Linskey A, Quintero-Salinas R, et al. Depressive symptoms, drug use and suicidal ideation among youth in the Rio Grande Valley: a bi-national school survey. *J Am Acad Child Adolesc Psychiatry.* 1992;31: 669–678.

9. Pumariega A, Swanson J, Holzer C, et al. Cultural context and substance abuse in Hispanic adolescents. *J Child Fam Stud.* 1992;11:75–92.

10. Walker RL. Acculturation and acculturative stress as indicators for suicide risk among African-Americans. *Am J Orthopsychiatry.* 2007;77:386–391.

11. Brown J, Cohen P, Johnson J, et al. Childhood abuse and neglect: specificity of effect on adolescent and young depression and suicidality. *J Am Acad Child Adolesc Psychiatry.* 1999;38:1490–1496.

12. Borowski I, Resnick M, Ireland M, et al. Suicide attempts among American Indian and Alaska Native youth: risk and protective factors. *Arch Ped Adolesc Med.* 1999;153:573–580.

13. Olvera R. Suicidal ideation in Hispanic and mixed ancestry adolescents. *Suicide Life Threat Behav.* 2001;31:416–427.

14. Willis L, Coombs D, Cockerham W, et al. Ready to die: a post-mortem interpretation of the increase of African-American adolescent male suicide. *Soc Sci Med.* 2002;55:907–920.

15. Hunter E, Milroy H. Aboriginal and Torres Strait Islander suicide in context. *Arch Suicide Res.* 2006;10:141–157.

16. Silviken A, Kvernmo S. Suicide attempts among indigenous Sami adolescents and majority peer in Arctic Norway: prevalence and associated risk factors. *J Adolesc.* 2007;30:613–626.

17. Pumariega AJ, Rothe E, Pumariega JB. Mental health of immigrants and refugees. *Community Ment Health J.* 2005;41:581–597.

18. Vazsonyi A, Trejos-Castillos E, Huang L. Are developmental processes affected by immigration? Family processes, internalizing behaviors, and externalizing behaviors. *J Youth Adolesc.* 2006;35:799–813.

19. Oppendal B, Rpysamb E. Young Muslim immigrants in Norway: an epidemiological study of their psychosocial adaptation and internalizing problems. *App Dev Sci.* 2007;11:112–125.

20. Oppendal B, Roysamb E, Heyerdahl S. Ethnic group, acculturation, and psychiatric problems in young immigrants. *J Child Psychol Psychiatry.* 2005;46:646–660.

21. Kataoka SH, Zhang L, Wells KB. Unmet need for mental health care among U.S. children: variation by ethnicity and insurance status. *Am J Psychiatry.* 2002;159:1548–1555.

22. Ruiz P, Langrod J. Hispanic Americans. In: Lowisohn J, Ruiz P, Millman R, et al., eds. *Substance Abuse: A Comprehensive Textbook.* 3rd ed. Baltimore, Md: Williams and Wilkins; 1997.

23. Gaw AC. Psychiatric care of Chinese Americans. In: Gaw AC, ed. *Culture, Ethnicity, and Mental Illness.* Washington, DC: American Psychiatric Press; 1993:245–280.

24. Kilgus M, Pumariega A, Cuffe S. Race and diagnosis in adolescent psychiatric inpatients. *J Am Acad Child Adolesc Psychiatry.* 1995;34:67–72.

25. DelBello M, Lopez-Larson M, Soutullo C, et al. Effects of race on psychiatric diagnosis of hospitalized adolescents: a retrospective chart review. *J Child Adolesc Psychopharmacol.* 2001;11:95–103.

26. Nguyen L, Arganza G, Huang L, et al. The influence of race and ethnicity on psychiatric diagnoses and clinical characteristics of children and adolescent in children's services. *Cultur Divers Ethnic Minor Psychol.* 2007;13:18–25.

27. Whaley A, Geller P. Towards a cognitive process model of racial/ ethnic bias in clinical judgment. *Rev Gen Psychol.* 2007;11:7–96.

28. Rost K, Smith R, Matthews D, et al. The deliberate misdiagnosis of major depression in primary care. *Arch Fam Med.* 1994;3:333–337.

29. Cooper L, Roter D, Johnson R, et al. Patient-centered communication, ratings of care, and concordance of patient and physician race. *Ann Intern Med.* 2003;139:907–916.

30. Zito J, Safer D, Dosreis S, et al. Racial disparity in psychotropic medications prescribed for youths with Medicaid insurance in Maryland. *J Am Acad Child Adolesc Psychiatry.* 1998;32:179–184.

31. Cuffe S, Waller J, Cuccaro M, et al. Race and gender differences in the treatment of psychiatric disorders in young adolescents. *J Am Acad Child Adolesc Psychiatry.* 1995;34:1536–1543.

32. Pumariega A, Glover S, Holzer C, et al. Utilization of mental health services in a tri-ethnic sample of adolescents. *Community Ment Health J.* 1998;34:145–156.

33. Hough R, Hazen A, Soriano F, et al. Mental health care for Latinos: mental health services for Latino adolescents with psychiatric disorders. *Psychol Serv.* 2007;53:1556–1562.

34. Rowland D. Lessons from the Medicaid experience. In: Ginzberg E, ed. *Critical Issues in U.S. Health Reform.* Boulder, Colo: Westview Press; 1994:190–207.

35. Malgady R, Rogler L, Dharma E. Cultural expression of psychiatric symptoms: idioms of anger amongst Puerto Ricans. *Psychol Assess.* 1996;8:265–268.

36. Glover S, Pumariega A, Holzer C, et al. Anxiety symptomatology in Mexican-American adolescents. *J Child Fam Stud.* 1999;8:47–57.

37. Chentsova-Dutton Y, Tsai J, Chu J, et al. Depression and emotional reactivity: variation among Asian Americans of East Asian descent and European-Americans. *J Abnorm Psychol.* 2007;116:776–785.

38. Jaycox L, Stein B, Kataoka S, et al. Violence exposure, posttraumatic stress disorder, and depressive symptoms among recent immigrant schoolchildren. *J Am Acad Child Adolesc Psychiatry.* 2002;41:1104–1110.

39. McFarlane J, Groff J, O'Brien J, et al. Behaviors of children who are exposed and not exposed to intimate partner violence: an analysis of 330 black, white and Hispanic children. *Pediatrics.* 2003;112:e202–e207.

40. Romero J, Carvajal S, Valle F, et al. Adolescent bicultural stress and its impact on mental well-being among Latinos, Asian-Americans, and European-Americans. *J Community Psychol.* 2007;35:519–534.

41. Kleinman A. *Rethinking Psychiatry.* New York: Free Press; 1988.

42. Vontress C. Cultural dysthymia: an unrecognized disorder among African Americans? *J Multicult Counsel Dev.* 2007;35:130–141.

43. Simons RC, Hughes CC. Culture bound syndromes. In: Gaw A, ed. *Culture Ethnicity and Mental Illness.* Washington, DC: American Psychiatric Press; 1993.

44. Freedenthal S, Stiffman A. "They might think I was crazy:" Young American Indian's reasons for not seeking help when suicidal. *J Adolesc Res.* 2007;22:58–77.

45. Suite D, LaBril R, Primm A, et al. Beyond misdiagnosis, misunderstanding, and mistrust: relevance of the historical perspective in the medical and mental health treatment of people of color. *J Nat Med Assoc.* 2007;99:879–885.

46. Constantine M. Perceived family conflict, parental attachment, and depression in African-American female adolescents. *Cultur Divers Ethnic Minor Psychol.* 2006;12:697–709.

47. Sagrestano L, Paikoff R, Holmbeck G, et al. Longitudinal examination of familial risk factors for depression among inner city African-American adolescents. *J Family Psychol.* 2003;17:108–120.

48. Lin K, Gray G. Ethnopharmacology in Asians. In: Ruiz P, ed. *Ethnicity and Psychopharmacology.* Washington, DC: American Psychiatric Press; 2000.

49. Lin K, Smith M. Pharmacotherapy in the context of culture and ethnicity. In: Ruiz P, ed. *Ethnicity and Psychopharmacology.* Washington, DC: American Psychiatric Press; 2000.

50. Pumariega AJ, Rogers K, Rothe E. Culturally competent systems of care for children's mental health: advances and challenges. *Community Ment Health J.* 2005;41:539–556.

51. Canino I, Spurlock J. *Culturally Diverse Children and Adolescents: Assessment, Diagnosis, and Treatment.* New York: Guilford Press; 1994.

52. Rothe EM. Hispanic adolescents in the United States: psychosocial issues and treatment considerations. *Adolesc Psychiatry.* 2004;28:251–278.

53. Rosello J, Bernal G. The efficacy of cognitive-behavioral and interpersonal treatments for depression in Puerto Rican adolescents. *J Consult Clin Psychol.* 1999;67:734–745.

54. Brown C, Schulberg H, Sacco D, et al. Effectiveness of treatments for major depression in primary care practice: a post-hoc analysis of outcomes for African-American and white patients. *J Affect Disord.* 1999;53:185–192.

55. Rosello J, Jimenez-Chafey M. Cognitive-behavioral therapy for depression in adolescents with diabetes: a pilot study. *Interam J Psychol.* 2006;40:219–226.

56. Mufson L, Dorta KP, Wickramaratne P, et al. A randomized effectiveness trial of interpersonal psychotherapy for depressed adolescents. *Arch Gen Psychiatry.* 2004;61:577–584.

57. Cardemil E, Reivich K, Beevers C, et al. The prevention of depressive symptoms in low-income minority children: two year follow-up. *Behav Res Ther.* 2007;45:313–327.

58. Kataoka S, Stein B, Jaycox L, et al. A school-based mental health program for traumatized Latino immigrant children. *J Am Acad Child Adolesc Psychiatry.* 2003;42:311–318.

59. Constantino G, Malgady R, Rogler L. Storytelling through pictures: culturally sensitive psychotherapy for Hispanic children and adolescents. *J Clin Child Psychol.* 1994;23:13–20.

60. De Rios M. Magical realism: a cultural intervention for traumatized Hispanic children. *Cult Divers Ment Health.* 1997;3:159–170.

61. Salvendy J. Ethnocultural considerations in group psychotherapy. *Int J Group Psychother.* 1999;49:429–464.

62. Curry J, Rohe P, Simons A, et al. Predictors and modifiers of acute outcome in the Treatment for Adolescents with Depression Study (TADS). *J Am Acad Child Adolesc Psychiatry.* 2006;45:1427–1439.

63. Richardson L, DiGiuseppe D, Garrison M, et al. Depression in Medicaid-covered youth: differences by race and ethnicity. *Arch Pediatr Adolesc Med.* 2003;157:984–987.

64. Olfson M, Gameroff M, Marcus S, et al. Outpatient treatment of child and adolescent depression in the United States. *Arch Gen Psychiatry.* 2003;60:1236–1242.

Childhood Depression: International Views and Treatment Practices

F. NESLIHAN INAL-EMIROGLU AND RASIM SOMER DILER

KEY POINTS

- An understanding of the complex role that cultural background, national medical traditions, and diverse experiences play in mental disorders is crucial for early diagnosis, treatment, and prevention.
- Only a small proportion of children and adolescents affected by mental disorders receive adequate care.
- The gap in meeting child mental health training needs worldwide is staggering.
- The lack of epidemiologic data related to child and adolescent mental disorders in the developing world is well documented.
- Reported prevalence rates of childhood depression across the world vary considerably.
- Depression in children is considered in many countries to be a "temporary reaction to a stressor" or a "spiritual problem."
- Despite suggestions that a higher incidence of guilt feelings in Western cultures is related to the influence of the Judeo-Christian religious tradition, religion is largely reported as protective against suicide. When different religions are compared, the presence or absence of guilt feelings is associated with the level of education and the degree of depression but not with religious background.
- In most countries, suicide in children and adolescents is considered to be "moderately" associated with depression.
- Although the *Classification of Mental and Behavioral Disorders* by the World Health Organization (WHO) and the U.S. *Diagnostic and Statistical Manual of Mental Disorders* are widely accepted as the standard for statistical reporting, clinical use, and research, local diagnostic systems remain in some regions.
- In nondeveloped countries, traditional healers, alternative medicine practitioners, and religious figures are consulted more readily than mental health professionals.
- Psychotherapies that have been found useful for the treatment of depression in youth, such as cognitive behavioral therapy and interpersonal psychotherapy, are largely unavailable, but most clinicians provide counseling as well as supportive therapy and sometimes play therapy for the child and family.
- Selective serotonin reuptake inhibitors (mostly fluoxetine), tricyclic antidepressants (such as imipramine and amitriptyline), and benzodiazepines (for comorbid anxiety and depression) are the most commonly used medications worldwide.

Introduction

An understanding of the complex role that cultural background, national medical traditions, and diverse experiences play in mental disorders is crucial for early diagnosis, treatment, and prevention. Children and adolescents younger than 18 years represent about half of the world's population, although this varies widely from country to country. For example, the proportion of people younger than 15 years is 14% in Japan, 20% in the United States, 30% in Colombia, and 42% in Nigeria.[1]

> *Current epidemiologic data indicate that one in five has a mental health problem, and 3% to 4% have a serious mental disorder requiring treatment, with depression one of the most frequent.*[2] *Only a small proportion of children and adolescents affected by mental disorders receive adequate care. The gap in meeting child mental health needs worldwide is staggering, with between a half and two-thirds of the need going unmet, with higher proportions in low- and middle-income countries.*[2]

A cross-national examination of depression raises many issues, including the following: Do all youth, regardless of their culture, experience emotions in similar ways? Does the description of the experience of an emotion and its response to treatment change from culture to culture, or is it similar? This chapter describes the available literature regarding differences regarding the diagnosis and treatment of childhood depression across the world. To this end, we reviewed the few studies published and briefly present the results of a survey among psychiatrists/child psychiatrists carried out to gather information about practices to diagnose and treat depression in different countries (unpublished results). It is acknowledged that "country" and "culture" are not synonymous (e.g., several countries may share a similar culture, whereas several cultures often coexist in one country), but separating country and culture is difficult and both terms are used. Irrespective of culture, within-country differences are minimized because of homogeneous health delivery systems, health funding, and so on, and are more meaningful because of the availability of statistical data. *Child* is used to mean both children and adolescents unless specified otherwise.

EPIDEMIOLOGY

The absence of epidemiologic data related to childhood mental disorders in the developing world is well documented and confirmed by the World Health Organization's ATLAS survey.[2] Among high-income countries, 8 out of 20 (40%) have some form of epidemiologic data available, compared with 1 in 16 (6%) in low-income countries.[2] Accordingly, research on cross-national aspects of depression in children is limited. Some of the difficulties in the cross-cultural study of depression stem from diagnostic conceptualization. Historically, psychiatrists in different countries have used different diagnostic concepts such as endogenous depression, reactive depression, depressive psychosis, neurotic depression, major depression, and dysthymic disorder, making it difficult to compare cross-cultural data. Standardized methods and uniform diagnostic criteria are crucial for cross-country epidemiologic study.

Reported prevalence rates of childhood depression across the world vary considerably from 1% to 14% (Australia, 14.2%; China, 13%; Brazil, 1%; Italy, 3.8%; Japan, 2.7%; Russia, 11%; Trinidad and Tobago, 14%; Turkey, 8%; and United Kingdom, 10%).[3–11] However, studies used different samples, methodologies, and diagnostic instruments. A European study that sought to estimate the prevalence of childhood psychiatric disorders in four ethnic groups (Dutch, Moroccan, Turkish, and Surinamese) using best-estimate diagnoses reported an overall prevalence of psychiatric disorder of 11%; externalizing disorders (9%) were more common than mood disorders (2%). They also reported that the prevalence of childhood disorders did not differ between natives and immigrant children of low socioeconomic status from inner-city neighborhoods.[12]

CHILDHOOD DEPRESSION FROM A CULTURAL PERSPECTIVE

A symptom is a communication, an interpretation, and an experience, which is also a signal and a changing set of expectations and demands.[13] Symptoms reveal the culture and its influences, whether they are expressed idiomatically or in conventional Western medical terms.[13] Cultural considerations in the assessment, diagnosis, and treatment of childhood disorders are always necessary[14] (see also Chapter 23); however, it is very difficult to disentangle what is nature (e.g., genetics, biology) and what is nurture (e.g., environment, society, culture). A universalistic orientation tries to incorporate both biologic or genetic factors and cultural or environmental factors in the understanding of human behavior. As detailed by Choi,[15] this orientation assumes the existence of common features in human development and mental health across ethnocultural groups, and it considers observable behaviors, expressions of emotion, and the manifestations of mental illness as shaped by culture.[15] A recent study suggests that people from different cultures may weight facial cues in different parts of the face differently when interpreting emotional expressions: Americans focused on the mouth, whereas Japanese gave more weight to the eyes.[16]

It has been suggested the reported increase in rates of childhood depression in North America and Europe may reflect a lowering of the threshold for diagnosis.[17] A recent meta-analysis reviewed studies between 1965 and 1996 that had used at least one structured diagnostic interview, finding no evidence for an increase in the prevalence of childhood depression over the past 30 years.[18] It is possible that public perceptions of an *epidemic* may be the consequence of heightened awareness of a disorder that was long underdiagnosed, or the availability of better measures, screening programs, and new treatment options, resulting in more depressed children seeking help.[18,19]

There are many case reports about cross-cultural differences in the manifestation of depression. For example, it was reported that depressive symptoms in Afghanistan are similar to those in other countries, but in Afghanistan the majority of depressed patients express "passive death wishes" rather than active suicidal thoughts. Despite suggestions that a higher incidence of guilt feelings in Western countries is related to the influence of the Judeo-Christian religious traditions, religion is largely reported as protective against suicide.[20] When different religions are compared, the presence or absence of guilt feelings is associated with the level of education and the degree of depression but not with religious background.[21]

The Indian value system is not based on the dichotomous view of the world central to Western thought (such as individual versus collective, humankind versus nature, body versus mind). Characteristics such as interdependence, interpersonal harmony and cooperation, and nonverbal and indirect communication are more valued in India and in other Eastern countries. These cultures are weary, if not critical, of the value placed by Western cultures on individualism and of the priority given to individual needs above those of the group.[22]

To explore variations in the meaning and subjective experience of depression, Tanaka-Matsumi and Marsella[23] asked Japanese, Japanese American, and white American college students to associate a word with "depression." They reported that Japanese do not describe (mild or ordinary) depression in the same way as Americans, nor do they express feelings in the same way. For the Japanese, concrete images from nature allow personal emotions to be expressed impersonally; as a result, they largely lack a personal reference or connection when expressing emotions.[23]

Asians generally experience greater family and social connections and support than do people in Western cultures. However, this could also be a result of poverty and need for survival. For example, growing problems in Singapore are associated with development and increasing wealth (e.g., family breakdown, not looking after elders), similar to those in many Western countries.[24] It has been suggested that family support is protective against depression; rates of depression in Asian countries such as Japan, China, and Taiwan are reported to be lower than in the Western world.[25] It is, however, questionable whether the prevalence of depression is truly lower in Asian countries or simply an artifact of cultural biases.[15] Clinicians' training and practice could also influence the reported rates of depression in those populations. For example, Israeli clinicians tend to give one primary diagnosis, whereas in the United States multiple diagnoses are very common. A study reported a significantly higher percentage of diagnoses of depression in U.S. adolescent psychiatric inpatients compared with Israeli ones (78% versus 24%); depression was mostly assigned as a secondary diagnosis in the U.S. sample but not in the Israeli sample.[26]

Hispanic cultures also place a greater emphasis on family than other Western cultures. Although support from the family is protective, poverty and lack of resources loom large in some of these countries.[27] Rather than as feelings of guilt or low mood, depression is frequently experienced in somatic terms in Hispanic populations. Clinicians must be aware that depressed Hispanic youth may present with headaches, gastrointestinal and cardiovascular symptoms, or complaints of "nerves"[28] (see Chapter 23). In this context, the use of "somatic" to refer to melancholic or endogenous aspects of the depressive syndrome can be confusing.[28] It should be noted that presentations with somatic symptoms are not limited to Hispanic depressed children but are frequent in adolescents from other countries as well, such as Italians.[29]

SUICIDE

Adolescent suicide, a very common problem in all countries, is linked to depression.[30] However, this association is often overlooked outside the developed world, where accurate suicide data are rarely collected. Further, because of guilt, shame, or religious disapproval, suicides are not always reported or are recorded as accidents. Research is still needed to ascertain risk factors for youth suicide in different cultures.[31] For example, suicide, particularly self-poisoning with pesticides, is the leading cause of death among 14- to 24-year-olds in China. Contrary to what happens in Western countries, suicide in China is much more common among women and in rural areas. Whereas youth suicide is strongly associated with depression in the West, this is less so for women in China, where stressors, impulsivity, easy access to pesticides—stored at home in rural areas—and lack of access to medical care largely explain the high female suicide death rate. At the contrary, psychiatric disorder is associated with suicide in Chinese males. The implication is that reducing access to pesticides would be a key issue to lessen youth suicide in China.[32] A large multinational study concluded that per capita income is of more relevance for suicidal behavior than culture: The strongest diagnostic risk factor in high-income countries was a mood disorder, whereas impulse control disorders were the main risk in low- and middle-income countries.[33]

PERSPECTIVES ON CLASSIFICATION

Although the WHO's *Classification of Mental and Behavioral Disorders* (ICD) and the U.S. *Diagnostic and Statistical Manual of Mental Disorders* (DSM) are widely accepted as the standard for statistical reporting, clinical use, and research,[34,35] local diagnostic systems remain in some regions, such as in China and South America. Similarities and differences between the ICD and DSM classifications were highlighted in Chapter 1. These classifications have traditionally ignored cross-cultural issues, although an attempt was made to include them in *DSM-IV-TR*,[36] a crucial innovation. The outline for a cultural formulation and glossary of culture-bound syndromes is presented in Appendix I of *DSM-IV TR*.[34] It includes cultural identity of the individual, cultural explanations of the illness, cultural factors related to the psychological environment and levels of functioning, cultural elements of the relationship between the individual and the clinician, and overall cultural assessment of diagnosis and care.

China issued the first edition of the *Chinese Classification of Psychiatric Disorders* (CCPD) in 1986. The third edition of the *CCPD* (CCPD-3) was published in 2001. Familiarity with CCPD-3 would allow better communication with Chinese psychiatrists.[37] Mood disorders used to be a major area of disagreement between the Chinese and international classifications, but differences have lessened. *CCPD-3* recognizes depression and mild depression ("hypodepression"), but it does not specify them further according to the presence of somatic, psychotic, catatonic, atypical, or postpartum features. For the first time, chronic low-grade depression is classified as dysthymia (duration criterion of 6 months) in the section of mood disorders, rather than as depressive neurosis (duration criterion of 3 months) in the section of neurosis. *CCPD-3* also includes a diagnosis of "emotional disorders with onset specific to childhood" in Section 8 (hyperkinetic, conduct, and emotional disorders with onset usually occurring in childhood and adolescence). There are problems about translating *DSM* terms into Chinese. For example, major depression translates as "severe, severe depression." Chinese psychiatrists are concerned that diagnosing a patient with "major depression" has negative, undesirable connotations.

Two adaptations of the international classification to the Latin American context have emerged: the *Cuban Glossary of Psychiatry* and *La Guía Latinoamericana de Diagnóstico Psiquiátrico* (GLADP), a project of the Section on Diagnosis and Classification of the Latin American Psychiatric Association. Although GLADP is broadly based on *ICD-10*, there are differences, including the classification of childhood depression.[28] A number of child psychiatrists proposed that childhood depression should be included in the sections devoted to childhood disorders to do justice to the specific features in this age group.[28]

Russian psychiatrists generally refer to *ICD-10*. However, they distinguish several types of depressive disorder that are different: asthenic, adynamic, boring, melancholic, psychopathic, dysphoric, somatic, and depression in the context of anorexia.[38]

TREATMENT

As detailed in other chapters of this book, there are effective pharmacotherapy[39] and psychotherapy[40] interventions for childhood depression. Clinicians need to keep up to date and change their practice according to new information in this rapidly evolving field.[41] Treatment of mood disorders needs to be culturally and biologically sensitive to be effective and ensure adherence. For example, the cytochrome P450 (CYP) allele is known to vary among ethnic groups.[42] As already highlighted in Chapter 14, different CYP systems are involved in the metabolism of different drugs; as a result, effectiveness and drug–drug interactions may vary from one population to another. Patients from cultures who tend to present with somatic rather than emotional symptoms—perhaps because of difficulties expressing feelings or lack of mind/body distinctions—may find it hard to discuss feelings and personal problems during therapy (e.g., some Asian patients).[25] This may also be related to the fact that emotional problems are viewed as more stigmatizing in some cultures than others. When assessing and managing childhood depression, it is recommended to (1) appraise the patient's interpretation and understanding of the symptoms, (2) discuss somatic symptoms in the context of the child's life situation, (3) remain sensitive to the cultural idioms regarding specific somatic symptoms, and (4) listen to them with empathy and compassion[43] (see Chapter 23).

Barriers to care exist in all countries and at all levels. The most important include transportation, limited financial resources, and stigma. The last is a more significant barrier in high-income (80.0%) than in low-income countries (37.5%).[2] Another barrier is the availability of child psychiatrists and other trained professionals. For example, it is estimated that up to 30 million children and adolescents in China have significant mental disorders, but there are only 150 physicians trained in child psychiatry.[44] Japan, with a population of 126 million, only has 100 child and adolescent psychiatrists. The rate of child and adolescent psychiatrists varies tenfold among European countries, from 1 per 5,300 people in Switzerland to 1 per 51,800 people in Serbia. With few exceptions, the number of child and adolescent psychiatrists is negligible in most African, Eastern Mediterranean, Southeast Asian, and Western Pacific countries, ranging from 1 to 4 per million population.[2] For example, one study estimated the number of child psychiatrists per million people in 2006 to be 21 in the United States, 2.8 in Singapore, 2.5 in Hong Kong, and 0.5 in Malaysia.[24] Although psychiatric nurses are a resource throughout the world, specialization to work with children is rare.[2]

The public's knowledge and attitudes toward depression may lead to delayed or inappropriate help seeking or may impair adherence to clinicians' recommendations. An Australian telephone survey sought to assess young people's (12 to 25 years of age) ability to recognize clinically defined depression and psychosis, the types of help they thought appropriate for these problems, their knowledge of suitable treatments, and their perceptions regarding prognosis. Depression was far more readily recognized than psychosis by the young people surveyed, but belief in the helpfulness of recommended interventions was generally greater for psychosis. Younger respondents were more likely to consider seeking help from family and friends.[45] In a similar survey, antidepressants were the most favorably viewed psychiatric medication, but still less than half of the respondents thought they would be helpful for depression. Interestingly, parents were less favorable toward antidepressants in adolescents than in young adults.[46] Another survey in Turkey sought to assess the public's knowledge and attitudes toward depression and associated sociodemographic factors. The results suggest that Turks identified depression as an illness, tended to perceive depression as a social problem, believed that depression could be treated with drugs (but had little knowledge about drugs and treatment), and were doubtful about society's acceptance of depressed patients.[47]

There is no essential drug list for pediatric psychotropic medications in >70% of the countries surveyed by WHO, and national systems for monitoring their prescription rarely exist.[2] Less than half of the countries provide some form of subsidy for medication.[2]

Antidepressant use also varies widely. In 2000, the use of antidepressants among insured youth younger than 20 years in the United States (1.63%) was more than three times higher than in Denmark, Germany, and the Netherlands (range, 0.11% to 0.54%). Tricyclic antidepressant use predominated in Germany, whereas selective serotonin reuptake inhibitors (SSRIs) predominated in the United States, Denmark, and the Netherlands.[48] In Germany, SSRIs represented only 15% of antidepressants prescribed, but there had been a doubling of its use from 2000 to 2003.[49] This may have changed after the "black box" warning of suicide risk by the Food and Drug Administration (FDA).

There are evidence-based psychotherapy treatments for childhood depression available,[40,50] but replication studies in different countries and cross-cultural studies are needed.

INTERNATIONAL SURVEY OF PSYCHIATRISTS

To our knowledge, there are no studies describing the views of psychiatrists regarding the nature, symptoms, and treatment of childhood depression across countries. Thus the authors performed a preliminary survey through e-mail. To obtain a picture of childhood depression around the world, we tried to reach as many psychiatrists and child psychiatrists as possible by searching PsychInfo, MedLine, and other Internet resources (e.g., scholar.google.com) for local scientific publications on childhood depression. We e-mailed the survey to the authors and asked them to complete it. Given the scarcity of child psychiatrists in many countries, we also e-mailed three World Psychiatric Association (WPA) young psychiatrists in each country—from the Educational Liaisons Network listed at the World Psychiatric Association's website (http://www.wpanet.org/home.html)—and asked their help to refer us to the local experts in their region. Of the 63 surveys mailed, 44 (70%) were returned completed by psychiatrists from 28 countries, including Argentina, Azerbaijan, Belgium, Bosnia, Bolivia, Brazil, Canada, China, Czech Republic, Egypt, France, Germany, Guatemala, Jordan, Latvia, India, Iran, Israel, Italy, Lithuania, Nigeria, Pakistan, Russia, Spain, Taiwan, Turkey, United States, and Uruguay. The survey included items such as "What are medical practitioners' main sources of information about childhood depression?" and "Are there culturally bound presentations of childhood depression in your country/region?" (The survey is available on request from the first author.)

Readers should take into account the limitations of this survey before drawing conclusions. For example, the results summarized here are largely anecdotal, reflecting the opinions of the respondents, which may or may not represent the views of most psychiatrists in the countries mentioned or what actually occurs.

EDUCATION AND TRAINING

The dearth of professionals, including allied health, trained in this area is a worldwide problem. Not only there are few child and adolescent psychiatrists, but also the profession is not formally recognized as specialty in many countries, even in some developed nations (e.g., Singapore, Spain). Many countries do not have a specific journal or association for child and adolescent mental health, and they lack research or review papers on assessment or treatment of childhood depression in their local scientific journals or language. Medical practitioners' main sources of information about childhood depression are medical schools, conferences, and international mental health journals. Some countries (e.g., Azerbaijan, Jordan, Uruguay) reported pharmaceutical representatives as their main source of information. The predominant orientation among psychiatrists and child psychiatrists was reported as biologic. However, learning theories (e.g., Bolivia) and psychoanalysis (e.g., Argentina, Russia, Uruguay) have a strong following in some countries.

PERCEPTIONS OF DEPRESSION

In many countries (e.g., Argentina, Azerbaijan, Bosnia, Bolivia, Brazil, China, Czech Republic, Egypt, India, Iran, Jordan, Latvia, Lithuania, Nigeria, Russia, Taiwan), the general public as well as teachers, parents, and sometimes health care professionals (e.g., by underreferring, underdiagnosing, and undertreating depression) still do not believe that depression exists in children. Childhood depression is considered in many countries to be a "temporary reaction to a stressor" or a "spiritual problem." Teachers and parents often attribute depressive symptoms to behavioral and adjustment difficulties, labeling these children as *problematic* instead of as suffering from a depressive disorder that could benefit from treatment.

DIAGNOSIS AND CLASSIFICATION

Practitioners in some countries (e.g., in Egypt, India, Jordan, Nigeria) sometimes regard "not respecting parents and not praying to God" as signs of depression. School refusal, aggression, and unexplained somatic complaints are reported frequently as symptoms associated with depression.

Clinicians in developing countries seem to give more weight to the physical/vegetative symptoms of depression than to unhappiness, anhedonia, or depressive cognitions. Irritability is widely accepted as a symptom for depression and chronic depression is recognized in many countries, but few professionals feel comfortable diagnosing children with dysthymia.

In most countries, suicide in children and adolescents is considered to be *moderately* associated with depression. When psychotic symptoms are present with depression, many clinicians around the world tend to diagnose "depression with psychotic symptoms" rather than schizophrenia, and some consider a diagnosis of bipolar disorder.

ICD-10 is more widely used for administrative and insurance purposes than *DSM-IV. DSM-IV* encourages multiple diagnoses when necessary; however, most clinicians around the world tend to make one diagnosis (the one considered primary or most important). Few depression scales for children (e.g., Children's Depression Inventory, Depression Self-Rating Scale) have been validated outside the West, are available, and in clinical use in local languages (see Chapter 3). Some countries (e.g., Argentina, Guatemala) use adult scales (e.g., Zung and Hamilton Depression Scales).

TREATMENT

Traditional healers, alternative medicine practitioners, and religious figures are consulted more readily than mental health professionals in nondeveloped countries. Cognitive behavioral therapy and interpersonal therapy are largely unavailable outside Western countries, but clinicians often provide counseling as well as supportive therapy and sometimes play therapy to the child and family.

Selective serotonin reuptake inhibitors (SSRIs), mostly fluoxetine, tricyclic antidepressants (TCAs), such as imipramine and amitriptyline, and benzodiazepines (for comorbid anxiety and depression) were reported as the most commonly used medications. Some countries (e.g., in Germany) use St. John's wort widely. Apart from the United States, there is little data (e.g., from France, India, Jordan, Spain) about changes in prescribing practices following the FDA warnings, although clinicians report an overall decrease in prescription of antidepressants. However, clinicians from other countries (e.g., Bolivia, China, Belgium, Egypt, Germany, Russia, Turkey) deny decreasing their prescription of SSRIs. Further, higher recognition and treatment of childhood depression may have offset any decrease in antidepressant prescription. Practitioners from some countries (e.g., China, Egypt, Nigeria, Russia) believe that iron deficiency is etiologically relevant; some clinicians from developed countries (e.g., Israel, United States) consider vitamin E or omega-3 deficiency also to be relevant.

In India, there is an inpatient facility where both child and caregivers are admitted for assessment and treatment; the practice is to always admit children with their caregivers who stay with the child during the entire inpatient treatment. In some clinics in China, Western practices (pharmacotherapy and psychotherapy) are applied concurrently with traditional Chinese medicine (e.g., acupuncture, auricular plaster therapy, herbal treatments); other clinics choose to use only one of them.

RESOURCES FOR PRACTITIONERS

World Psychiatric Association. *Atlas, Child and Adolescent Mental Health Resources, Global Concerns: Implications for the Future:* http://www.who.int/mental_health/resources/Child_ado_atlas.pdf .

Psychiatric Rating Scales Index for Depression: http://www.neurotransmitter.net/depressionscales.html.

World Health Organization, Child and Adolescent Mental Health and Policies: http://www.who.int/mental_health/policy/Childado_mh_module.pdf.

National Member Organizations of the International Association for Child and Adolescent Psychiatry and Allied Professions: http://iacapap.ki.se/members_national.htm

References 2, 3, 36, 44, 48, 49.

Kolch M,. Schnoor K, Fegert JM. The EU-regulation on medicinal products for paediatric use: impacts on child and adolescent psychiatry and clinical research with minors. *Eur Child Adolesc Psychiatry.* 2007;16:229–235.

REFERENCES

1. Source 2008 World Factbook, CIA. Available at: https://www.cia.gov/library/publications/the-world-factbook/.
2. World Psychiatric Association. *Atlas, Child and Adolescent Mental Health Resources, Global Concerns: Implications for the Future.* World Health Organization and International Association for Child and Adolescent Mental Health and Allied Professions; 2005.

3. Boyd CP, Gullone E, Kostanski M, et al. Prevalence of anxiety and depression in Australian adolescents: comparison with world wide data. *J Genet Psychol.* 2000;161:479–492.

4. Charman T, Pervova I. Self-reported depressed mood in Russian and UK schoolchildren. A research note. *J Child Psychol Psychiatry.* 1996;37:879–883.

5. Diler RS, Kocak E. Childhood psychiatric problems at the primary health care. In: Narlı N, Karatas Y, eds. *General Medicine Handbook for General Practitioners.* Adana, Turkey: Nobel Medical Publications; 2004: 105–114.

6. Fleitlich-Bilyk B, Goodman R. Prevalence of child and adolescent psychiatric disorders in Southeast Brazil. *J Am Acad Child Adolesc Psychiatry.* 2004;43:727–734.

7. Frigerio A, Pesenti S, Molteni M, et al. Depressive symptoms as measured by the CDI in a population of Northern Italian children. *Eur Psychiatry.* 2001;16:33–37.

8. Ikawa T, Okubo T, Koda R, et al. Depression in the general population: telephone survey. *Abstracts XIIth World Congress of Psychiatry.* Vol. 2. Yokohama, Japan, 2002:181.

9. Maharijah HD, Ali A, Konings M. Adolescent depression in Trinidad and Tobago. *Eur Child Adolesc Psychiatry.* 2006;15:30–37.

10. Ollendick TH, Yule W. Depression in British and American children and its relation to anxiety and fear. *J Consult Clin Psychol.* 1990;58:126–129.

11. Shek DTL. Depressive symptoms in a sample of Chinese adolescents: an empirical study using the Chinese version of the Beck Depression Inventory. *Int J Adolesc Med Health.* 1991;5:1–16.

12. Zwirs BWC, Burger H, Wiznitzer M, et al. Prevalence of psychiatric disorders among children of different ethnic origin. *J Abnorm Child Psychol.* 2007;35:556–566.

13. Marsella AJ, Yamada AM. Culture and mental health: an introduction and overview of foundations, concepts, and issues. In: Cuéllar I, Paniagua FA, eds. *Handbook of Multicultural Mental Health.* San Diego, Calif: Academic Press; 2000:3–24.

14. Canino I, Canino G, Arroyo W. Cultural considerations for childhood disorders: how much was included in DSM-IV? *Transcult Psychiatry.* 1998;35:343–355.

15. Choi H. Understanding adolescent depression in ethnocultural context. *Adv Nurs Sci.* 2002;25:71–85.

16. Yuki M, Maddux WW, Masuda T. Are the windows to the soul the same in the East and West? Cultural differences in using the eyes and mouth as cues to recognize emotions in Japan and the United States. *J Exper Soc Psychol.* 2007;303–311.

17. Rutter M, Smith D. *Psychosocial Disorders in the Young: Time Trends and Their Causes.* Chichester, UK: John Wiley; 1995.

18. Costello J, Erkanli E, Angold A. Is there an epidemic of child or adolescent depression? *J Child Psychol Psychiatry.* 2006;47:1263–1271.

19. Thomsen PH. The treatment of child and adolescent depression: a matter of concern? *Acta Psychiatr Scand.* 2007;115:169–170.

20. Weaver AJ, Samford JA, Morgan VJ, et al. Research on religious variables in five major adolescent research journals: 1992 to 1996. *J Nerv Ment Dis.* 2000;188:36–44.

21. Tseng WS. Culture and psychopathology: disorders of depression. In: Tseng WS, ed. *Handbook of Cultural Psychiatry.* Gainesville, Fla: Academic Press; 2001:335–343.

22. Banhatti R, Dwivedi K, Maitra B. Childhood: an Indian perspective. In: Timimi S, Maitra, eds. *Critical Voices in Child and Adolescent Mental Health.* London: Free Association Books; 2006:75–97.

23. Tanaka-Matsumi J, Marsella AJ. Cross cultural variations in the phenomenological experience of depression: I. Word association studies. *J Cross Cult Psychol.* 1976;7:379–396.

24. Tan SMK, Fung D, Hung S-F, et al. Growing wealth and growing pains: child and adolescent psychiatry in Hong Kong, Malaysia, and Singapore. *Australasian Psychiatry.* 2008;16:204–209.

25. Tsai JL, Chentsova-Dutton Y. Understanding depression across cultures. In: Gotlib IH, Hammen CL, eds. *Handbook of Depression.* New York: Guilford Press; 2002:467–491.

26. Cohen Y, Spirito A, Apter A, et al. A cross-cultural comparison of behavior disturbance and suicidal behavior among psychiatrically hospitalized adolescents in Israel and the United States. *Child Psychiatry Hum Dev.* 1997;28:89–102.

27. Hovey J. Acculturative stress, depression, and suicidal ideation in Mexican immigrants. *Cultur Divers Ethnic Minor Psychol.* 2000;6:134–151.

28. Berganza CE, Mezzich JE, Otero-Ojeda AA, et al. The Latin American guide for psychiatric diagnosis: a cultural overview. *Psychiatry Clin N Am.* 2001;24:433–445.

29. Masi G, Millepiedi S, Mucci M. Somatic symptoms in children and adolescents referred for emotional behavioral disorders. *Psychiatry.* 2000;63:140–159.

30. Birmaher B, Ryan ND, Williamson DE, et al. Childhood and adolescent depression. *J Am Acad Child Adolesc Psychiatry.* 1996;35:1427–1439.

31. Anonymous. Adolescent suicide. Report from the Group for the Advancement of Psychiatry. 1996; 140:1–184.

32. Li XY, Phillips MR, Zhang YP, et al. Risk factors for suicide in China's youth: a case-control study. *Psychol Med.* 2008;38:397–406.

33. Nock MK, Borges G, Bromet EJ, et al. Cross-national prevalence and risk factors for suicidal ideation, plans, and attempts. *Br J Psychiatry.* 2008;192:98–105.

34. American Psychiatric Association. *Diagnostic and Statistical Manual of Mental Disorders, 4th Edition, Text Revision.* Washington, DC: APA Press; 2000.

35. World Health Organization: The ICD-10 *Classification of Mental and Behaviour Disorders—Clinical Descriptions and Diagnostic Guidelines.* Geneva: WHO; 1992.

36. Mezzich JE, Berganza CE, Ruiperez MA. Culture in DSM-IV, ICD-10, and evolving diagnostic systems. *Psychiatry Clin N Am.* 2001;24:407–419.

37. Lee S. From diversity to unity: the classification of mental disorders in 21st-century China. *Psychiatry Clin N Am.* 2001;24:421–431.

38. Grebchenko Y, Evgeny K. Pediatric bipolar disorder: from the perspective of Russia. In: Diler RS, ed. *Pediatric Bipolar Disorder: A Global Perspective.* New York: Nova Sciences Publications; 2007:179–192.

39. Hughes CW, Emslie GJ, Crismon ML, et al. Texas Children's Medication Algorithm Project: update from Texas Consensus Conference Panel on Medication Treatment of Childhood Major Depressive Disorder. *J Am Acad Child Adolesc Psychiatry.* 2007;46:667–686.

40. Watanabe N, Hunot V, Omori IM, et al. Psychotherapy for depression among children and adolescents: a systematic review, *Acta Psychiatr Scand.* 2007;116(2):84–95.

41. Rey JM, Martin A. Selective serotonin reuptake inhibitors and suicidality in juveniles: review of the evidence and implications for clinical practice. *Child Adolesc Psychiatry Clin N Am.* 2006;15:221–237.

42. Bradford LD. CYP2D6 allele frequency in European Caucasians, Asians, Africans, and their descendants. *Pharmacogenomics.* 2002;3:229–243.

43. Lewis-Fernández R, Das AK, Alfonso C, et al. Depression in US Hispanics: diagnostic and management considerations in family practice. *J Am Board Family Pract.* 2005;18:282–296.

44. Jiao F, Jiao W, Yen TG. Pediatric bipolar disorder: from the perspective of China. In: Diler RS, ed. *Pediatric Bipolar Disorder: A Global Perspective.* New York: Nova Sciences Publications; 2007:71–90.

45. Wright A, Harris MG, Wiggers JH, et al. Recognition of depression and psychosis by young Australians and their beliefs about treatment. *Med J Aust.* 2005;183:18–23.

46. Jorm AF, Wright A. Beliefs of young people and their parents about the effectiveness of interventions for mental disorders. *Aust N Z J Psychiatry.* 2007;41:656–666.

47. Ozmen E, Ogel K, Boratav C, et al. The knowledge and attitudes of the public towards depression: an Istanbul population sample. *Türk Psikiyatri Dergisi.* 2003;14:89–100.

48. Zito JM, Tobi H, de Jong-van den Berg LT, et al. Antidepressant prevalence for youths: a multi-national comparison. *Pharmacoepidemiol Drug Safety.* 2006;15:793–798.

49. Fegert JM, Kolch M, Zito JM, et al. Antidepressant use in children and adolescents in Germany. *J Child Adolesc Psychopharmacol.* 2006;16:197–206.

50. Weisz JR, McCarty CA, Valeri SM. Effects of psychotherapy for depression in children and adolescents: a meta-analysis. *Psychol Bull.* 2006;132:132–149.

Index

Page numbers in *italics* refer to figures; those followed by t refer to tables.

AACAP practice parameter, for treatment of depression, 49–50, 52

Abnormal Involuntary Movement Scale (AIMS), 182

Abuse. *See* Physical abuse; Sexual abuse

Acamprosate, for alcohol dependence, 247

Accommodations, by school, 202

Achenbach System of Empirically Based Assessment (ASEBA), 36, 36t

Activation, 52, 79, 163, 184

Active monitoring, 49, 258

Activity module, CBT, 104–106, *106*

Acute (phase of treatment), 45t

Acute depressive episodes, managing, 162–173
  encouragement of youth and parents, 166–167
    chain analysis, 167
    confidentiality and trust, 166
    interviews, 166–167
    misperceptions arising as consequences of depression, 167t
  overview, 162–163
  STAU (specialist treatment as usual)
    activation, 163
    case management, 163
    complexity of case, 164
    developmental considerations, 164
    formulation, 163
    organization of session, 168–169
    rating scales, 164
    risk assessment and management, 164, 165t–166t
    severity, 163–164
    specific psychotherapy input into, 169
  treatment
    exercise, sleep, and diet, 170
    frequency of sessions, 168
    length of sessions, 168–169
    medications, 169–170
    NICE stepped care approach, 170, 171t
    outcomes, 171
    outpatient *versus* inpatient, 168
    planning and delivery, 167–168
    psychoeducation, 168

Acute treatment
  algorithm, 72, 74
  definition, 71

Adderall, for comorbid ADHD and depression, 225t

ADDICTD mnemonic, 239

ADHD. *See* Attention deficit hyperactivity disorder

Adjunctive agents, 45t, 81–82, 303t. *See also* Augmentation

Adjustment disorder with depressed mood, 12t, 32

Adolescent Obsessive-Compulsive Drinking Scale (A-OCDS), 240–241, 246, 247

Adolescents, engaging and supporting, 55–57, 56t

Advice and praise, verbal technique in dynamic psychotherapy, 146t

Affectionless control (parenting type), 20

Affiliative needs, gender differences in, 18

African American children and youth, 322–326, 328
  See also Minority children and youth

Age of onset, 6–7

Aggression, comorbid with depression, 231–234
  algorithm for treatment, *233*
  medications, 227t, 232–233
  rating scales, 231–232
  TRAAY guidelines, 232, 234

Agree to disagree, learning to, 137

AIMS (Abnormal Involuntary Movement Scale), 182

Alcohol, interaction with antidepressants, 261

Alcohol abuse. *See also* Substance use/abuse
  consequences and treatment, 165t
  pharmacotherapy, 246–247
  as risk factor for acute depressive episodes, 165t

Alcohol Use Disorders Identification Test (AUDIT), 241

All in the timing (IPT-A technique), 122–123

Alternative medicine. *See* Complementary and alternative medicine (CAM)

Alternative treatments, 78–79, 82

Ambiguous messages, in family therapy, 137

American Academy of Child and Adolescent Psychiatry (AACAP) practice parameter, for treatment of depression, 49–50, 52

American Indian children and youth, 322–323, 326
  See also Minority children and youth

Amitriptyline, 338

Amphetamines, for comorbid ADHD and depression, 225t

Anaclitic line, of personality development, 143, 143t

Anger, in minority youth, 324

Anhedonia, 167t

Anticholinergics, 180

Anticoagulant drugs, interaction with essential fatty acids, 154

Anticonvulsants
  for depression comorbid with chronic physical illness, 303t
  for depression comorbid with pain, 305
  interaction with St. John's wort, 156t

Antidepressants. *See also* Medication; *specific drugs*
  adding to STAU, 170
  black box warnings, 260

Antidepressants (*Cont.*)
for depression comorbid with chronic physical
illness, 301–302
for depression comorbid with substance
abuse, 245
for depression in intellectually disabled patients, 315
discontinuation, 82
drug interactions, 261–262
alcohol, 261
herbal remedies, 262
over-the-counter medications, 261
prescription medications, 262
street drugs, 262
indications for use, 259t
media stories, effect of, 5
monitoring treatment, 261
primary care setting, use in, 260–262
response of children and adolescents to, 6
safety, 78–79
side effects, 184–185, 189, 261
variation in use internationally, 336
Antidepressant Treatment History Form, 71
Antipsychotics
adverse effects, 178
cardiovascular, 303–304
metabolic syndrome, 184–185
seizures, 305
for depression comorbid with chronic physical
illness, 303t
Anxiety
comorbid with depression, 222–229
algorithm for treatment, 224
cognitive behavior therapy, 224, 228–229, 228t
incidence, 221
medications, 225t, 228
rating scales, 222, 223t, 224
systematic desensitization, 228–229
of patients about medication, 180
rating scales, 222, 223t, 224
as risk factor for depression, 19
school refusal and, 202
symptom overlap with other disorders, 222t
A-OCDS (Adolescent Obsessive-Compulsive
Drinking Scale), 240–241, 246, 247
Appetite loss, 167t
Areas of influence, pie chart, 131
Aripiprazole, 80t
Aristolochic acid, 153
ASEBA (Achenbach System of Empirically Based
Assessment), 36, 36t
Asians. *See also* Minority children and youth
availability of mental health professionals, 336
depression in children and youth, 324–326
family support, 334
Asperger's disorder, 316
Assent, 47, 91
Assessment, 23–38
of children *versus* adults, 23–24
comorbidity, 37
conflicting data, reconciling, 25
of depressive episodes, 27

detecting depression, 25–27
behavior problems, 26
bullying or abuse, 27
common presentations, 26t
drop in school performance, 26
drug abuse, 27
excessive somatic complaints, 26
family history, 27
relationship problems, 27
suicidality, 26
sustained negative mood change, 26
developmental differences in presentation, 30
differential diagnosis, 31–33
adjustment disorder, 32
bereavement, 32
bipolar disorder, 31
medical conditions, 32–33
ODD, ADHD, and pervasive developmental
disorder, 32
posttraumatic stress disorder, 32
of functioning, 36–37, 37t
general recommendations, 24–30
goals, 23
interview, conducting, 24–25
parental psychopathology, 38
rating scales, 33, 34t, 35, 36–37, 36t–37t
referral to child psychiatrist, 38
SIGECAPS mnemonic, 27, 28t–29t
structured diagnostic interviews, 35–36, 35t
treatment history, 38
treatment location, 38
Asthma, 305
Atomoxetine, for comorbid ADHD and depression,
226t, 229–230
Attachment deficits, as risk for depression, 20
Attention deficit hyperactivity disorder (ADHD)
comorbid with depression, 229–231
algorithm for treatment, 230
behavioral programs, 231
individualized therapy, 231
medications, 225t–226t, 229
rating scales, 229
treatment guidelines, 231
differential diagnosis for depression, 32
psychoeducation, 231
symptom overlap with other disorders, 222t
Atypical antipsychotics
adverse effects
cardiovascular, 303–304
seizures, 305
aggression inhibition by, 232
augmentation of therapy with, 81, 216–217
for comorbid aggression and depression,
232–233
for comorbid anxiety with pulmonary disease, 305
formulations and dosing, 80t
AUDIT (Alcohol Use Disorders Identification
Test), 241
Augmentation
atypical antipsychotics, 81
bupropion, 81

definition, 45t
formulations and dosing, 80t
lithium, 79–80, 80t
triiodothyronine (T3), 81
Authenticity, teen reaction to, 137
Autistic disorder, 316, 317
Autistic spectrum disorder, 316–318
Autonomy, informed consent and, 47
Ayurveda, 152

Barriers, to cognitive behavior therapy, 110–111
BASC (Behavioral Assessment System for
    Children), 221
Beck Depression Inventory (BDI), 33, 34t, 35,
    116, 255, 312
Behavioral activation
    during antidepressant treatment, 79
    medication-associated, 184
    SSRIs and, 52
Behavioral Assessment System for Children
    (BASC), 221
Behavior problems, as symptom of depression, 26
Benefit versus risk, appraisal of, 46
Benzodiazepines
    for anxiety comorbid with pulmonary disease, 305
    for depression comorbid with chronic physical
      illness, 303, 303t
    international use, 338
Bereavement, 32
Berkson effect, 13
Best estimate diagnosis, 25
Best Pharmaceuticals for Children Act (2002), 70
Bias, of clinician, 131
Bibliotherapy, 157
Biofield therapy, 152
Bipolar disorder
    comorbid with substance abuse, 240
    description, 12t
    as differential in depression diagnosis, 31
    electroconvulsive therapy for, 88–89
    family history of, 72
    manic/hypomanic switching during antidepressant
      treatment, 79
    sudden deterioration and, 202
    symptom overlap with other disorders, 222t
    treatment, 52
    treatment-resistant depression, 212
Black box warnings, 47, 70, 72, 78, 260
Bleeding, as medication side effect, 185
Breastfeeding, medication side effects and, 185
Brief psychodynamic therapy, adding to STAU, 169
Bullying
    antibullying measures by school, 168
    consequences and treatment, 165t
    link to depression, 27
    as risk factor for acute depressive episodes, 165t
Bupropion
    as augmenting agent, 81
    for depression comorbid with chronic physical
      illness, 302
    for depression comorbid with substance abuse, 245

efficacy, pharmacodynamics and
    pharmacokinetics, 77t
formulations and dosing, 77t, 80t
mechanism of action, 302
renal failure and, 301
side effects, 79, 304
for Stage 3 treatment, 77–78
Burden of disease, 14–15
Burton, Robert, 4
Buspirone
    for anxiety comorbid with pulmonary disease, 305
    as augmenting agent, 81
    formulations and dosing, 80t
    serotonin syndrome and, 302

CAM. See Complementary and alternative
    medicine (CAM)
Cannabis Youth Treatment (CYT) study, 247–249
Carbamazepine, 177
Carbohydrate-deficient transferrin (CDT), 241
Cardiovascular disease, drug effects on, 303–304
Case formulation. See Formulation
Case management, STAU, 163
Causality
    circular, 129
    establishing with treatment-emergent adverse
      events, 182
    reciprocal influence versus, 130
CBCL (Child Behavior Checklist), 141, 229, 312
CBT. See Cognitive behavior therapy
C-CASA (Columbia Classification Algorithm for
    Suicide Assessment), 196, 206–208
CDI (Children's Depression Inventory), 34t, 35
CDRS-R (Children's Depression Rating Scale-
    Revised), 33, 34t
CDT (carbohydrate-deficient transferrin), 241
CESD (Center for Epidemiological Studies
    Depression Scale), 33, 34t, 286
CES-DC (Center for Epidemiological Studies
    Depression Scale for Children), 33, 34t
CGAS. See Children's Global Assessment Scale
CGI (Clinical Global Impression Scale), 36, 37t
Chain analysis, 167
Checklist for Carers, 312t
Child Behavior Checklist (CBCL), 141, 229, 312
Child maltreatment, as depression risk factor, 18
Children, engaging and supporting, 55
Children's Depression Inventory (CDI), 34t, 35
Children's Depression Rating Scale-Revised
    (CDRS-R), 33, 34t
Children's Global Assessment Scale (CGAS), 36, 37t,
    141, 164, 245–246
Children's Yale-Brown Obsessive-Compulsive
    Scale, 223t
China
    availability of mental health professionals, 336
    suicide in, 335
Chinese Classification of Psychiatric Disorders
    (CCPD), 335
Chiropractic, 152
Chlorpromazine, 305

Circle of closeness, 118, *118*

Circular causality, 129

Citalopram
  for depression comorbid with pain, 304
  efficacy, pharmacodynamics, and
      pharmacokinetics, 75t
  formulations and dosing, 76t
  as second-line treatment, 76, 170
  for Stage 1 treatment, 75

Clarification, verbal technique in dynamic
      psychotherapy, 146, 146t

Classification
  cultural perspective on, 335
  systems, 9, 24

Clinical assessment. *See* Assessment

Clinical characteristics, 7, 7t–8t, 9

Clinical Global Impression Scale (CGI), 36, 37t

Clomipramine, for treatment-resistant
      depression, 217

Clozapine
  adverse effects, 305
  formulations and dosing, 80t

CMAP. *See* Texas Childhood Medication Algorithm
      Project

Cocaine, 238, 262

Cognitive behavior therapy (CBT), 100–112
  adding to STAU, 169
  augmentation of medication by, 216–217
  barriers to, 110–111
  for depression comorbid with anxiety, 224,
      228–229, 228t
  for depression comorbid with physical illness, 299
  for depression in intellectually disabled patients, 315
  for depression in minority or immigrant children
      and youth, 328
  depression prevention programs, 282–283t, 284
  developmental considerations, 111
  for early intervention in subclinical
      depression, 286
  evidence base and practice parameters, 101–102
    CBT and medication, 101–102
    effectiveness under routine practice
        conditions, 102
    monotherapy, 101
  interpersonal psychotherapy (IPT) compared, 114
  nondirective supportive therapy compared, 129
  phases of program, 103–104
    conceptualization, 103
    relapse prevention, 103–104
    skills and application training, 103
  planning individual sessions, 104–110
    activity module, 104–106, *106*
    cognitive module, 106–108, *108*
    communication and problem-solving module,
        109–110
  in primary care setting, 258, 260
  principles, 103
  response rates, 50–51, *51*
  for substance use disorder, 248–249
  systemic behavioral family therapy compared, 129
  for treatment-resistant depression, 210, 211, 215

Cognitive module, CBT, 106–108, *108*

Cognitive restructuring exercise, 108, *108*

Cognitive symptoms, 9

Columbia Classification Algorithm for Suicide
      Assessment (C-CASA), 196, 206–208

Columbia Depression Screen, use in primary care
      settings, 255

Communication
  with families, 58–59
  improving with cognitive behavior therapy (CBT),
      109–110
  with schools, 62

Communication analysis (IPT-A technique), 121

Communication and problem-solving module, CBT,
      109–110

Community resources, locating, 260

Comorbidity, 220–235
  aggression/disruptive behavior disorders, 227t,
      231–234, *233*
  anxiety, 222–229, 223t, *224*, 225t, 228t
  assessment, 37
  attention deficit hyperactivity disorder (ADHD),
      225t–226t, 229–231, *230*
  chronic physical illness, 295–306
  incidence, 221
  overview, 12–14, 220–222, 222t
  personality disorder, 14
  substance use/abuse, 237–252
  suicidal behavior, 14
  symptom overlap, 222t

Complementary and alternative medicine (CAM),
      151–161
  malpractice liability, 153
  medicines and homeopathic remedies, list of,
      160–161
  omega-3 fatty acids, 152–155
    dosage and administration, 154–155
    efficacy, 154, 154t
    overview, 153–154, 154t
    safety and side effects, 154
  overview, 151–152
    categories of CAM, 152
    reasons for interest in CAM, 152
  physical exercise, 157
  physical treatments, list of, 161
  S-adenosyl methionine (SAMe), 156–157
    dosage and administration, 157
    efficacy, 154t, 157
    overview, 154t, 156
    safety and side effects, 157
  safety, 153
  St. John's wort
    dosage and administration, 156
    efficacy, 154t, 155
    overview, 154t, 155
    safety and side effects, 155, 156t

Complexity, case, 164

Concerta, for comorbid ADHD and depression, 226t

Condom, 243

Conduct disorder, comorbid with substance
      abuse, 240

Confidentiality
    breach of, 166, 238–239
    discussions with patient concerning, 166
    substance abuse and, 238–239
Conflicting data, reconciling, 25
Confrontation, verbal technique in dynamic
    psychotherapy, 146t, 147
Conners Parent and Teacher Rating Scale,
    229, 232
Consent, informed, 47, 91
Continuation treatment
    definition, 45t, 71
    with fluoxetine, 82
Coping strategies, 104
Coping with Depression Course, 276, 277t–278t,
    282, 283t, 284
Cost of depression, 14–15
Course of disease, 6–7
CRAFFT mnemonic, 241
Crises and emergencies, 194–205
    family instability, 195t, 203
    nonadherence to treatment, 195t, 200–201
    nonsuicidal self-injury, 197–199, 207
    overview, 194–195, 195t
    school, 195t, 202–203
    substance abuse, 203–204
    sudden deterioration, 195t, 201–202
    suicidal behavior, 195t, 196–197
    telephone management of, 195
    violent behavior, 195t, 199
Cuban Glossary of Psychiatry, 335
Cultural competence, 325–327
Cultural perspectives. *See* International perspectives;
    Minority children and youth
Culture
    family therapy and, 132
    influence on treatment and engagement,
    60–61
Cutting of self, 197–199
Cytochrome P450 (CYP)
    activation by St. John's wort, 155
    enzyme inhibition
        implications for treatment, 73t
        of SSRIs, 75t
    genotype, 214
    polymorphism, 179, 325, 336
    system, 177
CYT (Cannabis Youth Treatment) study,
    247–249

Data sources, resolving discrepancies between, 25
Day-patient admission, 168
Daytrana, for comorbid ADHD and depression, 226t
DBC (Developmental Behaviour Checklist), 312t
DBT. *See* Dialectical behavior therapy
Decision analysis (IPT-A technique), 121
Defensive displacement, metaphor as form
    of, 146
Definition, of depression, 4
Denial, defense exhibited in psychodynamic
    therapy, 142t

Depressed mood
    adjustment disorder with, 32
    misperceptions concerning depression
        consequence, 167t
    SIGECAPS mnemonic, 27, 28t–29t
Depression Self-Rating Scale (DSRS), 33, 34t
Depressive equivalents, 5
Developmental assistance, verbal technique in
    dynamic psychotherapy, 146–147, 146t
Developmental Behaviour Checklist (DBC), 312t
Developmental differences, in clinical presentation
    of depression, 30
Developmental disabilities, 310–320
    intellectual disability, 310–315
    pervasive developmental disorder (PDD),
        316–318
Developmental transitions, cognitive behavior
    therapy and, 111
Dexedrine, for comorbid ADHD and depression, 225t
Dextromethorphan, serotonin syndrome and, 302
DextroStat, for comorbid ADHD and depression, 225t
DHA (docosahexaenoic acid), 154, 155
Diabetes, 33
Diagnosis, 9–11. *See also* Assessment
    algorithm, *10*
    best estimate, 25
    classification systems, 9, 24
    cultural challenges to, 324–325
    informant and, 11
    medication treatment and, 70–71
    reliability, 10–11
    severity, 11
Diagnostic and Statistical Manual of Mental Disorders,
    4th edition *(DSM-IV)*
    comorbidity and, 12–13
    depression diagnosis, 9, 24
    international use, 338
    symptoms of depression, 5
Diagnostic and Statistical Manual of Mental Disorders
    3rd edition *(DSM-III),* 5
Diagnostic Criteria for Psychiatric Disorders for Use
    with Adults with Learning Disabilities/Mental
    Retardation (DM-LD), 311
Diagnostic Interview for Children and Adolescents
    (DICA), 221
Diagnostic Interview Schedule for Children
    Version-IV (DISC-IV), 35–36, 35t
Diagnostic Manual-Intellectual Disability (DM-ID), 311
Dialectical behavior therapy (DBT)
    engagement strategies, 64
    for self-injury behavior, 199
Diary, mood and activities, 104–106, *106*
Diet, negative effects of unhealthy, 170
DIGFAST (mnemonic), 31, 31t
Disappointment and loss event
    consequences and treatment, 165t
    as risk factor for acute depressive episodes, 165t
Discontinuation syndrome, 82, 201–202
Discrepancies between data sources, resolving, 25
Displacement, defense exhibited in psychodynamic
    therapy, 142t

Disputes
  interpersonal psychotherapy problem area,
      116, 120t
  stages of, 120t
Disrupted attachments, as depression risk factor, 18
Disruptive behavior disorders
  comorbid with depression, 231–234
  as risk factor for depression, 19
  symptom overlap with other disorders, 222t
Dissolution, stage of dispute, 120t
Disulfiram, aversive agent for alcohol
      consumption, 246
Docosahexaenoic acid (DHA), 154, 155
Documenting adverse reactions, 185–186
Dosage, optimal, 51
Dosage Records Treatment Emergent Scale
      (DOTES), 182
Double depression, 12t
Down syndrome, 313
Drug abuse. *See also* Substance use/abuse
  consequences and treatment, 165t
  as risk factor for acute depressive episodes, 165t
  as symptom of depression, 27
Drug Use Screening Inventory (DUSI), 241
*DSM-IV. See Diagnostic and Statistical Manual of
      Mental Disorders,* 4th edition
DSRS (Depression Self-Rating Scale), 33, 34t
Duloxetine
  for depression comorbid with chronic physical
      illness, 302
  efficacy, pharmacodynamics and
      pharmacokinetics, 77t
  formulations and dosing, 77t
  mechanism of action, 302
  for Stage 3 treatment, 77–78
Dynamic formulation, 143–144
Dynamic psychotherapy, 140–150
  basic principles, 142–143
  case formation, 143–144
  comorbid disorders, 147–148
  defenses exhibited by children in, 142t, 146
  for depression comorbid with physical illness, 299
  dynamics of depression, 143, 143t
  evidence of efficacy, 141–142
  referrals to dynamic therapist, 148
  resistant depression, 148
  skills needed by therapist, 142
  structuring therapy, 144–145
    combining with medications, 145
    expressive therapy, 144
    frequency of sessions, 144
    group therapy, 145
    length of treatment, 145
    parent and child together in session, 144–145
    phases of therapy, 145
    room environment, 144
  techniques, 145–147
    clarification, 146, 146t
    confrontation, 147
    developmental assistance, 146–147
    emphatic validation, 146, 146t

  encouragement to elaborate, 146, 146t
  interpretation, 147
  play, 145–146
  reconstructions, 147
  verbal, 146–147, 146t
Dysthymia
  description, 12t
  introduction of concept, 5
  prevalence, 5–6, 6t
  reliability of diagnosis, 11
  SIGECAP mnemonic, 27, 30t

Early intervention with subclinical depression,
      285–286
Eco-maps, 134
Economic burden of depression, 14–15
ECT. *See* Electroconvulsive therapy
Education
  about medications, 72
  comorbid physical illness with depression,
      298–299
  of family members, 59
  information about ECT for young patients
      and their families, 98–99
  information handout for adolescents and parents
      about suicide, 267–268
  medication side effects, 180–181, *181*
  pervasive development disorder (PDD) patients
      and, 316–317
  in primary care setting, 257–258
  of psychiatrists internationally, 337
  of teachers and school personnel, 62
  treatment-resistant depression and, 214
EFAs (essential fatty acids), 154–155
Eicosapentaenoic acid (EPA), 154, 155
Electroconvulsive therapy (ECT), 88–92, 88t
  attitudes toward, 90
  cognitive effects of, 90
  for depression in intellectual disabled patients, 315
  effectiveness and indications, 88–89
  follow-up, 91–92
  information for young patients and families, 98–99
  legislation, 90
  practical aspects of treatment, 91
    assessment, 91
    informed consent and consultation, 91
    procedure, 91
  side effects, 89–90
    cognitive effects, 90
    death, 90
    prolonged seizures, 90
    structural abnormalities, 90
  for treatment-resistant depression, 217
EMEA (European Medicines Evaluation Agency), 174
Emergency. *See* Crises and emergencies
Emotionality, high
  consequences and treatment, 165t
  as risk factor for acute depressive episodes, 165t
Emotions
  emotional deprivation as depression risk factor, 18
  as signals in dynamic therapy, 143

Emphatic validation, verbal technique in dynamic psychotherapy, 146, 146t
Enactment, use in family therapy, 135
Encouragement to elaborate, verbal technique in dynamic psychotherapy, 146, 146t
Energy medicine, 152
Engagement strategies, 54–64
  family, 57–61, 131
  schools, 61–64, 61t
  in special mental health services, 64
  for young patients, 55–57, 56t
EPA (eicosapentaenoic acid), 154, 155
Ephedra, 153
Epidemiology, 5–6, 6t
Epilepsy, 33
  depression comorbidity with, 305
  vagus nerve stimulation for, 93
Escitalopram
  efficacy, pharmacodynamics, and pharmacokinetics, 75t
  formulations and dosing, 76t
  as second-line treatment, 76
Essential fatty acids (EFAs), 154–155
Estrogen, effects of recurrent withdrawal, 18
Ethical issues
  informed consent, 47
  off-label prescribing, 47–48
  primun non nocere, 46–47
Ethnicity. See also Minority children and youth
  family therapy and, 132
  treatment-resistant depression, 211
Ethnopharmacology, 325
European Medicines Evaluation Agency (EMEA), 174
Exercise, antidepressant effect of, 157
Externalization, defense exhibited in psychodynamic therapy, 142t

Family
  assessment interview and, 24–25
  conflict
    consequences and treatment, 165t
    between parents, 165t
    as risk factor for depression, 19–20, 129, 165t
    treatment-resistant depression and, 213
  depression in parents, 19, 27, 38, 129
  depression prevention programs, 285
  engagement in treatment, 57–61
    communication, 58–59
    education, 59
    out-of-home situation, 58
    risk management, 60
    social and cultural context, 60–61
    in specialist mental health services, 64
    support, 59–60
  history of depression
    consequences and treatment, 165t
    as risk factor for acute depressive episodes, 165t
    treatment-resistant depression and, 213
  information handout for adolescents and parents about suicide, 267–268
  instability, crisis precipitation by, 195t, 203

  involvement in treatment, 52, 115
  overprotectiveness of parents, 59
  support, 57–61
    action plan, 273
    goal setting, 273
  what to discuss concerning depression, 269–270
Family Bereavement Program (FBP), 278t, 285
Family therapy, 128–139
  adding to STAU, 169
  assessment tools, 133–134
    eco-maps, 134
    genogram, 133
    structural maps, 134
    timeline, 133–134
  for depression comorbid with physical illness, 299
  for depression in intellectually disabled patients, 315
  for depression in minority or immigrant children and youth, 328
  evidence of effectiveness, 129
  indications for, 203
  reciprocal influence versus causality, 130
  skills for family intervention
    areas of influence pie chart, 131
    balancing treatment and safety, 133
    core beliefs, 131–132
    culture and ethnicity, understanding of, 132
    engagement, 131
    positive assumptions, 132–133
    reframing, 132
  for substance use disorder, 247–248
  systems theory, 129–130
  therapy outline, 134–137
    challenges and solutions, 136–137
    inviting key players, 134–135
    phase one: orientation and assessment, 135
    phase three: review and disposition, 136
    phase two: intervention, 135–136
    prevention of relapse and recurrence, 136
  treatment-resistant depression and, 215
FBP (Family Bereavement Program), 278t, 285
FDA Modernization Act, 70
Fear Survey Schedule for Children, 223t
FEAST (focal electrically administered seizure therapy), 93
First line treatment, 45t
Fish oil capsules, 155, 170
Fluoxetine
  cognitive behavior therapy (CBT) combined with, 101–102
  for continuation treatment, 82
  for depression comorbid with anxiety, 225t, 228
  for depression comorbid with epilepsy, 305
  for depression comorbid with substance abuse, 245
  discontinuation, 82
  efficacy, pharmacodynamics, and pharmacokinetics, 75t
  as first-line treatment for acute depressive episode, 170
  formulations and dosing, 76t
  international use, 338

Fluoxetine (*Cont.*)
    response rates, 50–51, *51*
    as second-line treatment, 76
    for Stage 1 treatment, 74–75
Fluvoxamine
    for comorbid anxiety and depression, 225t
    efficacy, 78
Focal electrically administered seizure therapy
        (FEAST), 93
Focalin, for comorbid ADHD and depression, 226t
Food and Drug Administration, 174
Forgetfulness, treatment nonadherence and, 200
Formulation
    dynamic formulation, 143–144
    STAU, 163
    substance use disorder, 239–240
Foster care, 58
Fragile X syndrome, 313
Frequently asked questions about treatment
        of depression, 271–272
FRIENDS program, 280t, 284

Gamma-glutamyltransferase (GGT), 241
Gender, risk differences and, 18
Generic drugs, 46t
Genetic risk factors, 17–18
Genogram, 133
GGT (gamma-glutamyltransferase), 241
Give to get (IPT-A technique), 122
Goals of treatment, 49
Goodness of fit of interventions, 137
Grapefruit juice, effect on medications, 325
Grief, interpersonal psychotherapy and, 116, 120t
Group therapy
    for depression comorbid with physical illness, 299
    for depression in minority or immigrant children
        and youth, 328
    psychodynamic, 145
    for substance use disorder, 248
*Guía Latinoamericana de Diagnóstico Psiquiátrico
        (GLADP)*, 335
Guidelines for Adolescent Depression in Primary
        Care (GLAD-PC), 286

Half-life
    meaning and practical implications
        for treatment, 73t
    of SSRIs, 75t
Hamilton Rating Scale for Depression, 116
Harm minimization, 168
HEADS interview (mnemonic for Home,
        Education/employment/eating, Activities,
        Drugs, cigarettes, alcohol, Sexuality,
        Suicidality/depression, Safety), 55, 67–68
Health Canada, 174
Health of the Nation Outcome Scales for Children
        and Adolescents (HoNOSCA), 36–37, 37t
Health Professional's Antidepressant Communication
        Tool, 181, *181*
Helpful/unhelpful thoughts, 106
Herbal medicine, 152, 153, 262

Heritability, of depression, 17–18
Heroin, 238
Heterotypic continuity, 14, 19
Hierarchal rapport, 135
Hispanics. *See* Latino children and youth
History, of depression, 4–5
HIV, substance use disorder and, 243
Homeopathic medicine, 152
Homeostasis, within family system, 129
Homicidal behavior/ideation
    assessment of, 199
    initial interventions, 195t
Homotypic continuity, 14
HoNOSCA (Health of the Nation Outcome Scales
        for Children and Adolescents), 36–37, 37t
Hopelessness, assessment with treatment-resistant
        depression, 211–212
Humor, teen reaction to, 137
Hypericum perforatum, 154t, 155–156
Hypnotics, 81
Hypomanic switching, 79

ICD-10. *See International Classification of Diseases,
        10th edition*
Illness, chronic. *See* Physical illness, chronic
Imipramine
    international use, 338
    side effects, 78
Immigrant children and youth, 321–331
    diagnosis and treatment
        biological factors, 324–325
        cultural challenges, 324–325
        cultural competence, 325–327
        ethnopharmacology, 325
        rating scales, 325–326
        stigma, 324
        summary of strategies, 327t–328t
    epidemiology, 322–323
    evidence-based interventions, 328
    family therapy, 132
    mental health disparities, 323
    overview, 321–322
    risk factors, 322–323
Impasse, stage of dispute, 120t
Independence, issues in family therapy, 137
Indian culture, value system in, 334
Indicated preventive interventions, 275, 276,
        277t–279t, 281
Information, providing families with, 47
Informed consent, 47
    for electroconvulsive therapy, 91
    patients with intellectual disability, 314
Insomnia, treatment for, 81
Institute of Medicine (IOM) classification
        of prevention programs, 275
Integrative medicine, 152
Intellectual disability and depression, 310–315
    assessment of depression, 311–312, 312t
    causes of intellectual disability, 313
    diagnosis, 311
    presentation and diagnosis, 312–313

prevalence, 311
psychosocial risk factors, 313
rating scales, 312, 312t
treatment
    cognitive behavior therapy, 315
    electroconvulsive therapy, 315
    family therapy, 315
    informed consent, 314
    medications, 315
    psychosocial management, 314–315
    supportive management, 314
Intellectual Disability Mood Scale, 312t
Intelligence quotient (IQ), 311
Intergenerational conflict, in family therapy, 132
Internal representations, in dynamic
        psychotherapy, 142
International Classification of Diseases, 10th edition
        (ICD-10)
    comorbidity and, 12–13
    depression diagnosis, 24
    diagnosis and, 9
    international use, 338
    recognition of depression, 5
International perspectives
    classification of disorders, 335
    cultural perspective on childhood depression,
        333–334
    epidemiology, 333
    prevalence rates, 333
    psychiatrists, survey of
        diagnosis and classification, 337–338
        education and training, 337
        perception of depression, 337
        treatment, 338
    suicide, 334, 335
    treatment, 336–337
    unmet needs, 333
Interpersonal deficits, interpersonal psychotherapy
        and, 116, 120t
Interpersonal disputes, interpersonal psychotherapy
        and, 116, 120t
Interpersonal formulation, 119
Interpersonal inventory, 118
Interpersonal psychotherapy (IPT). *See also*
        Interpersonal psychotherapy for adolescents
        (IPT-A)
    adding to STAU, 169
    augmentation of medication by, 216
    for depression comorbid with physical
        illness, 299
    for depression in minority or immigrant
        children and youth, 328
    depression prevention program, 284–285
    for treatment-resistant depression, 210,
        211, 215
Interpersonal Psychotherapy—Adolescent Skills
        Training Program (IPT-AST), 279t, 281
Interpersonal psychotherapy for adolescents
        (IPT-A), 114–127
    adaptations, 116
    cognitive behavior therapy (CBT) compared, 114

efficacy and effectiveness, 125, 126t
evidence for, 125, 126t
interpersonal problem areas, 116, 120t
maintenance treatment, 125
overview, 114
parental involvement, 115
phases of treatment
    initial phase (sessions 1–4), 116–119
        session 1, 116–117
        session 2, 117–118
        session 3, 118–119
        session 4, 119
        troubleshooting, 119
    middle phase (sessions 5–8), 119–123
        all in the timing (technique), 122–123
        being specific (technique), 123
        communication analysis (technique), 121
        compromise and negotiation, 123
        decision analysis (technique), 121
        description, 119–120
        do not give up (technique), 123
        give to get (technique), 122
        link mood to event and event to mood
            (technique), 121
        parental session, 119
        role playing (technique), 121–122
        strike while iron is cold (technique), 122
        using I statements (technique), 122
        work at home (technique), 122
    termination phase (sessions 9–12), 123–125
        session 11, 124
        session 12, 124–125
        sessions 9 and 10, 123–124
    in primary care setting, 258, 260
    suitability for, 115
Interpersonal role transitions, interpersonal
        psychotherapy and, 116, 120t
Interpersonal vulnerability, link to depression, 20
Interpretation, verbal technique in dynamic
        psychotherapy, 146t, 147
Interpreters, 325
Intervention
    early with subclinical depression, 285–286
    prevention of depression, 274–292
Interview
    adolescent alone, 167
    conducting assessment, 24–25
    joint (patient-parent), 166
    motivational interviewing strategies, 56,
        56t, 249
    in primary care settings, 256
    structured diagnostic, 35–36, 35t
    substance abuse, 238–239
Introjective line, of personality development,
        143, 143t
IPT. *See* Interpersonal psychotherapy
IPT-A. *See* Interpersonal psychotherapy
        for adolescents
IQ. *See* Intelligence quotient
Irritability, 167t
I statements, using, 122

Japan
  availability of mental health professionals, 336
  emotional expression by Japanese, 334

Kinetics
  definition, 73t
  pharmacokinetics
    drug interactions, 177
    ethnopharmacology, 325
    in treating depression comorbid with physical
      illness, 300–301
    of SSRIs, 75t
Kraepelin, Emil, 4
Kutcher Adolescent Depression Scale (KADS),
    34t, 35, 255, 264–265

Laboratory tests, for substance use disorder (SUD),
    241–242
Lactation, medication side effects and, 185
Lamotrigine
  adverse effects, 303
  for depression comorbid with chronic physical
    illness, 303
Language barriers, 325
Lateral rapport, 135
Latino children and youth, 322–326, 328, 334
    See also Minority children and youth
Legal problems, substance abuse and, 243
Liability, alternative medicine treatments
    and, 153
Light therapy, 88t, 93–94, 217
Link mood to event (IPT-A technique), 121
Liothyronine sodium, 80t
Lisdexamfetamine, for comorbid ADHD and
    depression, 225t
Lithium
  augmentation of therapy with, 79–80,
    216–217
  for depression comorbid with chronic physical
    illness, 303, 303t
  for depression comorbid with epilepsy, 305
  for depression comorbid with substance abuse,
    245–246
  drug interactions, 177
  formulations and dosing, 80t
  renal failure and, 301, 303
  side effects, 178, 303, 304
Liverpool University Neuroleptic Side Effects
    Scale (LUNSERS), 182
Loss event
  consequences and treatment, 165t
  as depression risk factor, 18, 20, 165t
Loss of concentration, 167t
LUNSERS (Liverpool University Neuroleptic
    Side Effects Scale), 182

Magnetic seizure therapy (MST), 93
Maintenance treatment
  definition, 45t
  duration of, 82
  electroconvulsive therapy, 92
Major depression with seasonal pattern, 12t

Major depressive disorder (MDD)
  comorbid conditions, 221–234
  course, 6–7
  prevalence, 5–6, 6t
  reliability of diagnosis, 10–11
  risk factors, 129
  treatment-resistant depression, 209–217
Major depressive episode, SIGECAPS mnemonic
    for, 27, 28t–29t
Malpractice liability, alternative medicine treatments
    and, 153
Manic episode, DIGFAST mnemonic for, 31, 31t
Manic switching, 79, 184
MAOIs. See Monoamine oxidase inhibitors
Marijuana use, 262
Marital discord, as risk factor for depression, 19–20
MASC (Multidimensional Anxiety Scale for
    Children), 223t, 224
Masked depression theory, 5
MASS (Mood and Anxiety Semi-Structured)
    interview, 312t
MDD. See Major depressive disorder
MedED, 181
Medical conditions, presenting with depressive
    symptoms, 13t, 32–33
Medication, 69–83. See also specific drug classes;
    specific drugs
  adding to STAU, 169–170
  adverse effects
    minimizing in physically ill youth, 300t
    racial/ethnic sensitivities, 325
  alternative treatment options, 78–79, 82
  augmenting (adjunctive agents), 81–82,
    215–217, 216t
    atypical antipsychotics, 81
    bupropion, 81
    formulations and dosing, 80t
    lithium, 79–80, 80t
    triiodothyronine (T3), 81
  checking blood levels of, 214
  cognitive behavior therapy (CBT) combined
    with, 101–102
  continuation and maintenance treatment, 82
  for depression comorbid with physical illness,
    300–303, 300t, 303t
  for depression comorbid with substance use
    disorder, 244–247
  for depression in intellectual disabled patients, 315
  for depression in pervasive development disorder
    (PDD) patient, 317–318
  discontinuation, 79, 82
  drug clearance, influences on, 301
  dynamic psychotherapy combined with, 145
  general management issues, 70–72
    diagnosis, 70–71
    education of families, 72
    measurement of outcomes, 72
    previous treatment, 71
    psychotherapy integration with medication, 71
    safety assessment, 71–72
  initiating, 49–50
  microdose initiation, 180

off-label use, 174–175
optimization, 215
patient anxiety about, 180
pharmacological issues, 73t, 75t, 77t
in primary core setting, 260–262
regulatory agencies, 174
safety, 78–79
switching, 215–217, 216t
therapeutic index, 300
treatment-resistant depression and, 210, 211,
    215–217, 216t
treatment strategies, 72–78
  acute treatment, 72
  algorithm, 74
  Stage 1, 74–76
  Stage 2, 76
  Stage 3, 76–78, 77t
use and avoidance of antidepressants, 175t
variation in use internationally, 336
volume of distribution, 301
Medication side effects, 174–189
  classification, 176
  definition, 176
  depression induction, 33
  detecting, 182–183
  discontinuation of medication, 183
  documenting, 185–186
  dose-related, 178, 179, 180, 183
  education of patient/caregiver, 180–181, 181
  emotional, 178
  examples
    activation syndrome, 184
    bleeding, 185
    cardiovascular, 184
    metabolic syndrome, 184–185
    pregnancy and lactation, 185
    serotonin syndrome, 184
    sexual, 185
    suicidality and SSRIs, 184
  incidence with Prozac use, 176t
  managing, 183
  Mental Health Therapeutic Outcomes Tool (TOT),
      182–183, 190–193
  patient anticipation of, 180
  pharmacodynamic interactions, 177
  pharmacokinetic interactions, 177
  physical, 178
  placebo treatments, 178, 180
  polypharmacy and, 179
  prevention, 178–181
  rating scales, 182–183, 189
  self-reporting by patient, 182, 189
  start low, go slow approach, 178, 180
Medicines and Healthcare Products Regulatory
    Agency (MHRA), 174
Melancholic depression, 9, 12t
Mental health screening programs, in schools, 63
Mental Health Therapeutic Outcomes Tool (TOT),
    182–183, 190–193
Mental retardation. See Intellectual disability
    and depression
Meperidine, serotonin syndrome and, 302

Metabolic syndrome, 184–185
Metadate, for comorbid ADHD and depression, 226t
Metaphor, as form of defensive displacement, 146
Methylin, for comorbid ADHD and depression, 226t
Methylphenidate, for comorbid ADHD and
    depression, 226t
MFQ (Mood and Feelings Questionnaire), 34t, 35,
    164, 255
MHRA (Medicines and Healthcare Products
    Regulatory Agency), 174
Migraine, 33
Mind-body medicine, 152
Minor depression. See also Subsyndromal
    depression
  description, 12t
  prevalence, 5
Minority children and youth, 321–331
  diagnosis and treatment
    biological factors, 324–325
    cultural challenges, 324–325
    cultural competence, 325–327
    ethnopharmacology, 325
    rating scales, 325–326
    stigma, 324
    summary of strategies, 327t–328t
  epidemiology, 322–323
  evidence-based interventions, 328
  family therapy, 132
  mental health disparities, 323
  overview, 321–322
  risk factors, 322–323
Mirtazapine
  for depression comorbid with chronic physical
      illness, 302
  drug interactions, 262
  efficacy, pharmacodynamics and
      pharmacokinetics, 77t
  formulations and dosing, 77t
  mechanism of action, 302
  for Stage 3 treatment, 77–78
Misdiagnosis, treatment failure and, 212
Misperceptions, as consequence of depression, 167t
Monoamine oxidase inhibitors (MAOIs)
  augmentation of therapy with, 216–217
  for depression comorbid with chronic physical
      illness, 302
  diet management and, 78
  discontinuation, 82
  drug interactions, 262
  serotonin syndrome and, 302
  side effects, 79
Mononucleosis, 33
Mood
  charts, 27
  disorders
    electroconvulsive therapy for, 89
    mood disorder not otherwise specified
        (NOS), 12t
    SIGECAPS mnemonic, 27, 28t–29t
  linking to event in IPT-A therapy, 121
  sustained negative problem, 26
  symptoms, 9

Mood and activities diary, 104–106, *106*
Mood and Anxiety Semi-Structured (MASS)
    interview, 312t
Mood and Feelings Questionnaire (MFQ), 34t, 35,
    164, 255
Motivational enhancement therapy, for substance
    use disorder, 249
Motivational interviewing
    strategies, 56, 56t
    substance use disorder, 249
Motivational symptoms, 9
MST (magnetic seizure therapy), 93
MTA (Multimodal Treatment of ADHD)
    study, 230
Multidimensional Anxiety Scale for Children
    (MASC), 223t, 224
Multimodal Treatment of ADHD (MTA)
    study, 230
Multiple symptom domains, scales for, 36, 36t

Naltrexone, for alcoholism, 246
National Association for the Dually Diagnosed, 311
National Center for Complementary and Alternative
    Medicine (NCCAM), 152
National Institute for Clinical Excellence (NICE),
    11, 49–50, 71, 89, 170
National Institute of Drug Abuse (NIDA), 242
National Runaway Switchboard, 203
Native American children and youth, 322–323, 326
    See also Minority children and youth
Native populations, depression in, 322–323
Naturopathic medicine, 152
NCCAM (National Center for Complementary and
    Alternative Medicine), 152
Nefazodone, 78
Negative cognitions, as depression risk factor, 18–19
Negative explanatory style, 18
Neuroleptic malignant syndrome (NMS), 90
Neuroticism
    consequences and treatment, 165t
    as risk factor for acute depressive episodes, 165t
Neurovegetative symptoms, 9
New Beginnings program, 279t, 285
NICE. *See* National Institute for Clinical Excellence
NICE stepped care model, 170, 171t
NIDA (National Institute of Drug Abuse), 242
NMS (neuroleptic malignant syndrome), 90
Nonadherence to treatment
    comorbidity and, 201
    initial interventions, 195t
    reasons for, 200
    refusal of treatment, 201
    ways to lessen occurrence, 200
Nonmaleficence, 46
Non-SSRIs
    efficacy, pharmacodynamics, and pharmacokinetics
        of, 77t
    formulations and dosing, 77t
    in Stage 3 treatment, 77–78
Nonsuicidal self-injury (NSSI), 197–199, 207
    See also Self-injury behaviour

Normalization, 137
Number needed to harm (NNH), 45t
Number needed to treat (NNT), 44t

ODD
    differential diagnosis for depression, 32
    symptom overlap with other disorders, 222t
Off-label prescribing, 47–48
Olanzapine
    for comorbid aggression/disruptive behavior
        disorders, 227t
    formulations and dosing, 80t
Omega-3 fatty acids, 152–155
    dosage and administration, 154–155
    efficacy, 154, 154t
    overview, 153–154, 154t
    safety and side effects, 154
Ondansetron, for alcohol dependence, 246–247
Optimal dosage, 51
Optimization, 45t, 215
Oral contraceptives, interaction with St. John's
    wort, 156t
Osteopathy, 152
Out-of-home situations, children in, 58
Overt Aggression Scale, 231
Over-the-counter medications, interaction
    with antidepressants, 261

Pain
    depression comorbidity with, 304–305
    neuropathic, 305
Panic disorder, SSRIs for, 225t, 228
Parenting
    definition, 20
    role in depression development, 19–20
Parent medication guide, 72
Parents
    assessment interview and, 24–25
    conflict between
        consequences and treatment, 165t
        as risk factor for acute depressive episodes, 165t
    depression in, 27
        assessment of, 38
        as risk factor for depression, 19, 129
    engaging and supporting families, 57–61
    information handout for adolescents and parents
        about suicide, 267–268
    involvement in treatment, 52, 115
    overprotectiveness of, 59
    what to discuss concerning depression, 269–270
Paroxetine
    for comorbid anxiety and depression, 225t
    discontinuation, 82
    efficacy, pharmacodynamics, and
        pharmacokinetics, 75t
    formulations and dosing, 76t
    renal failure and, 301
    as second-line treatment, 76
    side effects, 185
PARS (Pediatric Anxiety Rating Scale), 223t, 224
Partial response, 44t

Patient preference for management, determining, 258–260, 259t
PATS (Preschool ADHD Treatment Study), 230
Pediatric Anxiety Rating Scale (PARS), 223t, 224
Pediatric Quality of Life Enjoyment and Satisfaction Questionnaire (PQ-LES-Q), 37, 37t
Penn Prevention Program (PPP), 276, 277t, 282
Penn Resiliency Program (PRP), 286
Personality development, line of, 143, 143t
Personality disorder, depression comorbidity with, 14
Pervasive developmental disorder (PDD), 316–318
    diagnosis of depression, 316
    differential diagnosis for depression, 32
    prevalence, 316
    risk factors, 316
    treatment
        education, 316–317
        medications, 317–318
        psychosocial management, 317
Pessimism, as depression risk factor, 18–19
Pharmacodynamics
    drug interactions, 177
    ethnopharmacology, 325
Pharmacokinetics
    drug interactions, 177
    ethnopharmacology, 325
    in treating depression comorbid with physical illness, 300–301
Pharmacology
    definitions, 73t
    ethnopharmacology, 325
    non-SSRIs, 77t
    SSRIs, 75t
Phobia, systematic desensitization for, 228–229
Phototherapy, 93–94
Physical abuse
    consequences and treatment, 166t
    link to depression, 18, 27
    notification of authorities, 203
    as risk factor for acute depressive episode, 166t
Physical exercise, antidepressant effect of, 157
Physical illness, chronic, 295–309
    assessment and diagnosis, 297–298
    definition, 296
    impact of depression on, 296
    prevalence, 296
    psychopharmacologic treatment
        adjunctive agents, 303
        antidepressants, 301–302
        cardiovascular disease, 303–304
        choice of medication, 300–301
        diabetes, 304
        epilepsy, 305
        general considerations, 300–301
        minimization of adverse events, 300
        pain, 304–305
        premenstrual syndrome (PMS)/premenstrual dysphoric disorder, 306
        pulmonary disease, 305
        selective serotonin reuptake inhibitors, 301–302

    treatment
        education, 298–299
        medications, 300–303, 300t, 303t
        psychotherapy, 299
Pie chart of the areas of influence, in family therapy, 131
Placebo
    response, 48
    run-in strategy, 180
    side effects, 178, 180
Play, in dynamic psychotherapy, 145–146
Poison control centers, 180
Polymorphism, 179, 325, 336
Polypharmacy, side effects of, 179
Positive assumptions, in family therapy, 132–133
Posttraumatic stress disorder
    depression comorbidity with, 14
    differential diagnosis for depression, 32
    SSRIs for, 228
PPP (Penn Prevention Program), 276, 277t, 282
PQ-LES-Q (Pediatric Quality of Life Enjoyment and Satisfaction Questionnaire), 37, 37t
Prader-Willi syndrome, 313
Pregnancy
    medication side effects and, 185
    substance use disorder and, 243
    testing for, 244
Premenstrual syndrome (PMS)/premenstrual dysphoric disorder, 306
Preschool ADHD Treatment Study (PATS), 230
Prescription, definition, 46t
Prescription medications, interactions with antidepressants, 262
Prevalence, of depression, 5–6, 6t
Prevention, 274–292
    definitions, 275
    programs
        cognitive behavioral therapy (CBT), 282, 283t, 284
        context, structure, and content, 281–282
        Coping with Depression Course, 276, 277t–278t, 282, 283t, 284
        efficacy, 276, 276t, 277t–280t, 281
        Family Bereavement Program (FBP), 278t, 285
        family-focused, 285
        features of effective, 281, 285
        FRIENDS program, 280t, 284
        group format, advantages of, 282
        indicated, 275, 276, 277t–279t, 281
        interpersonal psychotherapy (IPT), 284–285
        Interpersonal Psychotherapy-Adolescent Skills Training (IPT-AST) program, 279t, 281
        New Beginnings, 279t, 285
        Penn Prevention Program (PPP), 276, 277t, 282
        Problem Solving for Life (PSFL) program, 278t–279t, 281, 284
        Resourceful Adolescent Program (RAP), 276, 278t, 281, 284
        school-based, 281, 284
        selective, 275, 276, 277t–279t, 281, 285
        universal, 275, 276, 277t–280t, 281
    reasons for focus on, 274

Prevention effect, 275
Primary care, managing depression in, 253–270
    assessment, 256–257, 257t
        comorbid disorders, 256–257
        medical conditions, 257
        symptoms, 256
        tips for assessing suicidality, 257t
    management
        active monitoring, 258
        antidepressants, 260–262
        choice of therapy, 258–260, 259t
        initial, 257–258
        locating resources in community, 260
        of mild depression, 258
        of moderate and severe depression, 258–262
        patient preference, determining, 258–260, 259t
        psychotherapy, 258–260
    procedures for suicidal adolescent, 255–256
    rate of depression in primary care, 253
    screening in primary care settings, 254–256, 254t
Primary prevention, 275
Primum non nocere, 46–47
Privacy, issues in family therapy, 137
Problem Solving for Life program (PSFL), 278t–279t,
        281, 284
Problem-solving skills, improving with cognitive
        behavior therapy (CBT), 109–110
Progressive muscle relaxation, 229
Projective testing, 148
Prozac, 176t
PRP (Penn Resiliency Program), 286
Psychiatrist
    international survey, 337–338
    referral to, 38
Psychoanalysis, definition, 143
Psychoanalytic theories, depression and, 5
Psychoeducation. *See also* Education
    acute depressive episodes, 168
    attention deficit hyperactivity disorder
        (ADHD), 231
    cognitive behavior therapy program, 104
    comorbid physical illness with depression,
        298–299
    depression prevention, 285
    in family therapy, 130
    of school personnel, 202
Psychosis
    sudden deterioration and, 202
    treatment-resistant depression, 212
Psychosocial management
    for depression in intellectual disabled patients,
        314–315
    for depression in pervasive development disorder
        (PDD) patients, 317
    HEADS interview (mnemonic for Home,
        Education/employment/eating, Activities,
        Drugs, cigarettes, alcohol, Sexuality,
        Suicidality/depression, Safety), 55,
        67–68
    for substance abuse, 247–249
Psychostimulant, as augmenting agent, 81

Psychotherapy. *See also specific therapy modalities*
    augmentation of medication by, 216
    for depression comorbid with physical illness, 299
    indications for use, 259t
    integration with medication, 71
    in primary care setting, 258–260
    treatment-resistant depression and, 215
PTSD. *See* Posttraumatic stress disorder
Public perception of childhood depression, 4
Pulmonary disease, depression comorbidity with, 305
Punishment, therapy perceived as, 136

Quetiapine, 80t
Quick Inventory of Depressive Symptoms, 72

RADS/RCDS (Reynolds Adolescent/Child Depression
        Scales), 34t, 35
Randomized controlled trials (RCTs), 47, 70
RAP (Resourceful Adolescent Program), 276, 278t,
        281, 284
Rapport, in family therapy, 135
Rating scales. *See also specific scales*
    aggression, 231–232
    anxiety, 222, 223t, 224
    attention deficit hyperactivity disorder
        (ADHD), 229
    depression, 33, 34t, 35, 36, 36t–37t
    depressive symptoms in people with intellectual
        disability, 312, 312t
    for functioning, 36–37, 37t
    international use, 338
    in management of acute depressive episodes, 164
    medication side effects, 182–183, 189
    for multiple symptom domains, 36, 36t
    self-reporting, 164
    substance use disorder, 240–241
    translation and validation for ethnic/racial
        populations, 325–326
Rauwolfia serpentina, 152
Reaction formation, defense exhibited in
        psychodynamic therapy, 142t
Reciprocal influence *versus* causality, 130
Reconstructions, 147
Recovery, definition, 44t, 71
Recurrence
    definition, 44t, 71
    rate in TADS trial, 51
Recursive feedback loops, 129
Referral
    child psychiatrist, 38
    dynamic therapist, 148
    educational specialist, 202
    family therapy and, 136
    minority or immigrant children and youth, 327
    NICE stepped care model, 170, 171t
    substance abuse, 242
Reframing
    in family therapy, 132
    substance use as health-compromising
        behavior, 244
Refusal of treatment, 201

Relapse
  definition, 44t, 71
  prevention, cognitive behavior therapy and,
      103–104
  rate in TADS trial, 51
Relational/anaclitic depressions, 143, 147
Relational line, of personality development, 143
Reliability, of depression diagnosis, 10–11
Remission, 44t, 71
Renegotiation, stage of dispute, 120t
Repercussions, in family therapy, 136–137
Repetitive TMS (rTMS), 92–93
Repression, defense exhibited in psychodynamic
      therapy, 142t
Reserpine, 153
Resistant depression. *See* Treatment-resistant
      depression
Resourceful Adolescent Program (RAP), 276, 278t,
      281, 284
Response, definition, 44t, 71
Response rates, to treatment in TADS trial,
      50–51, *51*
Reynolds Adolescent/Child Depression Scales
      (RADS/RCDS), 34t, 35
Risk factors, 17–21
  attachment deficits, 20
  familial
    family functioning, 19–20
    marital discord, 19–20
    parental depression, 19
    parenting, 19–20
  individual
    anxiety, 19
    attachments and early childhood, 18
    cognitive styles, 18–19
    gender, 18
    genetic, 17–18
    stressful life events, 18
  interpersonal vulnerability, 20
  social, 20–21
Risk management
  consequences and treatment of common risk
      factors for depression, 164, 165t–166t
  family engagement and, 60
  school engagement and, 62
  talking about suicide and self-harm, 57
Risk *versus* benefit, appraisal of, 46
Risperidone
  adverse effects, 317
  for comorbid aggression/disruptive behavior
      disorders, 227t
  formulations and dosing, 80t
Ritalin, for comorbid ADHD and depression, 226t
Role playing (IPT-A technique), 121–122
Role reversal, in dynamic psychotherapy, 146
Role transitions, interpersonal psychotherapy
      and, 116, 120t
Ruminating cognitive style
  consequences and treatment, 166t
  as risk factor for acute depressive episode, 166t
Runaways, 203

SAD. *See* Seasonal affective disorder
S-adenosyl methionine (SAMe), 156–157
  dosage and administration, 157
  efficacy, 154t, 157
  overview, 154t, 156
  safety and side effects, 157
Safety
  balancing treatments with in family therapy, 133
  complementary and alternative medicine (CAM),
      153, 154, 155, 156t, 157
  dynamic psychotherapy and, 144
  planning in primary care setting, 258
Safety and Monitoring Uniform Report Form
      (SMURF), 182
SAICA (Social Adjustment Inventory for Children
      and Adolescents), 37, 37t
SAMHSA (Substance Abuse and Mental Health
      Services Administration), 242
SBFT. *See* Systemic behavioral family therapy
Scales. *See* Rating scales
Schedule for Affective Disorders and Schizophrenia
      for School Age Children, Present and
      Lifetime Version (KSADS-PL), 35, 35t
Scheduling, flexibility in, 137
Schools
  accommodations, 202
  antibullying measures, 168
  communication with, 62, 202
  coordinating care, 63–64
  depression prevention programs, 281, 284
  intellectual disabled patients, 315
  managing crises, 195t, 202–203
  minority or immigrant children and youth,
      326, 328
  performance drop as symptom of depression, 26
  psychoeducation, 62, 168, 202
  risk management, 63
  school refusal, 202–203
  shootings, school-based, 63
  working with, 61–64, 61t
Screen for Anxiety-Related Emotional Disorders
      (SCARED), 223t, 224
Screening, in primary care settings, 254–256, 254t
SDQ (Strengths and Difficulties Questionnaire),
      36, 36t
Seasonal affective disorder (SAD)
  description, 12t
  light therapy for, 93–94
Seasonal depression, 12t
Secondary prevention, 275
Second line treatment, 45t
Seizures, 305
  prolonged as side effect of electroconvulsive
      therapy, 90
  as side effect of transcranial magnetic
      stimulation, 92
Selective norepinephrine reuptake inhibitor.
      See Serotonin norepinephrine reuptake
      inhibitors (SNRIs)
Selective preventions, 275, 276, 277t–279t,
      281, 285

Selective serotonin reuptake inhibitors (SSRIs)
adverse effects, 301
activation, 317
extrapyramidal, 317
in pervasive development disorder (PDD)
patient, 317–318
for anxiety comorbid with pulmonary disease, 305
behavioral activation and, 52
cognitive behavior therapy (CBT) combined
with, 102
for depression comorbid with anxiety, 224,
225t, 228
for depression comorbid with chronic physical
illness, 301–302
for depression comorbid with diabetes, 304
for depression comorbid with epilepsy, 305
for depression comorbid with pain, 304–305
for depression in intellectual disabled patients, 315
for depression in pervasive development disorder
(PDD) patient, 317–318
discontinuation, 82
drug interactions, 178
efficacy, pharmacodynamics, and
pharmacokinetics, 75t
formulations and dosing, 76t
interaction with S-adenosyl methionine, 157
interaction with St. John's wort, 156t
international use, 338
for posttraumatic stress disorder, 228
for premenstrual syndrome (PMS)/premenstrual
dysphoric disorder, 306
side effects, 78–79, 177, 178, 262
bleeding, 185
reproductive, 185
sexual, 185
in Stage 1 treatment, 74–76
in Stage 2 treatment, 76
suicidal behavior and, 47
suicidality decrease with treatment, 184
switching to different, 216
variation in use internationally, 336
Selegiline, 78
Self-critical/introjective depressions, 143, 147
Self-esteem line, of personality development, 143
Self-injury behavior
assessment prior to medication, 72–73
association with suicidal behavior, 198
crisis, 197–199
definitions, 207
in developmentally disabled patients, 311
dialectical behavior therapy (DBT) for, 199
emotion regulation as reason for, 197, 198
incidence and prevalence, 198
misperceptions concerning depression
consequence, 167t
parental watchfulness for warning signs, 60
risk management
by families, 60
by schools, 63
talking to young patients, 57
talking with adolescents about, 57

Sequenced Treatment Alternatives to Relieve
Depression (STAR*D) study, 72, 78,
216–217
Serotonin norepinephrine reuptake inhibitors
(SNRIs)
adverse cardiovascular effects, 304
for depression comorbid with ADHD, 226t
for depression comorbid with chronic physical
illness, 302
for depression comorbid with pain, 304–305
mechanism of action, 302
Serotonin syndrome
description, 184
in pervasive development disorder (PDD) patient,
317–318
S-adenosyl methionine and, 157
St. John's wort and, 155, 179, 262
symptoms, 262, 301
Serotonin transporter gene, 18
Sertraline
for comorbid anxiety and depression, 225t
discontinuation, 82
efficacy, pharmacodynamics, and
pharmacokinetics, 75t
formulations and dosing, 76t
as second-line treatment, 76, 170
for Stage 1 treatment, 75
for substance abuse comorbid with
depression, 245
Severity
acute depressive episodes, 163–164
evaluation of, 11, 27, 30t
Sexual abuse
link to depression, 18, 27
notification of authorities, 203
treatment-resistant depression and, 213
Sexually transmitted diseases (STDs)
substance use disorder and, 243
testing for, 244
Sexual risk behavior, substance use disorder
and, 243–244
Short-term psychodynamic psychotherapy
(STPP), 141
Side effects. *See* Medication side effects
SIGECA (mnemonic), 27, 30t
SIGECAPS (mnemonic), 27, 28t–29t
Sleeping aids, 81–82
Sleep problems, depression and, 170
SMURF (Safety and Monitoring Uniform Report
Form), 182
Social Adjustment Inventory for Children
and Adolescents (SAICA), 37, 37t
Social Anxiety Scale for Children, 223t
Social capital, 20
Social context, influence on treatment and
engagement, 60–61
Social risk factors, for depression, 20–21
Society for Prevention Research (SPR), 276, 276t
Somatic complaints, 9
excessive as symptom of depression, 26
in schools, 62

Somatization
  defense exhibited in psychodynamic therapy, 142t
  in minority youth, 324
Specialist mental health services, engaging patients
    and families in, 64
Specialist treatment as usual. See STAU
SPR (Society for Prevention Research), 276, 276t
SSRIs. See Selective serotonin reuptake inhibitors
St. John's wort
  dosage and administration, 156
  efficacy, 154t, 155
  international use, 338
  overview, 154t, 155
  safety, 155, 156t
  side effects, 155, 156t, 177, 179, 262
Stage whisper, 146
STAR*D (Sequenced Treatment Alternatives to
    Relieve Depression) study, 72, 78, 216–217
STAU (specialist treatment as usual), 49
  activation, 163
  case management, 163
  complexity of case, 164
  developmental considerations, 164
  formulation, 163
  organization of session, 168–169
  outcomes, 171
  rating scales, 164
  risk assessment and management, 164, 165t–166t
  severity, 163–164
  specific psychotherapy input into, 169
STDs
  substance use disorder and, 243
  testing for, 244
Stigma
  cultural beliefs and, 324, 336
  influence on treatment, 48
  as therapy challenge, 136
Stimulants
  adverse effects, 304
  for depression comorbid with ADHD, 229–230
  for depression comorbid with chronic physical
    illness, 303t
STPP (short-term psychodynamic psychotherapy), 141
Strengths and Difficulties Questionnaire (SDQ),
    36, 36t
Stressful life events, as risk factors, 18
Strike while the iron is cold (IPT-A technique), 122
Structural maps, use in family therapy, 134
Structured diagnostic interviews, 35–36, 35t
Subclinical depression, early intervention with,
    285–286
Substance Abuse and Mental Health Services
    Administration (SAMHSA), 242
Substance-induced depression, ruling out, 33
Substance use/abuse
  assessment of, 203–204
  consequences and treatment, 165t
  as risk factor for acute depressive episodes, 165t
  symptom overlap with other disorders, 222t
  symptoms, 239
  violent criminal offense risk and, 243

Substance use/abuse, with comorbid
    depression, 237–252
  assessment and monitoring, 238–242
    ADDICTD mnemonic, 239
    assessment instruments, 240–241
    CRAFFT mnemonic, 241
    experimental use, 239
    formulation, 239–240
    information from multiple sources, 238–239
    infrequent use, 239
    laboratory tests, 241–242
    referrals, 242
    subthreshold use, 239
    symptoms, 239
    treatment setting, factors influencing, 242
    WILD mnemonic, 239
  medications
    acamprosate, 247
    benzodiazepines, 247
    bupropion, 245
    disulfiram, 246
    fluoxetine, 245
    lithium, 245–246
    naltrexone, 245–246
    ondansetron, 246–247
    sertraline, 245
    stimulants, 247
  overview, 237–238
  prevalence of, 238
  psychosocial interventions
    cognitive behavior therapy, 248–249
    family therapy, 247–248
    group therapy, 248
    motivational interviewing, 249
  risk behaviors, 242–243
    sexual, 243–244
    suicidality, 242–243
    violent criminal offenses, 243
  treatment
    goals, overall, 244
    pharmacologic, 244–247
    psychosocial, 247–249
    reframing use as health-compromising
      behavior, 244
Subsyndromal depression, 5
Subtypes of depression, 11–12, 12t
Sudden deterioration
  discontinuation syndrome, 201–202
  initial interventions, 195t
  reasons for, 201–202
SUDs (substance use disorders). See Substance
    use/abuse
Suicidal behavior
  antidepressant use and, 261
  assessment
    access to lethal means of suicide, 197
    Columbia Classification Algorithm for Suicide
      Assessment (C-CASA), 196, 206–208
    prior to medication, 72–73
    of risk s, 196–197
    tips for assessing in primary care, 257t

Suicidal behavior (*Cont.*)
  association with self-injurious behavior, 198
  classifications and definitions, 206–208
  cultural perspectives on, 334, 335
  death rates from suicide, 196
  decrease with SSRI treatment, 184
  depression comorbidity with, 14, 26
  in developmentally disabled patients, 311, 316
  family history of, 72
  flowchart for approach to patient, *198*
  hospitalization, 197
  information handout for adolescents and parents,
      267–268
  initial intervention, 195t
  in minority and immigrant children and youth,
      322, 323
  misperceptions concerning depression
      consequence, 167t
  monitoring during antidepressant treatment, 79
  onset during course of treatment, 197
  parental watchfulness for warning signs, 60
  patient care and, 196, 197
  prevention of suicide, 266
  procedures for in primary care settings,
      255–256
  questions concerning during assessment
      interview, 25
  risk management
    by families, 60
    risk assessment, 196–197
    risk factors, 196
    by schools, 63
    talking to young patients, 57
  SSRIs and, 47
  substance use as risk factor, 242–243
  suicide attempts
    emergency assessment, 196
    prevalence, 14
  talking with adolescents about, 57
Suicidal ideation
  definition, 207
  flowchart for approach to patient, *198*
  HEADS interview (mnemonic for Home,
      Education/employment/eating, Activities,
      Drugs, cigarettes, alcohol, Sexuality,
      Suicidality/depression, Safety), 55, 67–68
  homicidal ideation compared, 199
  monitoring during antidepressant treatment, 79
  questions for assessing, 197
Sumatriptan
  drug interactions, 262
  serotonin toxicity and, 302
Support, of family members, 59–60
Supportive management (treatment option), 49
Suppression, defense exhibited in psychodynamic
      therapy, 142t
Sustained response
  definition, 44t
  rate in TADS trial, 51
Susto, 324
Switching treatment, definition, 45t

Symptoms
  behavior problems, 26
  bullying or abuse, 27
  cognitive, 9
  common presentations, 26t
  drop in school performance, 26
  drug abuse, 27
  excessive somatic complaints, 26
  family history, 27
  mood, 9
  motivational, 9
  neurovegetative, 9
  relationship problems, 27
  severity evaluation and, 11
  SIGECAPS mnemonic, 27, 28t–29t
  somatic, 9
  suicidality, 26
  sustained negative mood change, 26
  table of characteristic, 7t–8t
Systematic desensitization, for phobia, 228–229
Systemic behavioral family therapy (SBFT), 129.
      See also Family therapy
Systems theory, 129–130

TADS (Treatment for Adolescents with Depression
      Study), 50–51, *51*, 71, 101, 328
Talk therapy, 261. *See also* Dynamic psychotherapy
TBI (traumatic brain injury), 33
TCAs. *See* Tricyclic antidepressants
Technology, use to enhance engagement, 57
Templates, in dynamic psychotherapy, 142
Tertiary prevention, 275
Texas Childhood Medication Algorithm Project
      (CMAP)
    for depression, 72, 74
    for depression and ADHD, *230*
    for ADHD and anxiety, *224*
    for depression with aggression, *233*
Therapeutic Goods Administration, 174
Therapeutic index, 300
Therapeutic Outcomes Tool (TOT), 182–183,
      190–193
Therapy as punishment, perception of, 136
Thyroid disorders, 33
Timeline Follow-Back (TLFB), 241
Timelines, use in family therapy, 133–134
Time pressures, influence on treatment, 48
Time to steady state
  meaning and practical implications
      for treatment, 73t
  of SSRIs, 75t
TMS. *See* Transcranial magnetic stimulation
TORDIA (Treatment of Resistant Depression
      in Adolescents study), 102, 210, 216
Toronto Side Effects Scale (TSES), 182
TOT (Therapeutic Outcomes Tool), 182–183, 190–193
TRAAY, 232, 234
Traditional Chinese medicine, 152, 153, 338
Traditional healers, 327, 338
Tramadol, 79, 305
Transcranial direct current stimulation (tDCS), 93

Transcranial magnetic stimulation (TMS),
88t, 92–92
procedure, 93
side effects, 92
for treatment-resistant depression, 217
Transference, 142
Translation, 325–326
Traumatic brain injury (TBI), 33
Traumatic event/stress
consequences and treatment, 166t
depression comorbidity with, 14
as risk factor for acute depressive episode, 166t
Treatment. *See also specific modalities*
bipolar depression, 52
discontinuation, 82
engaging young patients, 55–57
adolescents, 55–57, 56t
children, 55
motivational interviewing, 56, 56t
risk management, 57
technology use, 57
family engagement and support, 57–61
communication, 58–59
education, 59
out-of-home situation, 58
risk management, 60
social and cultural context, 60–61
in specialist mental health services, 64
support, 59–60
frequently asked questions, 271–272
managing crises and emergencies, 194–204
measurement of outcomes, 72
medications, 69–83
nonadherence to, 200–201
nonpharmacolic biological, 87–99, 88t
electroconvulsive therapy (ECT),
88–92, 98–99
light therapy, 93–94
transcranial magnetic stimulation (TMS),
92–93
vagus nerve stimulation (VNS), 93
optimal dosage, 51
overview, 43–52
definition, 44, 44t–46t
ethical issues, 46–48
goals of treatment, 49
level of treatment, 50–52
monitoring treatment, 50
parental involvement, 52
placebo response, 48
stigma, 48
time pressures, 48
when to treat, 49–50
refusal of, 201
response rates, 50–51, *51*
schools, working with, 61–64, 61t
communication, 62
coordinating care, 63–64
education, 62
risk management, 63
undertreatment, 50–51

when to treat
initiating medication, 49–50
supportive management, 49
watchful waiting, 49
where to treat, 38
Treatment effect, 275
Treatment-emergent adverse events. *See* Medication
side effects
Treatment for Adolescents with Depression Study
(TADS), 50–51, *51*, 71, 101, 328
Treatment history, assessment of, 38
Treatment of Resistant Depression in Adolescents
study (TORDIA), 102, 210, 216
Treatment-resistant depression, 209–219
definition of, 44t, 210–211
dynamic psychotherapy, 148
example vignettes, 213–214
factors associated with, 211–214, *212*
clinician, 212
environment, 213–214
family, 213
individual, 211–212
incidence of, 210
treatment, 214–217
augmentation *versus* switching, 215–217, 216t
education, 214
electroconvulsive therapy, 217
general issues, 214
light therapy, 217
pharmacotherapy, 215
psychotherapy, 215
Tricyclic antidepressants (TCAs)
for bipolar depression, 52
for depression comorbid with chronic physical
illness, 302
for depression comorbid with pain, 305
drug interactions, 262
efficacy, 78
international use, 338
lithium as augmenting agent, 79–80
renal failure and, 301
side effects, 79, 178
cardiovascular, 184, 304
variation in use internationally, 336
Triiodothyronine (T3), as augmenting agent, 81
Truancy, 202
Trust
confidentiality and, 166
gaining during assessment interview, 25
Tryptophan, serotonin syndrome and, 302
TSES (Toronto Side Effects Scale), 182
Turning passive to active, defense exhibited in
psychodynamic therapy, 142t, 146

UKU Side Effects rating Scale, 182
Undertreatment, 50–51
Unipolar depression, 12t
Universal preventive interventions, 275, 276,
277t–280t, 281
Urinary drug screens, for substance use
assessment, 241

Vagus nerve stimulation (VNS), 88t, 93, 217
Venlafaxine
    for depression comorbid with chronic physical
        illness, 302
    efficacy, pharmacodynamics and
        pharmacokinetics, 77t
    formulations and dosing, 77t
    mechanism of action, 302
    renal failure and, 301
    side effects, 216
    for Stage 3 treatment, 77–78
Violent behaviors
    assessment of, 199
    initial interventions, 195t
    substance abuse comorbid with
        depression, 243
VNS (vagus nerve stimulation), 88t,
        93, 217

Volume of distribution, 301
    meaning and practical implications
        for treatment, 73t
    of SSRIs, 75t

Ward of the state, 58
Warning signs, of recurrence, 136
Watchful waiting, 49, 222
WILD mnemonic, 239
Williams syndrome, 313
Work at home (IPT-A technique), 122
World Health Organization ATLAS survey, 333
World Psychiatric Association (WPA), 337

Young Mania Rating Scale, 231
Youth Partners-in-Care (YPIC) study, 102, 286

Ziprasidone, 80t